THE COMPLETE & UP-TO-DATE

FAT
BOOK

THE COMPLETE & UP-TO-DATE

FAT

BOOK

Reduce the Fat in Your Diet with This Guide to the Fat, Calories, and Fat Percentages in Your Food

Newly Revised
5th Edition

Karen J. Bellerson

AVERY
a member of Penguin Group (USA) Inc.
New York

AVERY

Published by the Penguin Group

Penguin Group (USA) Inc., 375 Hudson Street, New York, New York 10014, USA ◦ Penguin Group (Canada), 90 Eglinton Avenue East, Suite 700, Toronto, Ontario M4P 2Y3, Canada (a division of Pearson Penguin Canada Inc.) ◦ Penguin Books Ltd, 80 Strand, London WC2R 0RL, England ◦ Penguin Ireland, 25 St Stephen's Green, Dublin 2, Ireland (a division of Penguin Books Ltd) ◦ Penguin Group (Australia), 250 Camberwell Road, Camberwell, Victoria 3124, Australia (a division of Pearson Australia Group Pty Ltd) ◦ Penguin Books India Pvt Ltd, 11 Community Centre, Panchsheel Park, New Delhi–110 017, India ◦ Penguin Group (NZ), Cnr Airborne and Rosedale Roads, Albany, Auckland 1310, New Zealand (a division of Pearson New Zealand Ltd) ◦ Penguin Books (South Africa) (Pty) Ltd, 24 Sturdee Avenue, Rosebank, Johannesburg 2196, South Africa

Penguin Books Ltd, Registered Offices: 80 Strand, London WC2R 0RL, England

Most Avery books are available at special quantity discounts for bulk purchase for sales promotions, premiums, fund-raising, and educational needs. Special books or book excerpts also can be created to fit specific needs. For details, write Penguin Group (USA) Inc. Special Markets, 375 Hudson Street, New York, NY 10014.

Library of Congress Cataloging-in-Publication Data

Bellerson, Karen J.
    The complete & up-to-date fat book: reduce the fat in your diet with this guide to the fat, calories, and fat percentages in your food / Karen J. Bellerson.—New rev. 5th ed.
      p.   cm.
    ISBN 1-58333-247-2
    1. Food—Fat content—Tables. I. Title: The complete & up-to-date fat book. II. Title.

TX551.B39   2006   2005044491
613 2'4—dc22

Printed in the United States of America
10 9 8 7 6 5 4

While the author has made every effort to provide accurate telephone numbers and Internet addresses at the time of publication, neither the publisher nor the author assumes any responsibility for errors, or for changes that occur after publication. Further, the publisher does not have any control over and does not assume any responsibility for author or third-party websites or their content.

Every effort has been made to ensure that the information in this book is complete and accurate. However, neither the publisher nor the author is engaged in rendering professional advice or services to the individual reader. The ideas, procedures, and suggestions herein are not intended as a substitute for consulting with a physician. All matters regarding health require medical supervision. Calories, fat content, and fat percentages for processed foods are subject to change, and might in the future vary from listings in this book, which are based on research conducted in 2005. Neither the author nor the publisher shall be liable or responsible for any loss, injury, or damage allegedly arising from any information or suggestion in this book.

SOURCES OF NUTRITION INFORMATION
United States Department of Agriculture Handbook No. 8 (revised), "Composition of Foods Raw, Processed, Prepared," sections 8–1 through 8–22; Handbook No. 456, "Nutritive Value of American Foods in Common Units"; Home and Garden Bulletin No. 232, "Nutrition and Your Health: Dietary Guidelines for Americans"
Food manufacturers and processors, as well as their product labels
Individual fast-food chains

In memory of my beloved sister . . .

Valerie Dee Rushing
1952–2003

. . . always a piece of my heart

Contents

Acknowledgments

As always, my appreciation goes to those food manufacturers who make nutritional information about their products available and who have listened to consumers' requests for tastier healthful food choices.

For all of you who take the time to write me (whether to ask questions, make comments, or offer suggestions), I want you to know that your letters are of great help to me. Thank you very much for allowing me to play a small part in your endeavors to pursue a healthier, nutritionally sound lifestyle.

Preface

Look to your health; and if you have it,
praise God. Value it next to a good con-
science; for health is the second blessing
that we mortals are capable of; a blessing
that money cannot buy!   —Unknown

Hello, and thank you, once again, for joining me in our never-ending quest for healthy eating habits. So much has happened since the last edition of The Complete & Up-to-Date Fat Book. *We have endured much tragedy in our country, with 9/11, the war in Iraq, and ongoing unrest, not only here in the United States of America but throughout the world. We have become a stronger, closer-than-ever nation in facing those who wish us harm. We celebrated the 2004 Olympics, awash with athletic excellence and victories. Baseball fans celebrated an incredible World Series, in which the Boston Red Sox were unstoppable in their quest to go home to Boston with a World Series trophy! As I began this most current revision, we were in the process of electing yet another president of the United States. Now, two years later, this edition nears completion. I remain in awe of what wonders the future has in store for all of us. Life goes on. . . . Life is good. . . . Life can be great!*

What also continues is my desire to bring you the most complete and up-to-date nutritional data available. With that goal in mind, I continue to educate not only you but myself as well. By this I mean that the constantly changing food industry keeps me on my toes with its ingenuity in manufacturing new food products. It is an endless challenge, which I gladly accept, to keep up with the extraordinary abundance of food products making their debut on our grocery shelves.

Many food manufacturers, along with nutritional watchdogs such as the Center for Science in the Public Interest, the National Cancer Institute, the American Heart Association, and the publishers of numerous nutrition and health newsletters, take our nutritional habits very seriously. They persevere in proving the direct relationship between a high-fat diet (in which more than 30 percent of daily calories comes from fat) and a higher risk of developing cancer, heart disease, stroke, diabetes, high blood pressure (hypertension), and other life-threatening diseases. Along these same lines, professionals throughout the health field promote the very real health benefits of a low-fat nutritional lifestyle.

In their endeavors to bring their findings to the public's attention, some of these groups publish dietary guidelines, which seem almost to be clones of one another. I offer you the guidelines of one such group, the National Cancer Institute. They are geared to cancer prevention, but they are consistent with the Dietary Guidelines for Americans below.

NATIONAL CANCER INSTITUTE DIETARY GUIDELINES

- *Reduce daily fat intake to 30 percent of calories or less.*
- *Increase fiber to 20–30 grams/day, with an upper limit of 35 grams.*
- *Include a variety of fruits and vegetables in the daily diet.*
- *Avoid obesity.*
- *Consume alcoholic beverages in moderation, if at all.*
- *Minimize consumption of salt-cured, salt-pickled, and smoked foods.*

As much as I agree with the recommendations of the National Cancer Institute, there is one that is, sadly, missing from this list and others published in this country. I am referring to the proven fact that healthful eating habits encompass more than just sustained physical well-being, and involve more than just what you eat. The following recommendations, found in published dietary guidelines from some other countries, reinforce that fact:

- *Britain's number one dietary guideline is "Enjoy your food."*
- *Japanese dietary advice includes "Avoid too much salt," and furthermore: "Happy eating makes for happy family life. Sit down and eat together and talk. Treasure family taste and home cooking."*
- *The Norwegian government tells its people that "food and joy equal health."*
- *Vietnam advocates preparing "a healthy family meal that is delicious" and serving it "with affection."*

As charming as the above advice is, it also makes perfect sense. Why? As you will find, following it often leads to a welcome bonus of more harmony within the family circle. And those of you who have teenagers may very well enjoy a double bonus by following any of these guidelines. Research strongly indicates that teenagers who eat with adult family members an average of five times a week tend to be more mentally alert, more motivated to do well in school, and less likely to use drugs or experience depression than those who eat with their parent/parents only three times a week or less.

As you read this book and plan your meals, keep in mind that it is your total diet that counts, not the nutrient content of a single food. Educating yourself in how much and what kind of dietary fat is in the foods you eat will enable you to make wise choices and keep your eating habits balanced and in moderation to make room for all your favorite foods. Remember, too, that small, gradual changes can add up to lifelong eating habits. Choose foods that fit in with your personal tastes and preferences, balancing good nutrition, variety, and great taste!

I wish you health, I wish you happiness, I wish all of us peace. Until next time,

THE COMPLETE & UP-TO-DATE

FAT
BOOK

Introduction

Only saturated fats and dietary cholesterol raise blood cholesterol. A high level of cholesterol in the blood is a major risk factor for coronary heart disease, which leads to heart attack.—American Heart Association

The single most influential dietary change one can make to lower the risk of these diseases [cardiovascular disease, diabetes, and certain forms of cancer] is to reduce intake of foods high in fats and to increase the intake of foods high in complex carbohydrates and fiber.
                    —The Surgeon General's Report on Nutrition and Health, 1988

More than half of all adults in the United States are overweight or obese, and the rates of obesity in children and teens have doubled since the late 1970s. Obesity increases the risk of diabetes, heart disease, stroke, and other health problems. Each year in this country, obesity causes tens or even hundreds of thousands of premature deaths, and *costs the public tens of billions of dollars.*
                    —Centers for Disease Control and Prevention

Health specialists are calling it a "fat epidemic," and no wonder, with the latest numbers showing that more than half of Americans are overweight and one out of three adults is obese. The fat-and-fatter trend has initiated more research into obesity than ever, focusing on its causes and effects. This is especially significant in light of findings that link higher fat intake to a myriad of serious health problems, including heart and respiratory disease, diabetes, osteoarthritis, and some forms of cancer.

For decades, studies have shown the influence of diet on the development of such diseases. Much of what we know today about the diet-disease relationship dates back to World War II, during which the incidence of death from heart attacks among Western Europeans declined greatly. The cause of this dramatic decline was found to lie in the wartime rationing of foods such as meat, dairy products, and eggs. Once the war was over and high-fat foods were once again available, the incidence of heart disease rose. In-depth studies were begun in earnest to investigate the negative effects of these foods.

Today we know that populations with low-fat diets tend to have a lower occurrence of heart disease, stroke, and diabetes, and countless studies prove that there is a very real relationship between diet and the risk of developing a life-threatening disease.

The Food Guide Pyramid, designed by the United States Department of Agriculture, can help you plan a healthy, balanced diet that meets your individual nutrition needs and caloric intake, while taking into consideration your particular food likes and dislikes. When making choices based on the Food Pyramid's recommendations, remember to balance your choices by including foods from all six categories every day. In doing so, you will be eating a variety of foods. Bear in mind moderation, in order to keep your consumption of calories, fat, sodium, and sugar in line.

To practice moderation, you need to know what the USDA considers a serving size for each category of food in the pyramid. If you eat a portion of a certain food that is larger than the indicated serving size, that portion should be counted as more than one serving for that particular group.

What exactly does a serving size look like? The following should help you to visualize a standard recommended serving:

A golf ball = 1-ounce meatball

A deck of cards = 3 ounces cooked lean meat

A baseball = 1 cup milk or other liquid dairy product

3 stacked dominoes = 1½ ounces cheese

Table 1.   Serving Sizes

Food Group	Amount
Bread, cereal, rice, and pasta (6–11 servings daily)	1 slice bread ½ hamburger roll, bagel, or English muffin 1 ounce ready-to-eat cereal (be sure to check labels, as 1 ounce may equal anywhere from ¼ cup to 2 cups, depending on the cereal) ½ cup cooked cereal, rice, or pasta 3 or 4 plain crackers (small)
Vegetables (3–5 servings daily)	1 cup raw leafy vegetables ½ cup other vegetables, cooked or chopped raw ¾ cup vegetable juice
Fruit (2–4 servings daily)	1 medium apple, banana, orange, nectarine, or peach ½ cup chopped raw, cooked, or canned fruit ¾ cup fruit juice
Milk, yogurt, and cheese (2–3 servings daily)	1 cup milk or yogurt 1½ ounces natural cheese 2 ounces processed cheese
Meat, poultry, fish, dry beans, eggs, and nuts (2–3 servings daily)	2–3 ounces cooked lean meat, poultry, or fish 1½ cups cooked dry beans 2–3 eggs 4–6 tablespoons peanut butter

Table 1 on page 2 shows the UDSA's recommended serving sizes for the various types of food in the pyramid.

Other USDA dietary guidelines include these:

1. Eat a variety of foods.

2. Balance the food you eat with physical activity and maintain or improve your weight.

3. Choose a diet low in fat, saturated fat, and cholesterol.

4. Choose a diet with plenty of grain products, vegetables, and fruits.

5. Choose a diet moderate in salt and sodium.

6. If you drink alcoholic beverages, do so in moderation. Children, adolescents, and pregnant women should abstain.

Okay, you're convinced that you need to get the fat out of your diet, but where do you begin? Before we go into some simple guidelines, let's look at a few basic facts about dietary fat.

FAT: A NECESSARY NUTRIENT

The fact is that we need some fat in our diets. *Adults need a minimum daily intake of 15 to 25 grams of dietary fat to meet the body's needs.* Children under age two should not have their dietary fat restricted, because that may interfere with their development.

Our bodies use fat in numerous ways—ways most of us are unaware of. We use fat in manufacturing antibodies to fight disease. Fat acts as carriers for the fat-soluble vitamins (A, D, E, and K). Fat is one of the body's three nutrient energy sources, and it aids in digestion by slowing down the stomach's secretions of hydrochloric acid. This is what produces that satisfying feeling of fullness after a meal. Fat deposits in the body cushion, protect, and hold in place vital organs such as the kidneys, heart, and liver, and also give the body its shape. Fat is the body's insulation against environmental temperature changes. As you can see, fat is a vital nutrient, and should not be totally eliminated from our diets.

All fats are composed of building blocks called fatty acids. There are two types of fatty acids: nonessential, which our body is able to manufacture, and essential, which we cannot make and must obtain through our diets. Essential fatty acids are necessary for normal growth; for healthy skin, blood, arteries, and nerves; and for a smoothly running metabolism.

CHOLESTEROL AND LIPOPROTEINS (LDL AND HDL)

The main reason to be concerned with the fat in your diet is that fat—both the amount and the type—affects blood cholesterol. Cholesterol is a white, waxy, fatty substance found in all foods that come from animal sources, particularly organ meats such as brains, kidney, and liver. Because plants do not manufacture cholesterol, there is no cholesterol in them; this applies as well to oils that come from vegetable sources. While cholesterol is not a fatty acid, it is a fatlike substance and is often referred to as a fat.

Cholesterol, too, is essential to our well-being. We need it to help build cell membranes, to produce hormones (estrogen, progesterone, and testosterone), and to manufacture bile acids needed for eliminating excess cholesterol from the body. If we have more cholesterol than we need in our blood, however, it clogs the arteries. For the average person, about 75 percent of the cholesterol found in the body—all the body needs—is manufactured in the liver, even if that person eats no animal products; the other 25 percent comes from the diet.

Cholesterol is carried through the bloodstream by molecules called lipoproteins. The cholesterol manufactured by the liver is carried to the cells that need it by low-density lipoproteins (LDLs). High levels of LDLs in the bloodstream can result in clogged arteries, causing high blood pressure, stroke, and heart disease. This is why LDL is referred to as "bad cholesterol"—or, as I call it, "lethal cholesterol." *LDL levels can be reduced through a proper diet.*

Now we come to the high-density lipoproteins (HDLs), or "good cholesterol," which I refer to as "healthy cholesterol." HDLs pick up excess cholesterol from various body tissues and carry it to the liver. It is then metabolized by the liver, processed through the intestines, and eliminated from the body. High levels of HDL are associated with a decreased risk of coronary heart disease. HDL levels can be raised through regular exercise. Total cholesterol, the sum of LDL plus HDL, is also important, because it allows us to see the ratio of LDL to HDL.

TYPES OF DIETARY FATS IN INDIVIDUAL FOODS

Because of differences in their chemical structure, the fatty acids in the foods we eat fall into three categories: polyunsaturated, monounsaturated, and saturated. Most foods contain a combination of all three kinds of dietary fat, usually with a higher content of one of them. The relative percentage of each type of fat in any one food is what makes it a healthier or less healthy choice than another.

Polyunsaturated Fats

Polyunsaturated fats are found in most foods. Omega-3 polyunsaturated fats are found primarily in certain fish, while omega-6 polyunsaturated fats are found mainly in nuts, plant oils, seeds, and soybeans. These fats are liquid at room temperature. Polyunsaturated fats reduce blood cholesterol, but if eaten in excess they may lower the level of protective "good cholesterol," or HDL. Some studies indicate a link between a high consumption of polyunsaturated fats and breast cancer.

Foods in which polyunsaturated fats are the main type of fat include those listed below. Note that the foods listed here are **not** necessarily high in fat. They are simply higher in polyunsaturated fats than in the other two types of fats.

Bagels
Barbecue sauce
Bluefish
Brazil nuts
Chickpeas (garbanzo
  beans)
Cod
Corn chips
Cornmeal
French bread
Haddock
Herring
Italian bread
Lentils
Mackerel
Mussels

Oatmeal bread
Oysters
Pine nuts
Popcorn (air-popped)
Potato chips
Potato salad (made
  with mayonnaise)
Pumpernickel
Pumpkin seeds
Rainbow trout
Raisin bread
Refried beans
Rye bread
Salad dressings (most
  types)
Salmon

Sardines
Scallops
Sesame seeds
Soybeans
Squash
Squash seeds
Sunflower seeds
Sweet potatoes
Tofu
Tuna salad (made with
  mayonnaise)
Vegetable and nut oils
  (see table, page 480)
Walnuts
Whitefish

Monounsaturated Fats

Monounsaturated fats are found in most foods, but mainly in vegetable and nut oils such as canola (rapeseed), olive, and peanut. These fats, too, are liquid at room temperature. They reduce total blood cholesterol while not lowering the protective "good cholesterol," HDL.

The following foods are higher in monounsaturated fats than in the other two types of fats. Those marked with an asterisk are also high in saturated fats.

Almonds
Animal fats* (most
  types)
Avocados
Beef* (leaner cuts)
Biscuits
Bread* (most types)
Brownies
Cake* (most types)
Cashews
Chestnuts
Chicken
Cookies* (most
  types)
Croissants*

Doughnuts* (most
  types)
Eggs*
Fruitcake
Gingerbread
Hazelnuts
Lard*
Macadamia nuts
Margarine (stick types)
Muffins*
Oatmeal
Ocean perch
Pastry (including pie
  crust)
Peanut butter

Peanuts
Pecans
Pies* (most types)
Pistachios
Popcorn (popped in
  vegetable oil)
Pork*
Sausage* (most types)
Spaghetti (with tomato
  sauce)
Taco*
Veal* (leaner cuts)
Vegetable and nut oils
  (see table, page 480)
Vegetable shortening

Saturated Fats

All meat and dairy products contain saturated fats. Coconut, palm, and palm kernel oils, although of plant origin, are also high in saturated fat, as is cocoa butter, which is used in making chocolate. (This is why I recommend substituting powdered cocoa in recipes that call for chocolate.) Saturated fats are generally solid at room temperature. *Saturated fats—even more than dietary cholesterol—raise total blood cholesterol.*

The following foods are higher in saturated fats than in the other two types of fats. Other foods high in saturated fats appear in the list of foods high in monounsaturated fat. Those foods are marked with an asterisk, and while monounsaturated fats predominate, they contain significant amounts of saturated fats as well.

Remember, the essential fatty acids—the ones that must be obtained through the diet—are unsaturated. This means we can get all the fat we need from unsaturated fats; there is no biological need for saturated fat.

The American Heart Association points out that the body can use all three types of fats, but it recommends, for the average person, that:

- total daily fat intake (saturated, monounsaturated, polyunsaturated) should be limited to no more than 30 percent of total calories.

- daily saturated fat intake should be limited to 7 to 10 percent of total calories.

- daily polyunsaturated fat intake should be no more than 10 percent of total calories.

- daily monounsaturated fat intake should be no more than 15 percent of total calories.

The American Heart Association further recommends a total daily fat intake equivalent to between 5 and 8 teaspoons of fats and oils, to reduce the possibility of an excess of transfats.

Beef (fattier cuts)	Coconut products	Gravy (brown,
Beef tallow	Cottage cheese (4% fat)	packaged)
Boston brown bread	Cream	Hot dogs
(canned)	Cream soups (most	Ice cream
Butter	types)	Lamb
Cheese (most types)	Custard (baked)	Luncheon meats
Cheesecake	Duck	Malts
Chili (with beef)	Eggnog	Milk (whole, 2%, and
Chocolate	Fried foods (fried in	1%)
Cocoa butter	saturated oils)	Nondairy creamer
Cocoa mixes	Garlic spread	Nondairy whipped
Coconut	Granola	topping

Pies (cream types)
Pizza
Pompano
Popcorn (most microwave types)
Pork (fattier cuts)
Puddings
Quiche
Sauces (butter-, egg-,

milk-based, such as béarnaise, hollandaise, white, or cheese sauce)
Seaweed
Shakes
Snack cakes (most types, those with chocolate frosting)

Sour cream
Turkey (dark meat or self-basting)
Veal (fattier cuts)
Vegetable and nut oils (especially coconut, palm, and palm kernel; see table page 480)

Table 2. Recommended Daily Fat Gram Budget per Caloric Intake*

Total Daily Calories	Total Daily Fat (in grams†)	Daily Saturated Fat Calories (in grams†)
1,200	40	9–12
1,500	50	11–15
1,800	60	13–18
2,000	67	14–20
2,200	73	15–22
2,500	83	18–25
3,000	100	21–30

*For healthy people over age two
†There are 9 calories in 1 gram of fat. To calculate your maximum allowable total daily fat, see the formula on page 13.

Hydrogenated Fats and Trans-Fatty Acids

You may have read of, and been confused by, the term "trans-fatty acids." These are simply types of fats formed when liquid polyunsaturated or monounsaturated oils are subjected to a process called hydrogenation, in which hydrogen is added to an oil to convert it to a solid or semisolid at room temperature, so that it can be used in baked goods, non-dairy creamers, whipped toppings, and other processed foods. The hydrogenation of unsaturated fats causes them to act like saturated fats in the bloodstream, raising blood cholesterol and LDL. On the labels of such products as margarine, shortening, chips, and baked goods, the amount of trans-fatty acids is included in the amount of total fat, but not in the amount of saturated fat. Be aware that both polyunsaturated and monounsaturated fats can be hydrogenated. While some trans fats occur naturally in dairy products and other foods of animal origin, most are formed by hydrogenation. When you read product labels, watch for the words "hydrogenated" or "partially hydrogenated," which indicate the presence of trans-fatty acids.

The Food and Drug Administration is currently proposing that trans fat be listed as part of the saturated fat content on food labels. Under this proposal, food products advertised as "low in saturated fat" could contain more than 0.5 grams of trans fat, aside from the current requirement of less than 1 gram of saturated fat per serving, and a food labeled as "low cholesterol" could contain no more than 2 grams of saturated fat and trans fat combined per serving size. The American Heart Association recommends using liquid vegetable oil and liquid or soft margarines whenever possible. The harder and more solid a margarine is, the more trans-fatty acids it contains.

"Fake Fats"

For years we have heard about ongoing research in the area of "fake fats," or fat substitutes. Manufacturers have been eager to develop low- or no-calorie substitutes for fat that would have the characteristics of fat: the texture, "mouth feel," and flavor, as well as the ability to stand up under a wide range of manufacturing processes.

Even the United States Department of Agriculture has scientists working on the development of an acceptable fat replacement. Dr. George Inglett, a research chemist at the department's Agricultural Research Service National Center for Agricultural Utilization Research in Peoria, Illinois (and developer of Oatrim-10, an earlier fat substitute), has developed a fat substitute known as Z-Trim. This is a purified insoluble fiber made from seed hulls of oats, soybeans, peas, and rice, or corn or wheat bran and dried to a white powder. Since Z-Trim is made of natural dietary fiber, it does not upset the digestive system when consumed in ordinary amounts. Fantesk, which uses biopolymers and water to mimic fat in food products, is another fat substitute developed at the National Center for Agricultural Utilization Research. It has been licensed for use in ice cream and processed meat products.

Simplesse is one of the better-known fake fats. Made of egg whites and milk protein, it has been on the market for several years. Whereas fat has 9 calories per gram, Simplesse has only 1 to 2 calories per gram. Because it consists largely of protein and contains only the fat found in skim milk, its safety, like that of Z-Trim and Fantesk, has not been questioned by the FDA.

Procter & Gamble scientists have been working on their fake fat, Olestra, for twenty-five years or so. Finally, after P&G had spent more than $200 million in research and produced more than 150,000 pages of supporting data, the FDA gave the green light for Olestra (marketed under the trade name Olean) in January 1996.

Olestra is a chemically engineered variation of natural fat made from sugar and vegetable oil. It is reported to be virtually fat-free and can withstand cooking at high temperatures without breaking down. Although Olestra has the taste and consistency of fat, it cannot be digested or absorbed by the body like fat. Its ability to "pass through the body undigested" has made Olestra controversial among health care professionals and others within the public health community.

When the FDA cleared Olestra for use in the manufacture of salty, savory snack foods only (until studies of long-term effects can be done), there were both cheers and boos to be heard across the nation. Enthusiasm came from those who focused on new and improved low-fat and fat-free products they hoped to see on grocery shelves, while opposition came from nutritional watchdogs who focused on the possible side effects of consuming foods containing Olestra. Their very real concerns included the fact that since Olestra cannot be absorbed by the body, some of the fat-soluble vitamins (A, D, E, and K), when eaten at the same time as Olestra, will be dissolved in the Olestra and will also pass through the body. Vitamins eaten at least two hours before or after the Olestra should not be affected. Also, Olestra sharply decreases the levels of some carotenoids in the bloodstream. Carotenoids, a group of more than 500 related compounds found in fruits and vegetables (beta-carotene and lycopene are the best known) are also fat-soluble. Large quantities of carotenoids from fruits and vegetables are associated with lower rates of cancer; lower levels of carotenoids in the bloodstream are associated with heart disease and stroke. Further, because Olestra is not digested or absorbed, it may have negative gastrointestinal side effects.

Because of the concerns suggested above, and so that consumers will know if any foods they purchase contain Olestra (Olean), the FDA is requiring P&G to make sure that all foods containing Olestra are packaged in containers that carry the following statement: "This product contains Olestra. Olestra may cause abdominal cramping and loose stools. Olestra inhibits the absorption of some vitamins and other nutrients. Vitamins A, D, E, and K have been added."

The American Heart Association discourages the use of substitute (fake) fats or sugars, particularly in children's diets. In the absence of evidence for overall health benefits, it feels that people, especially children, are better off developing a taste for fruits, vegetables, and whole-grain foods instead of foods containing fat or sugar substitutes and, as is often the case, little nutritional value.

FOOD LABELS: "NUTRITION FACTS"

As you walk down the aisles of your supermarket, make it a practice to look at the array of foods offered. You will see hundreds of new food products flooding the market each year from our industrious food manufacturers. Before you buy, read nutrition labels to decide whether a particular food will fit in with your ultimate goal of a healthy eating lifestyle.

Although the standard food nutrition label offers a lot of information (see Figure 2), people often tell me they are confused by it. The "% Daily Value" column especially causes confusion. Some consumers make the mistake of assuming that the percentage across from "Total Fat" represents the percentage of calories that come from fat. Don't be misled; it has nothing to do with the percentage of calories from fat. Rather, "% Daily Value" indicates what part of a 2,000-calorie-a-day diet is constituted by the corresponding nutrient. Thus, in the label in Figure 2, the "5%" opposite "Total Fat" means that one serving of the product provides 5 percent of daily fat intake. Of course, if you eat more or less than 2,000 calories a day, the "% Daily Value" listed will not reflect the true percentage for you. However, you can still use these numbers to get a general idea of a particular food's nutritional values relative to an average daily diet and thus determine whether or not to include the food in your eating plans. *Remember that the guidelines shown on food labels are for healthy adults and children two years of age or older.* A low-fat diet may be harmful to children younger than two years of age.

Also potentially confusing are the many descriptive words that appear on food labels, words such as "lite," "reduced calorie," "low fat," and "no sodium." I offer the following definitions in hopes they will help clarify matters:

- *Cholesterol-free.* Containing less than 2 milligrams of cholesterol and 2 grams or less of saturated fat per serving. This in no way indicates that a product is fat-free.
- *Extra-lean.* Containing less than 5 grams of total fat, less than 2 grams of saturated fat, and less than 95 milligrams of cholesterol per serving.
- *Fat-free.* Containing less than 0.5 grams of fat per serving.
- *High-fiber.* Containing 5 grams or more of fiber per serving.
- *Lean.* Containing less than 10 grams of total fat, less than 4 grams of saturated fat, and less than 95 milligrams of cholesterol per serving (but not as little as extra-lean).
- *Less.* Referring to a food, altered or not, containing 25 percent less of a nutrient or of calories than other comparable foods.
- *Light* or *lite.* Containing one-third fewer calories or no more than half the fat of the higher-calorie, higher-fat version; or containing no more than half the sodium of the higher-sodium version.
- *Low-saturated-fat.* Containing 1 gram or less of saturated fat per serving.
- *Low-calorie.* Containing 40 or fewer calories per serving.
- *Low-fat.* Containing 3 grams of fat or less per serving.
- *Reduced-fat.* Referring to nutritionally altered product containing 25 percent less of a nutrient or of calories than the regular product.

Figure 2 offers a sample of the most widely used nutrition information label. Other, smaller styles of label are used when the larger ones do not fit on the packaging. The smaller labels show the same nutritional information as the larger version, but in a different format. If a package is too small for any type of readable label (as, for example, certain candy wrappers), the manufacturer must list an address or telephone number from which consumers may request nutritional information.

Another style of label is used for food products that are to have ingredients added to them by the consumer during preparation. Boxed pancake mix is an example of such a product. This type of label shows the nutritional information for one serving of the packaged contents "as packaged" and separate nutritional information for one serving of the finished product with the added ingredients included.

Recently, a bill was introduced in Washington mandating that the Department of Agriculture require, within one year, the same nutritional label on fresh meat and poultry that is now required for processed meat and poultry. This would be particularly beneficial to the consumer, as red meat is one of the largest sources of artery-clogging saturated fat.

Nutrition Facts

Serving Size ½ cup (114g)
Servings Per Container 4

Amount Per Serving

Calories 90   Calories from Fat 30

	% Daily Value*
Total Fat 3g	**5%**
Saturated Fat 0g	**0%**
Cholesterol 0mg	**0%**
Sodium 300mg	**13%**
Total Carbohydrate 13g	**4%**
Dietary Fiber 3g	**12%**
Sugars 3g	
Protein 3g	

Vitamin A	80%	Vitamin C	60%
Calcium	4%	Iron	4%

* Percent Daily Values are based on a 2,000 calorie diet. Your daily values may be higher or lower depending on your calorie needs:

	Calories	2,000	2,500
Total Fat	Less than	65g	80g
Sat Fat	Less than	20g	25g
Cholesterol	Less than	300mg	300mg
Sodium	Less than	2,400mg	2,400mg
Total Carbohydrate		300g	375g
Fiber		25g	30g

Calories per gram:
Fat 9 • Carbohydrate 4 • Protein 4

More nutrients may be listed on some labels.

Caution: "Fat-Free" Products Can Be Hazardous to Your Weight!

Grocery shelves carry more and more fat-free products, and average fat consumption in the United States decreased from 40 percent of daily calories in the 1960s to 34 percent in 1990. Yet these changes have not had the expected effect on people's weight. Why? A clue may lie in the following statistics: The percentage of Americans concerned about their fat intake climbed from 16 in 1987 to 65 in 1995, according to the Food Marketing Institute, while only 13 percent of us appeared to be concerned about calorie intake. Is it any wonder, then, that the National Center for Health Statistics reports that 33 percent more of us are obese (defined as 30 percent or more over healthy weight) than just fifteen years before?

Studies by the Department of Nutrition and Food Studies at New York University indicate that while Americans are consuming more calories than ever, we are not compensating with an increase in physical activity. Along these same lines, Dr. Marion Nestle, a professor in and chair of the department, remarks: "The ubiquity of fast-food outlets and soda vending machines, the huge increase in portion sizes at restaurants, the decline in school physical education programs, and the many hours spent on the Internet and watching television are all contributing to the obesity epidemic."

Although the biggest culprit behind the obesity statistics seems to be lack of exercise, it is becoming increasingly evident that consumers see fat-free products as being totally healthful. They forget the fact that fat-free foods still contain calories—in some cases, as many as (if not more than) their higher-fat counterparts. (Sugar, it should be remembered, is sometimes used to make up for the flavor lost in cutting out fat.) Studies show that some people use the absence of fat as a license to binge on fat-free and low-fat foods.

Remember: Both the amount of fat and the number of calories are important. Don't buy the myth that "calories don't count." If you eat more calories than you burn, regardless of the source, you will gain weight. Whether the extra calories come from fat, carbohydrates, or protein, you will store them as body fat.

So while fat-free products may be of a higher quality than they were a few years ago, and while they will offer a viable way to cut the amount of fat we consume, portion control is still very much in order. You might try keeping things in perspective by reminding yourself that while a one-and-a-half-ounce serving of "fat-free" cake has less than 0.5 grams of fat, it still has almost the same number of calories as a tablespoon of butter.

GUIDELINES FOR REDUCING THE FAT IN YOUR DIET

As mentioned earlier, fat is needed for healthy body functions and should not be eliminated from the diet. According to a Surgeon General's Report on Nutrition and Health: "Adults need a minimum daily intake of 15 to 25 grams of fat to meet these necessities." The American Heart Association, the American Health Foundation, the American Cancer Society, the National Heart, Lung, and Blood Institute, the National Center for Nutrition and Dietetics, the American Diabetes Association, and the Surgeon General all recommend that no more than 30 percent of daily calories come from fat, and that no more than a third of those fats (or 10 percent of daily calories) be saturated fats. Below you will see how to calculate these percentages.

The Fat Gram Budget Formula

Fortunately, since you have decided to reduce your dietary fat, a simple formula will let you know the exact maximum number of fat grams you can allow yourself every day. To calculate your maximum daily allowance, multiply your daily calorie intake by .3, and divide that total by 9 (there are 9 calories in each gram of fat). For a daily intake of 1,500 calories, your calculation would be:

$$1,500 \times .3 = 450$$
$$450 \div 9 = 50$$

So you should have a maximum of 50 grams of fat per day.

To make things even easier, I have listed the fat gram budgets for specific daily calorie intakes in Table 3. It shows 10 percent, 20 percent, 30 percent maximum daily fat gram budgets for diets of 1,200 to 3,000 calories per day. (Note that the data are rounded; decimal fractions have been dropped.) The table opens with a daily intake of 1,200 calories; it is not recommended that anyone eat fewer than 1,200 calories (for women) or 1,500 calories (for men), in order to ensure that daily nutritional needs are met. In using your daily fat gram budget, remember that the fact that you have budgeted X amount of fat grams for the day doesn't mean you have to eat that entire amount. Just make sure not to go over budget!

Table 3. Maximum Daily Fat Gram Budget

Daily Calorie Intake	Fat Grams Allowed			Daily Calorie Intake	Fat Grams Allowed		
	10%	20%	30%		10%	20%	30%
1,200	13	27	40	2,200	24	49	73
1,300	14	29	43	2,300	26	51	76
1,400	16	31	46	2,400	27	53	80
1,500	17	33	50	2,500	28	56	83
1,600	18	36	53	2,600	29	58	86
1,700	19	38	56	2,700	30	60	90
1,800	20	40	60	2,800	31	62	93
1,900	21	42	63	2,900	32	64	96
2,000	22	44	66	3,000	33	67	100
2,100	23	47	70				

Of course, to calculate your daily fat gram budget, you need to know your daily calorie intake. If you don't already know this, keep a diary for three or four days. Write down the calorie amounts for everything you eat and drink for these days, add the daily totals, then divide by the number of days you kept track.

People often wonder how many calories they should be consuming on a daily basis. Table 4 gives you a general idea of what your daily calorie consumption should be, making it easier for you to figure your fat gram budget. Keep in mind, though, that everyone has a different metabolism, so the appropriate amount of daily calories for you may vary slightly, above or below the amount listed.

Table 4.   Daily Calorie Requirements

Age / Sex / Activity Level	Requirements
Minimum calories for adequate nutrition (women)	1,200
Minimum calories for adequate nutrition (men)	1,500
Sedentary women	1,600
Moderately active women; children 4–6 years; women 51 and over	1,800
Active women; sedentary men; teen girls; children 7–10 years	2,000–2,200
Very active women; average men 50 and over; boys 11–14 years	2,200–2,600
Active men; teen boys	2,600–2,800
Active to very active men 25–50; athletes in training	3,000–4,000

Source: U.S. Department of Health and Human Services, Food and Drug Administration, FDA Special Report, May 1993.

Making Smarter, Healthier Choices

Here are some tips to follow as you take stock of your eating habits and improve your nutrition by reducing your intake of dietary fat:

• Beef and pork have become leaner than ever because the animals are fed a less fattening diet and are taken to market sooner, before they have a chance to build up a store of fat. You can now choose cuts of beef or pork that have little more fat than a skinless breast of chicken. Stay with the following cuts, boneless and trimmed of visible fat, and keep your cooked portions to 3 ounces (trimmed of all visible fat), prepared without added fat:

Beef (USDA Select)	*Pork*	*Veal*
Chuck arm pot roast	Cured ham (lean)	Cutlets
Eye of round	Loin roast	Sirloin
Flank steak	Sirloin chops	Tenderloin
Top round	Tenderloin	
Top sirloin	Top loin	

• Familiarize yourself with the number of grams of fat and the percentage of calories from fat in the foods you eat most often, so that it becomes second nature to compute your fat consumption.

• Once you are familiar enough with where the fat is in the foods you eat, make your fat gram budget an average covering three to four days instead of focusing on each meal. This allows some flexibility, which is important for healthy lifelong habit changes.

• When putting together a macaroni, potato, tuna, or turkey salad, don't forget fat-free and reduced-fat mayonnaise on the market today.

• Use a reduced-fat or fat-free margarine or spread instead of butter or regular margarine or spread. Either comes in spreadable, squeezable, and sprayable forms.

• Use canned evaporated skim milk as a substitute for heavy cream, and low-fat or skim milk in place of whole milk or cream in your recipes.

• There is quite a selection of low-fat and fat-free salad dressings available now, in many flavors and styles. Try them until you find one or more to your taste. You can avoid as many as 6 to 10 grams of fat per tablespoon by not using regular salad dressings.

• For desserts, go ahead and splurge on occasion, but more often indulge in the wide range of frozen yogurt desserts in your grocery store's freezer section. Again, because of the wide range, you may have to try more than one or two to find a favorite or favorites. There are also "lighter" ice creams, even in such gourmet flavors as caramel nut fudge sundae and mocha almond fudge. Low-fat and fat-free bakery goods give almost unlimited choices for anyone's sweet tooth. Remember, though: moderation and portion control!

• Substitute low-fat, reduced-fat, or fat-free cheeses for cheeses that are higher in fat. The fat avoided here is between 6 and 10 grams per ounce!

• Most breads are low in fat (1 gram per slice), but be careful when you reach for a croissant to make that sandwich. One butter croissant can have 20 or more grams of fat and 360 calories!

• Dry cereals make a great-tasting snack. Most of them have 0 to 3 grams of fat per serving. Read the labels on granola-type cereals, though, as most of them are higher in fat.

• Canadian bacon is a tasty lower-fat substitute for bacon. Bacon bits also have less fat, and can be used as a pizza topping, too.

• When contemplating potato snacks, consider this: While ten French fries have 8 grams of fat, a 1.5-ounce package of potato chips has a whopping 15 grams!

• You can thicken sauces without fat by substituting puréed vegetables for cream or whole milk.

• Make your own bread coatings with plain bread crumbs and your choice of spices. Dip food into skim milk, buttermilk, or egg whites before coating in the bread crumbs and baking.

• Use powdered low-fat or skim milk instead of non-dairy creamer.

• Reduce the amount of oil or melted butter in your recipes by a third to a half, and replace the subtracted amount with water, fruit juice, or yogurt. If you buy commercial mixes, buy only those to which you add the fat or oil, so you can control the amount.

• Instead of pan-frying or deep-frying, bake or broil meat, fish, or poultry and baste it with wine, lemon or tomato juice or another juice, broth, or low-fat or fat-free salad dressing to keep it from drying out.

• Instead of using whole eggs, replace each yolk with two egg whites, or use a low-fat egg substitute. Omelets can be made with one whole egg and an additional egg white or two.

• Use partly skimmed ricotta instead of full-fat cream cheese for a luscious cheesecake.

• When using oil, make sure it's the least saturated type available. Although an oil may be low in saturated fat, all oils have 14 grams of fat per tablespoon. (See Oil, pages 480–481.)

• Cocoa powder is an excellent low-fat substitute for baking chocolate, which is high in fat. Use a mixture of 3 tablespoons cocoa, 2 teaspoons sugar, and 1 tablespoon water or other liquid for each 1-ounce square baking chocolate. If the recipe absolutely requires baking chocolate, use a smaller amount than called for.

• Coconut-flavored extract and coconut milk (the liquid found inside the coconut, which has only 0.5 gram of fat per cup) are excellent substitutes for coconut when you want that taste. Add shredded carrots and you can have the texture of coconut without the fat.

• Instead of preparing a pan with cooking oil or shortening, use a nonstick pan sprayed with a small amount of cooking spray. Or spread a small amount of oil over the surface of the pan with a paper towel.

    These changes can be made easily. Learn the low-fat substitutes to use in your home cooking, and stay away from high-fat store-bought products. Read your labels. Once you have learned from this book how to recognize the fat content of the foods available to you, making healthier eating choices will become a way of life.

LET'S GET STARTED!

Remember, knowledge is power! Therefore, by following the suggestions in this book, even just a little at a time, and educating yourself about the sources of dietary fat, you will be on your way to a healthy, low-fat lifestyle. Check the fat content of the foods you usually eat against your daily fat gram budget and see what foods you may need to change or replace with lower-fat choices. Then find appropriate low-fat substitutes for these higher-fat foods to bring you in line with your budget. Sound easy? With the variety of lower-fat foods available, it's easier than ever!

You may be startled by exactly how much dietary fat you have been eating. Moreover, you may find that if a favorite food takes a big enough bite (no pun intended) out of your daily fat gram budget, you will want that favorite food less often and will automatically begin to make more nutritionally sound food selections. It will become a way of life for you . . . a wonderful, *healthy* way of life!

Food for Thought

According to the USDA, the following are America's top ten fat sources:

1. Margarine
2. Whole milk
3. Shortening
4. Mayonnaise and salad dressing
5. American cheese
6. Ground beef
7. Reduced-fat milk
8. Eggs
9. Butter
10. Vanilla ice cream

Write It Down

In the beginning, you will find that keeping a daily account of your food intake cannot be overrated. Keep track of *everything* you eat and drink, so you can accurately total the fat grams and calories for each day. This way, you will have a precise idea of what you are eating and where you need to make adjustments. Your diary will be invaluable also in keeping track of your eating habits and help you form new, healthier ones. It will, furthermore, help you:

- recognize your eating patterns and reevaluate your food choices,
- remember what you have eaten throughout the day,

- gain control over what you eat,
- budget your fat grams and calories more realistically,
- think twice about straying from a healthy low-fat lifestyle,
- take pride in seeing your progress in writing.

At the back of this book you will find a Personal Food Diary to help you start recording your new eating habits.

GET ACQUAINTED WITH *THE COMPLETE & UP-TO-DATE FAT BOOK*

This is a well-researched, in-depth, and comprehensive nutritional guide. As you shop for and prepare low-fat foods, it will be a valuable source of information for your healthy eating lifestyle. Although extreme care has been taken in recording the data in this book, you may come across occasional discrepancies between the information here and the nutritional data on product labels or other sources of nutritional information. There are a number of possible reasons for this.

First, manufacturers are given a little flexibility, so they may round off their data and still be in accordance with governmental regulations on product labeling. If a certain product contains 2.3 grams of fat, for example, the manufacturer may list the fat content as 2 grams, dropping the .3. The same is done with data on calories. If a product serving has 134 calories, the manufacturer may list the calorie content as either 130 or 135. Wherever possible, I have kept nutritional data intact, rounding off neither fat nor calorie content.

Second, when I gathered data from product labels and compared this with data I received directly from manufacturers, there was at times a difference between the two because the labels listed the nutritional data of old product formulas while the manufacturer provided up-to-date information reflecting a change in the formulas. In these cases, the book gives the more recent data obtained directly from the manufacturer. Also, product serving sizes may change and in turn alter the nutritional data. Be sure, when comparing products, that you are comparing them in the same serving size—that is, a quarter-cup of one product against a quarter-cup of another.

Other discrepancies may be due to differences in the analytical methods and sampling techniques used by various food manufacturers.

As you can see, data in this book are listed in four columns. "Amount" means the serving size of food served or used in a recipe. Any deviation in serving size will mean a change in the data in all the other columns. The fat content of each food is expressed as the number of fat grams (the measurement used for dietary fat) per serving. The calorie column needs no explanation.

In the fourth column, under "% Fat Calories," I have given the percentage of calories from fat for all foods listed. To figure the percentage of fat in the rare food that is not listed:

1. Multiply the number of fat grams by 9 (calories per gram) to get total fat calories (TFC).
2. Divide TFC by the total calorie content of your chosen food.

EXAMPLE: 1 ounce cheddar cheese contains 9 fat grams and 110 calories
9 (fat grams) x 9 (calories per gram) = 81 (TFC)
81 (TFC) ÷ 110 (total calories) = 0.73, or 73 percent

Since a high-fat food is defined as any food in which 30 percent or more of the calories come from fat, this cheddar cheese would be considered high-fat.

Some of the figures in the "% Fat Calories" column have been rounded, as mentioned, and the percentage might be off slightly, but not so much that it matters. For example, 100 percent of the calories in oils and fats comes from fat. But if you look at the listing for butter and calculate the percentage of calories from fat (11 fat grams x 9 calories per gram ÷ 100 calories = 99 percent), the result differs slightly from the "% Fat Calories" listed (100 percent). Because we know that all oils and fats contain 100 percent fat calories, I did not want to mislead you by listing the calculated 99 percent instead of the absolute 100 percent.

You will find both generic and brand-name products in these tables. The listing of a product by brand name is not an endorsement. If certain brand-name products are not listed, it means that there was no nutritional data available at the time the list was compiled, and they were not included for that reason only. Data are given for food products available in wholesale clubs and through wholesale distributors; these are identified as "food service products."

Serving size, fat grams, total calories, and percentage of calories from fat are provided for most products listed. In most cases, the entries are given alphabetically for easy reference. Where appropriate, some types of foods are presented in groups, such as "Frozen Entrée/Dinner," "Mexican Food," and "Asian Food." After the A-to-Z list is a separate section on fast foods, organized alphabetically by individual franchise name.

Since cereals and soups are frequently prepared with milk, quick-reference charts for adding milk can be found in the cereal and soup sections. And because it is important to choose the least saturated oil available when using oil in food preparation, charts on pages 480–481 show the percentages of saturated, polyunsaturated, and monounsaturated fats contained in the most commonly used fats and oils.

The book features main headings for foods in uppercase boldface letters. In some instances, subheadings (smaller and bold) with solid boxes before them have been added for clarity. Descriptions of foods are in upper/lowercase, with brand names in parentheses.

If you are unable to find a particular food, look for the entry of a similar food. The nutritional data should be similar, if not exactly the same. When comparing foods, make sure you are comparing the same serving size, weight measure, and/or volume. The Table of Equivalent Measures (page 22) should help you not only in comparing serving sizes but in making exchanges as well. Finally, note that all servings of cooked vegetables are drained of liquid, unless otherwise specified.

Your copy of *The Complete and Up-to-Date Fat Book* will be a treasured companion as you take control of your eating habits. You will discover that by adopting a low-fat lifestyle you will reap many rewards—rewards such as more energy, better sleep, lower grocery bills, more control over your weight, and perhaps most important, vibrant health and a more satisfying quality of life as a whole!

Abbreviations and Symbols

~	=	approximately
<	=	less than
"	=	inch
–	=	trace amount or less
dia	=	diameter
lb	=	pound
oz	=	ounce
pkg	=	package
pkt	=	packet
sec	=	second
Tbs	=	tablespoon
tsp	=	teaspoon
w/	=	with
w/o	=	without

For dishes described as "homemade," the data assume the use of standard ingredients in preparation—no low-fat substitutes. The data given are guidelines for the dishes as you might make them in your own kitchen. Data on dishes made from packaged mixes assume that they are prepared according to package directions and, unless noted otherwise, without low-fat substitute ingredients.

Table of Equivalent Measures

VOLUME

1 tablespoon	=	½ fluid ounce
		3 teaspoons
1 fluid ounce	=	2 tablespoons
¼ cup	=	2 fluid ounces
		4 tablespoons
⅓ cup	=	5⅓ tablespoons
½ cup	=	4 fluid ounces
		8 tablespoons
⅔ cup	=	10⅔ tablespoons
¾ cup	=	6 fluid ounces
		12 tablespoons
1 cup	=	½ pint
		8 fluid ounces
		16 tablespoons
1 pint	=	2 cups
		16 fluid ounces
1 quart	=	2 pints
		4 cups
		32 fluid ounces
1 gallon	=	4 quarts
		8 pints

WEIGHT

1 ounce	=	28.35 grams
100 grams	=	3.5 ounces
4 ounces	=	¼ pound
8 ounces	=	½ pound
12 ounces	=	¾ pound
1 pound	=	16 ounces
		454 grams

A

Food and Description	Amount	Fat Grams	Total Calories	% Fat Calories
ABALONE				
fried	3 oz	5.8	161	32%
raw	3 oz	1.0	90	10%
ACORN				
dried	1 oz	8.9	145	55%
raw	1 oz	6.8	105	58%
ACORN FLOUR (*See* FLOUR)				
ADUKI/ADZUKI BEAN				
(Arrowhead Mills) raw	1½ cup	0.5	160	3%
(Eden)	1½ cup	–	110	–
generic				
boiled	½ cup	<1.0	147	3%
raw	½ cup	<1.0	325	1%
sweetened/canned	½ cup	<1.0	351	1%
Yokan	¼" slice	–	35	–
AGAR (*See* SEAWEED)				
ALBACORE (*See* TUNA)				
ALE (*See* BEER, ALE & MALT LIQUOR)				
ALEWIFE/HERRING/raw	4 oz	5.6	144	35%
ALFALFA SPROUTS/raw	1 cup	<1.0	10	–
ALLIGATOR /raw	3 oz	3.0	200	14%
ALLSPICE	1 tsp	–	6	–
ALMOND (*See also* SALAD TOPPINGS)				
(Azar)..all styles	1 oz	15.0	170	79%
(Beer Nuts) Sweet & Salty	1 oz	14.0	170	74%
whole	1 oz	15.0	190	71%
(Blue Diamond)				
barbecue	1.1 oz	15.0	170	79%
blanched/whole	1 oz	15.0	190	71%
chopped/natural	1 oz	15.0	180	75%
dried/whole	1 oz	15.0	180	75%
dry-roasted	1 oz	15.0	170	79%
honey-roasted	1 oz	14.0	170	74%
roasted/salted	1 oz	17.0	190	81%
slivered	1 oz	16.0	200	72%
(Diamond of California)				
sliced	¼ cup	15.0	190	71%
slivered	¼ cup	15.0	190	71%
whole	¼ cup	15.0	190	71%

Food and Description	Amount	Fat Grams	Total Calories	% Fat Calories
slivered blanched	⅓ cup	15.0	180	75%
whole				
blanched	¼ cup	15.0	170	79%
natural	¼ cup	15.0	170	79%
(Fisher)				
Chef's Naturals				
almond bark				
chocolate-flavored	1.6 oz	15.0	240	56%
vanilla-flavored	1 oz	14.0	250	50%
ground/fine	1 oz	14.0	170	74%
sliced natural	1 oz	13.0	170	69%
slivered	1 oz	14.0	170	74%
Snack'n Serve Nut Bowl				
chocolate-covered	1.42 oz	16.0	220	65%
(Planters)	1 oz	15.0	170	79%
Gold Measure/slivered	2 oz	31.0	340	82%
honey-roasted	1 oz	14.0	160	79%
ALMOND BUTTER				
(Arrowhead Mills)	2 Tbs	20.0	210	86%
(Erewhon)	1 Tbs	8.0	90	80%
	1 cup	74.0	790	84%
(Hain)				
natural/raw	2 Tbs	18.0	190	85%
toasted-blanched	2 Tbs	19.0	220	78%
(Kettle) Roaster Fresh	1 oz	16.0	184	72%
(Westbrae Natural)				
crunchy	2 Tbs	17.0	190	80%
smooth	2 Tbs	17.0	190	80%
ALMOND FILLING				
(Odom) marzipan	2 Tbs	4.0	500	7%
(Solo)	2 Tbs	2.5	120	19%
ALMOND MEAL/partially defatted	1 oz	5.0	116	39%
ALMOND PASTE	1 Tbs	7.7	127	55%
	1 cup	62.0	1010	55%
ALMOND POWDER				
full-fat	1 oz	15.0	168	80%
	1 cup	34.0	385	80%
partially defatted	1 oz	5.0	112	40%
	1 cup	10.0	255	35%
ALOE VERA JUICE	2 oz	–	5	–
AMARANTH				
(Arrowhead Mills) seeds	¼ cup	2.0	170	11%
AMARANTH FLOUR (See FLOUR)				
ANASAZI BEAN				
(Arrowhead Mills) dry	¼ cup	0.5	150	3%
(Bean Cuisine) dry	½ cup	1.0	115	8%
ANCHOVY, EUROPEAN				
canned/in oil	5 fish	1.9	42	41%
fresh/raw	3 oz	4.0	62	58%
ANCHOVY PASTE	1 tsp	0.8	14	51%

Food and Description	Amount	Fat Grams	Total Calories	% Fat Calories
ANISE	1 tsp	–	7	–
APPLE (*See also* APPLE, CARAMEL)				
canned/jar				
(Luck's) fried				
plain	½ cup	–	130	–
w/cinnamon	½ cup	–	120	–
(Lucky Leaf)				
Dutch baked	5 oz	–	170	–
fried	4.6 oz	–	170	–
rings/red spiced	1.5 oz	–	35	–
sliced	4 oz	–	50	–
(Musselman's)				
chips	4 oz	–	50	–
crab/spiced	2 oz	–	35	–
diced	4 oz	–	50	–
Dutch baked	5 oz	–	170	–
rings/green or red	4 oz	–	100	–
sliced				
dessert	4 oz	–	70	–
sweetened				
in syrup or water	4 oz	–	50	–
whole				
baked	1 apple	–	110	–
sweetened				
peeled-cored	1 apple	–	90	–
(S&W)				
rings	2 pieces	–	25	–
spiced crab	1 piece	–	35	–
dried				
(Del Monte) sliced	⅓ cup	–	80	–
(Mariani)	¼ cup	–	150	–
(Nature's Favorite) apple chips				
cinnamon	1 oz	5.0	120	38%
golden delicious	1 oz	5.0	120	38%
original	1 oz	5.0	120	38%
(Seneca) apple chips				
1-ounce bags				
cinnamon	1 oz	7.0	140	45%
golden delicious	1 oz	7.0	140	45%
Granny Smith	1 oz	8.0	150	48%
honey apple	1 oz	7.0	140	45%
original	1 oz	7.0	140	45%
pink lady	1 oz	9.0	160	51%
sour apple	1 oz	7.0	140	45%
1.5-ounce bags				
caramel	1.5 oz	11.0	210	47%
Granny Smith	1.5 oz	11.0	210	47%
honey apple	1.5 oz	11.0	210	47%
original	1.5 oz	11.0	210	47%

Food and Description	Amount	Fat Grams	Total Calories	% Fat Calories
(Sun Maid) Washington	1.25 oz	–	110	–
(Tree Top)/fat-free				
caramel	1 oz	–	110	–
cinnamon	1 oz	–	110	–
Red Delicious	1 oz	–	110	–
fresh				
cooked/w/o skin	1 cup	0.6	91	6%
microwaved/sliced				
peeled	½ cup	0.5	65	7%
unpeeled	½ cup	0.5	50	9%
raw				
(Dole)	1 medium	1.0	80	11%
(Tree Top) crisp natural slices	2 oz	–	35	–
w/skin				
sliced	1 cup	–	64	6%
whole	1 medium	0.5	81	6%
w/o skin				
sliced	1 cup	–	62	–
whole	1 medium	–	72	–
APPLE, CARAMEL				
(Classic Kettle)				
almond chocolate	¼ apple	16.0	320	45%
peanut chocolate	¼ apple	12.0	260	42%
pecan chocolate	¼ apple	17.0	320	48%
toffee walnut chocolate	¼ apple	14.0	310	41%
triple chocolate chunk	¼ apple	12.0	300	36%
APPLE BUTTER				
(Dutch Girl)	1 Tbs	–	35	–
(Eden)	1 Tbs	–	25	–
(Kozlowski Farms)	1 Tbs	–	30	–
(Lucky Leaf) Old-Fashioned Spiced	1 Tbs	–	30	–
(R. W. Knudsen) Organic	1 Tbs	–	35	–
(Smucker's)				
cider	1 Tbs	–	45	–
Simply Fruit	1 Tbs	–	45	–
spiced	1 Tbs	–	45	–
(Welch's) Bama				
original recipe	1 Tbs	–	40	–
(Whitehouse) old-fashioned	1 Tbs	–	35	–
APPLE CIDER (See CIDER)				
APPLE DUMPLING (See PASTRY)				
APPLE FRITTERS/Frozen				
Mrs. Paul's Homestyle	4 oz	11.0	240	41%
APPLE JUICE/NECTAR				
bottled, boxed, or canned				
(Apple & Eve)	8 fl oz	–	110	–
(Knouse) Apple Time				
100% from concentrate	8 fl oz	–	120	–
original/unsweetened	8 fl oz	–	120	–
premium	8 fl oz	–	120	–

Food and Description	Amount	Fat Grams	Total Calories	% Fat Calories
(Libby's)				
Juicy Juice	4.23 fl oz	–	60	–
Juicy Pouch	4.23 fl oz	–	60	–
(Lucky Leaf)	5.5 oz	–	80	–
(Martinelli's) 100% pure				
natural/unfiltered	8 fl oz	–	140	–
not from concentrate	8 fl oz	–	140	–
sparkling	10 fl oz	–	180	–
apple-cranberry	8 fl oz	–	110	–
apple-grape	8 fl oz	–	120	–
from fresh apples	8 fl oz	–	150	–
(Minute Maid)	8 fl oz	–	110	
apple pure	12 fl oz	–	170	–
box	6.75 oz	–	90	–
100% pure	11.5 oz	–	160	–
(Mott's)				
natural	8 fl oz	–	120	–
	9.5 fl oz	–	140	–
	10 fl oz	–	150	–
(Odwalla) Essentials				
organic	8 fl oz	–	110	–
pressed	8 fl oz	–	140	–
(Tropicana)				
chilled	6 fl oz	–	80	–
	8 fl oz	–	110	–
	10 fl oz	–	140	–
	11.5 fl oz	–	160	–
(Walnut Farms)	8 fl oz	–	110	–
(Welch's)				
juice	5.5 fl oz	–	80	–
	8 fl oz	–	120	–
	10 fl oz	–	140	–
	11.5 fl oz	–	160	–
frozen				
(Minute Maid)	8 fl oz	–	110	–
(Seneca)	8 fl oz	–	120	–
country-style	8 fl oz	–	120	–
Granny Smith	8 fl oz	–	110	–
(Sunkist)	8 fl oz	–	80	–
(TreeTop)				
country-style	8 fl oz	–	120	–
original	8 fl oz	–	120	–

APPLE JUICE BLEND/DRINK
(NOTE: Unless stated otherwise, data are for prepared serving amounts.)
bottled, boxed, or canned

(Dole)				
Apple Berry Burst	8 fl oz	–	120	–
apple-cranberry	10 fl oz	–	160	–
(Hi-C) Jammin' Apple	8.45 fl oz	–	120	–

Food and Description	Amount	Fat Grams	Total Calories	% Fat Calories
(Knudsen)				
apple-boysenberry juice	8 fl oz	–	120	–
Thirst Quencher/apple-cranberry	8 fl oz	–	130	–
(Libby's) Juicy Juice				
apple-grape	8 fl oz	–	100	–
	8.45 fl oz	–	130	–
(Minute Maid) apple-grape	8 fl oz	–	125	–
(Mott's)				
apple juice drink	9.5 fl oz	–	150	–
	10 fl oz	–	160	–
apple-cranberry juice	8 fl oz	–	120	–
	9.5 fl oz	–	150	–
apple-grape juice	8 fl oz	–	120	–
apple-raspberry juice	6 fl oz	–	85	–
	8.45 fl oz	–	125	–
	9.5 fl oz	–	135	–
(Welch's)				
apple-cranberry drink	11.5 fl oz	–	210	–
apple-orange-pineapple drink	11.5 fl oz	–	210	–
Cocktail-in-a-Box				
apple-grape-cherry	8.45 fl oz	–	150	–
apple-grape-raspberry	8.45 fl oz	–	150	–
Juice Cocktail				
apple	8 fl oz	–	140	–
apple-cranberry				
low-cal	8 fl oz	–	15	–
regular	8.45 fl oz	–	180	–
apple-orange-pineapple	10 fl oz	–	150	–
frozen				
(Dole) Apple Berry Burst	8 fl oz	–	120	–
(Mott's) Fruit Basket Juice Cocktail				
apple	8 fl oz	–	120	–
apple-raspberry	8 fl oz	–	130	–
(TreeTop)				
apple-cranberry juice	8 fl oz	–	130	–
apple-raspberry juice	8 fl oz	–	110	–
(Welch's) Orchard Juice Blend				
apple-grape-cherry	8 fl oz	–	140	–
apple-grape-raspberry	8 fl oz	–	150	–
APPLESAUCE				
(Del Monte)				
light	½ cup	–	50	–
sweetened	½ cup	–	90	–
(Knouse) Apple Time				
unsweetened	4 oz	–	50	–
unsweetened cinnamon	4 oz	–	50	–
(Lucky Leaf)				
cherry	4 oz cup	–	90	–
chunky	4.8 oz	–	100	–
cinnamon	4 oz cup	–	80	–
	4.8 oz	–	100	–

Food and Description	Amount	Fat Grams	Total Calories	% Fat Calories
light	4.6 oz	–	50	–
old-fashioned natural	4.6 oz	–	50	–
orange-mango	4 oz cup	–	100	–
raspberry	4 oz cup	–	80	–
(Mott's)				
chunky	5 oz	–	110	–
cinnamon	5 oz	–	120	–
Dutch apple spice	4 oz	–	70	–
strawberry	4 oz	–	80	–
sweetened	4 oz	–	90	–
(Musselman's)				
chunky home-style	4.5 oz	–	100	–
cinnamon				
deluxe	4.5 oz	–	120	–
lite	4.3 oz	–	50	–
regular	6 oz cup	–	130	–
	4 oz cup	–	80	–
Fruit & Sauce/Lite				
cups..sweetened	4 oz cup	–	60	–
premium	8 oz	–	120	–
regular	½ cup	–	50	–
	6 oz cup	–	70	–
unsweetened	4.3 oz	–	50	–
(Santa Cruz) Organic				
cups..flavored..sweetened	4 oz cup	–	50	–
apple-cinnamon	4 oz cup	–	80	–
(Seneca)				
cinnamon	4.5 oz	–	100	–
Golden Delicious	4.5 oz	–	100	–
McIntosh	4.5 oz	–	60	–
100% natural	4.5 oz	–	60	–
	4 oz cup	–	50	–
regular	4.5 oz	–	100	–
wild berry	4 oz cup	–	80	–
(TreeTop)				
cinnamon	4 oz	–	90	–
	½ cup	–	100	–
natural/no sugar added/cups	4.6 oz	–	80	–
original	4 oz	–	90	–
	½ cup	–	100	
unsweetened	4 oz	–	70	–
	½ cup	–	70	–
(Walnut Acres) Kids' Snack				
Fruit Squeezies				
berry wild	2 oz	–	40	–
wild apple	2 oz	–	35	–
APRICOT				
candied	1 oz	–	96	–
canned				
(Del Monte) halves/unpeeled				
almond-flavored	½ cup	–	90	–

Food and Description	Amount	Fat Grams	Total Calories	% Fat Calories
in heavy syrup	½ cup	–	100	–
light	½ cup	–	60	–
Orchard Select	½ cup	–	80	–
(Libby's) unpeeled/light	½ cup	–	60	–
(S&W)				
almond in light syrup	½ cup	–	90	–
whole/peeled				
in heavy syrup	½ cup	–	120	–
dried				
(Ann's House of Nuts) Turkish	5 pieces	–	90	–
(Del Monte) sun-dried	⅓ cup	–	80	–
(Dole) Sun Giant Turkish	6 pieces	–	90	–
(Mariani)..all types	¼ cup	–	140	–
(Sun Maid)				
California	1.5 oz	–	110	–
Mediterranean	1.4 oz	–	100	–
fresh	3 medium	0.5	51	9%
	1 cup	0.6	74	7%
(Dole)	3 medium	–	60	–
APRICOT FILLING (Solo)	2 Tbs	–	80	–
APRICOT JUICE/NECTAR/bottled, boxed, or canned				
(Del Monte)	6 fl oz	–	100	–
(Goya)	6 fl oz	–	120	–
(Kern's)	5.5 oz	–	100	–
	6 fl oz	–	110	–
	12 fl oz	–	200	–
(Knudsen)	8 fl oz	–	105	–
(Libby's)	6 fl oz	–	110	–
	11.5 fl oz	–	220	–
(S&W)	12 fl oz	–	210	–
(Walnut Acres)	8 oz	–	130	–
APRICOT JUICE/NECTAR BLEND/bottled or canned				
(Kern's)..all apricot blends	11.5 oz	–	220	–
(Seneca) apricot nectar cocktail	8 fl oz	–	140	–
ARMADILLO/raw	3 oz	4.0	150	24%
ARROWHEAD/plant				
cooked	medium corm	0.5	9	50%
raw	medium corm	0.5	12	38%
ARTICHOKE (*See also* JERUSALEM ARTICHOKE)				
canned or jarred				
(Cara Mia)				
in water	1 oz	–	15	–
marinated				
crowns	1 oz	–	12	–
hearts	1 oz	1.5	25	54%
(Progresso) hearts				
in brine	3 oz	–	30	–
marinated	1.1 oz	5.0	50	90%
regular	2 pieces	–	35	–

Food and Description	Amount	Fat Grams	Total Calories	% Fat Calories
(Reese)				
bottoms	2 pieces	–	35	–
hearts	3 pieces	–	30	–
(S&W)				
bottoms/in water	3 pieces	–	25	–
hearts				
in water	3 pieces	–	30	–
marinated	2 pieces	2.0	20	90%
(Sun of Italy)/marinated	1 oz	1.5	25	54%
fresh				
(Dole) (Dole)	1 medium	–	25	–
frozen				
(Birds Eye) hearts/deluxe	½ cup	–	30	–
(C&W) hearts	½ cup	–	25	–
ARTICHOKE HEART (*See* ARTICHOKE)				
ARUGULA				
fresh/chopped	½ cup	<1.0	2	13%
	1 lb	1.5	105	13%

ASIAN FOOD (*See also* APPETIZERS; FROZEN ENTRÉE/DINNER; PASTA ENTRÉE/DINNER; RICE DISH; VEGETARIAN FOODS; individual listings)

■ **BEEF DISHES** (*See also* Chow Mein; Fried Rice; Sweet & Sour in this section)

(Chung King)				
Canned/				
beef pepper Oriental/divider pak entrée/prepared	1 cup	2.5	100	23%
frozen				
(LaChoy) prepared				
beef pepper/bi-pack	¾ cup	2.0	80	23%
beef pepper Oriental entrée/ prepared	¾ cup	4.0	100	36%

■ **CHICKEN DISHES** (*See also* Chow Mein; Fried Rice; Sweet & Sour in this section)

(Chun King) frozen entrée				
imperial chicken	13 oz	10.0	460	20%
walnut chicken	13 oz	19.0	460	37%
(La Choy) canned/prepared				
chicken teriyaki/bi-pack	¾ cup	2.0	85	21%
sweet & sour				
bi-pack	¾ cup	2.0	120	15%
entrée	¾ cup	2.0	240	8%

■ **CHOP SUEY**

homemade/USDA Standard Home Recipe				
w/beef & pork	1 cup	17.0	300	51%
w/beef w/o noodles	1 cup	17.0	300	51%

■ **CHOW MEIN** (*See also* Vegetables in this section)

beef				
(Chun King) canned/prepared				
divider pack entrée	1 cup	1.5	110	12%
stir-fry entrée	6 oz	19.0	290	59%
chicken				
(Chun King) canned/prepared				
divider pack entrée	1 cup	4.5	110	37%

Food and Description	Amount	Fat Grams	Total Calories	% Fat Calories
stir-fry entrée	1 cup	11.0	220	45%
homemade/USDA Standard	¾ cup	10.0	255	35%
(La Choy)				
bi-pack/canned/prepared	¾ cup	4.5	110	37%
dinner	¾ pkg	17.0	300	51%
entrée	¾ cup	4.0	70	51%
pork				
(Chun King) canned/prepared	1 cup	4.5	110	37%
(La Choy)				
bi-pack/canned/prepared	¾ cup	4.0	80	45%
shrimp				
(Chun King) canned/prepared	1 cup	2.5	110	37%
homemade/USDA Standard Home				
Recipe w/noodles	¾ cup	3.9	141	25%
(La Choy) canned/prepared	¾ cup	1.0	70	13%
■ EGG ROLL				
(Chun King) frozen				
chicken				
mini	6 pieces	9.0	210	39%
restaurant-style	1 piece	9.0	190	43%
pork & shrimp/mini	6 pieces	9.0	210	39%
shrimp				
mini	6 pieces	6.0	190	28%
restaurant-style	1 piece	7.0	180	35%
(La Choy) frozen				
bite-size				
pork & shrimp	12 pieces	10.0	210	43%
mini				
chicken	6 pieces	9.0	210	39%
pork & shrimp	6 pieces	9.0	210	39%
shrimp	6 pieces	6.0	190	28%
vegetable w/lobster	6 pieces	7.0	190	33%
restaurant-style/6 oz				
chicken	1 piece	9.0	210	39%
pork	1 piece	11.0	220	45%
shrimp	1 piece	7.0	180	35%
sweet & sour	1 piece	9.0	220	37%
(Minh) frozen				
chicken white meat	3 oz	5.0	150	30%
pork	3 oz	8.0	170	37%
pork & shrimp	3 oz	4.5	140	29%
seafood	3 oz	4.5	140	29%
vegetable	3 oz	4.5	140	29%
(Pagoda Cafe) frozen				
chicken				
sweet & sour	2.75 oz	6.0	160	34%
white meat	2.75 oz	6.0	160	34%
white meat/mini	3.2 oz	7.0	180	35%
pork/savory				
& vegetable	3.6 oz	8.0	170	42%

Food and Description	Amount	Fat Grams	Total Calories	% Fat Calories
mini	1.6 oz	9.0	200	41%
pork & shrimp	2.75 oz	8.0	170	42%
vegetable	2.75 oz	7.0	150	42%
(Schwan's) frozen				
chicken	2 pieces	12.0	240	45%
pork	2 pieces	11.0	240	41%
Southwest chicken	2 pieces	9.0	260	31%
won ton pizza-flavored	2 pieces	18.0	410	40%
(Yu Sing) frozen				
chicken	6 rolls	7.0	180	35%
pork & shrimp	6 rolls	9.0	200	41%
shrimp	6 rolls	7.0	180	35%
sweet & sour chicken	6 rolls	7.0	190	33%
sweet & sour pork	6 rolls	9.0	210	39%
■ EGG ROLL WRAPPER				
(Azumaya Pasta)	2 wrappers	–	130	–
(Nasoya)	2 wrappers	–	120	–
■ FORTUNE COOKIE				
(La Choy)	4 cookies	–	112	–
■ FRIED RICE (*See also* RICE DISH and YU SING in this section)				
(Chun King) frozen				
w/chicken	8 oz	6.0	270	20%
w/pork	8 oz	5.0	290	19%
(Kan Tong) dry				
chicken	2 oz	3.5	190	17%
pork	2 oz	1.0	190	5%
shrimp	2 oz	1.0	190	5%
spicy chicken	2 oz	1.0	190	5%
traditional	2 oz	3.0	190	14%
vegetable	2 oz	0.5	190	2%
(Ling Ling) frozen				
vegetable	1 cup	4.0	140	26%
■ NOODLE (*See also* PASTA; PASTA ENTRÉE/DINNER)				
(China Bowl)				
cellophane/cooked	1 cup	–	200	–
Chinese/cooked	1 cup	<1	210	2%
rice sticks/dry	2 oz	<1	200	2%
(China Boy)/dry				
chow mein				
classic	~1 oz	5.0	125	36%
wide	~1 oz	5.0	130	35%
rice/thin	~1 oz	5.0	130	35%
(Chun King) chow mein/dry	1 oz	7.0	140	45%
(La Choy)				
chow mein	½ cup	6.0	140	39%
crispy wide	½ cup	8.0	150	35%
rice	½ cup	3.0	120	23%
■ POTSTICKERS (See also APPETIZERS)				
(Ling Ling) frozen				
chicken & vegetable dumplings				
dumplings only	5 pieces	7.0	280	23%

Food and Description	Amount	Fat Grams	Total Calories	% Fat Calories
w/1 Tbs sauce	1 serving	7.0	300	21%
(Pagoda Cafe) frozen				
savory pork	3.25 oz	13.0	240	49%

■ **SAUCES & SEASONINGS** (*See also* SAUCE; SEASONINGS)

Food and Description	Amount	Fat Grams	Total Calories	% Fat Calories
(China Bowl)				
chili paste w/garlic	2 Tbs	–	15	–
hoisin	1 tsp	–	10	–
oyster	½ tsp	–	5	–
soy	½ tsp	–	<5	–
(Chun King)				
hot teriyaki sauce	1 Tbs	–	17	–
soy sauce	1 Tbs	–	10	–
(Contadina) Sweet & Sour Sauce	2 Tbs	1.0	40	23%
w/pineapple				
(House of Tsang)				
oil				
hot chili sesame	1 tsp	5.0	45	100%
Mongolian Fire Oil	1 tsp	5.0	45	100%
pure sesame	1 tsp	5.0	45	100%
Singapore curry	1 tsp	5.0	45	100%
wok	1 Tbs	14.0	130	100%
sauce				
Bangkok padang	1 Tbs	2.5	45	50%
classic stir-fry	1 Tbs	0.5	25	18%
hibachi grill sauce				
Hunan Smokehut	1 Tbs	0.5	40	11%
Kobe steak	1 Tbs	4.0	50	72%
sweet ginger sesame	1 Tbs	–	40	–
teriyaki	1 Tbs	–	40	–
Thai peanut	1 Tbs	3.0	50	54%
Hong Kong BBQ	1 tsp	–	10	–
Imperial citrus stir-fry	1 Tbs	–	17	–
Korean teriyaki	1 Tbs	0.5	30	15%
mandarin marinade	1 Tbs	–	25	–
oyster-flavored stir-fry	1 Tbs	–	30	–
Saigon sizzle	1 Tbs	1.0	40	23%
soy sauce				
dark	1 Tbs	–	17	–
ginger-flavored				
low-sodium	1 Tbs	–	10	–
regular	1 Tbs	–	20	–
light	1 Tbs	–	5	–
low-sodium	1 Tbs	–	5	–
spicy brown bean	1 tsp	–	15	–
sweet & sour concentrate	1 tsp	–	10	–
sweet & sour stir-fry	1 Tbs	–	35	–
Szechuan spicy stir-fry	1 Tbs	0.5	20	23%
vegetables & sauce				
Hong Kong sweet & sour	½ cup	1.0	160	6%
Szechaun hot & spicy	½ cup	1.0	70	13%

Food and Description	Amount	Fat Grams	Total Calories	% Fat Calories
Tokyo teriyaki	½ cup	–	100	–
(Kame) soy/dark	1 Tbs	–	5	–
(Kikkoman)				
chow mein seasoning				
light	1 Tbs	–	10	–
regular	1 pkg	–	100	–
soy sauce				
light	1 Tbs	–	10	–
regular	1 Tbs	–	10	–
stir-fry	1 Tbs	–	20	–
sukiyaki	1 Tbs	–	20	–
sweet & sour	1 Tbs	–	35	–
teriyaki				
baste & glaze	2 Tbs	–	50	–
light	1 Tbs	–	15	–
roasted garlic	1 Tbs	–	25	–
(La Choy)				
bead molasses	1 Tbs	–	50	–
brown gravy sauce	¼ cup	–	275	–
plum	1 Tbs	–	25	–
soy sauce/light	1 Tbs	–	10	–
stir-fry				
mandarin soy sauce	½ cup	–	70	–
sauce & marinade	½ cup	–	30	–
sweet & sour	½ cup	–	140	–
Szechwan	½ cup	–	80	–
teriyaki	½ cup	–	95	–
sweet & sour				
duck sauce	2 Tbs	–	60	–
original	2 Tbs	–	60	–
teriyaki				
light	1 Tbs	–	18	–
original	1 Tbs	–	40	–

■ **SEASONINGS** (*See* SAUCES & SEASONINGS in this section)
■ **STIR-FRY** (*See also* VEGETABLES, MIXED)

Food and Description	Amount	Fat Grams	Total Calories	% Fat Calories
(Birds Eye) Gourmet Meal Starter/Frozen/As packaged				
Oriental lo mein	2¼ cups	3.5	230	14%
sesame ginger teriyaki	2¼ cups	1.5	140	10%
spicy Szechuan w/cashews	2¼ cups	4.5	180	23%
sweet & sour w/pineapple tidbits	2¼ cups	0.5	200	2%
(C&W) frozen/vegetable stir-fry dinner				
w/basmati rice	1 cup	–	220	–
w/Oriental noodles	1 cup	2.5	200	11%
(Green Giant) frozen/Create A Meal!/as packaged				
garlic & ginger	1⅔ cups	1.5	130	10%
lo mein	2⅓ cups	1.5	170	8%
sweet & sour	1½ cups	–	180	–
Szechuan	1¾ cups	5.0	150	30%
teriyaki	1¾ cups	0.5	100	5%

Food and Description	Amount	Fat Grams	Total Calories	% Fat Calories
■ SUSHI				
homemade/USDA Standard Home				
Recipe/w/vegetables	4.5 oz	–	181	–
■ SWEET & SOUR				
(La Choy) canned/prepared				
chicken entrée	¾ cup	2.0	240	8%
pork entrée	¾ cup	4.0	250	14%
■ VEGETABLES/VEGETABLE DISHES (*See also* Chow Mein; Fried Rice; Stir-Fry in this section)				
(Birds Eye) Frozen stir-fry vegetables/as packaged				
asparagus	2 cups frozen	0.5	90	5%
broccoli	1 cup frozen	–	30	–
pepper	3 oz frozen	–	25	–
sugar snap	¾ cup frozen	–	35	–
whole bean	5.4 oz frozen	0.5	100	5%
(Chun King)				
Chinese pea pods	3 oz	1.5	35	38%
chow mein vegetables/divider pack entrée/prepared	⅔ cup	–	15	–
water chestnuts				
sliced	16 slices	–	10	–
whole	8.5 oz	0.5	190	2%
(Empress)				
bamboo shoots/sliced	2 oz	–	13	–
water chestnuts				
sliced	2 oz	–	14	–
whole	2 oz	–	14	–
(Geisha)				
bamboo shoots	4 oz	–	25	–
bean sprouts	~2 oz	–	25	–
water chestnuts				
sliced	5.3 oz	–	50	–
whole	5.3 oz	–	45	–
(La Choy)				
bamboo shoots	3 oz	–	10	–
	¼ cup	–	6	–
bean sprouts	6 oz	–	15	–
Chinese/mixed/fancy	4.6 oz	–	10	–
chop suey vegetables	4.6 oz	–	15	–
water chestnuts				
sliced	2 Tbs	–	10	–
	¼ cup	–	18	–
whole	2 medium	–	10	–
■ WON TON SOUP (*See* SOUP)				
■ WON TON WRAPPER				
(Azumaya)	1 wrapper	–	23	–
(Nasoya)	1 wrapper	–	23	–
■ (YU SING) (*See also* EGG ROLL in this section)				
Frozen Bowls				
beef				
spicy beef & broccoli	1 bowl	5.0	380	12%

Food and Description	Amount	Fat Grams	Total Calories	% Fat Calories
teriyaki steak	1 bowl	3.0	370	7%
chicken				
honey ginger	1 bowl	6.0	350	15%
sesame	1 bowl	6.0	390	14%
shrimp-fried rice	1 bowl	7.0	430	15%
sweet & sour w/rice	1 bowl	4.0	420	9%
teriyaki	1 bowl	3.0	400	7%
vegetables & white chicken	1 bowl	9.0	360	15%
frozen entrées				
beef				
Cantonese w/rice	1 meal	7.0	270	23%
Oriental beef & peppers w/rice	1 meal	7.0	290	22%
Pepper steak w/green peppers				
ginger beef w/rice	1 meal	9.0	290	28%
teriyaki w/rice	1 meal	2.5	260	8%
chicken				
chow mein w/rice	1 meal	6.0	270	20%
fried rice	1 meal	8.0	360	20%
garlic w/rice	1 meal	2.5	240	9%
ginger w/rice	1 meal	5.0	250	18%
lo mein	1 meal	4.0	230	16%
mandarin w/rice	1 meal	4.0	300	12%
sweet & sour w/rice	1 meal	3.5	340	9%
pork				
-fried rice	1 meal	12.0	440	25%
& shrimp-fried rice	1 meal	12.0	440	25%
fried rice	1 meal	13.0	450	26%
shrimp				
-fried rice	1 meal	6.0	350	15%
lo mein	1 meal	1.5	210	6%
ASPARAGUS				
canned				
(Del Monte) tender green				
all styles	½ cup	–	20	–
(Green Giant)..all cuts	½ cup	–	20	–
(LeSueur) extra-large spears	4.5 oz	–	20	–
(Native Forest				
all styles	4.5 oz	–	20	–
(Reese) white spears	⅓ can	–	20	–
(S&W)				
blended	6 pieces	–	15	–
colossal	3 pieces	–	10	–
no salt or sugar added	½ cup	–	20	–
(Stokely)				
cut green	½ cup	–	25	–
(Thank You) whole spears	½ cup	–	25	–
cooked				
cuts w/tips	½ cup	–	22	–
(Dole) spears	5 spears	–	25	–
spears	4 spears	–	15	–

Food and Description	Amount	Fat Grams	Total Calories	% Fat Calories
fresh				
(Chiquita) Walla Walla				
cuts & tips	½ cup	–	25	–
whole	½ cup	–	15	–
raw				
cuts w/tips	½ cup	–	15	–
spears	4 spears	–	13	–
AVOCADO				
fresh/raw				
(Calavo) medium avocado				
Fuerte	⅕ fruit	5.0	55	82%
Gwen	⅕ fruit	5.0	55	82%
Hass	⅕ fruit	5.0	55	82%
Lamb Hass	⅕ fruit	5.0	55	82%
Pinkerton	⅕ fruit	5.0	55	82%
Reed	⅕ fruit	5.0	55	82%
Zutano	⅕ fruit	5.0	55	82%
California				
mashed	1 cup	36.0	407	80%
whole/medium	1 fruit	30.8	324	86%
Florida/medium	1 fruit	27.0	340	72%

B

Food and Description	Amount	Fat Grams	Total Calories	% Fat Calories
BACON (*See also* BACON, CANADIAN STYLE; BACON BITS, CHIPS & PIECES; BACON SUBSTITUTE; LUNCHEON MEAT)				
(Armour) Ready				
crisp/fully cooked	2 slices	6.0	70	77%
hickory-smoked				
original	2 slices	7.0	70	90%
regular	2 slices	4.0	60	60%
(Boar's Head) fried				
domestic	2 slices	6.0	70	77%
imported	2 slices	5.0	60	75%
(Bob Evans) thick-sliced				
hickory-smoked	2 slices	7.0	80	79%
(Bryan)				
pre-cooked/pan-fried				
extra thick	2 slices	7.0	90	70%

Food and Description	Amount	Fat Grams	Total Calories	% Fat Calories
single pan-fried slices				
extra thick	2 slices	8.0	90	80%
quality	2 slices	8.0	90	80%
thick	2 slices	7.0	90	70%
thin	4 slices	8.0	90	90%
slab pan-fried slices	2 slices	8.0	90	80%
(Farmer John)				
lower-sodium	2 slices	7.0	80	79%
maple-flavored	2 slices	7.0	80	79%
regular	2 slices	7.0	80	79%
thick-sliced	1 slices	5.0	60	75%
(Gwaltney)..cooked				
Aberdeen	2 slices	5.0	60	65%
brown sugar	2 slices	5.0	60	65%
regular	2 slices	5.0	60	65%
(Hillshire Farm) country				
smoked	1 slice	12.0	120	90%
(Hormel) cooked				
Black Label				
center cut	3 slices	5.5	70	71%
low-salt	2 slices	7.0	80	79%
regular	2 slices	7.0	80	79%
Canadian style	2 oz	3.0	70	39%
microwave	4 slices	5.0	70	64%
Old Smokehouse	2 slices	7.0	80	79%
original	2.5 slices	5.0	70	64%
Range	2 slices	9.0	110	74%
Red Label	2 slices	7.0	80	79%
(Jimmy Dean)				
pre-cooked center piece				
regular-sliced	3 slices	7.0	80	79%
thick-sliced	2 slices	7.0	80	79%
shingle/sliced/cooked				
hotel shingle	1 slice	5.0	60	75%
original shingle	1 slice	5.0	60	75%
single-sliced				
applewood	1 slice	4.5	50	81%
heavy smoke				
(Kahn's)				
lower-sodium	2 oz	5.0	60	75%
regular	2 oz	5.0	60	75%
slab sliced/no				
sugar added	2 oz	6.0	60	90%
(Louis Rich) cured				
dark and light	1 slice	2.5	35	64%
(Oscar Mayer) cooked				
⅛" thick cut	1 slice	5.0	60	75%
center cut	2 slices	4.5	60	68%
lower sodium	2 slices	5.0	70	64%
original	2 slices	6.0	70	77%

Food and Description	Amount	Fat Grams	Total Calories	% Fat Calories
Ready Crisp/shelf	3 slices	6.0	70	77%
(Smithfield)..fried..all types	2 slices	6.0	70	77%
BACON, CANADIAN STYLE				
(Boar's Head) Extra Lea	2 oz	2.0	70	26%
(Dak) 98% fat-free	2 oz	6.0	60	90%
(Hormel)..cooked..1 oz slices	2 slices	3.0	70	39%
(Jones)/uncooked	3 slices	3.0	70	39%
(Oscar Mayer) cooked	2 slices	1.5	50	27%
BACON, VEGETARIAN (See VEGETARIAN FOODS)				
BACON BITS, CHIPS & PIECES				
imitation				
(Betty Crocker) BacOs				
bits	1½ Tbs	1.5	30	45%
chips	1½ Tbs	1.5	30	45%
(Durkee)				
bits	1 Tbs	1.0	25	36%
chips	1 Tbs	1.0	25	36%
(McCormick/Schilling)				
Bac'n Bits	1 Tbs	<1.0	25	18%
Bac'n Chips	1 Tbs	<1.0	25	18%
(Tone's) bits	1 Tbs	1.0	30	30%
real				
(Hormel)				
bits	1 Tbs	1.5	30	30%
bits/less fat	1 Tbs	2.5	35	64%
crispy real bacon				
chips	1 Tbs	3.0	45	60%
pieces	1 Tbs	1.5	25	54%
(Jimmy Dean)				
applewood ends				
& pieces	½ oz	7.0	80	78%
bits	1 Tbs	8.0	90	80%
diced	1 Tbs	8.0	90	80%
kettle-cooked	1 tsp	1.0	20	45%
(Oscar Mayer)				
Bits	1 Tbs	1.5	25	54%
Pieces	1 Tbs	1.5	25	54%
BACON SUBSTITUTE (See also BACON BITS, CHIPS & PIECES; VEGETARIAN FOODS)				
BAGEL				
(CarbXtract)				
blueberry	½ bagel	1.75	67	24%
chocolate chip	½ bagel	1.75	67	24%
cinnamon-raisin	½ bagel	2.0	95	19%
garlic-onion	½ bagel	1.75	67	24%
onion	½ bagel	1.75	67	24%
plain	½ bagel	2.0	86	21%
poppy seed	½ bagel	1.75	67	24%
sesame	½ bagel	1.75	67	24%
(Dunkin' Donuts)				
Bagels				
berry berry	1 bagel	3.0	340	8%

Food and Description	Amount	Fat Grams	Total Calories	% Fat Calories
blueberry	1 bagel	3.0	350	8%
cinnamon raisin	1 bagel	3.0	330	8%
everything	1 bagel	7.0	430	15%
garlic	1 bagel	3.5	410	8%
onion	1 bagel	4.0	370	9%
plain	1 bagel	3.0	360	8%
poppyseed	1 bagel	10.0	440	20%
salsa	1 bagel	3.0	320	8%
salt	1 bagel	3.0	360	8%
sesame	1 bagel	11.0	450	22%
sourdough	1 bagel	3.0	340	8%
wheat	1 bagel	4.5	350	12%
bagel spreads				
butter				
Shedd's Buttermatch Blend	1 Tbs	9.0	80	90%
cream cheese				
chive	2 oz	17.0	170	90%
garden vegetable	2 oz	15.0	170	79%
lite	2 oz	9.0	110	82%
salmon	2 oz	17.0	170	90%
strawberry	2 oz	17.0	190	81%
(Earth Grains) Premium/sliced				
apple cinnamon	1 bagel	1.5	240	6%
blueberry	1 bagel	1.5	240	6%
cinnamon raisin	1 bagel	1.5	230	6%
plain	1 bagel	1.0	240	4%
(Lender's)				
Bagel Shop/Fresh				
apple cranberry	1 bagel	2.0	310	6%
blueberry	1 bagel	2.5	270	8%
cinnamon raisin	1 bagel	4.0	280	13%
egg	1 bagel	3.5	280	11%
honey wheat	1 bagel	2.5	270	8%
onion	1 bagel	2.5	270	8%
plain	1 bagel	2.5	280	8%
standard tomato	1 bagel	2.5	300	8%
Bagel Shop/Refrigerated				
blueberry	1 bagel	1.0	200	5%
cinnamon raisin	1 bagel	2.5	230	10%
egg	1 bagel	2.5	220	10%
honey wheat	1 bagel	1.5	190	7%
onion	1 bagel	2.0	220	8%
plain	1 bagel	2.0	220	8%
Big 'n' Crusty/Frozen				
blueberry	1 bagel	1.0	250	4%
cinnamon raisin	1 bagel	2.5	260	9%
egg	1 bagel	1.5	260	5%
honey wheat	1 bagel	0.5	230	2%
onion	1 bagel	1.0	250	4%
plain	1 bagel	1.0	250	4%

Food and Description	Amount	Fat Grams	Total Calories	% Fat Calories
New York–style				
blueberry	1 bagel	1.0	250	4%
cinnamon raisin	1 bagel	2.5	160	14%
onion	1 bagel	1.0	250	4%
plain	1 bagel	1.0	230	4%
original/frozen				
blueberry swirl	1 bagel	0.5	160	3%
chocolate chip swirl	1 bagel	1.0	160	6%
cinnamon-raisin	1 bagel	1.0	160	6%
cinnamon swirl	1 bagel	0.5	150	3%
egg	1 bagel	1.0	160	6%
garlic	1 bagel	1.0	150	6%
onion	1 bagel	0.5	150	3%
plain	1 bagel	0.5	150	3%
plain bagelette	2 bagels	0.5	140	6%
poppy	1 bagel	1.0	150	6%
pumpernickel	1 bagel	1.0	150	6%
rye	1 bagel	1.0	150	6%
sesame seed	1 bagel	1.5	150	9%
soft original				
2.5 oz	1 bagel	3.5	210	15%
strawberry swirl	1 bagel	0.5	160	3%
(Otis Spunkmeyer) Thaw & Serve frozen				
3-oz bagels				
blueberry	1 bagel	1.0	210	4%
cinnamon raisin	1 bagel	1.0	210	4%
onion	1 bagel	1.0	210	4%
plain	1 bagel	1.0	210	4%
4-oz bagels				
blueberry	1 bagel	1.0	290	3%
cinnamon raisin	1 bagel	1.0	280	3%
onion	1 bagel	1.0	280	3%
(Pepperidge Farm) food service/Bountiful Bagels				
cinnamon raisin	1 bagel	0.5	280	2%
brown sugar cinnamon				
mini	1 bagel	0.5	120	4%
everything	1 bagel	2.0	310	6%
onion	1 bagel	1.5	290	5%
plain/mini	1 bagel	0.5	290	2%
(Sara Lee)				
blueberry	1 bagel	1.0	260	3%
cranberry orange	1 bagel	1.5	310	4%
egg	1 bagel	0.5	210	2%
honey wheat				
toaster size	1 bagel	1.0	170	5%
mini plain	1 serving	–	70	–
plain/sliced	1 bagel	1.0	250	4%
sun-dried tomato & basil	1 bagel	1.5.	300	5%

Food and Description	Amount	Fat Grams	Total Calories	% Fat Calories
the works	1 bagel	3.5	330	10%
(Thomas')				
Gourmet/pre-sliced				
cranberry orange	½ bagel	0.5	150	3%
wild blueberry	½ bagel	1.0	170	5%
New York–style				
blueberry	1 bagel	2.0	300	6%
carb counting				
plain	1 bagel	2.0	140	12%
whole wheat	1 bagel	2.0	140	12%
cinnamon raisin swirl	1 bagel	1.5	290	5%
cinnamon swirl	1 bagel	3.0	300	9%
multigrain	1 bagel	2.0	280	6%
oat bran	1 bagel	0.5	145	3%
onion	1 bagel	1.5	290	5%
plain				
6-count	1 bagel	1.5	280	5%
mini/pre-sliced	1 bagel	1.0	130	7%
sesame	1 bagel	3.5	300	11%
whole wheat	1 bagel	2.0	140	12%
BAGEL CHIPS				
(New York–style)				
chip mix/baked				
fat-free	1 oz	–	100	–
garlic	~1 oz	3.0	130	21%
original	1 oz	7.0	180	35%
chips.. garlic pita	7 chips	5.0	130	35%
crisps				
cinnamon raisin	7 pieces	5.0	130	35%
everything bagel	7 pieces	6.0	130	42%
plain pita	7 pieces	4.0	90	40%
roasted garlic	7 pieces	5.0	130	35%
sesame	7 pieces	7.0	140	45%
(Old London)..bagel snacks				
cinnamon	5 pieces	1.0	60	15%
others..All	5 pieces	3.0	60	45%
(Rondelé)				
cinnamon raisin w/honey	13 chips	4.0	130	28%
roasted garlic				
original	13 chips	5.0	140	32%
reduced-fat	13 chips	3.0	130	21%
roasted garlic				
original	13 chips	5.0	140	32%
reduced-fat	13 chips	–	130	–
toasted onion & parsley	13 chips	5.0	140	32%
very plain	13 chips	5.0	140	32%
(Sara Lee)..all types	6 chips	5.0	130	35%

BAKE & FRY MIX (*See also* SEASONINGS; TEMPURA BATTER)
(Arrowhead) all-purpose baking mix/dry

Food and Description	Amount	Fat Grams	Total Calories	% Fat Calories
regular	¼ cup	0.5	140	3%
wheat-free	¼ cup	0.5	120	4%
(Bisquick) Dry mix only				
original	⅓ cup	7.0	160	39%
reduced-fat	⅓ cup	3.0	140	19%
(Calhoun Bend Mill) mix only				
awesome onion coating	3 Tbs	–	100	–
chicken & shrimp fry	4 tsp	–	35	–
fish & seafood breading	4 tsp	–	35	–
fish fry	4 tsp	–	35	–
mild	4 tsp	–	35	–
spicy	4 tsp	–	30	–
(Golden Dipped) dry mix only				
Breaders & Batters				
Fry Easy/Mix				
all-purpose batter	¼ cup	1.0	120	8%
beer batter	¼ cup	–	100	–
Cajun-style	1⅓ Tbs	–	35	–
cracker meal fry	¼ cup	1.0	130	7%
extra crispy				
chicken fry	1½ Tbs	–	60	–
fish & chips batter	¼ cup	–	100	–
fish fry	1½ Tbs	–	35	–
funnel cake batter	¼ cup	1.0	120	8%
herbs & spices				
chicken fry	2 Tbs	–	70	–
hot n spicy				
chicken fry	2 Tbs	–	50	–
hush puppy w/onion	¼ cup	0.5	130	3%
onion ring batter	¼ cup	–	100	–
original home-style chicken fry	2 Tbs	–	50	–
seafood fry	1⅔ Tbs	–	50	–
tempura batter	1¼ cup	–	100	–
Oven Easy/coating				
Cajun-style	¼ cup	3.0	90	30%
garlic & herb	3 Tbs	2.5	100	23%
lemon & pepper	¼ cup	3.0	90	30%
shrimp & seafood	2 Tbs	2.0	70	26%
pre-dip egg & milk				
replacement	¼ cup	1.0	140	6%
(Hain) whole wheat/dry	⅓ cup	1.0	140	6%
(Jiffy) dry mix only	¼ cup	4.0	160	23%
(Krusteaz) dry mix only				
bake & fry mix	¼ cup	1.0	100	9%
baking mix	⅓ cup	6.0	180	30%
tempura mix	¼ cup	0.5	110	4%
(Martha White) Recip-Ease	½ cup	8.0	240	30%
BAKING BITS, CHIPS, CHUNKS & PIECES				
(Baker's) baking chocolate				
bars				

Food and Description	Amount	Fat Grams	Total Calories	% Fat Calories
bittersweet	½ square	6.0	70	77%
German sweet	2 squares	3.5	70	45%
semi-sweet	½ square	4.5	70	58%
unsweetened	½ square	7.0	70	90%
white	½ square	4.5	80	51%
chips				
chocolate-flavored				
semi-sweet	½ oz	3.5	70	45%
real				
milk chocolate	½ oz	4.0	70	51%
semi-sweet	½ oz	3.5	60	52%
chunks				
milk chocolate	½ oz	4.5	70	58%
real semi-sweet	½ oz	3.5	60	52%
white chocolate	½ oz	3.5	70	45%
dipping chocolate				
real milk	½ oz	5.0	80	56%
(Best Yet) bark coating				
chocolate	2 oz	16.0	300	48%
white	½ oz	16.0	300	48%
(Ghirardelli) baking chocolate				
bars				
bittersweet	3 sections	15.0	210	64%
classic white	3 sections	15.0	240	56%
dark w/mint	5 squares	11.0	190	52%
milk	3 sections	9.0	150	54%
blocks				
milk	1 section	8.0	140	51%
semi-sweet	3 sections	14.0	210	60%
sweet dark	3 sections	14.0	210	60%
unsweetened	3 sections	23.0	210	99%
chips				
classic white	2 Tbs	4.0	70	51%
milk chocolate	2 Tbs	3.5	70	45%
semi-sweet	2 Tbs	4.0	70	51%
(Hershey)				
bits for baking				
candy-coated holiday	1 Tbs	3.0	70	39%
chocolate & Reese's				
peanut butter	1 Tbs	3.0	70	39%
Skor English toffee	1 Tbs	4.5	70	58%
chips				
butterscotch	1 Tbs	4.0	80	45%
chocolate				
milk	1 Tbs	4.5	80	51%
mint	1 Tbs	4.0	80	45%
semi-sweet				
mini	1 Tbs	4.0	80	45%
regular	1 Tbs	4.0	80	45%
sweet	1 Tbs	4.5	80	51%

Food and Description	Amount	Fat Grams	Total Calories	% Fat Calories
Premier white milk	1 Tbs	4.0	80	45%
raspberry	1 Tbs	4.0	80	45%
Reese's peanut butter	1 Tbs	4.0	80	45%
Kisses/mini for baking	11 pieces	4.5	80	51%
(M&M * Mars) M&M Baking Bits				
milk chocolate	0.5 oz	3.0	70	39%
semi-sweet chocolate	0.5 oz	3.5	70	45%
(Nestlé)				
baking bars/chocolate				
Choco Bake	½ oz	8.0	80	56%
Premier white	½ oz	5.0	80	56%
semi-sweet	½ oz	4.0	70	51%
unsweetened	½ oz	7.0	80	79%
baking morsels				
butterscotch	1 Tbs	4.0	80	45%
chocolate				
milk	1 Tbs	4.5	80	50%
mint	1 Tbs	4.0	70	51%
peanut butter				
& milk chocolate	1 Tbs	4.5	80	50%
Nestlé Crunch				
baking pieces	1 Tbs	3.5	80	39%
Premier white	1 Tbs	4.0	80	45%
semi-sweet				
mega	1 Tbs	4.0	70	51%
mini	1 Tbs	4.0	70	51%
regular	1 Tbs	4.0	70	51%
Reese's				
peanut butter chips	1 Tbs	4.0	80	45%
peanut butter cup sprinkles	2 Tbs	7.0	150	42%
chunks/real				
semi-sweet	½ oz	3.5	70	45%
BAKING CHOCOLATE (*See* BAKING BITS, CHIPS, CHUNKS & PIECES)				
BAKING POWDER				
(Calumet)	1 tsp	–	4	–
(Davis)	1 Tbs	–	15	–
BAKING SODA	1 tsp	–	5	–
BALSAM PEAR/raw	1 cup	–	15	–
pods				
cooked	½ cup	–	12	–
raw	½ cup	–	8	–
BAMBOO SHOOT (*See also* ASIAN FOOD)				
canned	1 cup	<1.0	25	18%
fresh				
cooked	1 cup	–	15	–
raw	½ cup	–	21	–
BANANA				
dried	¼ cup	0.5	90	5%
freeze-dried/chips	½ cup	8.0	250	29%

Food and Description	Amount	Fat Grams	Total Calories	% Fat Calories
fresh				
red				
whole	1 medium	<1.0	120	2%
sliced	½ cup	<1.0	70	3%
yellow				
mashed	1 cup	1.0	210	4%
whole	1 medium	0.5	105	4%
(Chiquita)	1 medium	–	110	–
(Dole)	1 medium	1.0	120	8%
powdered	1 Tbs	–	20	–
BANANA, COOKING OR BAKING (*See* PLANTAIN)				
BANANA NECTAR/NECTAR BLEND				
(After the Fall)				
Banana Casablanca	8 fl oz	–	100	–
(Kern's/Libby's) nectar	11.5 oz	–	190	–
(R. W. Knudsen)				
strawberry-banana	8 fl oz	–	120	–
BARBECUE SAUCE (*See also* SAUCE; SEASONINGS)				
(Annie's Naturals) smokey maple	2 Tbs	1.0	45	20%
(Bill Johnson's)..all flavors	2 Tbs	–	40	–
(Bull's Eye)				
All styles & flavors	2 Tbs	–	60	–
(Chicken 'N Ribs)				
hickory smoke	1 Tbs	–	45	–
honey	1 Tbs	–	45	–
hot style	1 Tbs	–	45	–
original	1 Tbs	–	50	–
(Crystal)..all flavors	3.6 oz	–	45	–
(Heinz)				
chicken & rib	2 Tbs	–	45	–
garlic	2 Tbs	–	40	–
honey garlic	2 Tbs	–	45	–
original	2 Tbs	–	25	–
regular	2 Tbs	–	40	–
(Hunt's)				
hickory				
regular	2 Tbs	–	45	–
hickory & brown sugar	2 Tbs	–	70	–
honey				
hickory	2 Tbs	–	50	–
mustard	2 Tbs	–	50	–
hot & spicy	2 Tbs	–	45	–
light	2 Tbs	–	25	–
mesquite	2 Tbs	–	40	–
mild	2 Tbs	–	40	–
Oriental	2 Tbs	–	50	–
original				
bold	2 Tbs	–	45	–
regular	2 Tbs	–	50	–

Food and Description	Amount	Fat Grams	Total Calories	% Fat Calories
(K. C. Masterpiece)				
hickory	2 Tbs	–	60	–
hickory brown sugar	2 Tbs	–	60	–
honey				
smoke	2 Tbs	–	50	–
teriyaki	2 Tbs	–	60	–
mesquite	2 Tbs	–	60	–
original				
no salt	2 Tbs	–	60	–
regular	2 Tbs	–	60	–
spicy original	2 Tbs	–	60	–
steakhouse	2 Tbs	–	60	–
(Kraft)				
regular				
Char-Grill	2 Tbs	–	60	–
hickory smoke				
regular	2 Tbs	–	40	–
w/onion bits	2 Tbs	–	45	–
honey				
hickory smoke	2 Tbs	–	60	–
mustard	2 Tbs	–	60	–
roasted garlic	2 Tbs	–	50	–
hot				
hickory smoke	2 Tbs	–	40	–
regular	2 Tbs	–	40	–
Kansas City–style	2 Tbs	–	50	–
mesquite smoke	2 Tbs	–	40	–
onion bits	2 Tbs	–	45	–
original	2 Tbs	–	40	–
roasted garlic	2 Tbs	–	50	–
spicy				
Cajun	2 Tbs	–	50	–
honey	2 Tbs	–	60	–
Sweet Recipes				
brown sugar	2 Tbs	–	60	–
hickory smoke	2 Tbs	–	60	–
steakhouse style	2 Tbs	–	60	–
teriyaki	2 Tbs	–	60	–
Thick 'n' Spicy				
brown sugar	2 Tbs	–	60	–
hickory				
bacon	2 Tbs	1.0	60	15%
smoke	2 Tbs	1.0	60	15%
honey	2 Tbs	–	60	–
Kansas City–style	2 Tbs	–	60	–
mesquite smoke	2 Tbs	–	50	–
original	2 Tbs	–	50	–
(Maull's)..All flavors	2 Tbs	–	60	–
(Open Pit)..All flavors	1 Tbs	–	25	–

Food and Description	Amount	Fat Grams	Total Calories	% Fat Calories
(Sweet Baby Ray's)				
honey	2 Tbs	–	70	–
original	2 Tbs	–	70	–
(Texas Best)..all flavors	2 Tbs	–	50	–
(Walnut Farm)..all flavors	2 Tbs	–	0	–
BARLEY (*See also* CEREAL)				
(Arrowhead Mills)				
flakes/rolled	¼ cup	1.0	110	8%
flour	¼ cup	0.5	93	5%
hulless	¼ cup	1.0	140	6%
pearled	¼ cup	0.5	170	3%
(Quaker/Scotch)				
pearled/quick	⅓ cup	1.0	170	5%
regular/medium	¼ cup	1.0	170	5%
BARLEY MALT				
(Eden)	1 Tbs	–	60	–
BARRACUDA				
baked or broiled	3 oz	5.0	135	33%
breaded & fried	3 oz	7.5	169	40%
BASIL				
dried				
(McCormick/Schilling)	¼ tsp	–	1	–
fresh	2 Tbs	–	1	–
BASS				
black				
cooked—dry heat	3 oz	14.5	215	61%
raw	3 oz	1.0	80	11%
freshwater/raw	3 oz	3.0	97	28%
mixed species/raw	3 oz	3.0	97	28%
striped/cooked—dry heat	3 oz	2.0	82	22%
BAY LEAF/crumbled	1 tsp	–	5	–
BEAN (*See* individual bean listings)				
BEAN DISH (*See also* BEANS, BAKED & VARIETY; FROZEN ENTRÉE/DINNER; MEXICAN FOOD; individual bean listings)				
can, jar, or microwave container				
(Green Giant) 3-bean salad	½ cup	–	90	–
(Hanover) 4-bean salad	½ cup	–	80	–
(Luck's)				
beans w/sliced				
hot dogs	1 cup	16.0	390	37%
mixed-bean salad				
seasoned w/pork	7.25 oz	5.0	200	23%
(Read)				
4-bean salad	½ cup	3.5	110	29%
3-bean salad	½ cup	3.5	100	32%
(S&W) bean salad				
deli-style	½ cup	–	90	–
marinated				
dill garden	½ cup	–	50	–
mixed-bean	½ cup	–	90	–

Food and Description	Amount	Fat Grams	Total Calories	% Fat Calories
BEAN SPROUTS (*See also* individual bean listings)				
canned				
(LaChoy) drained	⅔ cup	–	15	–
fresh				
kidney				
boiled	4 oz	<1.0	37	12%
raw	1 cup	<1.0	53	8%
mung				
boiled	½ cup	–	13	–
raw	4 oz	–	40	–
stir-fried	½ cup	–	31	–
navy				
boiled	1 cup	<1.0	88	5%
raw	4 oz	<1.0	70	6%
pinto				
boiled	4 oz	–	25	–
raw	4 oz	1.0	70	13%
soy				
boiled	½ cup	2.0	38	47%
raw	10 sprouts	0.6	12	45%
stir-fried	4 oz	8.0	143	50%
BEANS, BAKED & VARIETY (*See also* BEAN DISH; MEXICAN FOOD)				
(B&M) baked beans				
bacon & onion	½ cup	2.0	190	9%
barbecue	½ cup	1.0	210	4%
maple	½ cup	1.0	150	6%
original	½ cup	2.0	170	5%
red kidney	½ cup	1.0	170	5%
vegetarian	½ cup	1.0	150	6%
w/honey	½ cup	1.5	170	8%
(Bush's Best)				
baked beans				
barbecue	½ cup	1.0	160	6%
bold & spicy	½ cup	1.0	120	8%
Boston recipe	½ cup	1.5	170	8%
country-style	½ cup	1.0	170	5%
home-style	½ cup	1.5	150	9%
maple-cured bacon	½ cup	1.0	150	9%
onions	½ cup	1.5	150	9%
vegetarian	½ cup	1.0	130	7%
(Campbell's)				
baked beans				
brown sugar & bacon	½ cup	3.0	160	17%
pork & beans	½ cup	1.0	140	6%
(Hanover)				
baked beans				
barbecue	½ cup	2.0	140	13%
brown sugar & bacon	½ cup	1.0	120	8%
honey mustard	½ cup	1.0	170	5%

Food and Description	Amount	Fat Grams	Total Calories	% Fat Calories
vegetarian	½ cup	–	130	–
pork & beans	½ cup	1.5	120	11%
(Hunt's)				
Big John's Beans & Fixin's	½ cup	3.0	150	18%
(Libby's)				
pork & molasses	½ cup	2.0	140	13%
pork & tomato sauce	½ cup	2.0	140	13%
vegetarian	½ cup	1.0	130	7%
(Life Choice) Country BBQ	½ cup	0.5	140	3%
(Muir Glen) Grill Chef				
All flavors & styles	2 Tbs	–	40	–
(S&W)				
baked				
barbecue				
Texas-style	½ cup	1.5	140	10%
ranch-style	½ cup	1.5	140	10%
brick oven	½ cup	0.5	160	3%
honey mustard	½ cup	–	130	–
maple syrup	½ cup	0.5	150	33%
sweet bacon	½ cup	1.5	140	10%
Pinquitos	½ cup	0.5	80	6%
(The Allen's)				
barbecue	½ cup	1.0	130	7%
maple-cured	½ cup	1.0	150	6%
onion	½ cup	1.0	150	6%
original	½ cup	1.0	150	6%
vegetarian	½ cup	–	130	–
(Van Camp's)				
baked				
w/chicken & brown sugar	½ cup	2.0	360	5%
w/ground beef & brown sugar	1 cup	7.0	370	17%
w/hot dogs & brown sugar	½ cup	6.0	340	16%
Beanee Weenee	7.75 oz	9.0	290	28%
honey-smoked ham	½ cup	1.0	140	6%
original/slow-cooked w/bacon & brown sugar	½ cup	1.0	160	6%
sweet hickory & bacon	½ cup	1.0	150	6%
sweet onion w/brown sugar	½ cup	0.5	140	3%
BEAR				
simmered	4 oz	15.0	295	46%
simmered/diced	½ cup	19.0	365	47%
BEAVER				
roasted	4 oz	6.0	190	28%
roasted/diced	½ cup	7.5	230	29%
BEECHNUT/dried	1 oz	14.0	164	77%
BEEF				

(NOTE: All serving sizes are for cooked portions, unless otherwise stated. "Lean" means beef trimmed of separable fat before cooking. "Lean & fat" means untrimmed

Food and Description	Amount	Fat Grams	Total Calories	% Fat Calories

and cooked or eaten as purchased. In most cases, 4 ounces of raw beef yields approximately 3 ounces cooked. Prime cuts have the most fat; choice cuts less; and select cuts the least amount of fat of all.

■ BEEF CUTS/FRESH

brisket/all grades/braised

Food and Description	Amount	Fat Grams	Total Calories	% Fat Calories
flat half				
lean				
0" fat	3 oz	5.0	160	28%
¼" fat	3 oz	8.0	190	38%
lean & fat				
¼" fat	3 oz	24.0	310	70%
whole				
lean				
0" fat	3 oz	9.0	185	44%
¼" fat	3 oz	11.0	210	47%
lean & fat				
¼" fat	3 oz	27.0	330	74%
chuck				
arm pot roast/braised				
lean				
0" fat				
choice	3 oz	7.5	187	36%
select	3 oz	5.0	170	26%
¼" fat				
choice	3 oz	8.0	190	38%
select	3 oz	6.0	175	31%
lean & fat				
¼" fat				
choice	3 oz	16.0	250	58%
select	3 oz	12.0	220	49%
blade roast/braised				
lean				
0" fat				
choice	3 oz	12.0	225	48%
select	3 oz	10.0	205	44%
¼" fat				
choice	3 oz	12.0	225	48%
select	3 oz	10.0	205	44%
lean & fat				
¼" fat				
choice	3 oz	24.0	310	70%
select	3 oz	20.0	280	64%
roast or steak/braised				
lean				
choice	3 oz	15.6	218	64%
select	3 oz	8.7	187	42%
lean & fat				
choice	3 oz	31.0	364	77%
select	3 oz	25.8	321	72%

Food and Description	Amount	Fat Grams	Total Calories	% Fat Calories
stew meat				
boneless/braised or stewed				
lean	3 oz	8.0	183	39%
lean & fat	3 oz	20.0	279	65%
corned beef				
boneless/roasted	3 oz	25.8	316	74%
flank/braised				
lean/0" fat/choice	3 oz	8.5	175	44%
lean & fat/0" fat				
/choice	3 oz	10.5	195	48%
ground				
extra-lean (17% fat)				
baked				
medium	3 oz	14.0	215	59%
well-done	3 oz	13.5	235	52%
broiled				
medium	3 oz	14.0	215	59%
well-done	3 oz	13.0	225	52%
pan-fried				
medium	3 oz	14.0	220	57%
well-done	3 oz	14.0	225	56%
lean (20% fat)				
baked				
medium	3 oz	15.5	230	61%
well-done	3 oz	15.5	250	56%
broiled				
medium	3 oz	15.5	230	61%
well-done	3 oz	15.0	240	56%
pan-fried				
medium	3 oz	16.0	235	61%
well-done	3 oz	15.0	235	57%
regular (27% fat)				
baked				
medium	3 oz	18.0	245	66%
well-done	3 oz	18.0	270	60%
broiled				
medium	3 oz	17.5	245	64%
well-done	3 oz	16.5	250	59%
pan-fried				
medium	3 oz	19.0	260	66%
well-done	3 oz	16.0	245	59%
loin/top/broiled				
lean				
¼" fat				
choice	3 oz	8.5	185	41%
select	3 oz	6.5	165	35%
lean & fat				
¼" fat				
choice	3 oz	18.0	255	64%
select	3 oz	14.5	225	58%

Food and Description	Amount	Fat Grams	Total Calories	% Fat Calories
London broil/100% lean				
choice/braised	3 oz	6.0	167	32%
porterhouse/braised				
lean/¼" fat/choice	3 oz	9.0	185	44%
lean & fat/¼" fat				
/choice	3 oz	19.0	260	66%
rib				
large end/roasted				
lean/0" fat				
choice	3 oz	13.0	215	54%
select	3 oz	10.0	190	47%
lean & fat				
¼" fat				
choice	3 oz	27.0	326	76%
select	3 oz	23.0	290	71%
small end/broiled				
lean				
0" fat				
choice	3 oz	10.0	190	47%
select	3 oz	7.5	170	40%
¼" fat				
choice	3 oz	11.0	200	50%
select	3 oz	8.0	180	40%
lean & fat				
¼" fat				
choice	3 oz	24.0	300	72%
select	3 oz	20.5	275	67%
whole/roasted				
lean				
¼" fat				
choice	3 oz	12.0	210	54%
select	3 oz	9.0	180	45%
lean & fat				
¼" fat				
choice	3 oz	26.0	320	73%
select	3 oz	22.5	290	70%
rib eye/broiled				
lean/0" fat/choice	3 oz	10.0	190	47%
lean & fat/0" fat				
/choice	3 oz	19.0	260	66%
ribs/short/braised				
lean/choice	3 oz	15.0	250	54%
lean & fat/choice	3 oz	36.0	400	81%
round				
bottom/roasted				
lean				
0" fat				
choice	3 oz	6.5	167	35%
select	3 oz	4.5	145	28%

Food and Description	Amount	Fat Grams	Total Calories	% Fat Calories
¼" fat				
choice	3 oz	7.0	170	37%
select	3 oz	5.0	155	29%
lean & fat				
0" fat				
choice	3 oz	8.0	175	41%
select	3 oz	5.0	150	30%
¼" fat				
choice	3 oz	14.0	220	57%
select	3 oz	11.0	200	50%
eye of/roasted				
lean				
¼" fat				
choice	3 oz	5.0	150	30%
select	3 oz	3.5	140	23%
lean & fat				
¼" fat				
choice	3 oz	12.0	205	53%
select	3 oz	9.5	185	46%
full cut/broiled				
lean				
¼" fat				
choice	3 oz	6.5	165	35%
select	3 oz	4.5	145	28%
lean & fat /¼" fat				
choice	3 oz	11.5	205	50%
rump roast/roasted				
lean				
choice	3 oz	7.9	177	40%
select	3 oz	6.0	162	33%
lean & fat				
choice	3 oz	23.0	295	70%
select	3 oz	19.9	269	67%
shank crosscuts/simmered				
lean/choice	3 oz	5.5	175	28%
lean & fat/¼" fat				
choice	3 oz	12.5	225	50%
sirloin				
top/broiled				
lean				
¼" fat				
choice	3 oz	7.0	175	36%
select	3 oz	5.5	160	31%
lean & fat				
¼" fat				
choice	3 oz	14.0	230	55%
select	3 oz	12.0	219	51%
wedge-bone/broiled				
lean				
choice	3 oz	6.0	178	30%

Food and Description	Amount	Fat Grams	Total Calories	% Fat Calories
prime	3 oz	10.0	201	45%
select	3 oz	7.0	170	37%
lean & fat				
choice	3 oz	16.0	240	56%
prime	3 oz	19.0	271	63%
select	3 oz	15.0	232	58%
steak/broiled				
club/choice				
lean & fat	3 oz	34.5	386	30%
porterhouse/choice				
lean	3 oz	9.0	185	44%
lean & fat	3 oz	18.0	254	64%
sirloin	3 oz	6.0	170	21%
tenderloin	3 oz	9.0	180	45%
T-bone/choice				
lean	3 oz	9.0	185	44%
lean & fat/¼" fat	3 oz	18.0	255	64%
tenderloin/roasted				
lean				
¼" fat				
choice	3 oz	14.5	265	49%
select	3 oz	9.0	180	43%
lean & fat				
¼" fat				
choice	3 oz	22.5	290	70%
select	3 oz	21.0	275	69%
tip/roasted				
lean				
0" fat				
choice	3 oz	5.5	155	32%
select	3 oz	4.5	145	28%
¼" fat				
choice	3 oz	6.0	160	34%
select	3 oz	5.5	155	32%
lean & fat				
¼" fat				
choice	3 oz	12.5	210	54%
select	3 oz	10.5	195	48%
top/broiled				
lean				
¼" fat				
choice	3 oz	5.0	160	28%
select	3 oz	3.5	145	22%
lean & fat				
¼" fat				
choice	3 oz	9.0	190	47%
select	3 oz	7.0	175	36%

Food and Description	Amount	Fat Grams	Total Calories	% Fat Calories
■ **BEEF CUTS/BRAND NAME**				
(Boar's Head)				
beef/Italian-style/choice	2 oz	2.0	80	23%
corned beef				
brisket/first cut				
cooked/choice	2 oz	4.0	80	45%
top round/choice cap-off	2 oz	2.5	80	28%
eye round roasted beef				
Cajun-style seasoned	2 oz	2.0	80	23%
pepper-seasoned	2 oz	3.0	90	30%
pastrami/choice				
brisket	2 oz	4.0	90	40%
round	2 oz	2.5	70	32%
red	2 oz	3.0	80	34%
top round/cap off	2 oz	2.5	70	32%
top round				
deluxe cap off	2 oz	2.5	80	28%
oven-roasted				
no salt added	2 oz	3.0	90	30%
(Briar Street Market)				
corned beef				
bottom round/flat	2 oz	3.0	70	39%
brisket/raw	4 oz	23.0	280	74%
chunked and formed	2 oz	1.5	50	27%
top round/whole	2 oz	2.5	60	38%
rib eyes/rare	3 oz	16.0	210	69%
roast beef/sliced	2 oz	1.5	70	19%
round/top				
chunked and formed	2 oz	1.5	60	23%
medium	2 oz	1.5	60	23%
medium rare	2 oz	3.0	70	39%
whole				
medium	2 oz	3.5	70	45%
medium rare	2 oz	2.0	70	26%
medium well	2 oz	1.5	60	23%
(Coleman Natural Meats) Fresh/uncooked				
bottom round steak	4 oz	17.0	250	61%
brisket/flat cut	4 oz	27.0	330	74%
chuck				
arm roast	4 oz	22.0	290	68%
blade roast	4 oz	25.0	310	73%
roast				
rib roast (large end)	4 oz	35.0	390	81%
tip roast	4 oz	16.0	240	60%
steak				
eye of round	4 oz	17.0	250	61%
rib steak (small end)	4 oz	31.0	360	78%
sirloin	4 oz	18.0	260	62%
tenderloin	4 oz	27.0	330	74%

Food and Description	Amount	Fat Grams	Total Calories	% Fat Calories
top loin	4 oz	23.0	300	69%
top round	4 oz	11.0	210	47%
(Dakota Lean) raw				
chuck roast	3 oz	2.0	80	23%
eye of round	3 oz	2.0	80	23%
flank	3 oz	1.0	80	11%
ground	3 oz	2.0	90	20%
rib eye	3 oz	2.0	90	20%
round/outside	3 oz	1.0	80	11%
round/top	3 oz	1.0	80	11%
sirloin tip	3 oz	3.0	90	30%
strip loin	3 oz	2.0	90	20%
tenderloin	3 oz	1.0	70	13%
(Hillshire Farm)				
corned beef brisket (cooked unless otherwise noted)				
choice/whole				
dry	2 oz	10.0	130	69%
raw	4 oz	18.0	240	68%
wet	3 oz	6.0	110	49%
mesquite/whole				
smoked/choice	3 oz	21.0	260	73%
	2 oz	10.0	130	69%
select				
bottom round	2 oz	4.5	90	45%
whole/raw	4 oz	17.0	230	67%
pastrami/choice				
eye of round	2 oz	6.0	100	54%
rib eye				
choice/rare	3 oz	20.0	240	75%
select/rare	3 oz	17.0	220	70%
round/bottom				
select				
medium	2 oz	4.5	90	45%
pot roast	3 oz	7.0	130	48%
round/top				
choice				
medium/split	3 oz	3.5	110	29%
medium-well/seasoned	3 oz	3.0	100	27%
medium/whole	3 oz	5.0	100	41%
rare	3 oz	3.5	100	32%
select				
medium	2 oz	1.5	60	23%
(Laura's Lean)..uncooked/unless noted otherwise				
ground beef				
92%	4 oz	9.0	160	51%
96%	4 oz	4.5	140	28%
pot roast w/au jus				
fully cooked	3 oz	3.5	100	32%
roasts..eye of round	4 oz	4.0	135	27%

Food and Description	Amount	Fat Grams	Total Calories	% Fat Calories
steaks				
flank	4 oz	5.0	140	32%
rib eye	4 oz	9.0	175	46%
rib eye w/separable fat	4 oz	6.0	155	23%
sirloin	4 oz	5.0	140	32%
strip	4 oz	5.0	150	30%
tenderloin filet	4 oz	5.0	145	32%
(Lean & Free) raw				
burger	4 oz	9.5	175	49%
cube steak	4 oz	1.0	110	8%
rib eye	4 oz	2.5	120	19%
round steak	4 oz	1.0	110	8%
sirloin steak	4 oz	1.5	110	12%
sirloin tip	4 oz	1.0	110	8%
strip steak/loin	4 oz	2.0	115	16%
T-bone	4 oz	2.5	125	18%
tenderloin steak/fillet	4 oz	2.5	120	19%
top round	4 oz	4.5	135	30%
■ BEEF CUTS, ORGAN/OTHER				
brain				
fried	3 oz	13.5	167	73%
simmered	3 oz	10.6	136	70%
heart/braised	3 oz	4.8	148	29%
kidney/simmered	3 oz	2.9	122	21%
liver				
braised	3 oz	4.0	137	26%
fried	3 oz	6.8	184	33%
lung/braised	3 oz	3.0	102	27%
pancreas/braised	3 oz	14.7	232	57%
spleen/braised	3 oz	4.0	123	29%
sweetbread/braised	3 oz	19.7	272	65%
thymus/braised	3 oz	21.0	273	69%
tongue				
braised/medium fat	3 oz	22.0	208	95%
simmered	3 oz	17.6	241	66%
tripe..(Armour Star) canned	3 oz	2.0	90	20%
BEEF BROTH (*See* SOUP)				
BEEF DISH/ENTRÉE (*See also* ASIAN FOOD; FROZEN ENTRÉE/DINNER; HAMBURGER; MEXICAN FOOD; PASTA ENTRÉE/DINNER; RICE DISH; individual listings)				
CANNED/POUCH				
(Armour Star)				
beef stew	1 cup	11.0	210	47%
corned beef hash	1 cup	30.0	440	61%
roast beef hash	1 cup	25.0	400	56%
(Castleberry's)				
beef stew	8 oz	26.0	340	69%
corned beef hash	7.5 oz	28.0	430	59%

Food and Description	Amount	Fat Grams	Total Calories	% Fat Calories
(Chef Boyardee)				
beefaroni	7.5 oz	9.0	260	31%
beef overstuffed ravioli	7.5 oz	4.5	280	14%
mini bites	7.5 oz	13.0	300	39%
(Dinty Moore)				
beef stew	1 cup	8.0	180	40%
individual servings	1 cup	10.0	190	47%
meatball stew	1 cup	15.0	250	54%
(Heinz)				
beef stew	7.5 oz	9.0	210	34%
goulash	7.5 oz	11.0	240	41%
(Hormel)				
beef goulash	7.5 oz	11.0	230	43%
corned beef	2 oz	7.0	120	53%
roast beef w/gravy	½ cup	4.0	150	24%
(Libby's) Corned beef	2 oz	7.0	120	53%
(Mary Kitchen)				
corned beef hash				
50% less fat	1 cup	12.0	280	39%
original/individual				
serving	7.5 oz	22.0	350	57%
	1 cup	24.0	390	55%
Fiesta hash	1 cup	23.0	410	50%
roast beef hash	7.5 oz	21.0	348	54%
	1 cup	24.0	390	55%
(Mountain House)				
canned				
chili mac w/beef	1 cup	8.0	250	29%
diced beef/cooked	⅔ cup	3.5	130	24%
spaghetti w/meat sauce	1 cup	7.0	230	27%
stew				
beef	1 cup	8.0	210	34%
vegetable w/beef	1 cup	8.0	230	32%
Stroganoff w/beef & noodles	1 cup	11.0	260	38%
pouch				
beef stew	1 pouch	12.0	330	33%
double-serve pouch	½ pouch	9.0	270	30%
chili mac w/beef	½ pouch	8.0	290	25%
flamed broiled beef patty				
w/bbq sauce/double-				
serve pouch	½ pouch	5.0	230	20%
lasagna w/meat sauce	1 pouch	15.0	380	36%
double-serve pouch	½ pouch	12.0	310	35%
spaghetti w/meat & sauce	1 pouch	10.0	340	26%
double-serve pouch	½ pouch	8.0	270	23%
Stroganoff w/beef & noodles	1 pouch	16.0	390	37%
double-serve pouch	½ pouch	13.0	320	37%
FROZEN				
(Schwan's)				
beef, broccoli & rice	1 cup	4.0	210	17%

Food and Description	Amount	Fat Grams	Total Calories	% Fat Calories
burgers				
cheeseburger	1 burger	19.0	360	48%
chopped beef steak	1 burger	16.0	260	55%
ground chuck	1 burger	22.0	320	62%
quarter pound	1 burger	12.0	200	55%
chopped BBQ beef..w/sauce	½ cup	8.0	220	22%
creamed chipped beef	1 cup	17.0	310	49%
diced beef tips w/gravy	1 cup	7.0	240	26%
goulash	1 cup	12.0	280	39%
lasagna/single serve	1 tray	19.0	500	34%
meatballs				
Italian-style	6 pieces	20.0	260	69%
Swedish	6 pieces	19.0	260	66%
shepherd's pie	1 cup	12.0	250	43%
sirloin beef potpie	1 potpie	33.0	600	50%
sliced				
beef w/chunky mashed				
potatoes	¼ tray	15.0	320	42%
pot roast w/noodles	1 cup	6.0	230	23%
steaks				
battered cubed	1 steak	23.0	320	65%
New York strip	1 steak	33.0	470	63%
(Tyson)				
Meals & Entrées				
beef strips/seasoned	3 oz	6.0	140	39%
meatballs				
home-style	6 pieces	18.0	240	68%
Itallan-style	6 pieces	20.0	240	75%
Swedish-style	6 pieces	20.0	240	75%
meat loaf/seasoned	5 oz	16.0	270	53%
roast beef				
in brown gravy	5 oz	6.0	150	36%
MICROWAVE CONTAINER				
(Dinty Moore)				
American Classics bowls				
beef ravioli	1 bowl	9.0	300	27%
beef stew	1 bowl	11.0	250	40%
lasagna	1 bowl	16.0	340	42%
pot roast	1 bowl	3.0	200	14%
roast beef				
w/mashed potatoes	1 bowl	5.0	240	19%
Salisbury steak	1 bowl	15.0	320	42%
spaghetti w/meatballs	1 bowl	7.0	290	22%
Microwavable cups				
beef stew	1 cup	7.0	160	39%
burger stew/hearty	1 cup	13.0	240	49%
corned beef hash	1 cup	22.0	350	57%
noodles & beef				
Stroganoff	1 cup	14.0	240	53%
spaghetti				
w/meatballs		7.0	290	22%

Food and Description	Amount	Fat Grams	Total Calories	% Fat Calories
MIX				
(Betty Crocker) Hamburger Helper..prepared				
bacon cheeseburger	1 cup	18.0	380	43%
beef pasta	1 cup	13.0	290	40%
beef Romanoff	1 cup	13.0	290	40%
beef stew	1 cup	11.0	270	37%
beef taco	1 cup	13.0	310	38%
cheddar and broccoli	1 cup	17.0	350	44%
cheddar cheese melt	1 cup	14.0	310	41%
cheeseburger macaroni	1 cup	16.0	350	41%
cheesy				
hash browns	1 cup	20.0	410	44%
cheesy shells	1 cup	15.0	330	41%
chili macaroni	1 cup	12.0	290	37%
double cheese pizza	1 cup	13.0	330	35%
fettuccine Alfredo	1 cup	13.0	310	38%
4-cheese lasagna	1 cup	15.0	330	41%
meat loaf & mashed potatoes				
Oven Favorites	⅙ loaf	19.0	360	48%
Philly cheese steak	1 cup	17.0	330	46%
pizza pasta w/cheese topping	1 cup	12.0	310	35%
potatoes Stroganoff	1 cup	14.0	290	43%
ravioli & cheese	1 cup	12.0	320	34%
rice Oriental	1 cup	11.0	300	33%
Salisbury	1 cup	12.0	280	39%
soft taco bake/Oven Favorites	⅙ cup	21.0	420	45%
REFRIGERATED				
(Lloyd's) in BBQ sauce	¼ cup	2.0	90	20%
BEEF, DRIED (*See* individual meats; MEAT SNACK)				
BEEF JERKY, STICKS & STRIPS (*See* MEAT SNACK)				
BEEF SAUSAGE (*See* LUNCHEON MEAT; SAUSAGE)				
BEEF TALLOW				
	1 Tbs	12.8	115	100%
	1 cup	205.0	1849	100%
BEER, ALE & MALT LIQUOR				
(Anheuser-Busch)				
Bacardi Silver	12 fl oz	–	220	–
Bud				
dry	12 fl oz	–	130	–
ice	12 fl oz	–	148	–
ice light	12 fl oz	–	110	–
light	12 fl oz	–	110	–
Budweiser	12 fl oz	–	145	–
Busch	12 fl oz	–	133	
ice	12 fl oz	–	169	–
light	12 fl oz	–	110	–
n/a (nonalcoholic)	12 fl oz	–	60	–
Doc's Hard Lemon	12 fl oz	–	165	–
Hurricane	12 fl oz	–	158	–

Food and Description	Amount	Fat Grams	Total Calories	% Fat Calories
King Cobra	12 fl oz	–	166	–
Michelob	12 fl oz	–	155	–
amber rock	12 fl oz	–	166	–
black and tan	12 fl oz	–	168	–
golden draft	12 fl oz	–	152	–
golden draft light	12 fl oz	–	110	–
Hefeweizen	12 fl oz	–	176	–
honey lager	12 fl oz	–	175	–
light	12 fl oz	–	134	–
Ultra	12 fl oz	–	95	–
Natural				
ice	12 fl oz	–	157	–
light	12 fl oz	–	110	–
O'Doul's				
amber	12 fl oz	–	90	–
original	12 fl oz	–	70	–
Tequiza	12 fl oz	–	127	–
(Beck's)				
dark	12 fl oz	–	156	–
light	12 fl oz	–	132	–
regular	12 fl oz	–	145	
(Budweiser) (*See* Anheuser Busch, in this section)				
(Carlsberg)				
regular	12 fl oz	–	40	–
special brew	12 fl oz	–	205	–
(Champale) extra dry	12 fl oz	–	170	–
(Cheers) nonalcoholic	12 fl oz	–	55	–
(Colt 45)	12 fl oz	–	150	
(Coors)				
Extra Gold	12 fl oz	–	145	–
light	12 fl oz	–	102	–
nonalcoholic	12 fl oz	–	65	–
original	12 fl oz	–	142	–
(Elephant) malt liquor	12 fl oz	–	208	–
(Elk Mountain)				
amber ale	12 fl oz	–	201	–
red	12 fl oz	–	159	–
(Foster's) lager	12 fl oz	–	140	–
(George Killian's) Irish Red	12 fl oz	–	163	–
(Guinness)				
extra stout	12 fl oz	–	192	–
regular	12 fl oz	–	160	–
(Heileman's)				
Black Label	12 fl oz	–	156	–
Old Style				
light	12 fl oz	–	110	–
regular	12 fl oz	–	147	–
Special Export				
dark	12 fl oz	–	155	–
light	12 fl oz	–	115	–

Food and Description	Amount	Fat Grams	Total Calories	% Fat Calories
regular	12 fl oz	–	152	–
special dark	12 fl oz	–	192	–
(Heineken)				
regular	12 fl oz	–	160	–
special dark	12 fl oz	–	165	–
(Killian's) Irish Red	12 fl oz	–	155	–
(King Cobra)	12 fl oz	–	175	–
(Knickerbocker)	12 fl oz	–	145	–
(Löwenbrau)				
Pils	12 fl oz	–	180	–
regular	12 fl oz	–	165	
special	12 fl oz	–	160	
(Meister Brau)	12 fl oz	–	145	–
(Michael Shea's)				
black & tan	12 fl oz	–	150	–
Irish amber	12 fl oz	–	145	–
(Miller)				
Genuine Draft	12 fl oz	–	145	–
High Life	12 fl oz	–	145	–
Lite	12 fl oz	–	95	–
Magnum	12 fl oz	–	165	–
(Old Milwaukee)				
ice	12 fl oz	–	180	
light	12 fl oz	–	110	–
nonalcoholic	12 fl oz	–	72	–
red	12 fl oz	–	136	–
lager	12 fl oz	–	145	–
(Pabst)				
Blue Ribbon	12 fl oz	–	135	–
lager	12 fl oz	–	133	–
low-calorie	12 fl oz	–	110	–
nonalcoholic	12 fl oz	–	55	–
Old English malt liquor	12 fl oz	–	150	–
(Piels)				
light	12 fl oz	–	127	–
regular	12 fl oz	–	133	–
(Rheingold)				
light	12 fl oz	–	95	–
regular	12 fl oz	–	145	–
(St. Pauli Girl)				
dark	12 fl oz	–	155	–
light	12 fl oz	–	135	–
(Schaefer)				
light	12 fl oz	–	115	–
regular	12 fl oz	–	155	–
(Scrumpy) rough cider beer	1 pint	–	210	–
(Stroh's)				
American lager	12 fl oz	–	145	–
light	12 fl oz	–	110	–
Signature	12 fl oz	–	155	–

Food and Description	Amount	Fat Grams	Total Calories	% Fat Calories
(Tiger Heat) Ale	12 fl oz	–	160	–
(Zima)				
cherry	12 fl oz	–	234	–
lemon-lime	12 fl oz	–	231	–
orange	12 fl oz	–	231	–
BEET				
CANNED or JARRED				
(Aunt Nellie's)				
Harvard	⅓ cup	–	60	–
pickled				
ruby red				
sliced	~1 oz	–	15	–
whole	~1 oz	–	20	–
sliced	½ cup	–	35	–
whole	½ cup	–	35	–
(Blue Boy)				
Harvard	½ cup	–	100	–
pickled				
sliced	½ cup	–	100	–
whole	~1 oz	–	25	–
(Del Monte)				
pickled	½ cup	–	80	–
sliced	½ cup	–	35	–
(Libby's) with or w/o onion				
pickled				
sliced	½ cup	–	20	–
whole	½ cup	–	35	–
regular/sliced	½ cup	–	35	–
(Lohmann)				
Harvard	⅓ cup	–	60	–
no salt added	½ cup	–	20	–
pickled				
crinkle cut	1 oz	–	15	–
shoestring	1 oz	–	15	–
sliced	4 slices	–	20	–
whole	2 beets	–	20	–
(S&W)				
pickled				
party sliced	1 oz	–	15	–
sliced	½ cup	–	30	–
whole	1 oz	–	15	–
regular				
julienne..French-style	½ cup	–	30	–
small & tender	½ cup	–	30	–
(Stokely)				
pickled				
canned	½ cup	–	100	–
jar	½ cup	–	90	–
sliced	~1 oz	–	25	–

Food and Description	Amount	Fat Grams	Total Calories	% Fat Calories
Harvard	~1 oz	–	25	–
marinated/sliced	~1 oz	–	25	–
regular				
cut	½ cup	–	40	–
diced	½ cup	–	40	–
sliced	½ cup	–	40	–
whole	½ cup	–	40	–
FRESH				
cooked				
sliced	½ cup	–	26	–
whole	2 medium	–	30	–
raw				
sliced	½ cup	–	38	–
whole	2 medium	–	70	–
BEET JUICE	6 oz	–	75	–

BERRY DRINK/BLEND (*See also* individual berry juices/juice blends; FRUIT PUNCH; SOFT DRINK; SOFT DRINK MIX; individual drink listings)

BOTTLED, BOXED, or CANNED

Food and Description	Amount	Fat Grams	Total Calories	% Fat Calories
(Fruitopia)				
Berry Lemonade	8 fl oz	–	110	–
Kiwi Berry Ruckus	8 fl oz	–	110	–
(Hawaiian Punch)				
Berry Blue Typhoon	8 fl oz	–	120	–
Bodacious Berry	8 fl oz	–	110	–
Green Berry Rush	8 fl oz	–	120	–
(Hi-C)				
Boppin' Berry				
can	7.7 fl oz	–	110	–
drink box	8.45 fl oz	–	130	–
pet	8 fl oz	–	120	–
wild berry				
pet	8 fl oz	–	120	–
FROZEN/PREPARED				
(After The Fall)				
Oregon berry	8 fl oz	–	100	–
(Minute Maid)				
berry punch	8 fl oz	–	110	–
mixed berry	6.5 fl oz	–	100	–
(Tropicana)				
smoothie/mixed berry	11 fl oz	–	250	–
(V8 Splash)				
berry blend				
diet	8 fl oz	–	10	–
original	8 fl oz	–	110	–
smoothie/wild				
berry crème	8 fl oz	–	130	–

BIRCH BEER (*See* SOFT DRINK)

BISCOTTI (*See* COOKIE)

BISCUIT (*See also* BAKE & FRY MIX; BREAKFAST SANDWICH)

Food and Description	Amount	Fat Grams	Total Calories	% Fat Calories
FROZEN				
(Bob Evans)				
buttermilk/restaurant				
recipe	1 biscuit	6.0	190	28%
(Mary B's)				
fresh-bake				
buttermilk	1 biscuit	10.0	190	47%
jumbo buttermilk	1 biscuit	16.0	300	48%
Southern-made	1 biscuit	8.0	190	38%
Mexican-style	1 biscuit	17.0	280	55%
tea/bite-sized	1 biscuit	9.0	173	47%
(Rhodes).. buttermilk	1 biscuit	10.0	200	45%
(White Lily)				
buttermilk	1 biscuit	9.0	190	43%
Southern-style	1 biscuit	9.0	190	43%
taste of butter	1 biscuit	9.0	190	43%
(Schwan's)				
cheese & herb	1 biscuit	6.0	110	33%
Southern-style	1 biscuit	10.0	200	45%
MIX				
(Arrowhead Mills) biscuit mix				
mix only	¼ cup	1.0	120	8%
(Betty Crocker) Gold Medal				
prepared	2 biscuits	6.0	180	30%
(Bisquick) mix only				
complete				
buttermilk	⅓ cup	6.0	150	36%
cheese garlic	⅓ cup	7.0	160	38%
cinnamon swirl	⅓ cup	4.0	150	24%
three cheese	⅓ cup	7.0	160	38%
original	⅓ cup	7.0	160	38%
pouch mix	½ cup	6.0	160	34%
reduced fat	⅓ cup	2.5	150	15%
(Jiffy) buttermilk..prepared	⅓ cup	4.0	160	23%
(Krusteaz)..all-purpose				
baking mix..prepared	2 biscuits	6.0	180	30%
(Martha White)..Quick & Easy				
cheddar garlic	⅓ cup	11.0	190	52%
extra-rich buttermilk	⅓ cup	11.0	190	52%
home-style butter	⅓ cup	10.0	190	47%
(White Lily) buttermilk	¼ pkt	9.0	190	43%
PACKAGED/READY-TO-SERVE				
(Arnold) old-fashioned				
buttermilk	3 biscuits	8.0	190	38%
(Awrey's)				
buttermilk..round				
1 ounce	2	8.0	190	38%
2 ounce	1	7.0	180	40%
buttermilk..sliced..2 ounce	1	7.0	180	40%

Food and Description	Amount	Fat Grams	Total Calories	% Fat Calories
REFRIGERATED				
(Pillsbury)				
1869/buttermilk	1 biscuit	5.0	100	45%
Big Country..all types	1 biscuit	4.0	100	36%
Biscuits				
buttermilk	3 biscuits	2.0	150	12%
country	3 biscuits	2.0	150	12%
tender layer	3 biscuits	4.5	160	25%
Grands!				
blueberry	1 biscuit	9.0	210	39%
butter tastin'	1 biscuit	9.0	190	43%
buttermilk				
original	1 biscuit	9.0	190	43%
reduced-fat	1 biscuit	6.0	170	34%
corn	1 biscuit	7.0	190	33%
crescent	1 biscuit	15.0	270	50%
extra rich	1 biscuit	11.0	220	45%
flaky	1 biscuit	9.0	200	9%
home-style	1 biscuit	8.0	180	40%
Southern-style	1 biscuit	9.0	190	43%
Wheat/reduced-fat	1 biscuit	7.0	190	33%
Home Baked Classics				
butter tastin'	1 biscuit	9.0	180	40%
buttermilk	1 biscuit	9.0	190	43%
cheddar garlic	1 biscuit	10.0	190	47%
Southern-style	1 biscuit	9.0	180	45%
BLACK BEAN				
(Bush's Best)	½ cup	0.5	100	5%
(Eden)				
black soy	½ cup	6.0	120	45%
original	½ cup	–	100	–
(Fantastic Foods) big cup				
spicy Jamaican				
w/black beans	½ pkg	1.0	190	5%
(Goya) frijoles negros	½ cup	0.5	90	5%
(Joan of Arc)	½ cup	–	100	–
(Knorr)	7.5 oz	3.0	190	14%
refried	7.5 oz	2.5	140	16%
(Progresso)	½ cup	1.0	110	8%
(S&W)				
50% less salt	½ cup	–	70	–
regular	½ cup	–	70	–
(Westbrae)..all types	½ cup	–	100	–
BLACK CHERRY JUICE/bottled, boxed, or canned				
(Knudsen) Thirst Quencher	8 fl oz	–	180	–
(Smucker's)	8 fl oz	–	130	–
BLACK TURTLE BEAN				
(Bean Cuisine) Mix	½ cup	1.0	115	8%
(Hain)	½ cup	1.0	100	9%
BLACKBERRY				

Food and Description	Amount	Fat Grams	Total Calories	% Fat Calories
CANNED				
in heavy syrup	½ cup	<1.0	94	5%
in juice	½ cup	<1.0	41	11%
in water	1 cup	1.5	60	23%
(Allen's) in light syrup	½ cup	0.5	60	8%
FRESH	½ cup	<1.0	40	7%
(Oregon) in light syrup	½ cup	–	130	–
	1 lb	2.0	240	7%
FROZEN				
(Big Valley) no sugar	⅔ cup	–	70	–
(Cascadian Farm)	1 cup	0.5	80	6%
BLACKBERRY JUICE				
generic/canned	8 fl oz	2.0	92	20%
(Smucker's)	8 fl oz	1.5	91	15%
BLACK-EYED PEA				
CANNED				
(Bush's Best)				
jalapeño	½ cup	2.5	120	18%
regular	½ cup	1.0	110	8%
seasoned w/bacon	½ cup	1.0	110	8%
w/snaps	½ cup	0.5	110	8%
(Eden) Organic	½ cup	1.0	90	10%
(Glory) Southern-style	½ cup	0.5	60	8%
(Green Giant)	½ cup	1.0	90	10%
(Luck's) seasoned				
w/pork	½ cup	3.0	130	21%
(Trappey's)				
w/bacon	½ cup	2.0	120	15%
w/bacon & jalapeño	½ cup	2.0	110	16%
DRIED				
mature				
boiled	½ cup	0.6	100	5%
raw	½ cup	1.0	131	7%
young pods w/seeds				
boiled	1 cup	–	32	–
raw	1 cup	–	42	–
FROZEN				
(Freshlike)	3.3 oz	1.0	130	7%
(Pictsweet)	½ cup	1.0	110	8%
(Veg-All)	3.3 oz	1.0	130	7%
BLINTZ (*See* FROZEN ENTRÉE/DINNER)				
BLUEBERRY				
CANNED				
generic				
in heavy syrup	1 cup	<1.0	225	2%
in water	2 cup	<1.0	94	5%
(S&W) wild Maine				
in heavy syrup	⅓ cup	–	70	–

Food and Description	Amount	Fat Grams	Total Calories	% Fat Calories
DRIED				
Frieda's	¼ cup	–	140	
Sonoma	¼ cup	–	140	–
FRESH	2 cups	<1.0	82	6%
FROZEN				
(Big Valley)	⅔ cup	–	70	–
(C&W)	¾ cup	–	70	–
(Cascadian Farm)	1 cup	0.5	90	5%
generic				
no sugar added	1 cup	<1.0	88	5%
	3.5 oz	<1.0	50	9%
sweetened	1 cup	<1.0	190	2%
BLUEBERRY JUICE				
(Knudsen) Thirst				
Quencher..Maine coast	8 fl oz	–	90	–
BLUEFISH/raw	3 oz	3.6	105	31%
BOLOGNA (*See* LUNCHEON MEAT)				
BORAGE/fresh				
cooked	½ cup	1.0	25	36%
raw	½ cup	<1.0	9	50%
BORSCHT (*See* SOUP)				
BOYSENBERRY				
CANNED				
in heavy syrup	1 cup	–	226	–
in water	1 cup	–	90	–
FRESH	½ lb	–	125	–
FROZEN				
no sugar added	1 cup	–	66	–
sweetened	1 cup	–	144	–
BOYSENBERRY JUICE/NECTAR				
(Knudsen) nectar	8 fl oz	–	110	–
(Smucker's) juice	8 fl oz	–	120	–
BRAN (*See* CEREAL)				
BRANDY (*See* LIQUEUR)				
BRATWURST (*See* SAUSAGE)				
BRAZIL NUT				
dried	1 oz	19.0	186	91%
shelled	1 oz	19.0	190	90%
	1 cup	93.0	920	91%
(Best Yet)	1.5 oz	26.0	260	90%
(Diamond)	1 oz	19.0	190	90%
BREAD (*See also* BAGEL; BISCUIT; BREADSTICK; CROISSANT; MUFFIN; ROLL)				
■ **BROWN & SERVE**				
(Arnold) Francisco sourdough	1 oz	0.5	70	6%
(Colombo) sourdough				
French				
round	½" slice	0.5	120	4%
sourdough	1½" slice	–	130	–

Food and Description	Amount	Fat Grams	Total Calories	% Fat Calories
garlic/plain	3" slice	9.0	190	43%
Luigi's loaves	1" slice	1.0	130	7%
(Earth Grains) bake & serve				
French bread..premium				
plain	1 slice	1.0	130	7%
roasted garlic	1 slice	1.0	130	7%
(Wonder) du jour				
Austrian	1 slice	1.0	70	13%
French/twin loaves	3" slice	1.0	140	6%
■ CANNED				
(B&M)..all styles	½ slice	0.5	130	3%
(Friends)..all styles	½ slice	0.5	130	3%
■ FROZEN				
(Bridgeford) dough/baked				
French	2 slices	1.0	150	6%
honey wheat	1 slice	1.0	75	12%
white	1 slice	1.0	75	12%
(Mama Bella)				
garlic bread				
home-style				
5 servings	1" slice	8.0	150	48%
10 servings	1" slice	9.0	160	39%
home-style Parmesan	1" slice	9.0	160	39%
garlic toast				
cheese/9-count	1 piece	12.0	190	57%
5-cheese/8-count	1 piece	12.0	200	54%
traditional/9-count	1 piece	7.0	140	45%
(Marie Callender's)				
cornbread	1 piece	3.0	150	18%
honey butter added	1 Tbs	5.0	50	90%
(Marzetti)..garlic				
breadstick	1 stick	5.0	180	25%
original	2-1" slices	7.0	190	33%
reduced-fat	2-1" slices	3.0	160	17%
Texas garlic toast				
6 carb	1 oz slice	9.0	120	68%
Parmesan	1" slice	11.0	190	52%
w/cheese	1" slice	11.0	180	55%
w/5 cheeses	1" slice	12.0	200	54%
w/o cheese	1" slice	10.0	170	53%
(Pepperidge Farm)				
garlic	⅙ loaf	10.0	160	56%
garlic & olive oil				
loaves/reduced-fat				
½" slice	2 slices	7.0	170	37%
garlic Parmesan	⅙ loaf	7.0	160	39%
Monterey Jack				
jalapeño cheese	⅙ loaf	10.0	200	45%
mozzarella garlic	⅙ loaf	10.0	200	45%

Food and Description	Amount	Fat Grams	Total Calories	% Fat Calories
sourdough garlic	⅙ loaf	9.0	180	45%
2-cheddar cheese	⅙ loaf	11.0	210	47%
(Rhodes) dough/baked				
honey wheat	1 slice	2.0	130	14%
Italian	1 slice	2.0	130	14%
raisin	1 slice	2.0	140	13%
sweet	1 slice	3.0	150	18%
wheat	1 slice	2.0	130	14%
white	1 slice	2.0	140	13%
(Schwan's)				
cheese-stuffed bread				
w/sauce	3" wedge	5.0	160	28%
dough/baked				
wheat/honey	2 oz	1.5	130	10%
white	2 oz	1.5	140	10%
French bread..5-cheese garlic	1 piece	20.0	330	55%
ready to heat..French baguette	¼ loaf	–	120	–
■ MIX				
(Arrowhead Mills) mix only				
cornbread	¼ cup	1.0	120	8%
multigrain	⅓ cup	1.0	160	6%
rye	⅓ cup	0.5	160	3%
spelt	⅓ cup	1.0	150	6%
white	⅓ cup	0.5	150	3%
whole wheat	⅓ cup	1.0	150	3%
(Aunt Patsy) mix only				
cornbread	¼ cup	–	130	–
sourdough beer	¼ cup	–	130	–
(Ballard)				
cornbread				
mix only	1/18 pkg	1.5	110	12%
prepared	1 piece	2.5	130	17%
(Betty Crocker) Quickbread Mixes/pouch..prepared				
banana	1 slice	7.0	170	37%
cinnamon streusel	1 slice	7.0	180	35%
cranberry	1 slice	4.0	160	23%
lemon poppyseed	1 slice	7.0	170	37%
(Calhoun Bend Mill)..mix only				
cornbread/country-style				
prepared	1 piece	<1.0	146	3%
cornbread & muffin	3 Tbs	–	100	–
honey butter				
cornbread	3 Tbs	1.0	108	8%
hush puppy	2 Tbs	–	150	–
Mexican	3 Tbs	1.0	110	8%
sopapilla mix	.3 oz	1.0	35	26%
(Classic Hearth) bread-machine mixes/prepared				
Bavarian				
pumpernickel	1 slice	2.0	170	11%
Hawaiian royal sweet	1 slice	2.5	170	13%

Food and Description	Amount	Fat Grams	Total Calories	% Fat Calories
Mediterranean				
black olive	1 slice	2.5	150	15%
Parisian				
toasted onion	1 slice	2.0	140	13%
Provençal/sun-dried				
tomato & basil	1 slice	2.0	150	12%
Southwestern				
jalapeño cheese	1 slice	2.5	160	14%
(Daily Bread Co.) Quick Loaf..mix only				
all types	3 Tbs	–	120	–
(Dromedary) mix only				
cheddar cheese	1/9 pkg	2.5	140	16%
cornbread	1/10 pkg	2.5	140	16%
date nut	1/12 pkg	7.0	180	35%
gingerbread	1/6 pkg	4.0	260	14%
Italian herb	1/9 pkg	2.5	140	16%
sourdough	1/9 pkg	2.0	140	13%
wheat/stone-ground	1/9 pkg	2.0	140	13%
white/country	1/9 pkg	1.0	140	6%
(Eagle Mills) bread machine/mix only				
breakfast				
apple walnut	1/12 pkg	3.5	150	21%
cinnamon sunrise	1/12 pkg	3.0	150	18%
harvest fruit	1/12 pkg	2.5	140	16%
classic Italian	1/9 pkg	2.0	160	11%
country French	1/9 pkg	2.0	160	11%
dessert				
chocolate nugget	1/12 pkg	3.5	150	21%
lemon poppyseed	1/12 pkg	3.0	140	19%
harvest wheat	1/11 pkg	2.0	140	13%
hearty multigrain	1/11 pkg	2.0	150	12%
home-style white	1/9 pkg	3.0	160	11%
honey oat	1/11 pkg	2.5	150	15%
Old World rye	1/11 pkg	2.5	150	15%
San Francisco				
sourdough	1/9 pkg	2.0	160	11%
(Krusteaz)				
bread machine mixes..prepared				
cinnamon raisin	1 slice	2.5	180	13%
honey wheat berry	1 slice	2.0	150	12%
Italian herb	1 slice	2.0	150	12%
oat bran	1 slice	2.5	150	15%
savory rye	1 slice	2.0	150	12%
sourdough	1 slice	2.0	150	12%
12-grain	1 slice	2.5	170	13%
wheat/cracked	1 slice	2.0	150	12%
white/country	1 slice	2.0	150	12%
CarbSimple..prepared				
classic wheat	1/12 loaf	3.0	140	19%
cornbread/home-style	2 slices	4.5	160	25%

Food and Description	Amount	Fat Grams	Total Calories	% Fat Calories
cornbread/honey.. prepared	1 piece	3.0	120	23%
cornbread & muffin/fat-free honey prepared	1 slice	–	120	–
country white	1/12 loaf	3.0	140	19%
(Marie Callender's) cornbread	1/4 cup	4.0	150	24%
(Martha White)..cornbread mix..prepared				
buttermilk	1 piece	3.5	130	24%
cheddar cheese	1 piece	6.0	130	42%
Cotton Pickin'				
buttermilk	1 piece	3.5	130	24%
enriched				
white self-rising	1 piece	1.0	110	8%
yellow self-rising	1 piece	1.0	110	8%
extra-rich buttermilk	1 piece	5.0	130	35%
gladiola yellow	1 piece	3.0	110	25%
Mexican	1 piece	3.0	110	25%
plain enriched yellow	1 piece	1.0	120	8%
sweet yellow	1 piece	3.5	140	23%
(Pillsbury)..mix only				
quick bread & muffin mix				
apple cinnamon	1/12 pkg	2.5	130	17%
banana	1/12 pkg	1.5	130	10%
blueberry	1/12 pkg	1.5	140	10%
cinnamon swirl	1/12 pkg	5.0	180	25%
cranberry	1/12 pkg	1.5	140	10%
lemon poppy seed	1/12 pkg	3.0	150	18%
pumpkin	1/12 pkg	1.5	130	10%
(White Lily) dry mix only				
corn muffin mix	1/3 pkt	5.0	190	24%
cornbread/white	1/3 pkg	3.0	130	21%
(Zia Foods) cornbread mix/prepared				
blue cornmeal	1 piece	6.0	110	49%
■ PACKAGED/READY TO SERVE				
(Alvarado Street)				
bakery sprouted				
barley	1 slice	0.5	70	6%
multigrain				
no salt added	1 slice	1.0	60	15%
regular	1 slice	1.0	60	15%
soy crunch	1 slice	1.0	70	13%
(Arnold)				
Arnold Brand				
cinnamon French toast	1 slice	3.0	100	27%
country				
buttermilk	1 slice	1.5	110	12%
potato	1 slice	1.0	110	8%
wheat	1 slice	1.5	110	12%
white enriched	1 slice	1.5	110	12%
Health Nut	1 slice	1.0	90	9%
healthy multigrain	1 slice	1.5	120	11%

Food and Description	Amount	Fat Grams	Total Calories	% Fat Calories
honey wheatberry	1 slice	1.0	110	8%
marble rye & pumpernickel	1 slice	1.0	90	9%
Master's Best				
3-seed	1 slice	0.5	100	5%
winter wheat	1 slice	3.0	100	27%
natural oat	1 slice	1.5	90	15%
100% whole wheat				
low-fat	1 slice	0.5	80	6%
9-grain	1 slice	I.5	100	13%
regular	1 slice	1.0	90	9%
pumpernickel	1 slice	1.0	80	11%
raisin cinnamon	1 slice	2.5	90	25%
rye				
Jewish caraway.. seeded	1 slice	1.0	80	11%
melba thin/real Jewish				
seeded	2 slices	1.5	110	12%
w/o seeds	2 slices	1.5	80	17%
sandwich..sesame	1 slice	3.0	130	21%
7-grain	1 slice	1.0	100	9%
12-grain				
regular	1 slice	2.0	110	16%
soft	1 slice	1.5	110	12%
Bran'nola				
country oat	1 slice	1.5	100	14%
honey wheat berry	1 slice	1.5	90	15%
nutty grains	1 slice	2.5	90	25%
original	1 slice	1.5	90	15%
7-grain white	1 slice	2.0	90	20%
12-grain	1 slice	2.0	90	20%
wheat				
dark	1 slice	2.0	90	20%
hearty	1 slice	3.0	90	30%
Francisco International				
French bread/sliced	1 slice	1.0	120	8%
French stick	1 oz	1.0	70	13%
Italian/sliced bread	2 slices	1.5	100	14%
Sheepherders	1 slice	1.0	110	8%
Levy's				
melba thin				
sliced rye	2 slices	1.0	90	10%
pumpernickel	1 slice	0.5	80	6%
Real Jewish Rye				
w/caraway seeds	1 slice	1.5	90	15%
w/o seeds	1 slice	1.5	90	15%
(Awrey) fruit breads				
blueberry	1 slice	14.0	250	50%
lemon poppyseed	1 slice	15.0	270	50%
orange walnut	1 slice	15.0	270	50%
(Brownberry)				
100% whole wheat	1 slice	1.0	90	10%

Food and Description	Amount	Fat Grams	Total Calories	% Fat Calories
Bran'nola				
country oat	1 slice	1.5	100	14%
honey wheat berry	1 slice	1.5	90	15%
nutty grains	1 slice	2.5	90	25%
original	1 slice	1.5	90	15%
7-grain white	1 slice	2.0	90	20%
12-grain	1 slice	2.0	90	20%
buttermilk	1 slice	1.5	110	12%
Francisco International				
French bread/sliced	1 slice	1.0	120	8%
French stick	1 oz	1.0	70	13%
Italian/sliced bread	2 slices	1.5	100	14%
Sheepherders	1 slice	1.0	110	8%
sourdough/24-oz loaf	1 slice	0.5	100	5%
Health Nut	1 slice	2.0	100	18%
Natural				
100% whole wheat	1 slice	1.5	90	15%
soft wheat	1 slice	2.0	90	20%
wheat	1 slice	1.0	90	10%
oatnut	1 slice	2.0	100	18%
(CarbXtract)				
cinnamon raisin	1 slice	1.6	76	18%
cinnamon raisin swirl	1 slice	2.0	51	35%
cornmeal-crusted	1 slice	1.0	42	21%
French	1 slice	1.0	42	21%
marble				
rye & pumpernickel	1 slice	1.0	42	21%
multigrain	1 slice	1.0	42	21%
pumpernickel	1 slice	1.0	42	21%
rye	1 slice	1.6	76	18%
sourdough	1 slice	1.0	42	21%
Xbread	1 slice	1.6	69	21%
wheat	1 slice	1.0	42	21%
(D'Italiano)				
enriched real Italian				
light	1.6 oz	–	40	–
original	1.6 oz	1.0	70	13%
(Earth Grains)				
barley bran	1 slice	1.0	70	13%
Canadian oat	1 slice	1.0	70	13%
French	1 slice	1.0	70	13%
gold'n bran	1 slice	1.0	70	13%
honey 'n' bran	1 slice	1.0	70	13%
honey oat & nut	1 slice	2.0	80	23%
honey oatberry	1 slice	1.0	70	13%
oat & nut	1 slice	2.5	120	19%
oat bran	1 slice	2.0	80	23%
raisin cinnamon swirl	1 slice	2.0	80	23%
rye				
dark	1 slice	1.0	70	13%

Food and Description	Amount	Fat Grams	Total Calories	% Fat Calories
deli	1 slice	1.0	70	13%
extra sour	1 slice	1.0	80	11%
Jewish	1 slice	1.5	80	17%
Russian-style	1 slice	1.0	80	11%
sourdough	1 slice	1.0	70	13%
wheat berry	1 slice	1.5	100	14%
(Father Sam's)..pocket bread				
onion	1 pita	–	130	–
wheat				
medium	½ pita	–	120	–
mini	1 pita	–	100	–
white				
medium	½ pita	–	110	–
mini	1 pita	–	110	–
wraps (10")				
spinach	1 wrap	4.5	160	25%
tomato	1 wrap	4.5	160	25%
wheat	1 wrap	5.0	160	28%
white	1 wrap	5.0	160	28%
(Freihofer's)				
100% whole wheat				
stone-ground	1 slice	1.5	90	15%
12-grain	1 slice	1.5	120	11%
Canadian white	1 slice	2.0	110	16%
hearty nut	1 slice	2.0	120	15%
Italian				
soft sourdough	1 slice	1.0	90	10%
unseeded	1 slice	1.0	80	11%
rye/no seeds	1 slice	1.0	70	13%
split top				
wheat	1 slice	1.0	70	13%
white	1 slice	1.0	70	13%
(Garden of Eatin')				
Bible Bread/pita				
original	1 pita	1.5	160	8%
very low salt	1 pita	2.0	160	11%
Chapati Indian Flat Bread	1 piece	2.5	120	19%
(Grant's Farm)				
buttermilk	1 slice	1.0	80	11%
honey cracked	1 slice	1.0	70	13%
oat bran	1 slice	1.0	70	13%
oatmeal				
& toasted almonds	1 slice	2.0	80	11%
pumpernickel rye	1 slice	1.0	70	13%
stone-ground wheat				
& 7-grain	1 slice	1.0	70	13%
wheat berry	1 slice	1.0	70	13%
(Kangaroo) pocket/pita bread				
bread wraps/white	1 wrap	3.0	190	14%

Food and Description	Amount	Fat Grams	Total Calories	% Fat Calories
breakfast pita				
4" mini/whole wheat	1 pita	1.0	70	13%
Greek pita flatbread				
white	1 pita	2.0	145	12%
whole wheat	1 pita	2.0	145	12%
pita pocket				
onion	1 pocket	–	90	–
wheat 'n honey	1 pocket	–	90	–
white	1 pocket	–	90	–
salad pockets				
wheat 'n honey	1 pocket	–	80	–
white	1 pocket	–	90	–
(King's Hawaiian).. center slice	½" slice	4.5	180	23%
(Labrea Bakery)				
country white				
sourdough	⅛ loaf	–	150	–
French				
baguette	2 oz	–	130	–
loaf	4" slice	–	130	–
Italian boule	⅛ loaf	–	130	–
organic wheat	1/12 loaf	0.5	150	3%
pain rustique	⅛ loaf	2.0	160	11%
pecan raisin	⅛ loaf	5.0	180	25%
roasted garlic	⅛ loaf	2.0	130	14%
rosemary olive oil	2 oz	1.0	140	6%
seeded rye	1/12 loaf	0.5	120	4%
sourdough baguette	⅕ loaf	–	150	–
Tuscan Italian	⅛ loaf	2.0	170	11%
whole grain	1/12 loaf	1.5	130	10%
Middle East pita pocket bread				
garlic	1 pita	2.0	160	11%
onion	1 pita	2.0	150	12%
white				
4" dia	1 pita	–	70	–
4 per pkg	1 pita	1.0	210	4%
6 per pkg	1 pita	0.5	140	3%
wheat/4" dia	1 pita	–	70	–
whole wheat				
4 per pkg	1 pita	1.5	200	7%
6 per pkg	1 pita	1.0	140	6%
(Monk's Bread)				
cinnamon	1 slice	2.0	70	26%
golden rice bran	1 slice	1.0	70	13%
Hi-Fibre	1 slice	1.0	50	18%
raisin	1 slice	2.0	70	26%
sunflower & bran	1 slice	1.0	70	13%
home-style butter top	1 slice	1.0	70	13%
(Nature's Path) manna bread				
carrot raisin	1 slice	–	130	–
cinnamon date	1 slice	–	150	–

Food and Description	Amount	Fat Grams	Total Calories	% Fat Calories
fruit & nut	1 slice	1.0	140	6%
milet rice	1 slice	–	130	–
multigrain	1 slice	–	130	–
sun seed	1 slice	2.0	160	11%
whole rye	1 slice	–	150	–
whole wheat	1 slice	–	150	–
(Oroweat)				
Master's Best				
deli rye	2 slices	1.5	130	10%
northern oat	1 slice	3.0	100	27%
3-seed	1 slice	3.5	90	35%
winter wheat	1 slice	3.0	90	30%
Oroweat				
carb counting				
100% whole wheat	1 slice	1.5	60	23%
multigrain	1 slice	1.5	60	23%
natural				
100% whole wheat	1 slice	1.0	100	9%
100% whole wheat & oat	1 slice	1.0	100	9%
carb counting				
100% whole wheat	1 slice	1.5	60	23%
multigrain	1 slice	0.5	60	8%
raisin cinnamon swirl	1 slice	3.0	120	23%
whole grain				
100% whole wheat	1 slice	1.0	90	10%
ambor grains	1 slice	1.5	90	15%
honey whole wheat	1 slice	2.0	100	18%
natural				
100% whole wheat	1 slice	1.0	100	9%
whole wheat & oat	1 slice	1.0	100	9%
Schwarzwalder dark rye	1 slice	1.0	70	13%
variety				
100% whole wheat	1 slice	1.0	90	10%
dark wheat	1 slice	1.0	100	9%
milk & honey	1 slice	1.5	110	12%
7-grain	1 slice	1.0	100	9%
(Panera) Breads				
9-grain	2 oz	2.5	150	15%
artisan breads				
3-cheese	2 oz	1.5	120	11%
3-seed	2 oz	2.0	130	14%
country	2 oz	–	120	–
French	2 oz	–	110	–
kalamata olive	2 oz	2.0	140	13%
multigrain	2 oz	0.5	120	4%
raisin pecan	1 oz	2.5	140	16%
sesame semolina	2 oz	–	120	–
stone mill rye	2 oz	–	110	–
Asiago cheese				
demi loaf	2 oz	3.5	140	23%

Food and Description	Amount	Fat Grams	Total Calories	% Fat Calories
ciabatta	6 oz	10.0	430	21%
cinnamon raisin	2 oz	3.0	160	17%
focaccia				
Asiago cheese	2 oz	6.0	150	24%
basil pesto	2 oz	6.0	150	24%
rosemary & onion	2 oz	4.5	140	29%
honey wheat berry	2 oz	2.5	140	16%
lower carb				
golden original	1.2 oz	1.0	80	11%
Italian herb	1.1 oz	1.0	80	11%
bread stick	1.2 oz	2.5	120	19%
rosemary walnut	1.1 oz	2.5	80	28%
rye	2 oz	2.5	140	16%
sourdough				
2-ounce slice	1 slice	–	120	–
baguette	2.5 oz	–	160	–
loaf	2.5 oz	–	160	–
soup bowl	8 oz	1.5	500	3%
sunflower	2 oz	5.0	160	28%
tomato basil	2 oz	0.5	130	3%
(Panne)..Provincio	⅛ loaf	–	130	–
(Pepperidge Farm)				
banana swirl	1 slice	2.0	90	20%
Canadian white	1 slice	1.0	80	11%
cinnamon				
raisin	1 slice	1.5	80	17%
swirl	1 slice	2.5	90	25%
deli swirl	1 slice	1.0	80	11%
Farmhouse				
buttermilk				
wheat	1 slice	1.5	110	12%
white	1 slice	1.0	110	8%
butter-topped				
wheat	1 slice	2.0	120	15%
white	1 slice	1.5	110	12%
crunchy oat	1 slice	1.5	100	14%
golden potato	1 slice	1.0	110	8%
hearty white	1 slice	1.0	110	8%
honey wheatberry	1 slice	1.5	110	12%
oat bran	1 slice	1.0	90	10%
oatmeal	1 slice	1.0	110	8%
sesame wheat	1 slice	2.0	110	16%
7-grain	1 slice	1.5	110	12%
sourdough	1 slice	1.5	110	12%
French toast swirl				
brown sugar & cinnamon	1 slice	3.5	140	23%
French vanilla	1 slice	3.5	140	23%
maple syrup & cinnamon	1 slice	2.0	130	14%
hot & crusty bread				
garlic	2" slice	8.0	170	42%

Food and Description	Amount	Fat Grams	Total Calories	% Fat Calories
Italian	2" slice	2.0	150	12%
thin-sliced French	2 slice	1.5	150	9%
twin French	4" slice	1.5	150	9%
Italian bread	1 slice	1.5	90	15%
Jewish rye party bread	5 slices	1.0	120	8%
Lifeworks wheat bread	2 slices	2.5	170	13%
Light Style				
7-grain	3 slices	1.0	140	6%
oatmeal	3 slices	0.5	140	3%
wheat	3 slices	0.5	130	3%
white	3 slices	1.0	140	6%
Natural Whole Grain				
9-grain	1 slice	1.0	90	10%
crunchy grains	1 slice	1.5	90	15%
honey oat	1 slice	1.5	90	15%
German dark wheat	1 slice	1.0	90	15%
hearty bran	1 slice	1.5	90	15%
sourdough wheat	1 slice	1.0	90	10%
oatmeal	1 slice	1.0	60	15%
party pumpernickel	5 slices	1.5	130	10%
rye				
seeded	1 slice	1.0	80	11%
seedless	1 slice	1.0	80	11%
whole wheat				
multigrain	1 slice	2.0	90	20%
(Roman Meal)..original				
(Rubschlager)				
cocktail breads				
honey whole grain	3 slices	1.0	80	11%
pumpernickel	3 slices	1.0	80	11%
rye	3 slices	1.5	80	17%
regular				
Komissbrot				
German-style	1 slice	1.0	70	13%
pumpernickel..Danish	1 slice	1.0	70	13%
Westphalian	1 slice	0.5	70	6%
rye				
Jewish deli	1 slice	1.0	70	13%
marble	2 slices	1.5	110	12%
sandwich	1 slice	2.0	90	20%
Swedish limpa	1 slice	1.0	60	15%
Rye-ola				
rye	1 slice	0.5	100	5%
sunflower	1 slice	2.0	100	18%
sandwich				
malt	1 slice	2.0	90	20%
pumpernickel	1 slice	1.5	90	7%
rye	1 slice	1.5	90	7%
stone-ground honey wheat	1 slice	1.5	90	7%
wheat	1 slice	2.0	90	20%

Food and Description	Amount	Fat Grams	Total Calories	% Fat Calories
whole-grain..European-style	1 slice	0.5	70	6%
(San Francisco) French bread				
breadsticks..all sticks	1 stick	1.0	110	8%
breadstix/sourdough	1 stick	0.5	140	6%
cheddar cheese	⅕ loaf	5.0	170	26%
ciabatta	⅐ loaf	1.0	140	6%
Fisherman's Wharf French Bread				
extra sour	1 slice	0.5	110	4%
sour	1 slice	1.0	110	8%
focaccia	⅛ loaf	2.0	150	12%
French, sweet				
Loaf/stick	⅒ loaf	1.5	120	11%
slices	2 slices	1.0	100	9%
Le Bout/sourdough	⅜ slice	0.5	140	3%
Luigi/sourdough	¼ loaf	0.5	140	3%
Old Italy				
bread stick	1/16 loaf	1.5	140	10%
sliced	1 slice	1.0	70	13%
pesto garlic	⅕ loaf	9.0	190	43%
Pugliese	⅕ loaf	1.0	140	6%
rye/light	2 slices	1.5	120	11%
sheepherder's	1 slice	1.0	110	8%
sourdough				
cracked wheat	1 slice	0.5	100	5%
cracked wheat batard	1 slice	0.5	120	4%
squaw bread	1 slice	1.5	120	11%
wheat bread				
cracked	1 slice	1.0	70	13%
regular	1 slice	1.0	70	13%
wheatberry	2 slices	1.5	130	10%
white bread	1 slice	1.0	80	11%
(Sara Lee)				
Delightful				
white	1 slice	–	45	–
	2 slices	1.0	90	10%
whole wheat	1 slice	–	45	–
	2 slices	1.0	90	10%
pita bread				
plain	1 pita	1.0	160	6%
whole wheat	1 pita	1.0	160	6%
Premium				
Classic				
wheat	1 slice	1.0	70	13%
white	1 slice	1.5	80	17%
home-style wheat	1 slice	1.0	100	9%
honey				
wheat	1 slice	1.0	70	13%
white	1 slice	0.5	100	5%
(Thomas')				
date nut loaf	1 slice	2.0	80	23%

Food and Description	Amount	Fat Grams	Total Calories	% Fat Calories
Sahara pita bread				
oat bran	1 pita	1.0	130	7%
onion	1 pita	0.5	140	3%
original				
large, 4 per pkg	1 pita	1.0	220	4%
mini, 8 per pkg	1 pita	–	70	–
regular				
6/12 per pkg	1 pita	1.0	150	6%
sourdough	1 pita	0.5	150	3%
whole wheat				
mini, 8 per pkg	1 pita	0.5	60	9%
regular, 6 per pkg	1 pita	1.0	130	7%
(Toufayan)				
breadsticks/Grissini-style				
garlic	3 sticks	0.5	50	9%
plain	3 sticks	0.5	50	9%
flat bread				
corn & jalapeño	1 flat	2.0	210	15%
Mediterranean	1 flat	0.9	270	3%
pita pockets..mini petites				
regular	4 pieces	–	70	–
whole wheat	4 pieces	–	70	–
(Wolferman's)				
English muffin breads				
cinnamon & raisin	1 slice	0.5	130	3%
cranberry citrus	1 slice	–	130	–
1910 original	2 slices	–	120	–
San Francisco				
sourdough	1 slice	–	120	–
tea breads				
apple strudel	1 slice	4.5	160	25%
banana nut	⅛ loaf	8.0	190	38%
gingerbread	⅛ loaf	12.0	230	47%
tangy lemon	⅛ loaf	6.0	150	36%
(Wonder)				
cinnamon raisin	1 slice	1.0	70	13%
Good Hearth				
honey wheat	1 slice	1.0	70	13%
multigrain	1 slice	1.5	70	19%
Home Pride				
wheat	1 slice	1.0	80	11%
white	1 slice	1.0	80	11%
potato	1 slice	1.0	70	13%
Italian				
Light	2 slices	1.0	80	11%
regular	1 slice	1.5	120	11%
seeded	1 slice	1.0	70	13%
Kid's	1 slice	1.0	70	13%
multigrain/fat-free	1 slice	–	70	–
Oat bran 'n' fiber	1 slice	1.0	100	9%

Food and Description	Amount	Fat Grams	Total Calories	% Fat Calories
Oatmeal Goodness				
oat & bran	1 slice	1.0	80	11%
oat & sunflower	1 slice	1.5	90	15%
potato				
fat-free	1 slice	–	70	–
regular	1 slice	1.0	70	13%
soft	1 slice	1.5	80	17%
Jewish	1 slice	1.5	80	17%
sourdough				
light	2 slices	1.0	80	11%
regular	1 slice	0.5	60	8%
Texas toast	1 slice	1.5	120	11%
■ REFRIGERATED				
(Bread du Jour)				
twin French loaves	3" slice	1.0	140	6%
(Pillsbury)				
breadsticks				
cornbread twists	1 twist	6.0	130	42%
crusty French loaf	⅛ pkg	2.0	150	12%
garlic w/herbs	2 pieces	7.0	160	39%
original	2 pieces	2.5	140	16%
Parmesan w/garlic	2 pieces	7.0	180	35%
French loaf	⅕ loaf	2.0	150	12%
home-style loaf				
wheat	⅛ loaf	2.5	150	15%
white	⅛ loaf	2.5	150	15%
BREAD COATING (See BAKE & FRY MIX; SEASONINGS)				
BREAD CRUMBS (See also BAKE & FRY MIX; SEASONINGS)				
(Contadina)				
roasted garlic				
& savory spices	¼ cup	1.5	110	12%
seasoned Italian-style	¼ cup	1.5	100	14%
3-cheese	¼ cup	1.5	110	12%
traditional unseasoned	¼ cup	1.5	110	12%
(Devonsheer)				
Italian	⅛ cup	1.5	110	12%
plain	⅛ cup	1.5	110	12%
(Golden Dipt)				
all-purpose breading				
fully seasoned	¼ cup	1.0	140	6%
light 'n' crunchy				
Modern Maid				
American-style/fine	¼ cup	1.0	140	6%
Oriental/fine	¼ cup	–	45	–
Panko				
plain	¼ cup	–	45	–
seasoned	¼ cup	–	45	–
(Kellogg's)..Corn Flake crumbs	2 Tbs	–	40	–

Food and Description	Amount	Fat Grams	Total Calories	% Fat Calories
(Old Bay) Seasoned				
Dip & Crisp	1/9 can	2.0	110	16%
(Old London)				
lemon pepper	1/8 cup	1.5	120	11%
plain	1/8 cup	1.5	110	12%
roasted garlic	1/8 cup	1.0	110	12%
seasoned	1/8 cup	1.5	110	12%
(Progresso)				
garlic herb	1/4 cup	1.5	100	14%
Italian	1/4 cup	1.5	110	12%
Parmesan	1/4 cup	1.5	110	12%
plain	1/4 cup	1.5	110	12%
BREAD CUBES (*See* CROUTONS; STUFFING/DRESSING)				
BREAD PUDDING (*See* PUDDING & MOUSSE)				
BREAD STUFFING (*See* STUFFING/DRESSING)				
BREADFRUIT/raw	1/4 small	–	99	–
	1 cup	0.5	227	2%
BREADSTICK (See also BREAD)				
(Angonoa)				
mini				
cheese	1 oz	2.0	110	16%
pizza	1 oz	2.0	120	15%
sesame	1 oz	4.0	120	30%
whole wheat	1 oz	4.0	120	30%
regular				
cheese	1 oz	2.0	110	16%
garlic	1 oz	2.0	120	15%
Italian	1 oz	2.0	120	15%
onion	1 oz	3.0	120	23%
sesame royal	1 oz	4.0	120	30%
(Bread du Jour) brown & serve				
original	1 piece	1.0	130	7%
sourdough	1 piece	1.0	130	7%
(Fattorie & Pandea)..all types	3 pieces	1.0	60	15%
(Oroweat)				
cheese	1 oz	2.0	110	16%
garlic	1 oz	2.0	113	16%
plain	1 oz	2.0	110	16%
sesame	1 oz	2.0	120	15%
(Pepperidge Farm)				
brown & serve	1 piece	1.5	150	9%
cheddar cheese/thin	7 pieces	2.5	70	32%
onion/thin	7 pieces	2.0	70	26%
sesame/thin	7 pieces	1.5	60	23%
(Pillsbury) soft/refrigerated				
cornbread twists	1 twist	6.0	130	42%
crusty French loaf	1/5 pkg	2.0	150	7%
garlic and herb	2 pieces	7.0	180	35%
Parmesan	2 pieces	7.0	180	35%

Food and Description	Amount	Fat Grams	Total Calories	% Fat Calories
plain	2 pieces	2.5	140	16%
(Stella D'Oro)				
cracked pepper				
mini	4 pieces	2.0	70	26%
oven-baked snacks	½ oz	2.0	70	26%
garlic				
deli/fat-free	5 pieces	–	60	–
Grissini/fat-free	3 pieces	–	60	–
roasted	1 piece	1.0	45	20%
traditional/fat-free	2 pieces	–	70	–
onion	1 piece	1.0	40	23%
original	1 piece	1.0	45	20%
deli/fat-free	5 pieces	–	60	–
mini	4 pieces	1.5	70	19%
Grissini/fat-free	3 pieces	–	60	–
traditional/fat-free	2 pieces	–	70	–
pizza	1 piece	1.0	43	21%
sesame				
low-fat	2 pieces	1.0	70	13%
mini	⅔ oz	3.5	80	39%
sodium-free	1 piece	2.0	50	36%
(Toufayan)				
Grissini-style				
cheese	3 sticks	1.0	50	18%
garlic	3 sticks	0.5	50	9%
plain	3 sticks	0.5	50	9%
soft				
cinnamon raisin	1 piece	2.0	110	16%
pizza	1 piece	2.0	110	16%
plain	1 piece	2.0	110	16%
BREAKFAST/CEREAL BAR (See also GRANOLA/GRANOLA-TYPE BAR)				
(Atkins)				
Breakfast bars/Morning Start				
apple crisp	1 bar	9.0	170	48%
(Barbara's Bakery)				
Multigrain Cereal Bars				
all flavors	1 bar	1.5	120	11%
Puffins Cereal & Milk Bars				
blueberry yogurt	1 bar	1.5	120	11%
French toast	1 bar	1.5	120	11%
peanut butter chocolate chip	1 bar	3.5	140	23%
strawberry yogurt	1 bar	2.0	120	14%
(General Mills)				
MILK 'N CEREAL BARS				
all flavors	1 bar	4.0	160	23%
OATMEAL CRISP FRUIT 'N CEREAL BARS				
all flavors	1 bar	2.0	150	12%
(Health Valley)				

Food and Description	Amount	Fat Grams	Total Calories	% Fat Calories
BAKES/FAT-FREE				
All flavors	1 bar	–	70	–
CAFÉ CREATIONS				
cinnamon Danish	1 bar	2.5	130	17%
chocolate				
espresso	1 bar	3.0	130	21%
raspberry	1 bar	3.0	130	21%
COBBLER CEREAL BARS				
regular..all flavors	1 bar	2.0	130	14%
low-fat..all flavors	1 bar	2.0	130	14%
FRUIT BARS/FAT-FREE				
all flavors	1 bar	–	140	–
TARTS/LOW-FAT				
(Hain's) Crisp Bars	1 bar	1.0	80	11%
(Hostess) Cereal Bars				
apple	1 bar	1.5	120	34%
banana nut	1 bar	2.0	120	15%
blueberry	1 bar	1.5	120	34%
raspberry	1 bar	1.5	120	34%
strawberry	1 bar	1.5	120	34%
(Kellogg's) Breakfast Bars				
CEREAL & MILK BARS				
Cocoa Rice Krispies	1 bar	2.5	95	24%
Fruit Loops	1 bar	3.0	100	27%
Frosted Flakes	1 bar	3.0	110	25%
NUTRI-GRAIN CEREAL BARS				
all flavors	1 bar	3.0	140	19%
NUTRI-GRAIN MUFFIN BARS				
banana	1 bar	4.0	160	23%
cinnamon raisin	1 bar	4.0	170	21%
NUTRI-GRAIN TWISTS				
all flavors	1 twist	3.0	140	19%
NUTRI-GRAIN YOGURT BARS				
mini yogurt icing..all flavors	1 pouch	3.0	160	17%
regular-size..all flavors	1 bar	3.0	140	19%
SPECIAL K BARS..all flavors	1 bar	1.5	90	15%
(Post) Cereal Bar				
Carb Well				
cinnamon				
crunch	1 bar	2.0	110	16%
raisin	1 bar	5.0	140	32%
cranberry almond	1 bar	5.0	140	32%
golden crunch	1 bar	1.0	110	8%
peanut butter	1 bar	5.0	140	32%
(Quaker)				
Breakfast Squares				
BITES..all flavors	1 pouch	2.5	140	16%
NUTRITION FOR WOMEN				
all flavors	1 bar	4.0	220	16%

Food and Description	Amount	Fat Grams	Total Calories	% Fat Calories
REGULAR				
apple crisp	1 bar	3.0	130	21%
baked apple	1 bar	4.0	220	16%
brown sugar cinnamon	1 bar	4.0	220	16%
cheesecake				
blueberry	1 bar	3.0	130	21%
strawberry	1 bar	3.0	140	19%
cherry cobbler	1 bar	3.0	130	21%
chocolate strawberry	1 bar	3.0	130	21%
iced raspberry	1 bar	2.5	130	17%
oatmeal raisin	1 bar	4.0	220	16%
very berry	1 bar	3.0	130	21%
(SunBelt) Cereal Bars.. Fruit & Grain				
apple	1 bar	3.0	140	19%
blueberry	1 bar	3.0	140	19%
raspberry	1 bar	3.0	140	19%
strawberry	1 bar	2.5	140	16%

BREAKFAST DRINK (*See also* NUTRITIONAL LIQUID SUPPLEMENT)
(NOTE: Unless otherwise noted, mixes are prepared according to package directions)

Food and Description	Amount	Fat Grams	Total Calories	% Fat Calories
(Alba) Dairy Shake				
all flavors	8 fl oz	–	70	–
(Carnation) Instant Breakfast				
liquid/ready-to-drink				
Carb Conscious..all flavors	10 fl oz	5.0	150	30%
original				
creamy				
milk chocolate	10 fl oz	5.0	250	18%
French vanilla	10 fl oz	5.0	250	18%
strawberry crème	10 fl oz	5.0	240	19%
powdered.. Carb Conscious				
classic French vanilla	1 pkt	–	70	–
rich milk chocolate	1 pkt	0.5	70	6%

BREAKFAST SANDWICH (*See also* FROZEN ENTRÉE/DINNER; individual FAST FOOD listings; VEGETARIAN FOODS)

Food and Description	Amount	Fat Grams	Total Calories	% Fat Calories
(Armour)				
Sausage 'n' Biscuits	1 sandwich	19.0	300	57%
(Bob Evans)..Snackwich				
ham & cheese bagel	2 bagels	6.0	240	23%
sausage biscuits				
12-count pkg	2 biscuits	23.0	370	56%
sausage cheese burgers				
4-count pkg..large	1 burger	16.0	270	53%
12-count pkg	2 biscuits	21.0	320	59%
sausage, egg &				
cheese burritos	2 burritos	11.0	330	30%
(Nestlé USA)				
Hot Pockets bacon,				
egg & cheese	1 sandwich	9.0	170	48%
Lean Pockets bacon, egg				
& cheese/low-fat	1 sandwich	4.0	140	26%

Food and Description	Amount	Fat Grams	Total Calories	% Fat Calories
(Owens)				
Border breakfasts/tacos				
bacon/egg/cheese	2 tacos	18.0	330	49%
chorizo/egg/cheese	2 tacos	21.0	350	54%
sausage/egg/cheese				
2-count	1 taco	21.0	350	54%
6-count	2 tacos	21.0	350	54%
12-count	2 tacos	21.0	350	54%
sandwiches				
biscuits				
bacon/egg/cheese				
large/5 count	1 biscuit	21.0	340	56%
egg/bacon/cheese				
large	1 biscuit	20.0	350	51%
sausage				
2-count	2 biscuits	27.0	380	64%
6-count	2 biscuits	27.0	380	64%
16-count	2 biscuits	22.0	330	60%
large	1 biscuit	21.0	320	59%
sausage cheeseburger				
2-count	2 biscuits	21.0	310	61%
12-count	2 biscuits	21.0	310	61%
large	1 biscuit	18.0	280	58%
sausage/egg/cheese	2 biscuits	30.0	430	63%
4-count	2 biscuits	30.0	430	63%
5-count/large	1 biscuit	23.0	370	56%
(Purnell's Old Folks) Microwaveable				
country	2 sandwiches	14.0	280	45%
country w/cheese	2 sandwiches	20.0	360	50%
whole hog country				
6-count	2 sandwiches	16.0	300	48%
12-count	2 sandwiches	21.0	333	57%
(Schwan's) frozen				
personal pouches/sausage				
breakfast bagel	1 bagel	11.0	300	33%
country sausage biscuit	2 biscuits	22.0	340	58%
pigs in a blanket	4 pieces	22.0	310	64%
(Swanson) Great Starts..frozen				
croissant w/sausage,				
egg & cheese	1 croissant	33.0	470	63%
muffin w/egg, Canadian-style				
bacon & cheese	1 muffin	11.0	270	37%
(Weight Watcher's) Smart Ones				
English muffin sandwich	1 muffin	5.0	210	21%
BREATH MINT (See CANDY)				
BREWER'S YEAST (See YEAST)				
BROAD BEAN				
canned	½ cup	<1.0	91	5%
fresh				
boiled	½ cup	<1.0	93	5%

Food and Description	Amount	Fat Grams	Total Calories	% Fat Calories
raw				
immature	8 oz	1.0	238	4%
mature	8 oz	3.8	766	5%
BROCCOLI (*See also* BROCCOLI DISH; VEGETABLES, MIXED)				
fresh				
(Dole)				
florets	3 oz	0.5	25	18%
spears	1 medium	0.5	45	10%
frozen				
(Birds Eye)				
chopped	½ cup	–	25	–
cuts	½ cup	–	25	–
florets	3 oz	–	25	–
spears				
baby deluxe	3 oz	–	30	–
regular	3 oz	–	25	–
(C&W)				
florets	5 florets	–	25	–
microwave Brocclettes	1 cup	–	30	–
(Cascadian Farm)	⅔ cup	–	20	–
generic				
chopped	10 oz	<1.0	75	10%
spears	10 oz	1.0	85	11%
(Green Giant)				
cuts/cooked	⅔ cup	–	25	–
chopped/cooked	½ cup	–	25	–
florets/Select	1⅓ cups	–	25	–
no sauce broccoli				
spears				
boil-in-bag	3.5 oz	–	25	–
Select	3 spears	–	25	–
(Pictsweet) spears	3.3 oz	–	25	–
(Seneca)	1 cup	–	25	–
(Stokely) cuts	3 oz	–	25	–
BROCCOLI DISH (*See also* FROZEN ENTRÉE/DINNER: VEGETABLES, MIXED; VEGETARIAN FOODS)				
frozen				
(Birds Eye)				
baby broccoli blend	¾ cup	4.5	70	58%
in cheese sauce	¾ cup	4.0	70	51%
(Cascadian Farm)				
w/cheddar cheese sauce	½ cup	2.5	60	38%)
(Green Giant)				
broccoli in cheese-flavored				
sauce	⅔ cup	3.0	80	34%
broccoli & 3-cheese sauce/				
family size	¾ cup	2.5	50	45%
spears in butter sauce	4 oz	2.0	50	36%

Food and Description	Amount	Fat Grams	Total Calories	% Fat Calories
BROWNIE/BROWNIE-LIKE BARS (*See also* CAKE; CAKE, SNACK; COOKIE)				
FROZEN				
(Atkins) Endulge				
iced chocolate				
w/o nuts	1 brownie	13.0	180	65%
(Sara Lee) Brownie Bites				
triple chocolate fudge	1 serving	4.0	90	40%
(Weight Watchers)				
à la mode	1 brownie	4.0	190	19%
double brownie parfait	1 brownie	3.0	260	10%
MIX				
(Arrowhead Mills) prepared				
fat-free	1 brownie	–	120	–
regular	1 brownie	–	110	–
wheat-free	1 brownie	2.0	120	15%
(Betty Crocker)				
dark chocolate fudge	1 brownie	7.0	170	37%
frosted	1 brownie	9.0	210	39%
German chocolate	1 brownie	8.0	190	38%
original	1 brownie	6.0	160	34%
peanut butter w/Reese's Pieces	1 brownie	9.0	180	45%
pecan	1 brownie	9.0	170	42%
triple chunk	1 brownie	9.0	180	45%
turtle	1 brownie	8.0	170	42%
walnut	1 brownie	9.0	180	45%
walnut chocolate chunk	1 brownie	4.5	140	29%
(Duncan Hines)				
chewy recipe fudge				
Dark 'n' chunky	1 brownie	7.0	160	37%
original	1 brownie	7.0	170	37%
Premium family-size	1 brownie	8.0	170	42%
Dark 'n' Fudgy Chocolate				
double fudge	1 brownie	6.0	170	32%
Lover's Premium	1 brownie	8.0	170	42%
milk chocolate chunk	1 brownie	7.0	170	37%
turtle	1 brownie	8.0	160	45%
walnut	1 brownie	10.0	190	47%
(Eagle Brand) Premium dessert kits				
decadent fudge bar	1 bar	17.0	190	81%
magic cookie bars	1 bar	6.0	130	42%
peanut butter passion	1 bar	8.0	170	42%
(Ghirardelli) mix only				
double chocolate	⅟₂₀ pkg	4.5	150	27%
(Jiffy) mix only	⅕ pkg	4.0	150	24%
(Krusteaz) prepared				
fudge brownie				
fat-free	1 brownie	–	120	–

Food and Description	Amount	Fat Grams	Total Calories	% Fat Calories
original	1 brownie	7.0	190	33%
(Martha White) mix only				
California walnut				
& chocolate chips	⅟₂₀ pkg	4.5	140	29%
semi-sweet & milk				
chocolate chips	⅟₂₀ pkg	2.5	170	13%
traditional chewy				
fudge	⅟₂₀ pkg	2.0	130	14%
(Pillsbury)				
Brownie Classics/mix only				
all flavors	⅟₂₀ pkg	2.5	120	19%
Fudge Supreme/mix only				
Chocolate				
chunk	⅟₁₆ pkg	3.5	120	26%
double	⅟₁₆ pkg	2.0	110	16%
extreme	⅟₁₆ pkg	3.0	120	23%
frosted	⅟₁₆ pkg	3.5	140	23%
fudge toffee	⅟₂₀ pkg	2.5	120	19%
vanilla frosted	⅟₁₆ pkg	4.0	140	26%
walnut	⅟₁₂ pkg	5.0	140	32%
white fudge chunk	⅟₁₆ pkg	3.5	120	26%
Snack Batch fudge..mix only	⅟₉ pkg	2.5	130	17%
Thick 'N Fudgy/prepared				
cheesecake swirl	1 brownie	7.0	150	42%
chocolate chunk	1 brownie	7.0	160	39%
double chocolate	1 brownie	6.0	150	36%
walnut	1 brownie	10.0	190	47%
(White Lily) mix only				
triple chocolate chunk	⅟₁₈ pkg	2.0	120	15%
READY-TO-SERVE				
(Awrey)				
chocolate decadent				
individual	1 brownie	10.0	210	43%
pre-cut	⅟₂₄ sheet	22.0	470	42%
chocolate peanut				
sensation	1 brownie	13.0	240	49%
home-style fudge nut	1 brownie	10.0	210	43%
no nut brownie	1 brownie	19.0	420	41%
(Better Low Carb) brownies				
traditional	1 brownie	2.0	47	38%
w/chocolate chips	1 brownie	2.0	47	38%
w/walnuts	1 brownie	2.0	47	38%
(Drake's) fudge nut				
reduced-fat	1 brownie	2.5	170	13%
(Eagle) fudge w/chocolate chips	1 brownie	11.0	260	38%
(Entenmann's) fudge/fat-free	⅟₁₀ strip	–	110	–
(Famous Amos) fat-free	1 brownie	–	130	–
(Gourmet Baker) Food Service				
Bengal	1 brownie	11.0	230	43%
Blondie Obsession	1 brownie	15.0	260	52%

Food and Description	Amount	Fat Grams	Total Calories	% Fat Calories
Caramel Rage	1 brownie	16.0	290	50%
caramel silk	1 bar	13.0	240	49%
chocolate macaroon	1 bar	16.0	280	51%
chocolate silk	1 bar	13.0	240	49%
Obsession	1 brownie	14.0	250	50%
Rocky Road	1 brownie	12.0	240	53%
(Hostess)				
brownie bites..all types	3 brownies	9.0	170	48%
fudge brownies	1 brownie	11.0	330	30%
low-fat	1 brownie	2.5	140	16%
(Little Debbie)				
Be My Valentine	1 brownie	9.0	200	41%
Christmas Tree	1 brownie	6.0	200	27%
Cosmic	1 pkg	12.0	280	39%
	2.5 oz	14.0	320	39%
Easter	1 pkg	12.0	280	39%
Fall	1 pkg	12.0	270	40%
fudge	1 pkg	13.0	280	42%
	2 oz	11.0	280	35%
	2.1 oz	12.0	270	40%
	2.5 oz	14.0	320	39%
reduced-fat	1 brownie	3.0	190	14%
loaves	1 loaf	15.0	270	50%
Stars & Stripes	1 pkg	13.0	290	40%
treats	2.1 oz	15.0	270	50%
(Otis Spunkmeyer)				
brownie-like bars (3.25 oz)				
double chocolate caramel				
bar w/Snickers	2.0 oz bar	11.0	240	41%
lemon bar	2.8 oz	11.0	260	38%
pecan pie	3.25 oz bar	18.0	390	42%
raspberry	3.25 oz bar	13.0	330	35%
brownies				
café au lait	3.25 oz	19.0	390	44%
double chocolate	2 oz	11.5	260	40%
turtle	33.25 oz	25.0	420	54%
(Sara Lee) Food Service				
Bakery				
brownie w/ nuts	1 brownie	8.0	170	42%
decadent chocolate w/o nuts	1 brownie	8.0	180	40%
iced fudge nut	1 brownie	9.0	180	45%
Bristo Collection				
blondie	1 brownie	8.0	180	36%
chocolate pecan	1 brownie	7.0	170	37%
chocolate raspberry cordial	1 brownie	8.0	180	36%
marbled chocolate				
caramel	1 brownie	10.0	180	50%
peanut butter & chocolate	1 brownie	7.0	170	37%
Seven Layers of Heaven	1 brownie	10.0	190	47%
ultimate brownie bar	1 brownie	9.0	190	43%

Food and Description	Amount	Fat Grams	Total Calories	% Fat Calories
(Tastykake)..fudge walnut	1 brownie	8.0	180	40%
BRUSSELS SPROUTS				
FRESH				
cooked	½ cup	–	30	–
raw	½ cup	–	20	–
(Dole)	½ cup	–	20	–
FROZEN				
(Birds Eye)..all styles	3 oz	–	35	–
(C&W) petite	10 sprouts	–	30	–
(Green Giant)	½ cup	–	25	–
(Pictsweet)				
regular	3.3 oz	–	35	–
express microwave	2.5 oz	–	30	–
(Stokely)	3 oz	–	35	–
BRUSSELS SPROUTS DISH				
(Green Giant) baby				
in butter sauce	⅔ cup	1.0	45	20%
(Stokely) singles, in butter sauce	4 oz	1.0	50	18%
BUCKWHEAT GROATS/KASHA				
(Arrowhead Mills) brown	¼ cup	1.0	140	6%
(Wolff's) roasted kernels/cooked	½ cup	1.0	170	5%
BUFFALO/BISON				
COOKED				
(Denver Buffalo Co.)				
buffalo burgers	4 oz	5.2	130	36%
ground	4 oz	17.0	250	61%
DRIED	4 oz	2.0	149	12%
RAW	4 oz	1.6	112	13%
New West				
buffalo & beef				
hot Polish sausage	1 link	16.0	210	69%
steak	4 oz	3.0	130	21%
ROASTED	3 oz	2.0	148	12%
BULGUR/HARD RED WINTER WHEAT				
COOKED				
(Arrowhead Mills)	¼ cup	0.5	150	3%
DRY/canned				
seasoned	1 cup	4.5	246	17%
unseasoned	1 serving	0.9	227	4%
UNCOOKED	1 cup	3.0	600	5%
BUN (*See* PASTRY; ROLL)				
BURBOT/raw	3 oz	0.7	76	8%

BURGER (*See* BEEF; BUFFALO/BISON; HAMBURGER; TURKEY; VEGETARIAN FOODS)
BURGER MIX (*See* BEEF DISH/ENTRÉE; VEGETARIAN FOODS)
BURRITO (*See* BREAKFAST SANDWICH; MEXICAN FOOD; VEGETARIAN FOODS)
BUTTER (*See also* BUTTER BLEND/SPREAD; BUTTER-FLAVORED SEASONING; MARGARINE, MARGARINE SPREAD & SPRAY)

(Breakstone) salted or unsalted				
stick	1 Tbs	11.0	100	100%
whipped	1 Tbs	7.0	60	100%

Food and Description	Amount	Fat Grams	Total Calories	% Fat Calories
(Challenge) salted or unsalted				
European-style	1 Tbs	11.0	100	100%
light	1 Tbs	6.0	50	100%
sweet	1 Tbs	11.0	100	100%
whipped	1 Tbs	7.0	70	100%
(Keller's)	1 tsp	4.0	35	100%
	1 Tbs	11.0	100	100%
(Land O'Lakes) salted or unsalted				
honey butter	1 Tbs	8.0	90	80%
light				
stick	1 Tbs	6.0	50	100%
whipped	1 Tbs	3.5	35	100%
regular				
stick	1 Tbs	11.0	100	100%
whipped	1 Tbs	7.0	70	100%
roasted garlic	1 Tbs	11.0	100	100%
soft baking w/canola oil	1 Tbs	11.0	100	100%
spreadable w/canola oil	1 Tbs	12.0	110	100%
sweet cream	1 Tbs	11.0	100	100%
ultra creamy	1 Tbs	12.0	110	100%
BUTTER BEAN (*See also* LIMA BEAN)				
canned				
(Aunt Nellie's) Reber	½ cup	1.0	140	6%
(Bush Bros)				
baby	½ cup	–	120	–
green	½ cup	–	110	–
large	½ cup	–	100	–
speckled	½ cup	–	110	–
(Green Giant)	½ cup	–	90	–
(Joan of Arc)	½ cup	–	90	–
(Luck's) speckled/seasoned w/pork	½ cup	3.0	140	19%
(S&W) tender cooked/dry	½ cup	–	70	–
(Trappey's) large white	½ cup	1.0	80	11%
(Van Camp's)	1 cup	1.0	160	6%
BUTTER BLEND/SPREAD (*See also* MARGARINE, MARGARINE SPREAD & SPRAY)				
(Blue Bonnet)				
stick w/tub	1 Tbs	11.0	90	100%
	4 oz	44.0	360	100%
(Buttery Blend) liquid	1 Tbs	14.0	120	100%
(Downey's) honey butter				
cinnamon	1 Tbs	1.0	50	18%
original	1 Tbs	1.0	50	18%
(Kraft) Touch of Butter				
bowl	1 Tbs	6.0	50	100%
squeeze bottle	1 Tbs	9.0	80	100%
stick/50% fat	1 Tbs	10.0	90	100%
(Land O'Lakes)				
Country Morning Blend				
stick				
light	1 Tbs	6.0	50	100%

Food and Description	Amount	Fat Grams	Total Calories	% Fat Calories
regular/salted or unsalted tub	1 Tbs	11.0	100	100%
light	1 Tbs	6.0	50	100%
regular	1 Tbs	11.0	100	100%
BUTTERBUR				
cooked	½ cup	<1.0	8	56%
raw	1 cup	<1.0	13	35%
BUTTERFISH/raw	3 oz	6.8	124	49%
BUTTER-FLAVORED SEASONING (*See also* SEASONINGS)				
(Best O' Butter)				
cheddar cheese flavor	½ tsp	<1.0	6	60%
garlic buttery	½ tsp	<1.0	4	90%
original	½ tsp	<1.0	4	90%
sour cream flavor	½ tsp	<1.0	4	90%
(Butter Buds) butter-flavored				
granules	1 tsp	–	5	–
mix	1 tsp	–	5	–
salt	any	–	–	–
(Molly McButter) sprinkles				
butter	1 tsp	–	5	–
cheese	1 tsp	–	5	–
garlic & herb	1 tsp	–	5	–
BUTTERNUT/dried	1 oz	16.0	174	83%

C

Food and Description	Amount	Fat Grams	Total Calories	% Fat Calories
CABBAGE (*See also* SWAMP CABBAGE)				
canned or jarred				
(Aunt Nellie's)				
pickled	1 cup	<1.0	260	2%
red/sweet & sour	2 Tbs	–	20	–
(Libby's) red/sweet & sour	2 Tbs	–	20	–
(S&W) red/sweet & sour	2 Tbs	–	15	–
fresh				
Chinese/bok choy/Napa				
cooked	½ cup	–	10	–
raw/shredded	½ cup	–	5	–
(Dole)	½ cup	–	5	–

Food and Description	Amount	Fat Grams	Total Calories	% Fat Calories
Danish				
shredded	½ cup	–	20	–
whole/2-lb head	1 head	2.0	225	8%
red/raw/shredded	½ cup	–	10	–
(Dole)	3 oz	–	25	–
Savoy/raw	1 cup	–	12	–
spoon/raw	1 cup	–	37	–
white				
cooked	½ cup	–	16	–
raw/shredded	½ cup	–	12	–
CACTUS				
(Embassa)	⅔ cup	–	5	–
(La Costena)				
Napolitos tender cactus	1 cup	–	20	–

CAKE (*See also* BROWNIE/BROWNIE-LIKE BARS; CAKE, SNACK; DONUT; MUFFIN; PASTRY; POPCORN BARS & CAKES; RICE CAKES)

■ **FROZEN OR REFRIGERATED**

Food and Description	Amount	Fat Grams	Total Calories	% Fat Calories
(Atkins) Endulge				
cheesecake				
dessert cup	3 oz	11.0	140	71%
New York–style	1 slice	23.0	290	71%
fudgy chocolate torte	1 slice	29.0	360	73%
(Banquet) Dessert bakes				
chocolate lava cake	1 slice	7.0	370	17%
(CEMAC) Cheesecake				
fat-free	1 slice	–	100	–
(Edward's)				
cheesecake				
caramel				
dulce de leche	1 cake	19.0	290	59%
chocolate marble	1 cake	19.0	290	59%
harvest pumpkin				
limited edition	⅙ cake	32.0	520	55%
original	1 cake	21.0	290	65%
strawberry marble	1 cake	18.0	280	58%
(Mrs. Smith's)				
carrot	1 piece	13.0	240	49%
Flip It cakes				
apple caramel	1 cake	13.0	480	24%
strawberry delight	1 cake	9.0	380	21%
(Pepperidge Farm)				
3-layer cake				
carrot	1 piece	16.0	280	51%
chocolate decadence	1 piece	18.0	300	54%
chocolate fudge	1 piece	11.0	250	40%
chocolate fudge stripe	1 piece	13.0	250	47%
chocolate supreme	1 piece	16.0	300	48%
coconut classic	1 piece	11.0	250	40%
devil's food	1 piece	12.0	250	43%

Food and Description	Amount	Fat Grams	Total Calories	% Fat Calories
German chocolate	1 piece	13.0	250	47%
golden	1 piece	12.0	250	43%
strawberry stripe	1 piece	12.0	250	43%
(Sara Lee)				
Retail				
cheesecake				
cherry cream	¼ cake	12.0	350	31%
chocolate chip	¼ cake	21.0	410	46%
chocolate mousse	⅕ cake	25.0	400	56%
cheesecake bites				
chocolate-dipped				
original	1 piece	7.0	100	63%
	5 pieces	34.0	500	61%
chocolate praline				
pecan	1 piece	6.0	100	54%
	5 pieces	31.0	480	58%
coffee cake				
butter streusel	⅙ cake	9.0	190	43%
crumb	⅛ cake	8.0	190	37%
pecan	⅙ cake	13.0	140	84%
pound cake				
all butter				
family-size	⅙ cake	15.0	220	61%
regular	¼ cake	16.0	330	42%
free & light	¼ cake	4.0	200	18%
strawberry swirl	¼ cake	11.0	290	34%
shortcake/strawberry/filled w/real strawberries	⅛ cake	7.0	180	35%
French				
classic	⅕ cake	25.0	410	55%
cream cherry				
original	¼ cake	18.0	340	48%
reduced-fat/25%	¼ cake	13.0	310	38%
strawberry/original	¼ cake	12.0	330	33%
strawberry French	⅙ cake	14.0	320	39%
Food Service				
breakfast cakes				
blueberry	1 slice	5.0	180	25%
French crumb cake	1 slice	4.0	180	20%
cheesecakes				
French cream				
home-style	1/14 cake	16.0	280	51%
round	1/16 cake	22.0	360	55%
New York–style				
creamy	1/16 cake	31.0	420	66%
high-profile	1/14 cake	38.0	530	65%
plain	1/16 cake	28.0	410	61%
Gourmet Desserts/Bristo Collection				
cheesecakes				

Food and Description	Amount	Fat Grams	Total Calories	% Fat Calories
caramel pecan	1 slice	37.0	520	64%
chocolate raspberry rumble	1 slice	27.0	450	54%
key lime breeze	1 slice	36.0	510	64%
mint chocolate chip	1 slice	38.0	560	61%
mocha swirl	1 slice	35.0	500	63%
white chocolate tuxedo	1 slice	28.0	420	60%
chocolate, chocolate gourmet dessert torte	1 slice	24.0	370	58%
home-style				
blueberry yogurt	1 slice	11.0	300	33%
lemon poppyseed	1 slice	10.0	300	30%
tarts/individual				
pecan	1 tart	37.0	860	39%
rustic apple	1 tart	26.0	540	43%
tiramisu desserts				
pan	4.5 oz	29.0	430	61%
Viva	5.5 oz	32.0	500	58%
(Schwan's)				
cinnamon streusel coffee cake	⅛ cake	18.0	330	48%
New York–style cheesecake	1 slice	20.0	290	62%
(Weight Watcher's) Smart Ones				
carrot cake	1 serving	3.5	220	14%
cheesecake				
French-style	1 serving	4.0	170	21%
New York–style	1 serving	5.0	150	30%
double fudge cake	1 serving	4.5	150	27%
■ MIX				
(Betty Crocker)..prepared				
Classic Dessert				
gingerbread cake & cookie	1/12 cake	6.0	230	23%
pineapple upside-down cake	⅙ cake	14.0	400	32%
pound cake	⅛ cake	18.0	260	28%
Snackin' Cake/prepared				
banana walnut	⅑ cake	5.0	180	25%
chocolate chunk	⅑ cake	5.0	80	25%
cinnamon swirl	⅑ cake	5.0	190	24%
German chocolate	⅑ cake	5.0	180	25%
SuperMoist..prepared				
angel food				
confetti	1/12 cake	–	150	–
one-step white	1/12 cake	–	140	–
butter chocolate	1/12 cake	12.0	250	43%
butter pecan	1/12 cake	10.0	240	38%
butter yellow	1/12 cake	11.0	250	40%
carrot cake	1/10 cake	15.0	320	42%
cherry chip	1/10 cake	13.0	300	39%
chocolate chip	1/12 cake	11.0	250	40%
chocolate fudge	1/12 cake	13.0	270	43%

Food and Description	Amount	Fat Grams	Total Calories	% Fat Calories
chocolate w/creamy swirls of fudge	⅛ cake	8.0	210	34%
devil's food	1/12 cake	13.0	270	43%
double chocolate swirl	1/12 cake	13.0	270	43%
French vanilla	1/12 cake	10.0	240	38%
fudge marble	1/10 cake	12.0	290	37%
German chocolate	1/12 cake	10.0	270	43%
golden vanilla	1/12 cake	10.0	240	38%
lemon	1/12 cake	10.0	240	38%
milk chocolate	1/12 cake	11.0	240	41%
party rainbow white	1/10 cake	13.0	300	38%
party swirl	1/12 cake	11.0	240	41%
pineapple	1/12 cake	10.0	250	36%
sour cream white	1/10 cake	12.0	280	39%
spice	1/10 cake	10.0	250	36%
strawberry	1/12 cake	10.0	250	36%
white	1/12 cake	10.0	230	39%
yellow	1/12 cake	10.0	250	36%
Supreme Dessert Bar				
Sunkist lemon	1 bar	4.5	140	29%
(Carb Watchers) Cake & muffin mix				
prepared..all flavors	1 slice	1.0	80	11%
(Dromedary) pound cake				
carrot	1/12 cake	15.0	232	58%
date nut	1/12 cake	8.0	183	39%
gingerbread	1 piece	2.0	100	18%
pound cake	1 slice	6.0	150	36%
(Duncan Hines)..prepared				
angel food	1/12 cake	–	140	–
banana supreme	1/12 cake	11.0	250	40%
butter recipe fudge	1/10 cake	17.0	320	48%
butter recipe golden	1/10 cake	16.0	320	45%
butterscotch	1/12 cake	11.0	250	40%
caramel deluxe	1/12 cake	11.0	250	40%
chocolate mocha	1/12 cake	15.0	290	47%
cinnamon crumb cake	1 piece	6.0	200	18%
dark chocolate fudge	1/12 cake	5.0	290	47%
devil's food	1/12 cake	15.0	290	47%
French vanilla	1/12 cake	11.0	250	40%
fudge marble	1/12 cake	11.0	250	40%
German chocolate	1/12 cake	12.0	240	45%
lemon supreme	1/12 cake	11.0	250	40%
orange supreme	1/12 cake	11.0	250	40%
pineapple supreme	1/12 cake	11.0	250	40%
red velvet	1/12 cake	11.0	240	41%
spice	1/12 cake	11.0	250	40%
strawberry supreme	1/12 cake	11.0	250	40%
Swiss chocolate	1/12 cake	15.0	290	47%
white	1/12 cake	10.0	240	38%
yellow	1/12 cake	10.0	240	38%

Food and Description	Amount	Fat Grams	Total Calories	% Fat Calories
(Jell-O) no-bake				
Chips Ahoy	⅙ pkg	9.0	260	28%
no-bake cheesecake				
cherry	⅛ pie	12.0	340	32%
real	⅙ cake	16.0	360	40%
strawberry	⅛ cake	12.0	340	32%
strawberry swirl/reduced-fat	⅛ cake	6.0	250	21%
Oreo	⅙ pkg	8.0	270	27%
peanut butter cup	⅛ pkg	15.0	290	47%
prepared				
double-layer desserts				
cookies & cream	⅙ dessert	19.0	390	44%
chocolate	⅛ dessert	12.0	260	42%
lemon	1 serving	12.0	260	42%
(Jiffy)/mix only				
devil's food	⅕ pkg	5.0	220	20%
golden yellow	⅕ pkg	4.5	210	19%
white	⅕ pkg	4.5	210	19%
(McCormick) Fry Easy				
funnel cake/mix only	⅑ pkg	1.0	120	8%
(Pillsbury) mix only, unless noted otherwise				
German chocolate	1/12 pkg	3.5	170	19%
lemon				
mix only	1/12 pkg	3.0	170	16%
Moist Supreme				
angel food/prepared	1/12 cake	–	140	–
banana	1/12 pkg	4.0	180	20%
butter recipe chocolate	1/12 pkg	4.0	180	20%
chocolate chip	1/12 pkg	5.0	190	24%
devil's food	1/12 pkg	2.5	170	13%
Funfetti	1/12 pkg	3.5	180	18%
Easter	1/12 pkg	4.5	190	21%
Halloween	1/12 pkg	4.5	190	21%
holiday	1/12 pkg	4.5	190	21%
spring	1/12 pkg	4.5	190	21%
Stars & Stripes	1/12 pkg	4.5	190	21%
Valentine's Day	1/12 pkg	4.5	190	21%
quick bread & coffee cake				
cinnamon swirl	1/12 pkg	6.0	180	20%
pecan swirl	1/12 pkg	6.0	180	20%
strawberry				
mix only	1/12 pkg	4.0	180	20%
white	1/12 pkg	3.5	180	18%
yellow				
cake	1/12 pkg	6.0	150	36%
Halloween cupcake	1/12 pkg	6.0	200	18%
(Royal) No-Bake cheesecake				
light/whipped	⅛ cake	3.0	130	21%
real/original	⅛ cake	3.0	160	17%

Food and Description	Amount	Fat Grams	Total Calories	% Fat Calories
(Vermont Country Maple) prepared				
chocolate	1 slice	2.0	290	6%
gingerbread	1 slice	1.0	270	3%
■ READY-TO-SERVE				
(Awrey)				
Food Service				
sheet cakes				
banana	1 slice	17.0	360	43%
carrot				
banquet	1 slice	14.0	270	47%
supreme	1 slice	22.0	410	48%
coconut butter	1 slice	24.0	420	51%
double chocolate	1 slice	15.0	340	40%
frosty orange	1 slice	18.0	370	44%
harvest apple	1 slice	10.0	230	39%
German chocolate	1 slice	19.0	360	48%
red velvet	1 slice	21.0	380	50%
sponge cake/uniced	1 slice	10.0	230	39%
International Marquise cakes				
Cajeta caramel	1 slice	16.0	340	42%
French mint	1 slice	14.0	300	42%
pistachio lime	1 slice	12.0	270	40%
strawberry guava				
snow puff	1 slice	13.0	270	43%
Marquise cakes				
banana				
chocolate chip	1 slice	15.0	320	42%
cherries cordial	1 slice	15.0	280	48%
chocolate peanut				
fantasy	1 slice	20.0	360	50%
killer chocolate	1 slice	15.0	320	42%
lemon whisper	1 slice	14.0	280	45%
French espresso	1 slice	22.0	330	60%
Georgia peach	1 slice	15.0	280	48%
nut	1 slice	17.0	310	49%
raspberries & crème	1 slice	14.0	270	47%
raspberry				
extraordinaire	1 slice	20.0	390	46%
red velvet layer	1 slice	21.0	340	56%
tropical chocolate	1 slice	13.0	270	43%
Retail				
bars				
date nut	1 bar	8.0	180	40%
date oatmeal	1 bar	8.0	180	40%
coffee cake/long john	1 slice	10.0	200	45%
French butter cream				
desserts cake	1 slice	12.0	250	43%
(Entenmann's)				
all-butter loaf	⅙ loaf	9.0	210	39%

Food and Description	Amount	Fat Grams	Total Calories	% Fat Calories
blackout	⅑ cake	12.0	260	42%
cheesecake				
deluxe French	⅕ cake	28.0	460	55%
no fat/raspberry-filled	⅕ cake	–	200	–
chocolate chip chewy				
snack bars	1 bar	9.0	180	45%
chocolate fudge	⅛ cake	12.0	260	42%
coffee/crumb cakes				
cheese	⅛ cake	8.0	190	38%
crumb	⅒ cake	12.0	250	43%
Danish ring				
pecan	⅙ cake	15.0	250	54%
walnut	⅙ cake	15.0	240	56%
fudge crumb	1/12 cake	10.0	210	43%
lemon twist/no fat	⅛ cake	–	130	–
light crumb delight	⅑ cake	6.0	210	17%
little bites				
crumb cakes	1 cake	14.0	280	45%
ultimate for				
crumb lovers	⅒ cake	13.0	250	47%
cupcakes/holiday	1 cupcake	14.0	280	45%
Deluxe Desserts				
Louisiana crunch				
no fat	⅙ cake	–	220	–
original	⅑ cake	14.0	330	38%
lemon coconut	⅙ cake	18.0	320	51%
lemon crunch	⅑ cake	13.0	320	37%
light loaf/fat-free cake				
golden	⅛ cake	–	120	–
marble	⅛ cake	–	120	–
Marshmallow/iced				
Devil's food	⅙ cake	14.0	280	45%
pineapple-topped/no fat	⅙ cake	–	170	–
sour cream				
chip & nut loaf	⅛ loaf	12.0	220	49%
(Formagg) Le Crème..all types	2 oz	6.0	115	47%
CAKE, SNACK				
■ READY TO SERVE				
(Dolly)..Zinger/raspberry	1 cake	7.0	160	39%
(Drake)				
all-butter pound cake	1 piece	12.0	280	39%
Boston cream	1 cake	8.0	180	40%
coffee cakes				
chocolate crumb	1 cake	6.0	150	36%
large	1 cake	12.0	270	40%
low-fat	1 cake	2.0	110	16%
mini	4 pieces	8.0	210	34%
original	1 cake	6.0	140	39%
Devil Dogs				
original	1 piece	7.0	180	35%

Food and Description	Amount	Fat Grams	Total Calories	% Fat Calories
reduced-fat	1 piece	4.0	160	23%
Funny Bones				
mini	5 pieces	10.0	290	31%
regular	2 cakes	13.0	300	39%
Ring Dings				
chocolate mousse	2 cakes	15.0	310	44%
mini	5 pieces	9.0	310	26%
original	2 cakes	18.0	340	48%
Sunny Doodles	2 cakes	8.0	220	33%
Swiss rolls	1 cake	15.0	340	40%
Yankee Doodles				
mini	4 pieces	7.0	190	33%
regular	2 cakes	8.0	220	33%
Yodels	2 cakes	16.0	290	50%
(Hostess)				
angel food cake	⅛ cake	1.5	160	8%
apple spice lights	1 cake	1.0	130	7%
Brownie Bites				
plain	5 pieces	14.0	260	48%
walnut	5 pieces	15.0	270	50%
Brownie/light	1 brownie	2.5	140	16%
Chocodiles	1 cake	11.0	240	41%
Chocolicious	1 cake	7.0	190	33%
coconut cakes	1 cake	13.0	260	45%
crumb coffeecake				
light	1 cake	0.5	90	5%
regular	1 cake	5.0	130	35%
cupcakes				
chocolate				
light	1 cupcake	1.5	140	10%
regular	1 cupcake	6.0	180	30%
golden	1 cupcake	7.0	200	32%
orange	1 cupcake	5.0	160	28%
Ding Dongs	2 cakes	19.0	360	48%
Ho Ho's	2 cakes	12.0	250	43%
Leopards	1 cake	8.0	210	34%
Shortcake Dessert Cups	1 cake	2.0	100	18%
Snoballs	1 cake	5.0	180	25%
Suzy Q's	1 cake	9.0	230	35%
Twinkies				
lights	1 cake	1.5	130	10%
original	1 cakes	5.0	150	30%
(Lance)..fig cake/low-fat	½ cake	2.0	110	16%
(Little Debbie)				
angel cake/low-fat				
raspberry	1 pkg	0.5	130	3%
apple flips	1.25 oz	5.0	150	30%
banana twins	2.2 oz	10.0	250	36%
Be My Valentine cake/boxed				
chocolate	1 cake	13.0	280	41%

Food and Description	Amount	Fat Grams	Total Calories	% Fat Calories
vanilla	1 cake	14.0	290	43%
blueberry loaves	1 loaf	10.0	220	41%
Boston Crème rolls	2.2 oz	12.0	270	40%
cherry cordial	1 pkg	8.0	170	42%
Christmas Tree cake	2 oz	13.0	270	57%
chocolate chip cake	1 pkg	15.0	310	44%
coconut rounds	1 pkg	7.0	150	42%
coffee cakes	1 cake	7.0	240	23%
cupcakes				
cream-filled				
chocolate	1 cake	10.0	200	45%
	3.1 oz	18.0	380	43%
lemon	1 cake	10.0	210	43%
strawberry	1 cake	10.0	210	43%
devil cream cake				
boxed	1 pkg	8.0	190	38%
package	3.25 oz	5.0	370	36%
devil squares	1 pkg	13.0	280	42%
fall party cakes				
chocolate	2.4 oz	14.0	300	42%
vanilla	2.5 oz	15.0	320	42%
fancy cakes	2.4 oz	15.0	310	44%
fig bars/low-fat	1 pkg	3.5	150	21%
frosted fudge cake	1 cake	12.0	250	43%
fudge rounds	1 pkg	6.0	150	36%
double-decker	1 pkg	18.0	490	33%
golden cremes cake..boxed	1 pkg	4.5	150	27%
holiday cake roll				
cherry creme	1 pkg	12.0	270	40%
chocolate	1 pkg	14.0	300	42%
vanilla	1 pkg	15.0	320	42%
Jelly Creme	1 pkg	7.0	150	42%
Nutty Bar	1 pkg	18.0	310	52%
oatmeal cream pie	1 pkg	7.0	170	48%
oatmeal lights/low-fat	1 pkg	2.5	130	17%
PB&J oatmeal	1 pkg	5.0	140	32%
peanut butter bar	1 pkg	15.0	280	48%
peanut cluster	1 pkg	11.0	200	50%
pound cake	1 pkg	9.0	220	37%
raisin cream pie	1 pkg	5.0	140	32%
snack cake/chocolate	1 pkg	15.0	320	42%
Star Crunch	1 pkg	6.0	150	36%
cosmic snacks	2.2 oz	12.0	290	37%
Stars & Stripes cakes	1 pkg	15.0	310	44%
strawberry shortcake roll..box	1 pkg	8.0	240	30%
Swiss cake roll				
boxed	1 pkg	12.0	270	40%
double chocolate	1 pkg	12.0	280	39%
	3.3 oz	20.0	430	42%

Food and Description	Amount	Fat Grams	Total Calories	% Fat Calories
Zebra Cake	1 pkg	16.0	340	42%
	2.1 oz	13.0	270	43%
	3.67 oz	22.0	460	43%
(Mrs. Field's)..Bundt cakes				
banana walnut	1 slice	21.0	350	54%
banana walnut				
w/chocolate chips	1 slice	22.0	370	54%
blueberry	1 slice	12.0	270	40%
raspberry	1 slice	12.0	270	40%
white cake..w/chocolate chips	1 slice	17.0	350	44%
(Otis Spunkmeyer)				
Café Collection				
cakes				
chocolate truffle	2.65 oz	21.0	320	59%
orange ginger spice	4 oz slice	20.0	420	43%
vanilla pound	4 oz slice	25.0	460	49%
yogurt lemon poppy	4 oz slice	23.0	440	47%
coffee cakes				
apple cinnamon	3.25 oz slice	18.0	370	44%
cheese	3.25 oz slice	16.0	340	42%
crumb cakes				
apple	4 oz cake	17.0	410	37%
blueberry	4 oz cake	17.0	400	38%
cheese	4 oz cake	21.0	450	42%
mini loaves..all types	3.75 oz	14.0	370	34%
pound cake	3.5 oz	20.0	390	46%
(TastyKake)				
Creamies				
banana	1 cake	9.0	180	45%
chocolate	2 cakes	10.0	190	47%
cupid	2 cakes	11.0	220	45%
Kringle Kake	2 cakes	11.0	220	45%
Sparkle Kake	2 cakes	11.0	220	45%
St. Patty	2 cakes	11.0	220	45%
witchy treats	1 cake	6.0	150	36%
cupcakes				
butter cream iced				
cream-filled	2 cakes	8.0	240	30%
chocolate..iced/cream-filled	2 cakes	9.0	240	34%
	3 cakes	14.0	370	34%
low-fat cream-filled				
chocolate	2 cakes	2.0	190	9%
vanilla	2 cakes	3.0	200	14%
plain	2 cakes	7.0	210	30%
	3 cakes	10.0	320	28%
Koffee Kake				
apple-filled	2 cakes	2.0	170	11%
cream-filled				
plain	2 cakes	9.0	240	34%

Food and Description	Amount	Fat Grams	Total Calories	% Fat Calories
raspberry/low-fat	2 cakes	2.0	170	11%
lemon-filled	2 cakes	3.0	180	15%
Kreepy Kakes	2 cakes	8.0	240	30%
Juniors				
chocolate	2 cakes	12.0	340	32%
coconut	2 cakes	22.0	400	50%
Koffee Kake	2 cakes	10.0	270	33%
orange	2 cakes	10.0	340	26%
lemon	2 cakes	10.0	310	29%
Pound Kake	2 cakes	14.0	350	36%
Kandy Kakes				
Boston cream	1 cake	9.0	180	43%
chocolate	1 cake	9.0	180	43%
coconut	1 cake	9.0	170	48%
mint	1 cake	9.0	180	43%
peanut butter	2 cakes	10.0	180	50%
peppermint	1 cake	10.0	180	50%
raspberry	1 cake	9.0	180	43%
strawberry	1 cake	9.0	180	43%
Kreme bars				
original	2 bars	13.0	270	43%
peanut butter bar	2 bars	13.0	270	43%
Krimpets				
butterscotch iced	2 cakes	6.0	210	26%
	3 cakes	9.0	320	25%
chocolate jelly-filled	2 cakes	4.0	180	20%
	3 cakes	6.0	270	29%
Kreme Krimpies	2 cakes	12.0	250	43%
	3 cakes	18.0	370	44%
strawberry iced	2 cakes	6.0	220	25%
	3 cakes	9.0	320	25%
Santa snacks	2 cakes	8.0	240	30%
Snowballs	1 cake	7.0	210	30%
Tasty Tweets	2 cakes	9.0	240	34%
Tropical Delights				
coconut	2 cakes	11.0	230	43%
guava	2 cakes	7.0	190	33%
papaya	2 cakes	7.0	190	33%
pineapple	2 cakes	7.0	200	32%
CAKE FROSTING/ICING				
(Betty Crocker)				
MIX..prepared				
creamy frosting				
coconut pecan	2 Tbs	8.0	160	45%
fluffy frosting/white	6 Tbs	–	100	–
READY-TO-SPREAD				
creamy deluxe				
butter cream	2 Tbs	8.0	150	48%
cherry	2 Tbs	8.0	150	48%

Food and Description	Amount	Fat Grams	Total Calories	% Fat Calories
chocolate	2 Tbs	8.0	150	48%
chocolate almond	2 Tbs	8.0	150	48%
coconut pecan	2 Tbs	8.0	140	51%
cream cheese	2 Tbs	8.0	150	48%
dark chocolate	2 Tbs	9.0	150	54%
dulce de leche	2 Tbs	8.0	150	48%
French vanilla	2 Tbs	5.0	140	32%
lemon	2 Tbs	8.0	150	48%
milk chocolate	2 Tbs	8.0	150	48%
rainbow chip	2 Tbs	5.0	140	32%
sour cream chocolate	2 Tbs	8.0	150	48%
sour cream white	2 Tbs	8.0	150	48%
strawberry cream cheese	2 Tbs	8.0	150	48%
triple chocolate fudge	2 Tbs	5.0	140	32%
vanilla				
chocolate chip	2 Tbs	5.0	140	32%
original	2 Tbs	8.0	150	48%
white chocolate	2 Tbs	5.0	140	32%
READY-TO-SPREAD/Whipped Deluxe				
butter cream	2 Tbs	6.0	110	49%
chocolate	2 Tbs	5.0	100	45%
cream cheese	2 Tbs	6.0	110	49%
fluffy white	2 Tbs	6.0	110	49%
lemon	2 Tbs	6.0	110	49%
milk chocolate	2 Tbs	5.0	100	45%
strawberry	2 Tbs	6.0	110	49%
vanilla..all types	2 Tbs	6.0	100	49%
Toppers/vanilla w/sprinkles	2 Tbs	8.0	160	45%
(Duncan Hines) Creamy Homestyle/ready to spread				
butter cream	2 Tbs	5.0	140	32%
dark chocolate	2 Tbs	5.0	130	35%
milk chocolate	2 Tbs	5.0	130	35%
wild cherry vanilla	2 Tbs	5.0	140	32%
(Estee) mix/all flavors/mix only	⅛ pkg	–	80	–
(Jiffy) mix/prepared				
fudge	¼ cup	4.0	150	27%
white	¼ cup	4.5	150	24%
(Pillsbury) ready to spread				
Creamy Supreme				
banana cream	2 Tbs	6.0	150	48%
chocolate	2 Tbs	6.0	140	39%
chocolate fudge	2 Tbs	6.0	140	39%
chocolate mocha	2 Tbs	6.0	140	39%
classic white	2 Tbs	3.5	180	18%
coconut pecan	2 Tbs	10.0	160	56%
cookies & cream	2 Tbs	6.0	150	36%
cream cheese	2 Tbs	6.0	150	36%
French vanilla	2 Tbs	6.0	160	34%

Food and Description	Amount	Fat Grams	Total Calories	% Fat Calories
Funfetti/Confetti w/candy bits				
Easter	2 Tbs	6.0	150	36%
Funfetti	2 Tbs	3.5	180	18%
Funfish	2 Tbs	6.0	150	36%
Hallowee	2 Tbs	6.0	150	36%
Holiday	2 Tbs	6.0	150	36%
pink vanilla	2 Tbs	6.0	150	36%
spring	2 Tbs	6.0	150	36%
Stars & Stripes	2 Tbs	6.0	150	36%
Valentines	2 Tbs	6.0	150	36%
vanilla	2 Tbs	6.0	150	34%
hot fudge	2 Tbs	6.0	140	39%
lemon cream	2 Tbs	6.0	150	36%
milk chocolate	2 Tbs	6.0	140	39%
milk chocolate swirl	2 Tbs	6.0	140	39%
strawberry cream	2 Tbs	6.0	150	36%
white	2 Tbs	5.0	140	32%
(Vermont Country Maple) mix/prepared				
delectable cocoa	1 Tbs	–	50	–
maple butter cream	1 Tbs	–	40	–
CALAMARI (See SQUID)				
CALIFORNIA RED BEAN/boiled	½ cup	–	109	–
CALZONE (See PIZZA)				
CANADIAN BACON (See BACON, CANADIAN STYLE)				
CANDY (See also FRUIT SNACK)				
■ (Allen Wertz)				
Coffee Time				
assorted	1 piece	1.0	30	30%
decaffeinated	1 piece	1.0	20	45%
■ **ALMOND JOY** (See (Hershey) in this section)				
■ **ALMOND ROCA** (See (Brown & Haley) in this section)				
■ (Andes)				
CDM Changemaker	3 pieces	13.0	190	57%
cherry jubilee thins	8 pieces	13.0	200	59%
crème de menthe wafers	8 pieces	11.0	190	52%
mint patties	3 pieces	3.0	180	15%
parfait thins	8 pieces	13.0	200	59%
toffee crunch thins	8 pieces	11.0	190	52%
■ (Andre Prost)				
Honees Bars..all types	1 piece	–	20	–
Swedish peppermint creams	14 pieces	3.0	70	16%
Zotz				
Lotz-A-Zotz	1 piece	–	40	–
Mega Zotz	1 piece	–	15	–
pops	1 pop	–	40	–
strings	1 piece	–	15	–
■ **BABY RUTH** (See (Nestlé) in this section)				

Food and Description	Amount	Fat Grams	Total Calories	% Fat Calories
■ (Beich)..Laffy Taffy chews				
all flavors	1 oz	1.0	110	8%
■ ATKINS				
Endulge				
caramel nut chew	1.23 oz	9.0	140	58%
peanut butter cups	3 cups	13.0	160	73%
wafer crisp bars				
chocolate cream	2 bars	9.0	120	68%
mint	2 bars	9.0	120	68%
peanut butter	2 bars	9.0	120	68%
■ BIT-O-HONEY (*See* (Concorde) in this section)				
■ (Black Cow)..Sucker	1 oz	3.0	127	21%
■ (Brach's)				
chocolate candy				
almond supremes	11 pieces	13.0	220	53%
bridge mix	16 pieces	8.0	190	39%
California raisins	35 pieces	6.0	170	32%
caramel clusters	3 pieces	13.0	210	56%
double dippers	15 pieces	12.0	210	51%
malts	15 pieces	7.0	190	33%
Milk Maid				
chocolate caramels	18 pieces	6.0	160	34%
mint patties	3 pieces	3.0	140	19%
mint pearls	24 pieces	2.0	160	11%
peanut butter				
meltaways	3 pieces	13.0	200	59%
peanut clusters	3 pieces	13.0	210	56%
rich & dreamy assorted				
creams	3 pieces	3.0	170	16%
sprinkles	17 pieces	9.0	200	41%
stars/chocolate	10 pieces	11.0	200	45%
sugar candy				
A&W root beer barrels	3 pieces	–	70	–
Abra Ca Bubble	1 piece	–	45	–
butterscotch hard candy	3 pieces	–	70	–
candy corn	26 pieces	–	140	–
cinnamon hard candy	3 pieces	–	70	–
circus peanuts	6 pieces	–	160	–
dessert mints	14 pieces	–	60	–
French burnt peanuts	31 pieces	6.0	170	32%
fruit slices	3 pieces	–	150	–
jelly beans	14 pieces	–	150	–
jelly nougats	5 pieces	2.5	160	14%
Kentucky mints	7 pieces	–	60	–
maple nut goodies	7 pieces	8.0	200	36%
Milk Maid				
caramels	4 pieces	4.5	160	25%
flavored caramel roll	5 pieces	3.5	140	23%
orange slices	2 pieces	–	130	–

Food and Description	Amount	Fat Grams	Total Calories	% Fat Calories
root beer barrels	3 pieces	–	70	–
Smucker's jelly beans	3 pieces	–	70	–
spearmint leaves	5 pieces	–	130	–
Special Treasures/toffees				
coffee-flavored	3 pieces	1.0	70	13%
fruit & cream	3 pieces	0.5	60	8%
golden butter	3 pieces	2.0	80	23%
spice drops	12 pieces	–	130	–
Star Brites disks..all flavors	3 disks	–	60	–
sundaes Neapolitan..coconuts	3 pieces	5.0	160	28%
sugar-free candy				
butterscotch hard candy	3 pieces	–	35	–
cinnamon hard candy	3 pieces	–	35	–
Star Brites peppermint	3 pieces	–	30	–
■ (Brown & Haley)				
Almond Roca	3 pieces	15.0	210	64%
Carbs In-Line..all flavors	1 bar	10.0	110	92%
■ BUNCHA CRUNCH (See (Nestlé in this section)				
■ (Cadbury)				
Bassett's/licorice				
all sorts	1.46 oz	1.0	120	8%
Caramello chocolate	1.23 oz	8.0	170	42%
chocolate wafer	6 blocks	9.0	200	41%
dairy milk chocolate bar	9 blocks	12.0	220	49%
fruit & nut bar/chocolate	10 blocks	10.0	100	45%
roasted almond bar				
chocolate	10 blocks	13.0	220	53%
■ (Carborite)				
At Last! 1g Net Carb				
chocolate bars				
almond	1 oz	10.0	120	75%
crisp	1 oz	9.0	110	74%
mint	1 oz	10.0	110	82%
truffle	1 oz	8.0	100	72%
chocolate-covered peanuts	1.25 oz	11.0	150	66%
other chocolate bars				
caramel nouget	1 oz	5.0	100	45%
chocolate almond	1 oz	10.0	130	69%
	1.75 oz	17.0	230	67%
chocolate crisp	1.75 oz	17.0	250	61%
chocolate peanut butter	1.75 oz	18.0	250	65%
chocolate truffle	1.75 oz	14.0	190	66%
dark chocolate	1.75 oz	17.0	230	67%
milk chocolate	1.75 oz	19.0	240	71%
sugar-free chocolate candy bars				
chocolate almond	1 oz	9.0	130	62%
chocolate crisp	1 oz	9.0	120	68%
chocolate mint	1 oz	10.0	140	64%
chocolate peanut butter	1 oz	10.0	140	64%
chocolate truffle	1 oz	8.0	122	59%

Food and Description	Amount	Fat Grams	Total Calories	% Fat Calories
dark chocolate	1 oz	11.0	130	76%
milk chocolate	1.75 oz	18.0	250	65%
	1 oz	10.0	140	64%
■ **(Caramello)** (*See* (Cadbury) in this section)				
■ **(Cella)** (See (Tootsie Roll) in this section)				
■ **(Charms)**				
Blow Pop				
Junior	1 pop	–	50	–
regular	1 pop	–	60	–
super	1 pop	–	130	–
Charm's Way/ w/Sour Blow Pop	junior	–	50	–
	regular	–	60	–
	super	–	140	–
Charm's Zip-A-Dee Doo-Da Pop	3 pops	–	50	–
Sour Balls	1 piece	–	20	–
Sour Pop/flat				
junior	1 pop	–	50	–
regular	1 pop	–	70	–
Squares	2 pieces	–	20	–
Sweet Pop/flat				
junior	1 pop	–	50	–
regular	1 pop	–	70	–
■ **CHUNKY** (*See* (Nestlé) in this section)				
■ **(CLARK)**..Clark Bar	1.75 oz	8.0	220	33%
■ **COFFEE TIME** (*See* (Allen Wertz) in this section)				
■ **(Concorde)**				
Bit-O-Honey				
bar	1 bar	4.0	200	18%
pieces				
jar	1 piece	0.6	32	17%
twist-wrap	1 piece	0.5	28	16%
Laffy Taffy	1 piece	0.5	38	12%
	4 pieces	2.0	150	12%
Shock Tarts	1 piece	–	8	–
	8 pieces	0.5	60	8%
Taffy Tarts	1 piece	–	2	–
	27 pieces	0.5	60	8%
■ **CRUNCH BAR** (*See* (Nestlé) in this section)				
■ **DOVE** (*See* (M&M * Mars) in this section)				
■ **(Edward & Sons)**				
Let's Do (organic)				
black licorice bears	1 bag	–	80	–
gummy bears/all flavors				
classic	1 bag	–	80	–
fruit juicy	16 pieces	–	130	–
jelly	1 bag	–	80	–

Food and Description	Amount	Fat Grams	Total Calories	% Fat Calories
super sour gummy	1 bag	–	80	–
gummy worms				
sour	7 pieces	–	130	–
hard "Organic" candies				
butterscotch				
old-fashioned	3 pieces	–	50	–
cool peppermints	6 pieces	–	50	–
exotic jelly fruits	15 pieces	–	130	–
fruit flavors/all	6 pieces	–	50	–
fruit flavors/sour	6 pieces	–	50	–
intense breath mints	1 piece	–	5	–
sour fruit flavors	6 pieces	–	50	–
■ (Estee)				
candy-coated peanuts	¼ cup	9.0	200	41%
caramel/chocolate				
& vanilla	5 pieces	5.0	115	39%
chocolate bar				
dark chocolate	7 squares	14.0	200	63%
milk chocolate				
w/almonds	7 squares	17.0	230	67%
crisp rice	1 bar	26.0	370	63%
w/fruit & nuts	7 squares	16.0	220	65%
mint	7 squares	14.0	200	63%
plain	7 squares	17.0	230	67%
chocolate-covered raisins	¼ cup	6.0	180	60%
fruit & nut mix	¼ cup	12.0	210	51%
peanut brittle	⅓ box	9.0	160	51%
peanut butter cups	5 candies	12.0	200	54%
sugar-free				
gourmet jelly beans	26 pieces	–	70	–
gumdrops				
fruit	23 pieces	–	80	–
licorice	11 pieces	–	90	–
toffee	5 pieces	–	30	–
■ (Ghirardelli)				
chocolate drops				
milk chocolate	11 pieces	9.0	190	43%
Premier chocolate bars				
Baby Premier/1.25 oz				
cookies 'n' cream	1 bar	11.0	190	52%
dark chocolate				
plain	1 bar	12.0	180	60%
w/almonds	1 bar	12.0	180	60%
w/raspberries	1 bar	12.0	180	60%
double chocolate mocha	1 bar	10.0	180	50%
milk chocolate				
plain	1 bar	11.0	190	52%
w/almonds	1 bar	12.0	190	57%
w/crisp	1 bar	10.0	180	50%

Food and Description	Amount	Fat Grams	Total Calories	% Fat Calories
w/macadamia	1 bar	13.0	190	62%
mint	1 bar	12.0	180	60%
Premier/2.5 oz				
cookies 'n' cream	1 bar	21.0	380	50%
milk..w/macadamias	1 bar	26.0	380	62%
Premier/3 oz				
cookies 'n' cream	1 bar	21.0	370	51%
dark chocolate				
plain	6 sections	14.0	210	60%
w/almonds	6 sections	16.0	220	65%
w/raspberries	6 sections	14.0	210	60%
double chocolate mocha	1 bar	19.0	350	49%
	4 sections	12.0	210	51%
milk chocolate				
plain	6 sections	14.0	220	57%
raspberries & cream	6 sections	14.0	230	55%
w/almonds	6 sections	15.0	230	59%
w/crisp	1 bar	21.0	360	53%
w/macadamias	1 bar	26.0	380	62%
mint chocolate	6 sections	14.0	220	57%
raspberries & cream	6 sections	14.0	230	55%
■ **(Godiva)**				
almond butter dome	3 pieces	17.0	240	64%
bouchée au chocolat	1 piece	11.0	210	47%
bouchée ivory raspberry	1 piece	9.0	160	51%
gold ballotin	3 pieces	10.0	210	43%
truffles				
Amaretto di Saronno	2 pieces	12.0	210	51%
deluxe liqueur	2 pieces	13.0	210	43%
■ **GOOBERS** (See (Nestlé) in this section)				
■ **GOOD & PLENTY** (See (Hershey) in this section)				
■ **(Guylian)**				
chocolate bars/no sugar added				
dark chocolate	8 squares	9.0	112	72%
milk chocolate				
plain	8 squares	9.0	125	65%
w/hazelnuts	8 squares	10.0	132	68%
■ **(Hershey)**				
Almond Joy	0.69 oz bar	5.0	90	50%
	0.48 oz bar	4.0	70	51%
Carmello	0.66 oz bar	4.0	90	40%
Cookies 'n' Crème				
Bites	18 pieces	11.0	210	47%
Cookies 'n' Mint				
bar/0.6 oz	1 bar	4.5	90	45%
nuggets/0.35 oz	1 piece	2.5	45	50%
Crispy rice snacks				
peanut butter	3 bars	7.0	180	35%
5th Avenue	0.58 oz bar	3.5	80	39%

Food and Description	Amount	Fat Grams	Total Calories	% Fat Calories
Golden Collection solitaires				
w/almonds	1 piece	1.0	15	60%
Good & Plenty	1 box	–	170	–
Gummi Bears/amazin' fruit	1 pouch	–	60	–
Heath Bar	1.32 oz	11.0	200	50%
snack bar	1 piece	3.0	50	54%
Heide Jujubes	45 pieces	–	100	–
Hershey's				
Bites				
Almond Joy	18 pieces	14.0	230	55%
Cookies 'n' Creme	18 pieces	11.0	210	47%
milk chocolate				
w/almond	17 pieces	14.0	220	57%
Reese's peanut butter	16 pieces	12.0	220	49%
York Peppermint Patty	15 pieces	3.0	160	17%
Miniatures/chocolate bars				
special dark	5 pieces	13.0	230	51%
milk chocolate	5 pieces	13.0	230	51%
1 gram sugar carb				
chocolate candy	1.1 oz	11.0	130	76%
chocolate candy				
w/almonds	1.1 oz	12.0	140	77%
w/soy crisps	1.1 oz	10.0	120	75%
sugar-free chocolate candy	5 pieces	13.0	170	69%
dark chocolate	5 pieces	13.0	170	69%
peanut butter cup				
miniatures	5 pieces	12.0	170	64%
w/almonds	5 pieces	14.0	180	70%
Hugs/chocolate	9 pieces	12.0	210	51%
Jolly Ranchers				
hard assorted candies	3 pieces	–	70	–
lollipops	1 piece	–	60	–
Juicyfruits	2 boxes	–	80	–
Kisses				
plain	9 pieces	13.0	230	51%
w/almonds	9 pieces	14.0	230	55%
Kit-Kat wafer bar	king size	21.0	410	46%
	regular size	11.0	220	45%
Krackel	0.6 oz bar	4.5	90	45%
	1.45 oz	10.0	210	43%
milk chocolate bar				
plain	0.3 oz	5.0	90	50%
	0.6 oz	5.0	90	50%
w/almonds	0.6 oz	6.0	90	60%
Milk Duds	13 pieces	6.0	170	32%
Mr. Goodbar	0.6 oz	6.0	100	54%
	1.75 oz	16.0	270	53%
Mounds	0.68 oz bar	5.0	90	50%
	1.75 oz	13.0	240	49%

Food and Description	Amount	Fat Grams	Total Calories	% Fat Calories
Nibs				
cherry	2.25 oz pkg	1.5	220	6%
licorice	2.25 oz pkg	1.5	210	6%
Pay Day	1.83 oz	12.0	240	45%
	snack bar	5.0	90	50%
Reese's Nutrageous	1.8 oz	16.0	28	51%
	0.6 oz	11.0	190	52%
Peanut butter				
cup/miniatures	5 pieces	12.0	210	51%
eggs	1 piece	5.0	90	50%
regular	1.5 oz	13.0	230	51%
Robin Eggs				
mini	24 pieces	5.0	170	26%
regular	8 pieces	5.0	170	26%
Rolo chocolate caramels				
in milk chocolate	7 pieces	9.0	210	39%
	1.7 oz	10.0	230	39%
Skor	1.4 oz	13.0	220	53%
Symphony/milk chocolate	1.5 oz	13.0	230	51%
Swoops				
Almond Joy	1 cup	12.0	200	54%
Hershey's milk chocolate	1 cup	12.0	190	57%
Reese's	1 cup	10.0	180	50%
York Peppermint Patty	1 cup	11.0	190	52%
Twizzlers				
cherry	3 pieces	0.5	130	3%
chocolate	5 pieces	1.5	160	8%
licorice	4 pieces	0.5	150	3%
strawberry	4 pieces	1.0	160	6%
Whatchamacallit	0.57 oz bar	4.0	80	45%
	1.6 oz	11.0	230	43%
Whoppers malted milk balls	18 pieces	7.0	190	33%
Wunderbeans/jelly beans	33 pieces	–	100	–
York Peppermint Patty				
bites	15 pieces	3.0	150	18%
patties	1.4 oz	3.0	160	17%
Patty	1.5 oz	3.0	170	16%
Zagnut	0.5 oz	3.0	70	39%
	1.75 oz	10.0	230	39%
Zeo	1.85 oz	8.0	230	31%
Snack	0.6 oz	2.5	70	32%
■ **(Jelly Belly) Jelly Beans**				
all flavors	35 pieces	–	140	–
■ **JOLLY RANCHERS** (*See* (Hershey) in this section)				
■ **JUNIOR MINTS** (*See* (Tootsie Roll) in this section)				
■ **KIT-KAT** (*See* (Hershey) in this section)				
■ **(Kraft)**				
caramels				
cappuccino	1.4 oz	3.5	160	20%
caramel apple	1.4 oz	3.5	160	20%
chocolate	1.4 oz	3.5	160	20%

Food and Description	Amount	Fat Grams	Total Calories	% Fat Calories
Crème Savers	½ oz	1.5	60	23%
chocolate & caramel	1.375 oz	3.5	170	19%
	1.6 oz	4.0	180	20%
orange & crème	½ oz	1.5	70	19%
	1.6 oz	4.5	180	23%
raspberries & crème	½ oz	1.5	60	23%
strawberries & crème	½ oz	1.5	69	19%
	1.6 oz	4.5	180	23%
Crème Savers/sugar-free				
chocolate & caramel	½ oz	1.5	45	30%
strawberries & crème	½ oz	1.5	45	30%
Life Savers				
assorted flavors	2 pieces	–	20	–
Christmas storybook	1.4 oz	–	20	–
Easter jelly beans	1.4 oz	–	150	–
Milka/Christmas winter krisps				
chocolate gingerbread	1.4 oz	10.0	210	43%
Snack Bites..chocolate-covered				
strawberry	1 oz	7.0	130	48%
Terry's chocolate				
orange				
dark	1.5 oz	13.0	240	49%
milk	1.5 oz	12.0	230	47%
pure milk	1.5 oz	12.0	230	47%
Toblerone candy				
Swiss bittersweet w/honey				
& almond nougat	1.16 oz	9.0	170	48%
Swiss milk chocolate.. w/honey				
& almond nougat	1.4 oz	11.0	210	47%
	1.16 oz	9.0	170	48%
	1.8 oz	13.0	260	45%
w/honey & almond				
nougat bow	1.4 oz	11.0	210	47%
Swiss white confection w/honey				
& almond nougat	1.16 oz	10.0	180	50%
truffle peaks	1.4 oz	15.0	240	56%
Trolli/Gummi				
all flavors	1.4 oz	–	130	–
■ KRACKEL (See (Hershey) in this section)				
■ KUDOS (See (M&M * Mars) in this section)				
■ (Labrada)				
gourmet sugar-free..all types				
chocolate bars	1 bar	5.0	80	56%
■ (La Nouba)				
Belgian chocolate bars				
coconut	1 bar	15.4	204	68%
dark/dairy-free	1 bar	15.0	190	71%
milk	1 bar	15.4	204	68%
mint	1 bar	15.4	204	68%
white/caffeine-free	1 bar	15.2	205	67%

Food and Description	Amount	Fat Grams	Total Calories	% Fat Calories
■ **LAFFY TAFFY** (*See* (Beich); (Concorde); (Nestle) in this section)				
■ **LIFE SAVERS** (*See* (Planters) in this section)				
■ **(M&M * Mars)**				
Celebrations/mixed				
3 Musketeers	1 piece	1.0	30	30%
Dove's				
dark chocolate	1 piece	2.5	40	56%
milk chocolate	1 piece	2.5	45	50%
milk chocolate				
caramel	1 piece	2.0	40	45%
Milky Way	1 piece	1.5	35	39%
Milky Way/midnight	1 piece	1.5	30	45%
Snickers	1 piece	2.0	40	45%
Twix	1 piece	2.5	50	45%
Celebrations/pkg/boxed/tin				
11-ounce box	5 pieces	9.0	190	43%
15-ounce box	5 pieces	9.0	150	43%
"Dorothy" box	5 pieces	9.0	190	43%
Stocking Stuffer	1 pack	15.0	300	45%
Tin				
12 ounce tin	5 pieces	9.0	190	43%
21 ounce tin	5 pieces	9.0	190	43%
cookie bars				
M&M's	1 bar	9.0	170	48%
Milky Way	1 bar	11.0	180	55%
Snickers	1 bar	11.0	180	55%
Twix	1 bar	10.0	180	50%
Dove				
dark chocolate				
Promises	5 pieces	13.0	210	56%
single	1.3 oz	12.0	200	54%
6-oz bar	¼ bar	14.0	230	55%
milk chocolate				
Promises	5 pieces	13.0	220	53%
single	1.3 oz	12.0	200	54%
6-oz bar	¼ bar	13.0	230	51%
Kudos				
chocolate chip	1 bar	4.5	120	34%
chocolate fudge	1 bar	4.5	120	34%
M&M's milk				
chocolate mini's	1 bar	2.5	90	25%
peanut butter	1 bar	5.0	130	35%
Snickers Bar	1 bar	3.5	100	32%
M&M's				
almond..singles	1 bag	11.0	200	50%
baking bits	0.5 oz	3.5	70	45%
crispy	singles bag	8.0	200	36%
mini's	singles bag	7.0	150	42%
peanut	singles bag	13.0	250	47%

Food and Description	Amount	Fat Grams	Total Calories	% Fat Calories
peanut butter	singles bag	14.0	240	53%
plain	singles bag	10.0	240	38%
Mars Bar/Singles	1 bar	13.0	240	49%
Milky Way candy bars				
chocolate				
covered caramels	2 oz	8.0	200	33%
Midnight	1.76 oz	8.0	220	33%
milk chocolate	2.05 oz	10.0	270	33%
Musketeers (see 3 Musketeers, this section)				
Skittles				
Fresh mint/bite size				
5.2-oz bag	1.5 oz	2.0	170	11%
large (12.4-oz bag)	1.5 oz	2.0	170	11%
singles (1.6-oz tube)	1 tube	2.0	180	10%
original				
king size (4-oz bag)	⅓ bag	1.5	150	9%
large (16-oz bag)	1.5 oz	2.0	170	11%
single (2.17-oz bag)	1 bag	2.5	240	9%
sour				
large (13.3-oz bag)	1.5 oz	1.5	160	8%
singles (1.8-oz bag)	1 bag	2.0	200	9%
tropical				
singles (2.17-oz bag)	1 bag	2.5	240	9%
wild berry				
large bag (16-oz bag)	1.5 oz	1.5	170	8%
single (2.17-oz bag)	1 bag	2.5	240	9%
Snickers/Singles				
almond	1.76 oz	11.0	240	41%
cruncher	1.66 oz	13.0	230	51%
Marathon				
multigrain crunch	2.94 oz	7.0	220	29%
original	1.94 oz	7.0	220	29%
munch bar	1 bar	15.0	230	59%
original	2.07 oz	14.0	280	45%
Starburst				
California fruits	1 pack	5.0	240	19%
chew pops..all flavors	1 pop	–	50	–
fruit & crème..all flavors	1 pack	5.0	240	19%
jelly beans				
original..all flavors	1.5 oz	–	150	–
original fruits	1 pack	5.0	240	19%
sour fruits	1 pack	5.0	240	19%
tropical fruits	1 pack	5.0	240	19%
3 Musketeers				
2.13 oz	1 bar	8.0	260	28%
Chewlicious/chocolate–				
flavored chews	1 bar	2.5	100	23%
fun size	2 bars	4.5	140	29%
miniatures	7 pieces	5.0	180	25%

Food and Description	Amount	Fat Grams	Total Calories	% Fat Calories
Twix/cookie bars				
caramel	2 bars	14.0	280	45%
peanut butter	2 bars	17.0	280	55%
■ MILK DUDS (See (Hershey) in this section)				
■ MILKY WAY (See (M&M * Mars) in this section)				
■ MR. GOODBAR (See (Hershey) in this section)				
■ MOUNDS (See (Hershey) in this section)				
■ (Nestlé USA)				
Baby Ruth				
Beast (5 oz)	1.25 oz	8.0	160	
full-size	2.1 oz	13.0	280	42%
fun-size	1.0 oz	11.0	210	47%
king-size	1.25 oz	8.0	160	45%
miniature/4 pieces	1.6 oz	11.0	210	47%
Bit O'Honey	1.7 oz	3.5	190	17%
	1.4 oz	3.0	170	16%
	1.3 oz	3.0	160	17%
Bottle Caps (See Wonka, in this section)				
Buncha Crunch	1.4 oz	10.0	200	45%
crunchy movie pack	1.28 oz	10.0	190	47%
Butterfinger				
BB's	1.7 oz	9.0	220	33%
king size	1.85 oz	8.0	190	38%
half pounder	1.6 oz	8.0	190	38%
snack pack	1.57 oz	8.0	190	38%
candy bars				
Beast (5 oz)	1.25 oz	6.0	160	34%
Bittyfinger	2 bars	7.0	170	37%
full size (6 oz)	1 oz	11.0	270	37%
fun size (.75 oz)	1 bar	4.0	100	36%
king size	1.85 oz	8.0	190	38%
mini half pounder	1.33 oz	7.0	180	35%
mini's/4 pieces	1.37 oz	7.0	180	35%
mini's on the go	1.33 oz	7.0	180	35%
single (2.14 oz)	1 bar	11.0	270	37%
snack pack (5.5 oz)	1.57 oz	8.0	190	38%
Chunky Bar	1.4 oz	11.0	200	50%
milk chocolate	1.6 oz	12.0	230	47%
beast (3.5 oz)	1.16 oz	9.0	160	51%
king (2.8 oz)	2.8 oz	21.0	400	47%
milk chocolate/extra crunchy/king (2.8 oz)	1 bar	21.0	400	47%
milk chocolate w/caramel	1.5 oz	11.0	210	47%
white chocolate	1.4 oz	13.0	220	53%
Crunch				
assorted mini's	4 pieces	12.0	210	51%
milk chocolate	1.5 oz	11.0	210	47%

Food and Description	Amount	Fat Grams	Total Calories	% Fat Calories
	1.85 oz	12.0	230	47%
fun-size bag	1.4 oz	10.0	200	45%
white chocolate/fun size	1 bar	3.0	50	54%
100 Grand Bar				
fun size	1.5 oz	8.0	200	36%
super size	2.8 oz	15.0	370	36%
Flipz/2-oz pkg				
milk chocolate	.5 oz	3.0	70	39%
white fudge pretzel	.5 oz	3.0	70	39%
Goobers/milk chocolate covered				
1.38 oz bag	1 bag	13.0	210	56%
On-the-Go box	1.4 oz	14.0	220	57%
milk chocolate bar	1.45 oz	13.0	220	53%
fun size				
1.5 oz	4 pieces	3.0	53	51%
2.5 oz	1 bar	10.0	210	43%
mocha crunch bar	1.3 oz	12.0	200	54%
Nips				
butter rum	2 pieces	1.5	60	23%
caramel-flavor	2 pieces	1.5	60	23%
chocolate	2 pieces	1.5	60	23%
chocolate parfait	2 pieces	2.0	60	30%
coffee	2 pieces	1.5	50	27%
dulce de leche	2 pieces	2.0	60	30%
mocha coffee				
w/chocolate parfait	2 pieces	2.0	60	30%
peanut butter parfait	2 pieces	2.0	60	30%
sugar-free & rich creamy hard candy				
caramel	1 pieces	1.5	60	15%
coffee	2 pieces	1.5	60	15%
Oh Henry!	1.8 oz	5.0	120	38%
Raisinets	1.58 oz	8.0	200	36%
	1.8 oz	8.0	200	36%
fun size	2 oz	12.0	280	39%
movie pack	1.75 oz	8.0	200	36%
On-the-Go	1.75 oz	8.0	200	36%
Sammy Strawberry &				
Hanna Banana	1.5 oz	3.5	160	20%
Signatures				
Treasures				
butterfinger	3 pieces	9.0	180	45%
chocolate crème	1.33 oz	10.0	170	53%
creamy caramel	3 pieces	9.0	160	51%
peanut butter	1.33 oz	13.0	190	62%
Sno Caps/box	2.3 oz	13.0	300	39%
semi-sweet chocolate				
7-ounce bag	1.40 oz	8.0	190	38%
On-the-Go	1.55 oz	8.0	180	40%
Sparkle Jerry Cherry	1.5 oz	3.5	160	20%
Stretchy & Tangy	1 bar	1.0	60	15%

Food and Description	Amount	Fat Grams	Total Calories	% Fat Calories
Turtles				
original	1.16 oz	9.0	160	51%
original/bite-size	1.4 oz	12.0	210	51%
peanut	1.76 oz	13.0	240	49%
peanut/sugar-free	1.3 oz	10.0	150	60%
Thousand Grand Bar	1.5 oz	8.0	200	36%
Toll House Candy Bars/chocolate				
brownie	1 oz	6.0	120	45%
cookie	1 oz	6.0	120	45%
Wonder Ball/milk chocolate				
Cartoon Network	1 oz	6.0	140	39%
Disney	1 oz	6.0	140	39%
Wonka				
bottle caps	10 pieces	–	60	–
fun dip	1 packet	–	75	–
gobstoppers				
chewy	9 pieces	–	50	–
regular	9 pieces	–	50	–
gumball	1 ball	–	45	–
nerds	1 Tbs	–	60	–
nerds rope	1 rope	–	100	–
shocktarts	9 pieces	–	60	–
gumball	1 gumball	–	30	–
mini	21 pieces	–	60	–
Wonka/Laffy Taffy	5 bars	2.0	170	6%
banana	.08 oz	1.0	80	11%
blue vanilla	.08 oz	1.0	80	11%
cherry	1.4 oz	2.0	170	11%
chocolate	1.4 oz	2.0	170	11%
	.08 oz	1.0	80	11%
chocolate mousse	1.5 oz	3.5	160	20%
flavor flippers	1.6 oz	5.0	180	25%
grape	1.4 oz	2.0	170	11%
rope (.82 oz)	1 pkg	1.0	80	11%
■ (Newman's Own Organics)				
Organics chocolate bars				
milk chocolate	½ bar	16.0	240	60%
butter toffee	½ bar	13.0	210	56%
crispy rice	½ bar	11.0	200	50%
sweet dark				
chocolate	½ bar	13.0	200	59%
espresso chocolate	½ bar	14.0	200	63%
orange chocolate	½ bar	13.0	200	59%
Organics cups				
peanut butter cups				
dark chocolate	1 pkg	12.0	280	60%
milk chocolate	1 pkg	12.0	180	60%
peppermint cups				
dark chocolate	1 pkg	11.0	170	58%

Food and Description	Amount	Fat Grams	Total Calories	% Fat Calories
■ (Nutcracker)				
chocolate				
caramel cups	1.25 oz	9.0	180	45%
covered almonds	1.4 oz	15.0	220	61%
covered cashews	1.4 oz	15.0	220	61%
dark				
w/peppermint center	1.25 oz	11.0	200	50%
peanut butter cups				
creamy white	1.25 oz	11.0	200	50%
dark	1.25 oz	12.0	200	54%
peanut caramel clusters	1.60 oz	11.0	220	50%
ultimate tropical	1 oz	8.0	160	45%
	1.43 oz	15.0	220	61%
■ NUTRAGEOUS (See (Hershey) in this section)				
■ (Old Dominion)				
cashew brittle	1.5 oz	6.0	190	28%
peanut brittle	1.5 oz	5.0	190	24%
peanut candy	1.5 oz	6.0	200	27%
■ OH HENRY! (See (Nestlé) in this section)				
■ PAY DAY (See (Hershey) in this section)				
■ (Pearson's)				
Bun Bars				
caramel	1.75 oz	11.0	240	41%
maple	1.75 oz	12.0	240	45%
vanilla	1.75 oz	12.0	240	45%
Mint Patties	5 pieces	2.5	150	15%
Nut Goodie	1.75 oz	12.0	240	45%
Salted Nut Roll	.75 oz	6.0	100	54%
	1.8 oz	11.0	240	41%
	2.5 oz	16.0	340	42%
	3.5 oz	22.0	470	42%
■ (Pez) all flavors	1 roll	–	30	–
■ (Planters)				
Life Savers				
candy cane, big tablet	4 pieces	–	60	–
cards 'n' candy	4 pieces	–	40	–
Gummy Savers..all flavors	11 pieces	–	130	–
Holes..all flavors	20 pieces	–	20	–
Life Savers/regular roll				
all flavors	2 pieces	–	20	–
lollipops/assorted	1 pop	–	40	–
Sack'it				
all flavors	4 pieces	–	60	–
peanut bar	1.6 oz	14.0	230	54%
peanut brittle	½ cup	7.0	180	35%
peanut butter chocolates	4 pieces	15.0	230	59%
sweet 'n' crunchy	1 oz	7.0	140	45%
■ PUR DE-LITE				
chocolate bars				
caramel crisp	1 oz	6.0	120	45%
caramel pecan	1 oz	7.0	130	48%

Food and Description	Amount	Fat Grams	Total Calories	% Fat Calories
chocolate bars/sugar-free				
caramel crisp	1 oz	6.0	120	45%
caramel nougat	1 oz	5.0	110	41%
caramel pecan	1 oz	7.0	130	48%
peanut butter	1 oz	6.0	120	45%
dark	1.33 oz	13.6	173	71%
milk	1.33 oz	13.9	187	67%
w/almonds	1.33 oz	14.0	190	66%
truffle bar				
milk chocolate				
caramel	1 oz	8.0	140	51%
peanut butter	1 oz	11.0	160	62%
■ RAISINETS (*See* (Nestlé) in this section)				
■ REGAL DYNASTY				
imported chocolate				
dark	4 pieces	12.0	200	54%
milk	4 pieces	12.0	200	54%
w/cashews	4 pieces	12.0	200	54%
■ REESE'S (*See* (Hershey) in this section)				
■ (Rapunzel)				
organic chocolate				
Swiss bittersweet				
70% cocoa	½ bar	19.0	224	76%
Swiss espresso				
chocolate	½ bar	16.0	218	66%
Swiss milk chocolate				
w/nut truffle				
crème bar	½ bar	16.0	230	63%
w/rum raisin bar	½ bar	13.7	217	57%
Swiss semisweet				
w/almonds	½ bar	16.0	222	65%
w/hazelnuts	½ bar	15.0	216	63%
Vivani Premium Organic				
dark chocolate				
72% cocoa	1.5 oz	18.0	228	71%
milk chocolate	1.5 oz	16.0	235	61%
w/hazelnuts	1.5 oz	17.0	239	64%
w/praline filling	1.5 oz	17.0	240	64%
white chocolate				
w/crispy rice	1.5 oz	15.0	236	57%
■ RIESEN (*See* (Storck) in this section)				
■ (Ross)				
low-carb/sugar-free chocolate bars				
almond	1.2 oz	13.6	180	68%
Belgian	1.2 oz	12.4	167	67%
milk	1.2 oz	12.4	170	66%
white	1.2 oz	12.4	170	66%
cherry	1.2 oz	12.4	167	67%
coconut delight	1.2 oz	13.4	152	79%
crunchy				

Food and Description	Amount	Fat Grams	Total Calories	% Fat Calories
delight	1.2 oz	13.4	152	79%
orange delight	1.2 oz	12.4	167	67%
dark/only 1 gram bar	1.2 oz	12.2	161	68%
raspberry delight	1.2 oz	12.4	167	67%
■ (Russell Stover)				
almond delights	2 pieces	12.0	210	51%
Ambassadors miniature				
chocolates	6 pieces	9.0	190	43%
candy jar chocolates	4 pieces	9.0	190	43%
caramels	3 pieces	7.0	170	37%
assorted	3 pieces	8.0	190	38%
English	6 pieces	6.0	180	30%
Santas	1 Santa	11.0	230	43%
cherry cordials	3 pieces	7.0	170	37%
chocolate assortments				
dark chocolate	3 pieces	8.0	190	38%
gift box				
gold bow	2 pieces	10.0	200	45%
regular	3 pieces	8.0	180	40%
milk chocolate	3 pieces	8.0	190	38%
low-carb/sugar-free candies				
low-carb				
butter nut toffee				
sticks	4 pieces	11.0	160	62%
chocolate-covered				
almonds	15 pieces	18.0	210	77%
peanuts	25 pieces	16.0	210	69%
mint patties	2 pieces	7.0	130	48%
mousse medallions	2 pieces	5.0	120	38%
peanut butter				
crunch	4 pieces	9.0	180	45%
cups	4 pieces	14.0	180	70%
medallions	2 pieces	10.0	130	69%
pecan delights	4 pieces	13.0	180	65%
	2 pieces	10.0	130	69%
solid dark chocolate				
medallions	2 pieces	8.0	130	55%
toffee squares	2 pieces	7.0	110	57%
	3 pieces	12.0	180	60%
truffle cups	4 pieces	11.0	170	58%
wafers	2 pieces	10.0	130	69%
sugar-free				
almond clusters	3 pieces	17.0	200	77%
coconut miniatures	5 pieces	15.0	190	71%
crispy miniatures	6 pieces	12.0	180	60%
dark chocolate/solid	5 pieces	15.0	220	61%
French mint				
miniatures	5 pieces	14.0	190	66%
Liberty Orchards				
fruit softees	3 pieces	3.0	140	19%

Food and Description	Amount	Fat Grams	Total Calories	% Fat Calories
milk chocolate & almond				
medallions	2 pieces	8.0	110	65%
miniatures	5 pieces	14.0	190	66%
milk chocolate				
& almonds	5 pieces	15.0	200	68%
solid	5 pieces	14.0	190	66%
mints				
French chocolate				
boxed	4 pieces	14.0	220	57%
individual	1 bar	15.0	240	56%
Mint Dream	1 bar	8.0	160	45%
patties/dark				
chocolate-covered	6 pieces	6.0	180	30%
mint patties	3 pieces	11.0	190	52%
	2 pieces	7.0	130	37%
orange cream				
miniatures	5 pieces	12.0	170	64%
peanut clusters	4 pieces	13.0	170	69%
peanut delights	2 pieces	10.0	140	64%
pecan delights	2 pieces	12.0	170	64%
strawberry cream	5 pieces	12.0	170	64%
pecan delights				
boxed	2 pieces	14.0	220	57%
individual	1 bar	20.0	310	58%
pecan roll	1.5 oz	20.0	300	60%
truffles	3 pieces	11.0	200	50%
whips/assorted	2 pieces	7.0	210	30%

■ **SHOCK TARTS** (*See* (Concorde) in this section)
■ **SKITTLES** (*See* (M&M * Mars) in this section)
■ **(Slo Poke)**

Slo Poke sucker	1 sucker	2.0	124	15%

■ **SNO CAPS** (*See* (Nestlé) in this section)
■ **STARBURST** (*See* (M&M * Mars) in this section)
■ **(Storck)**

Mamba/fruit chews				
all flavors	6 pieces	1.5	110	12%
Riesen/chocolate caramel				
in rich chocolate	1.25 oz	7.0	180	35%
	1.43 oz	8.0	200	36%
fall	1.25 oz	7.0	170	37%
snowman	4 pieces	7.0	170	37%
Toffifay hazelnut in				
caramel	1.43 oz	11.0	210	47%
w/chocolate	1.16 oz	9.0	170	48%
Werther's				
caramels chewy	8 pieces	5.0	170	26%
chocolate	5 pieces	7.0	180	35%
original	3 pieces	1.0	60	15%
toffee & milk chocolate	1.25 oz	14.0	220	57%

Food and Description	Amount	Fat Grams	Total Calories	% Fat Calories
■ **SUGAR BABIES** (*See* (Tootsie Roll) in this section)				
■ **SUGAR DADDY** (*See* (Tootsie Roll) in this section)				
■ **SYMPHONY** (*See* (Hershey) in this section)				
■ **TAFFY TARTS** (*See* (Concorde) in this section)				
■ **3 MUSKETEERS** (*See* (M&M * Mars) in this section)				
■ **(Tootsie Roll)**				
Cella				
chocolate-covered cherries	2 pieces	4.0	110	33%
Charleston Chew bar				
chocolate	1.9 oz	6.0	230	23%
strawberry	1.9 oz	6.0	230	23%
vanilla				
mini	13 pieces	6.0	170	32%
regular	1.9 oz	6.0	230	23%
Fluffy Stuff/small bag	1.06 oz	–	120	–
Junior Mints	16 pieces	3.0	170	16%
Pops				
candy cane	1 pop	–	60	–
caramel apple	1 pop	0.5	60	8%
fruit smoothie	1 pop	–	60	–
hot chocolate	1 pop	–	70	–
orange cream	1 pop	0.5	70	6%
Sugar Babies	30 pieces	1.5	180	8%
Sugar Daddy				
junior pop	3 pops	2.0	160	11%
large pop	1 pop	2.5	200	11%
Sugar Daddy Junior	3 pops	2.0	160	11%
Tootsie Flavor Rolls	6 pieces	3.0	160	17%
Tootsie Frooties	12 pieces	3.0	140	19%
Tootsie Pop				
miniature	3 pops	–	50	–
regular	1 pop	–	60	–
small	1 pop	–	45	–
Tootsie Roll				
3-cent pieces	6 pieces	3.0	140	19%
5-cent pieces	4 pieces	3.0	140	19%
bars				
1.1 oz	½ bar	2.5	110	20%
1.5 oz	½ bar	3.5	150	21%
midgets				
regular	6 pieces	3.0	140	19%
small	12 pieces	3.0	160	17%
snack bars	2 bars	2.0	100	18%
■ **WERTHER'S** (*See* (Storck) in this section)				
■ **(Whitman's)**				
assorted	3 pieces	8.0	190	38%
dark chocolate	3 pieces	10.0	200	45%
Little Ambassadors	7 pieces	9.0	190	43%
Pecan Delight Bar	1 bar	20.0	310	58%
Pecan Roll	1 bar	20.0	300	60%

Food and Description	Amount	Fat Grams	Total Calories	% Fat Calories
■ **WHATCHAMACALLIT** (*See* (Hershey) in this section)				
■ **WHOPPERS** (*See* (Hershey) in this section)				
■ **WONKA** (*See* (Nestlé) in this section)				
■ **YORK** (*See* (Hershey) in this section)				
■ **ZOTZ** (*See* (Andre Prost) in this section)				
CANDY APPLE (*See* APPLE, CARAMEL)				
CANNELLINI BEAN (*See* KIDNEY BEAN)				
CANTALOUPE/MUSKMELON				
fresh				
cubed	1 cup	<1.0	57	8%
whole/~ 9.5 oz	½ melon	0.7	94	7%
CAPERS				
(Crosse & Blackwell)	1 Tbs	–	5	–
(Peloponnese) wild	½ oz	–	–	–
(Progresso) drained	1 tsp	–	5	–
CAPON				
giblets/simmered	5 oz	7.8	238	30%
meat & skin/roasted	3.5 oz	11.7	229	46%
	~1.5 lb	74.0	1457	46%
meat only/roasted	3.5 oz	8.8	178	44%
CARAMBOLA (*See* STAR FRUIT)				
CARAWAY SEEDS	1 tsp	–	8	–
CARDAMOM SEEDS				
ground	1 Tbs	0.5	20	23%
whole	1 tsp	–	6	–
CARDOON				
cooked	3 oz	–	19	–
raw/shredded	1 cup	–	35	–
CARIBOU/boneless				
raw	3 oz	5.0	160	28%
roasted	4 oz	5.0	190	24%
roasted/diced	1 cup	6.0	235	23%
CARISSA/NATAL PLUM				
raw	1 medium	–	12	–
CAROB CHIPS				
regular	1 oz	7.0	140	45%
mini	1 oz	7.0	140	45%
CAROB POWDER				
(Chatfield's)	¼ cup	–	96	–
(El Molino)	¼ cup	–	110	–
CARP (*See* CARP ROE)				
breaded & fried	3 oz	12.0	226	48%
cooked-dry heat	3 oz	6.0	138	39%
raw	3 oz	4.8	108	40%
smoked	1 oz	1.8	50	32%
CARP ROE/raw	3 oz	1.7	111	14%
CARROT (*See also* VEGETABLES, MIXED)				
CANNED				
(Del Monte)				
honey-glazed	½ cup	–	70	–

Food and Description	Amount	Fat Grams	Total Calories	% Fat Calories
julienne French-style	½ cup	30	—	
sliced	½ cup	–	35	–
(Green Giant) sliced	½ cup	–	25	–
(LeSueur) whole baby	½ cup	–	35	–
(Libby's)..all styles	½ cup	–	25	–
(Old South) pickled baby	1 oz	–	15	–
(S&W)..all styles	½ cup	–	30	–
(Seneca) all styles	½ cup	–	30	–
(Stokely)..all styles	½ cup	–	30	–
FRESH				
(Dole)				
shredded	½ cup	–	24	–
whole/1¼" dia	7" long	–	35	–
FROZEN				
(Birds Eye)				
sliced	½ cup	–	35	–
whole baby	½ cup	–	40	–
(C&W)				
Parisienne	⅔ cup	–	40	–
whole baby	⅔ cup	–	35	–
(Cascadian Farm)				
honey-glazed baby	1 cup	–	60	–
(Green Giant)				
baby cut				
Harvest Fresh	⅔ cup	–	20	–
boil-in-bag				
honey-glazed	1 cup	3.5	90	35%
regular	¾ cup	–	30	–
(Schwan) maple-glazed	4.5 oz	10.0	140	64%
CARROT JUICE/canned				
(Hain)	1 cup	0.5	80	6%
(Hollywood)	12 fl oz	–	120	–
(Odwalla)				
carrot blend	8 fl oz	–	100	–
Essentials	8 fl oz	–	70	–
organic	8 fl oz	–	70	–
CASABA MELON/fresh				
cubed	1 cup	–	45	–
whole/8" melon	2" slices	–	45	–
CASHEW				
(Ann's House of Nuts)				
roasted/salted	¼ cup	16.0	210	69%
(Beer Nuts).. sweet & salty	1 oz	13.0	170	69%
(Eagle)				
honey-roasted	1 oz	14.0	180	70%
lightly salted	1 oz	14.0	190	66%
(Fisher)				
Gourmet Select	1 oz	13.0	160	73%
halves & pieces	1 oz	13.0	160	73%

Food and Description	Amount	Fat Grams	Total Calories	% Fat Calories
Holiday Selections deluxe mixed/premium whole cashews				
honey-roasted	1 oz	13.0	150	78%
oil-roasted	1 oz	15.0	170	79%
1-oz snack bag	1 bag	13.0	160	73%
Snack 'n' Serve Nut Bowl jumbo whole	1 oz	15.0	170	79%
whole/Premium	1 oz	13.0	160	73%
(Nutcracker)				
chocolate-covered	1.43 oz	15.0	220	61%
fancy/salted	1 oz	14.0	170	66%
pieces/salted	1.18 oz	16.0	190	76%
(Planters)				
Cashew Dreams/whole w/creamy caramel & milk chocolate	1 oz	11.0	170	58%
fancy	1 oz	13.0	170	69%
halves & pieces	1 oz	14.0	170	74%
honey-roasted				
Munch 'n' Go	2 oz	24.0	310	70%
regular	1 oz	12.0	150	72%
	2 oz	24.0	310	70%
rich roasted/whole in milk chocolate	1.4 oz	14.0	220	57%
whole	1 oz	14.0	170	74%
whole honey-roasted	1 oz	14.0	170	74%
CASHEW BUTTER				
(Arrowhead Mills)	2 Tbs	14.0	160	79%
(Hain)				
raw	2 Tbs	15.0	190	71%
toasted	2 Tbs	17.0	210	73%
unsalted	2 Tbs	19.0	210	81%
(Kettle) Roaster..fresh..no salt	1 oz	14.0	165	76%
CASSAVA				
raw/trimmed	3.5 oz	<1.0	120	3%
	1 lb	2.0	525	3%
CATFISH (See also SEAFOOD ENTRÉE/DINNER)				
channel/fresh/meat only				
baked or broiled	3 oz	7.0	149	42%
breaded & fried	3 oz	11.0	194	51%
raw	3 oz	3.6	99	33%
CATSUP/KETCHUP				
(Atkins)..Ketch-A-Tomato	1 Tbs	–	10	–
(Del Monte)..all styles	1 Tbs	–	15	–
(Hain) natural	1 Tbs	–	16	–
(Healthy Choice)	1 Tbs	–	10	–
(Heinz)				
hot	1 Tbs	–	15	–
light	1 Tbs	–	10	–
regular	1 Tbs	–	15	–

Food and Description	Amount	Fat Grams	Total Calories	% Fat Calories
w/onions	1 Tbs	–	20	–
(Hunt's)				
no salt added	1 Tbs	–	20	–
regular	1 Tbs	–	15	–
squeeze	1 Tbs	–	15	–
(Smucker's)	1 Tbs	–	25	–
(Westbrae)				
fruit-sweetened				
no salt	1 Tbs	–	10	–
regular	1 Tbs	–	10	–
squeeze	1 Tbs	–	20	–
unsweetened	1 Tbs	–	5	–
CAULIFLOWER				
fresh				
cooked	½ cup	–	17	–
raw				
chopped	½ cup	–	12	–
(Dole)	3 oz	0.5	20	23%
whole/medium head	⅙ head	–	25	–
frozen				
(Birds Eye)	½ cup	–	25	–
(Green Giant)..florets/cooked	⅔ cup	–	20	–
(Seneca)	1 cup	–	20	–
jarred				
(Arnold's) pickled	1 oz	–	10	–
(Mrs. Klein's) hot	1 oz	–	–	–
(Vlasic)				
hot & spicy	1 oz	–	4	–
sweet	1 oz	–	35	–
CAULIFLOWER SOUP (*See* SOUP)				
CAVIAR				
general/black or red				
granular	1 Tbs	3.0	40	68%
	1 oz	5.0	71	63%
pressed	1 Tbs	2.8	54	47%
	1 oz	4.7	90	47%
(Romanoff)				
beluga	2 Tbs	4.3	74	16%
black lumpfish	1 Tbs	1.0	15	60%
black whitefish	1 Tbs	1.5	25	54%
red lumpfish	1 Tbs	1.0	15	60%
salmon	1 Tbs	1.5	35	39%
(T. Marzetti)				
black				
lumpfish	1 Tbs	1.0	15	60%
whitefish	1 Tbs	1.5	25	54%
golden				
lumpfish	1 Tbs	1.0	15	60%
whitefish	1 Tbs	1.5	25	54%
red lumpfish	1 Tbs	1.0	15	60%

Food and Description	Amount	Fat Grams	Total Calories	% Fat Calories
salmon				
natural	1 Tbs	1.5	35	39%
red	1 Tbs	1.5	35	39%
CELERIAC/CELERY ROOT/WILD CELERY				
raw	½ cup	–	31	–
	4-5 med	–	40	–
CELERY				
Chinese/diced	1 cup	–	15	–
fresh/medium stalks				
cooked	½ cup	–	11	–
raw	1 stalk	–	6	–
diced	½ cup	–	9	–
(Dole)	2 stalks	–	20	–
frozen				
(Freshlike)	3.5 oz	–	14	–
(Seneca)	¾ cup	–	10	–
CELERY ROOT (*See* CELERIAC)				
CELERY SEED/whole	1 tsp	0.5	8	56%
	1 Tbs	1.5	25	54%
CELERY SOUP (*See* SOUP)				
CEREAL (*See also* BARLEY; BULGUR; CORN GRITS)				
■ **COLD/READY-TO-EAT**				
Alpha-Bits (*See* (Post) in this section)				
(Arrowhead Mills)				
amaranth flakes	1 cup	2.0	140	13%
bran flakes	1 cup	1.0	110	8%
corn flakes	1 cup	–	120	–
kamut flakes	1 cup	1.0	120	8%
maple buckwheat flakes	1 cup	1.0	170	5%
multigrain flakes	1 cup	2.0	170	11%
Nature O's	1 cup	2.0	130	14%
oat bran flakes	1 cup	2.5	140	16%
perfect harvest	1 cup	2.0	140	16%
puffed corn	1 cup	1.0	60	–
puffed kamut	1 cup	–	50	–
puffed millet	1 cup	0.5	60	8%
puffed rice	1 cup	–	60	–
puffed wheat	1 cup	–	60	–
raisin bran	1 cup	1.5	190	7%
rice flakes	1 cup	1.0	180	5%
shredded wheat				
sweetened	1 cup	1.0	200	5%
unsweetened	1 cup	1.0	190	5%
spelt flakes	1 cup	1.0	120	8%
wheat bran	¼ cup	0.5	30	15%
wheat germ/raw	3 Tbs	1.5	50	27%
(Atkins) Morning Start Breakfast Cereal				
banana nut harvest	~¾ cup	2.5	100	23%
crunchy almond crisp	~¾ cup	1.5	100	14%

Food and Description	Amount	Fat Grams	Total Calories	% Fat Calories
(Barbara's)				
2 Good	1 cup	0.5	120	4%
Alpen/Swiss-style				
no sugar or salt added	⅓ cup	3.0	200	14%
original	⅔ cup	3.0	200	14%
	⅔ cup	4.0	220	16%
Apple Cinnamon Toasted O's	¾ cup	1.0	110	8%
Breakfast O's	1¼ cups	<2	110	12%
Brown Rice Crisps	1 cup	1.0	120	8%
Corn flakes	1 cup	–	110	–
Fruity punch	¾ cup	0.5	120	4%
Grain Shop	⅔ cup	1.0	90	10%
Honey Crunch'n Oats	¾ cup	1.0	120	8%
Honey Nut Toasted O's	¾ cup	2.0	120	15%
Organic				
Crispy wheats	¾ cup	0.5	110	4%
Weetabix biscuits	2 biscuits	1.0	120	8%
Wild puffs	1 cup	0.5	100	5%
Puffins				
cinnamon	¾ cup	1.0	100	9%
honey rice	¾ cup	1.5	120	11%
original	¾ cup	1.0	90	10%
peanut butter	¾ cup	2.0	110	16%
shredded				
oats/bite-size	1¼ cups	2.5	220	10%
spoonfuls/multigrain	¾ cup	1.5	120	11%
wheat biscuits	2 biscuits	1.0	140	6%
Soy Essence	¾ cup	0.5	110	4%
(Breadshop)				
granola				
blueberries 'n' cream	½ cup	7.0	220	29%
cinnamon raisin	½ cup	6.0	220	25%
crunchy oat bran	½ cup	8.5	210	36%
Honey Gone Nuts	½ cup	10.0	240	38%
mocha almond crunch	½ cup	7.0	210	39%
pralines 'n' cream	½ cup	7.0	210	39%
raspberries 'n' cream	½ cup	7.5	220	31%
strawberries 'n' cream	½ cup	7.5	220	31%
super natural w/almonds	½ cup	9.0	220	37%
tripleberry crunch	⅔ cup	7.0	220	29%
Vermont maple	½ cup	7.0	210	39%
Kamut 'n' Honey	1 cup	0.5	110	4%
Puffs 'n' Honey	¾ cup	3.0	120	23%
Cap'n Crunch (*See* (Quaker) in this section)				
(Cascadian Farm) Organic				
Hearty Morning	¾ cup	2.5	200	11%

Food and Description	Amount	Fat Grams	Total Calories	% Fat Calories
Honey Nut O's	1 cup	1.5	120	11%
Multi Grain Squares	¾ cup	0.5	110	4%
Oats & Honey Granola	⅔ cup	6.0	230	23%
Raisin Bran	1 cup	1.0	180	5%
Wheat Crunch	¾ cup	0.5	110	4%
Cheerios (*See* (General Mills) in this section)				
Crispix (*See* (Kellogg's) in this section)				
(Erewhon)				
amaranth/Aztec Corn	1 cup	–	110	–
Apple Stroodles	¾ cup	0.5	110	4%
Banana O's	¾ cup	–	110	–
corn flakes	1-/4 cup	2.5	210	11%
crisp brown rice				
gluten-free	¾ cup	0.5	110	4%
no salt added	¾ cup	–	110	–
original	¾ cup	–	110	–
w/mixed berries	¾ cup	0.5	120	4%
Fruit 'n Wheat	¾ cup	1.5	170	8%
kamut flakes	⅔ cup	–	110	–
Poppels	1 cup	1.0	120	8%
raisin bran	1 cup	1.0	170	5%
wheat flakes	1 cup	1.0	110	8%
(General Mills) Big G Cereals				
Basic 4	1 cup	3.0	200	14%
Boo Berry	1 cup	1.0	120	8%
Cheerios				
apple cinnamon	¾ cup	1.5	120	11%
berry burst				
strawberry	1 cup	1.5	110	12%
strawberry banana	1 cup	1.5	110	12%
triple berry	1 cup	1.5	110	12%
frosted	1 cup	1.0	120	8%
honey nut	1 cup	1.5	120	11%
multigrain plus	1 cup	1.0	110	8%
original	1 cup	2.0	110	16%
Team	1 cup	1.0	110	8%
Chex				
corn	1 cup	–	110	–
frosted mini	¾ cup	–	110	–
honey nut	¾ cup	0.5	120	4%
morning mix				
banana nut	1 pouch	3.5	130	24%
cinnamon	1 pouch	3.5	130	24%
fruit & nut	1 pouch	3.5	130	24%
honey nut	1 pouch	3.0	130	21%
multi bran	1 cup	1.5	200	7%
rice	1¼ cups	-	120	–
wheat	1 cup	1.0	180	5%
Cinnamon Grahams	¾ cup	1.0	120	8%

Food and Description	Amount	Fat Grams	Total Calories	% Fat Calories
Cinnamon Toast Crunch	¾ cup	3.5	130	24%
Cocoa Puffs	1 cup	1.0	120	8%
Cookie Crisp	1 cup	1.0	120	8%
Count Chocula	1 cup	1.0	120	8%
Country Corn Flakes	1 cup	–	110	–
Fiber One	½ cup	1.0	60	15%
Frankenberry	1 cup	1.0	120	8%
French Toast Crunch	¾ cup	1.0	120	8%
Gold Medal Raisin Bran	1⅓ cups	1.5	170	8%
Golden Grahams	¾ cup	1.0	120	8%
Harmony	1½ cups	1.0	120	8%
Honey Nut Clusters	1 cup	2.5	210	11%
Kaboom	1¼ cups	1.0	120	8%
Kix				
berry berry	¾ cup	1.5	120	11%
original	1-⅓ cups	1.0	120	8%
Lucky Charms	1 cup	1.0	120	8%
Millenios	1 cup	1.0	120	8%
Multi-bran Chex	1 cup	1.5	200	7%
Nature Valley low-fat				
fruit granola	⅔ cup	2.5	210	11%
Nesquick chocolate	¾ cup	2.0	120	15%
Oatmeal Crisp				
almond	1 cup	4.5	220	19%
apple cinnamon	1 cup	2.0	210	9%
raisin	1 cup	2.0	210	9%
Peanut Butter				
Toast Crunch	3¾ cup	3.5	130	24%
Raisin Nut Bran	¾ cup	4.0	200	20%
Reese's Peanut				
Butter Puffs	¾ cup	3.0	130	21%
Rice Chex	1¼ cups	–	120	–
Total				
brown sugar & oats	¾ cup	0.5	110	4%
corn flakes	1½ cups	–	110	–
raisin bran	1 cup	1.0	170	5%
whole wheat	¾ cup	1.0	110	8%
Trix	1 cup	1.0	120	8%
Wheaties				
honey-frosted	¾ cup	–	110	–
original	1 cup	1.0	120	8%
raisin bran	1 cup	1.0	180	5%
(Golden Temple) Part Organic low-fat				
apple cinnamon raisin	½ cup	2.0	190	9%
strawberry/raspberry	½ cup	2.0	200	9%
granola				
cinnamon apple raisin	½ cup	8.0	220	33%
fruit & nut	½ cup	8.0	220	33%

Food and Description	Amount	Fat Grams	Total Calories	% Fat Calories
gingersnap	½ cup	7.0	220	29%
super nutty	½ cup	8.0	220	33%
wild blueberry	½ cup	9.0	230	35%
(Health Valley)				
LOW-FAT GRANOLA				
date almond flavor	⅔ cup	1.0	180	5%
raisin cinnamon	⅔ cup	1.0	180	5%
tropical fruit	⅔ cup	1.0	180	5%
NON-ORGANIC CEREAL				
Banana Gone Nuts	¾ cup	3.0	200	14%
Corn Crunch-ems!	1 cup	–	110	–
Cranberry Crunch	¾ cup	3.0	200	14%
Empower	1 cup	3.0	200	14%
HeartWise	1 cup	3.0	200	14%
Honey Crunches & flakes	¾ cup	–	130	–
Raspberry Rhapsody	¾ cup	3.0	200	14
Real Oat Bran Almond Crunch	¾ cup	3.0	200	14%
Rice Crunch-ems!	1 cup	–	110	–
Slender	1 cup	1.5	180	8%
Soy Flakes				
original	1¼ cup	1.5	190	7%
raisin	1 cup	1.0	190	5%
Soy O's				
apple cinnamon	1 cup	2.0	180	10%
honey nut	1 cup	2.0	180	10%
original	1 cup	2.0	180	10%
ORGANIC CEREAL				
amaranth flakes	¾ cup	–	100	–
blue corn flakes	¾ cup	–	100	–
Fiber 7/multigrain flakes	¾ cup	–	100	–
Golden Flax	¾ cup	3.0	190	14%
Healthy Fiber/multi– grain flakes	¾ cup	–	100	–
Honey Fiber/7 flakes	¾ cup	–	110	–
Just Flakes/#1 box				
multigrain	¾ cup	1.0	100	9%
oats	¾ cup	1.0	100	9%
Oat Bran Flakes	¾ cup	–	100	–
w/raisins	¾ cup	–	110	–
Oat Bran O's	¾ cup	–	100	–
raisin bran flakes	1¼ cups	–	190	–
raisin crunch bran	¾ cup	–	160	–
(Kashi)				
GOLEAN				
crunchy	¾ cup	1.0	120	8%
regular	1 cup	3.0	190	14%

Food and Description	Amount	Fat Grams	Total Calories	% Fat Calories
Good Friends				
Cinna-raisin	1 cup	1.0	120	8%
regular	¾ cup	1.0	90	10%
Heart to Heart	¾ cup	1.5	110	12%
Kashi				
Baby & Me/dry	4 Tbs	–	50	–
Medley	¾ cup	1.0	120	8%
Pilaf	¾ cup	3.0	170	16%
Puffed	1 cup	0.5	70	6%
Promise/organic				
Autumn Wheat	1 cup	1.0	190	5%
Cranberry Sunshine	1 cup	1.0	110	5%
Strawberry Fields	1 cup	–	120	–
Seven in the Morning	¾ cup	1.5	210	6%
(Kellogg's)				
All Bran				
Bran Buds	⅓ cup	1.0	70	13%
original	½ cup	1.0	80	11%
w/extra fiber	½ cup	1.0	50	18%
Apple Jacks	1 cup	0.5	130	3%
Cinnamon				
Crunch Crispix	½ cup	1.0	120	8%
Marshmallow Scooby-Doo	1 cup	4.0	140	26%
Cocoa Rice Krispies	½ cup	1.0	120	8%
Complete				
Oat Bran Flakes	¾ cup	1.0	110	8%
Wheat Bran Flakes	¾ cup	0.5	90	5%
Corn Pops	1 cup	–	120	–
Cracklin' Oat Bran	¾ cup	7.0	200	32%
Crispix	1 cup	–	110	–
Disney				
Hunny B's Honey-Graham	1 cup	0.5	110	4%
Mickey's Magix	¾ cup	0.5	110	4%
Mud & Bugs	1 cup	1.0	110	5%
Froot Loops				
marshmallow-blasted	1 cup	0.5	120	4%
original	1 cup	1.0	120	80%
Frosted Flakes	¾ cup	–	120	–
Fruit Harvest				
apple cinnamon	1 cup	2.5	190	11%
peach strawberry	¾ cup	–	110	–
strawberry blueberry	¾ cup	–	110	-%
Granola				
low-fat w/raisins	⅔ cup	3.0	220	12%
Honey Crunch				
corn flakes	¾ cup	1.0	120	8%
Just Right				
w/fruit & nuts	1 cup	2.0	200	9%

Food and Description	Amount	Fat Grams	Total Calories	% Fat Calories
Kellogg's				
Corn Flakes	1 cup	–	100	–
w/real bananas	¾ cup	2.0	110	16%
Frosted Flakes	¾ cup	–	120	–
Smorz	1 cup	2.0	120	15%
Mini-Wheats				
apple cinnamon	¾ cup	1.0	180	5%
blueberry	¾ cup	1.0	180	5%
frosted				
bite-size	~24 biscuits	1.0	200	5%
maple & brown sugar	~24 biscuits	1.0	190	5%
original	~5 biscuits	1.0	180	5%
raisin	¾ cup	1.0	180	5%
strawberry	¾ cup	1.0	170	5%
Mueslix w/raisins,				
dates & almonds	⅔ cup	3.0	200	14%
Product 19	1 cup	–	100	–
Raisin Bran	1 cup	1.5	190	7%
Raisin Bran Crunch	1 cup	1.0	190	5%
Rice Krispies				
original	1¼ cup	–	120	–
Razzle Dazzle	¾ cup	–	110	–
Treats	¾ cup	1.5	120	11%
Smacks	¾ cup	0.5	100	5%
Smart Start				
original	1 cup	0.5	190	2%
soy protein	1 cup	1.5	200	7%
Special K				
original	1 cup	–	110	–
Plus	1 cup	2.0	210	9%
Red berries	1 cup	–	110	–
SpongeBob Square Pants	1 cup	1.0	120	8%
Tony's Cinnamon				
Krunchers	1 cup	–	110	–
(Kretschmer)				
toasted wheat bran	¼ cup	1.0	30	30%
wheat germ				
honey crunch	5 tsp	1.0	50	18%
original	2 Tbs	1.0	50	18%
Life (*See* (Quaker) in this section)				
(Lifestream)				
berry granola	¾ cup	3.0	210	13%
8-grain flakes	¾ cup	1.0	130	7%
Flax Plus	¾ cup	2.0	120	15%
multigrain honey puffs	¾ cup	3.0	120	23%
SmartBran	½ cup	1.5	120	11%
Wild Berry Muesli	½ cup	3.0	210	13%
(Malt-O-Meal)				
Apple Zings	1 cup	1.0	130	7%
Balance w/berries	1 cup	0.5	110	4%

Food and Description	Amount	Fat Grams	Total Calories	% Fat Calories
Berry Colossal Crunch	¾ cup	1.5	120	11%
Cinnamon Toasters	¾ cup	3.5	130	24%
Cocoa Dyno-bites	¾ cup	1.0	120	8%
Cocoa Roos	¾ cup	1.0	190	5%
Corn Bursts	¾ cup	–	120	–
Crispy Rice	1¼ cups	-	130	–
frosted				
flakes	¾ cup	–	120	–
mini spooners	1 cup	1.0	190	5%
Fruity Dyno-bites	¾ cup	0.5	100	5%
Golden Puffs	¾ cup	–	100	–
Honey Buzzers	1⅓ cups	0.5	110	4%
Graham Squares	¾ cup	1.0	120	8%
Nut Toasty O's	1 cup	1.0	110	8%
Marshmallow Mateys	1 cup	1.0	110	8%
puffed rice	1 cup	–	60	–
puffed wheat	1 cup	–	50	–
raisin bran	1 cup	1.5	190	7%
toasted cinnamon twists	¾ cup	3.5	130	24%
toasty O's	¾ cup	2.0	110	16%
Tootie Fruities	1 cup	1.0	120	8%
Nature Valley (See (General Mills) in this section)				
(Nature's Path)				
EnviroKid				
Amazon Frosted Flakes	⅔ cup	1.0	120	8%
Cheetah Chomps	⅔ cup	2.0	130	14%
Gorilla Munch	⅔ cup	1.0	115	8%
Koala Crisp	⅔ cup	0.5	120	4%
Orangutan-O's	⅔ cup	1.0	120	8%
Peanut Butter				
Panda Puffs	¾ cup	2.5	130	17%
Organic				
flakes				
8-grain synergy				
multigrain	⅔ cup	1.0	100	9%
corn				
honey'd	¾ cup	–	120	–
original	¾ cup	–	120	–
Flax Plus				
original	¾ cup	1.5	100	14%
raisin bran	¾ cup	2.5	180	13%
Heritage	¾ cup	1.0	100	9%
Kamut Krisp	¾ cup	–	100	–
Mesa Sunrise	¾ cup	1.5	120	11%
millet rice oatbran	⅔ cup	1.0	100	9%
multigrain oatbran				
flakes	⅔ cup	1.0	100	9%
& raisins	⅔ cup	1.0	100	9%
raisin bran/honey'd	¾ cup	0.5	100	5%

Food and Description	Amount	Fat Grams	Total Calories	% Fat Calories
spelt	¾ cup	1.0	120	8%
Organic Eco Pacs				
cornflakes	¾ cup	–	120	–
Heritage	¾ cup	1.0	100	9%
Bites	¾ cup	1.0	100	9%
Honey'd				
cornflakes	¾ cup	–	120	–
raisin bran	¾ cup	0.5	100	5%
Kamut Krisp	¾ cup	–	100	–
Mesa Sunrise	¾ cup	1.5	120	11%
millet rice oatbran				
flakes	⅔ cup	1.0	100	9%
multigrain oatbran				
flakes	⅔ cup	1.0	100	9%
flakes & raisins	⅔ cup	1.0	100	9%
Oaty bites	⅔ cup	1.5	120	11%
Organic Granola				
Ginger Zing	⅔ cup	6.0	150	36%
Hemp Plus	⅔ cup	5.0	140	32%
Pumpkin Flax Plus	⅔ cup	6.0	140	38%
Raspberry Heritage	⅔ cup	3.0	130	21%
Soy Plus	⅔ cup	3.0	130	21%
Organic Muesli				
blueberry almond	½ cup	3.5	210	15%
Heritage	½ cup	4.0	220	16%
Organic Optimum				
Power breakfast	1 cup	2.5	190	12%
Slim cereal	1 cup	2.5	180	13%
Zen	¾ cup	2.5	200	11%
Organic Puffed				
corn	1 cup	–	60	–
kamut	1 cup	–	50	–
millet	1 cup	–	50	–
rice	1 cup	–	50	–
wheat	1 cup	–	50	–
Shredded Bites				
Oatie	¾ cup	1.5	120	11%
Heritage	¾ cup	1.0	100	9%
(New Morning)				
cocoa crispy rice	¾ cup	0.5	120	4%
Cocomotion	¾ cup	0.5	100	5%
cornflakes				
frosted	1 cup	1.0	120	8%
plain	1 cup	1.01	120	8%
w/strawberries	1 cup	1.0	120	8%
Cornfetti	¾ cup	1.0	110	8%
Fruit-e-O's	1 cup	1.5	120	11%
Oatios				
apple cinnamon	1 cup	1.0	120	8%
cocoa	¾ cup	1.0	110	8%

Food and Description	Amount	Fat Grams	Total Calories	% Fat Calories
honey almond	1 cup	1.0	120	8%
original	1 cup	–	110	–
Kamutios	1 cup	1.0	120	8%
Ultimate oat bran	⅔ cup	2.0	110	16%
Wafflers	⅔ cup	1.0	110	8%
(Post)				
Alpha-Bits				
original	1 cup	1.5	130	10%
w/marshmallows	1 cup	1.0	120	7%
bran flakes	¾ cup	0.5	100	5%
Cocoa Pebbles	¾ cup	1.0	120	8%
Fruit & Bran				
dates/raisins/walnuts	1 cup	3.0	200	14%
peaches/raisins				
/almonds	1 cup	3.0	190	14%
Fruity Pebbles	¾ cup	1.0	110	8%
Golden Crisp	¾ cup	–	110	–
Grape-Nuts				
flakes	¾ cup	1.0	110	8%
original	½ cup	1.0	200	5%
O's	¾ cup	–	120	–
Honey Bunches of Oats				
honey-roasted	¾ cup	1.5	120	11%
w/almonds	¾ cup	2.5	130	17%
w/real strawberries	¾ cup	2.0	120	15%
Honeycomb	1 cup	0.5	110	4%
strawberry-blasted	1 cup	1.0	120	8%
Hulk w/marshmallow bits	1 cup	–	110	–
Post Toasties	1 cup	–	100	–
Raisin Bran	1 cup	1.0	190	5%
Selects Cereal				
Banana Nut Crunch	1 cup	6.0	240	22%
Blueberry Morning	1¼ cups	3.5	230	13%
Cranberry Almond				
Crunch	1 cup	3.0	210	13%
Great Grains				
crunchy pecan	⅔ cup	6.0	220	25%
raisins, dates				
& pecans	⅔ cup	4.5	200	20%
Shredded wheat				
Frosted spoon-size	1 cup	1.0	180	5%
Honey nut spoon-size	1 cup	1.5	200	7%
Original				
spoon-size	1 cup	1.0	170	5%
regular	2 biscuits	1.0	160	6%
Wheat 'n bran	1¼ cups	1.5	200	7%
Waffle Crisp	1 cup	2.5	130	17%
(Quaker)				
Apple Zaps	1 cup	1.0	120	8%
Bran/unprocessed	⅓ cup	0.5	35	13%

Food and Description	Amount	Fat Grams	Total Calories	% Fat Calories
Cap'n Crunch				
Crunchberries	¾ cup	1.5	100	14%
Oops! Choco Donut	¾ cup	1.0	100	9%
peanut butter	¾ cup	2.5	110	20%
regular	¾ cup	1.5	110	12%
Cinnamon Crunch	1 cup	2.0	120	15%
Cocoa				
Blasts	1 cup	1.0	130	7%
Bronto Blasts	¾ cup	–	110	–
Cranberry Macadamia Nut	1 cup	6.0	240	
Crispy Corn Puffs	1 cup	1.0	110	8%
Crunchy Corn bran	¾ cup	1.0	90	10%
Frosted				
Flakes	¾ cup	–	120	–
Oats	1 cup	1.5	110	12%
Fruitangy Oh's	1 cup	1.0	120	8%
Fruity				
Bronto Blasts	¾ cup	0.5	110	4%
Ocean Adventure	2 cup	1.0	110	8%
Honey Crisp Corn Flakes	¾ cup	–	110	–
Honey Dipps	1¼ cup	1.5	130	10%
Honey Graham Oh's	¾ cup	2.0	110	16%
Honey Nut Oats	¾ cup	1.0	110	8%
King VitamaCorn	1½ cups	1.0	120	8%
Kretschmer				
wheat bran	¼ cup	1.0	30	30%
wheat germ				
Honey Crunch	1⅔ Tbs	1.0	50	18%
regular	2 Tbs	1.0	50	18%
Life				
cinnamon	¾ cup	1.0	120	8%
regular	¾ cup	1.5	120	11%
Marshmallow Safari	¾ cup	2.0	140	13%
Oat Bran High Fiber	1¼ cup	3.0	210	13%
Oat Squares				
cinnamon	1 cup	2.5	230	10%
original	1 cup	3.0	220	12%
100% Natural Granola				
low-fat w/raisins	½ cup	3.0	210	13%
regular				
oats & honey	½ cup	9.0	220	37%
w/raisins	½ cup	9.0	230	35%
Popeye Puffed				
rice	1¼ cup	–	50	–
wheat	1¼ cup	–	50	–
Quaker Oatmeal Cereals				
Brown Sugar Bliss	1 cup	2.5	190	12%
Honey Nut Heaven	1 cup	3.5	190	17%
Quaker Squares				
cinnamon	1 cup	2.5	230	10%

Food and Description	Amount	Fat Grams	Total Calories	% Fat Calories
regular	1 cup	2.5	210	11%
Quisp	1 cup	1.5	110	12%
Rice Crisps	1 cup	–	110	–
Shredded Wheat				
frosted	1 cup	1.0	190	5%
original	3 pieces	1.5	220	6%
Sugar Frosted Flakes	¾ cup	–	110	–
Sweet Crunch	1 cup	1.5	110	12%
Sweet Puffs	1 cup	1.0	130	7%
Toasted Oatmeal				
Honey Nut	1 cup	2.5	190	12%
original	1 cup	2.5	190	12%
Toasted Oatmeal Squares				
cinnamon	1 cup	2.5	210	11%
original	1 cup	2.5	230	10%
Toasted Oats	1 cup	1.5	110	12%
(Ralston)				
Bran Flakes/enriched	¾ cup	0.5	90	5%
Confruity Crisp	¾ cup	1.0	110	8%
Cocoa Crispy Rice	¾ cup	1.0	120	8%
Cocoa Crunchies	1 cup	1.0	120	8%
Corn Biscuits	1 cup	–	110	–
Corn Bran	1 cup	2.0	120	15%
Corn Flakes	1 cup	–	100	–
Crisp Crunch Berry	¾ cup	1.0	120	8%
Crisp Crunch Treets	1 cup	1.0	120	8%
Crisp Rice	1¼ cup	–	120	–
Crispy Hexacons	1 cup	–	110	–
Freaky Fruits	1 cup	1.0	120	8%
Frosted Flakes/Sugar	¾ cup	–	120	–
Fruit Rings	1 cup	1.0	120	8%
fruit muesli				
blueberry pecan	1 cup	3.0	200	14%
cranberry walnut	¾ cup	3.0	200	14%
peach pecan	¾ cup	3.0	200	14%
raspberry almond	¾ cup	3.0	200	14%
strawberry pecan	1 cup	3.0	200	14%
Magic Stars	¾ cup	1.0	120	8%
Oats & more				
w/almonds	¾ cup	1.5	130	10%
Raisin Bran	1 cup	1.5	200	7%
Rice Biscuits/natural	1¼ cup	–	110	–
Shredded wheat				
Frosted spoon-size	1¼ cup	1.0	200	5%
Silly Spheres	1½ cup	0.5	110	4%
Tasteeos				
apple cinnamon	¾ cup	1.5	120	11%
honey nut	1 cup	1.5	120	11%
original	1 cup	1.5	110	12%

Food and Description	Amount	Fat Grams	Total Calories	% Fat Calories
Rice Krispies (*See* (Kellogg's) in this section)				
(Skinner) Raisin Bran	1 cup	1.0	170	5%
Special K (*See* (Kellogg's) in this section)				
(Sunbelt)				
5 whole grains				
muesli	½ cup	2.0	210	9%
granola				
banana nut	½ cup	9.0	250	32%
berry basic	½ cup	6.0	240	23%
fruit & nut	½ cup	7.0	240	26%
low-fat cinnamon				
raisin	½ cup	3.0	220	12%
raisin almond crunch	½ cup	3.0	220	12%
(S. W. Graham)				
cinnamon	½ cup	–	100	–
plain	½ cup	–	100	–
Total (*See* (General Mills) in this section)				
(U.S. Mills) Uncle Sam	1 cup	1.0	110	8%
(Weetabix) (*See* (Barbara's) in this section)				
Wheaties (*See* (General Mills) in this section)				

■ HOT/COOKED

(NOTE: All cereals are either dry or prepared with water per directions on packaging. If milk is used, calorie and fat content increase accordingly. For additional information on milk, see MILK.)

Food and Description	Amount	Fat Grams	Total Calories	% Fat Calories
(Arrowhead Mills) Dry				
Bear Mush	¼ cup	1.0	150	6%
Bits of Barley	¼ cup	1.0	160	6%
bulgur	¼ cup	0.5	150	3%
corn grits				
white	¼ cup	–	150	–
yellow	¼ cup	–	130	–
couscous	¼ cup	–	170	–
cracked wheat	¼ cup	0.5	140	3%
4-grain plus flax	¼ cup	1.0	150	6%
old-fashioned oatmeal	⅓ cup	2.0	130	8%
oat				
bran	⅓ cup	2.5	130	17%
flakes	⅓ cup	2.0	130	8%
oats/oatmeal				
instant				
cinnamon raisin				
almond	1 pkg	3.0	140	19%
maple apple spice	1 pkg	2.0	140	13%
regular	1 pkg	2.0	110	16%
regular/steel-cut	¼ cup	3.0	160	17%
Rice & Shine	¼ cup	1.0	150	6%
7-grain cereal				
regular	⅓ cup	1.0	140	6%
wheat-free	¼ cup	2.5	150	15%
wheat bran	¼ cup	1.0	35	26%

Food and Description	Amount	Fat Grams	Total Calories	% Fat Calories
wheat germ/raw	3 Tbs	1.5	50	27%
(Cream of Rice) (*See* (Post) in this section)				
(Cream of Wheat) (*See* (Post) in this section)				
(Erewhon)				
Barley Plus/dry	¼ cup	1.0	170	5%
cream of brown rice/dry	¼ cup	1.0	170	5%
oat bran				
w/toasted wheat germ	1 pkg	2.5	170	13%
oatmeal/instant dry				
apple cinnamon	1 pkg	2.0	130	14%
apple raisin	1 pkg	2.0	140	13%
dates & walnuts	1 pkg	2.5	130	17%
maple spice	1 pkg	2.0	130	14%
oatmeal w/added bran	1 pkg	2.5	130	17%
raisins dates & nuts	1 pkg	2.5	130	17%
w/added oat bran	1 pkg	3.0	125	22%
(Fantastic Foods) Oatmeal Big Cup/Dry				
apple cinnamon/low-fat	1 pkg	3.5	270	12%
banana nut barley	1 pkg	3.5	270	12%
cranberry orange	1 pkg	4.0	300	12%
maple raisin 3-grain	1 pkg	2.0	270	7%
wheat 'n' berries	1 pkg	2.0	260	7%
(Farina)				
dry	3 Tbs	–	120	–
prepared	1 cup	–	120	–
(Highspire)				
Maltex	⅓ cup	0.5	170	3%
Wheatena	⅓ cup	1.0	150	6%
(Gram's Gourmet)				
cream of flax				
cinnamon toast	½ cup	5.0	140	32%
maple & brown sugar	½ cup	5.0	140	32%
vanilla almond	½ cup	5.0	140	32%
(H-O)				
farina/quick/dry	3 Tbs	–	120	–
oatmeal				
instant/dry				
apple cinnamon	1 pkg	2.0	130	14%
maple & brown sugar	1 pkg	2.0	160	11%
oats 'n' fiber				
apple & bran	1 pkg	2.0	130	14%
plain	1 pkg	2.0	110	16%
raisin & bran	1 pkg	2.0	150	12%
plain	1 pkg	2.0	110	16%
raisins & spice	1 pkg	2.0	150	12%
sweet 'n' mellow	1 pkg	2.0	150	12%
regular				
gourmet	⅓ cup	2.0	100	18%
quick	½ cup	3.0	150	18%

Food and Description	Amount	Fat Grams	Total Calories	% Fat Calories
(Health Valley) Hot Cereal Cups				
Amazing Apple	1 cup	2.0	210	9%
Banana Gone Nuts	1 cup	3.0	240	11%
Maple Madness!				
w/raisins	1 cup	2.0	240	8%
Terrific 10 Grain!	1 cup	2.5	220	10%
(Krusteaz)/dry				
Grain Gourmet Cracked				
Wheat Bulgur	¼ cup	0.5	150	3%
Zoom/100% whole wheat	⅓ cup	0.5	120	4%
(Lundberg Family) Purely Organic				
hot 'n' creamy rice cereal/prepared				
cinnamon & raisin	⅓ cup	1.5	190	7%
plain	⅓ cup	2.0	190	9%
w/almonds & nuts	⅓ cup	3.5	200	16%
(Malt-O-Meal)				
Hot Wheat cereal	1 serving	0.5	120	4%
chocolate	1 serving	0.5	120	4%
maple & brown sugar	1 serving	–	120	–
original	1 serving	0.5	120	4%
Instant Oatmeal/Big Bowl				
apples & cinnamon	1 serving	2.0	190	9%
cinnamon & spice	1 serving	3.0	250	11%
cinnamon roll	1 serving	3.0	240	11%
Deluxe variety	1 serving	3.0	225	12%
Fruit & Creamy/variety	1 serving	3.0	195	14%
maple & brown sugar	1 serving	3.0	230	12%
(Maypo)				
instant maple	½ cup	2.0	190	9%
Vermont-style	⅓ cup	2.0	150	12%
(McCann's) Irish Oatmeal				
oat bran	½ cup	1.0	80	11%
pinhead oatmeal	½ cup	2.0	150	12%
quick-cooking oatmeal	½ cup	2.0	150	12%
traditional oatmeal	½ cup	2.0	150	12%
(Mother's)/dry				
barley	⅓ cup	1.0	170	5%
multigrain	½ cup	1.0	130	7%
oat bran	½ cup	3.0	150	18%
oatmeal/instant	½ cup	0.5	150	3%
rolled oats	½ cup	3.0	150	18%
wheat germ	2 Tbs	1.0	50	18%
whole wheat/100% natural	½ cup	1.0	130	7%
(Nature's Path) Organic				
Instant Oatmeal				
apple cinnamon	1 pkt	2.0	190	9%
flax 'n' oats	1 pkt	4.0	200	9%
maple nut	1 pkt	4.0	200	9%
original	1 pkt	4.0	190	19%

Food and Description	Amount	Fat Grams	Total Calories	% Fat Calories
(Post) Instant				
Cream of Rice/dry	1 serving	–	170	–
Cream of Wheat/dry				
1 minute	1 serving	–	120	–
10 minute	1 serving	–	120	–
2½ minute	1 serving	–	120	–
Cream of wheat/flavored				
apples 'n' cinnamon	1 pkt	–	130	–
cinnamon swirl	1 pkt	–	130	–
maple brown sugar	1 pkt	–	120	–
original	1 pkt	–	90	–
peaches 'n' cream	1 pkt	1.5	130	10%
strawberries 'n' cream	1 pkt	1.5	130	10%
(Quaker)				
oat bran	½ cup	3.0	150	18%
oatmeal				
Express cups				
baked apple	1 cup	2.5	200	11%
cinnamon roll	1 cup	3.5	210	15%
golden brown sugar	1 cup	2.5	200	11%
instant				
apple & cinnamon	1 pkt	1.5	130	8%
apple crisp	1 pkt	2.0	150	12%
banana bread	1 pkt	2.0	150	12%
bananas & cream	1 pkt	2.5	140	16%
blueberries & cream	1 pkt	2.5	140	16%
cinnamon & spice	1 pkt	2.0	170	11%
cinnamon apple & brown sugar	1 pkt	2.0	160	12%
cinnamon roll	1 pkt	3.0	160	17%
dinosaur eggs brown sugar	1 pkt	4.0	200	18%
double raisin Danish	1 pkt	2.0	170	11%
French toast	1 pkt	2.0	160	12%
honey nut	1 pkt	3.5	170	19%
maple & brown sugar	1 pkt	2.0	160	11%
peaches & cream	1 pkt	2.5	140	16%
raisin/spice	1 pkt	2.0	150	7%
raisins, dates & walnuts	1 pkt	2.5	140	16%
regular	1 pkt	2.0	100	18%
strawberries & cream	1 pkt	2.5	140	16%
Nutrition for Women				
apple cinnamon	1 pkt	2.0	170	11%
golden brown sugar	1 pkt	2.5	160	14%
vanilla cinnamon	1 pkt	2.0	160	11%
oats/dry				
Crystal Wedding	½ cup	3.0	150	18%
old-fashioned	½ cup	3.0	150	18%
quick-cooking	½ cup	2.5	150	15%

Food and Description	Amount	Fat Grams	Total Calories	% Fat Calories
Sun Country				
iron-fortified	½ cup	3.0	150	18%
multigrain	½ cup	1.0	130	7%
whole wheat hot				
natural cereal	½ cup	1.0	130	7%
(Ralston) 3-Minute Brand				
instant hot Ralston	⅓ cup	1.0	150	6%
instant oatmeal				
cinnamon roll	1 pkg	2.0	160	11%
fruit & cream variety	1 pkg	2.0	100	18%
maple & brown sugar	1 pkg	1.5	160	8%
regular flavor	1 pkg	2.0	100	18%
variety pack	1 pkg	2.5	130	17%
oats/100% natural				
old-fashioned	1 serving	2.5	150	15%
quick	1 serving	2.5	140	16%
plus oat bran	1 serving	3.0	150	18%
raisin	1 serving	3.0	150	18%
(Roman Meal) dry				
cream of rye	⅓ cup	1.0	110	8%
oatmeal/instant				
hearty				
apple cinnamon	⅓ cup	1.0	120	8%
raisins, dates & almonds	⅓ cup	2.0	130	14%
original	⅓ cup	1.0	110	8%
(Skinners)..oat bran	1 serving	2.0	110	16%
(Spice Hunter) Cereal Cups/3-grain				
apple cinnamon	1 cup	1.5	210	6%
banana nut cream	1 cup	3.0	210	13%
maple cream	1 cup	1.5	200	7%
raisin nut	1 cup	3.0	220	12%
(Stone-Buhr)				
4-grain cereal mates	⅓ cup	2.0	140	13%
7-grain cereal	⅓ cup	2.0	140	13%
oat bran	⅓ cup	2.0	90	20%
oats				
rolled old-fashioned	¼ cup	3.0	150	16%
Scotch	¼ cup	4.0	150	24%
(Uncle Sam)..instant oatmeal	1 pkt	3.0	130	21%

CEREAL BAR (See BREAKFAST/CEREAL BAR; GRANOLA/GRANOLA-TYPE BAR)
CERVELAT (See SAUSAGE)
CHAMPAGNE (See WINE)
CHARD
fresh

cooked	½ cup	–	18	–
raw/chopped	½ cup	–	3	–
frozen				
(C&W) Swiss	3.3 oz	–	20	–

Food and Description	Amount	Fat Grams	Total Calories	% Fat Calories
CHAYOTE/fresh				
boiled	½ cup	–	19	–
raw/whole	1 medium	–	56	–
CHEESE (*See also* CHEESE ALTERNATIVE/IMITATION; CHEESE SPREAD; COTTAGE CHEESE; CREAM CHEESE)				
■ **(Alouette)**				
baby Brie				
plain	1 oz	8.0	100	72%
w/herbs	1 oz	8.0	100	72%
baby Swiss				
light	1 oz	6.0	90	60%
regular	1 oz	8.0	110	65%
smoked	1 oz	8.0	110	65%
baked Brie w/raspberries/almonds	2 oz	14.0	220	57%
MONTRACHET				
goat cheese..all styles	1 oz	6.0	70	77%
(Alpine Lace)				
*DELI SELF-SERVICE/*chunk cheese				
reduced-fat				
cheddar	1 oz	7.0	90	70%
feta	1 oz	3.0	50	54%
hot pepper	1 oz	7.0	90	70%
provolone	1 oz	6.0	90	60%
Swiss	1 oz	7.0	110	57%
*DELI COUNTER/*slicing cheese				
American	1 oz	7.0	90	70%
reduced-fat				
cheddar	1 oz	7.0	90	70%
mozzarella	1 oz	3.0	70	38%
Swiss	1 oz	7.0	110	57%
reduced fat/reduced sodium				
American				
hot pepper	1 oz	7.0	90	70%
white	1 oz	6.0	90	60%
yellow	1 oz	7.0	90	70%
provolone	1 oz	6.0	90	60%
reduced-sodium				
Muenster	1 oz	9.0	100	81%
PRE-SLICED SELF-SERVICE DELI CHEESE				
reduced-fat				
cheddar	1 oz	7.0	90	70%
Co-Jack semi-soft	1 oz	7.0	90	70%
low-moisture				
mozzarella	1 oz	5.0	70	64%
Swiss	1 oz	7.0	110	57%
reduced-fat/reduced-sodium				
American				
hot pepper	1 oz	6.0	90	60%

Food and Description	Amount	Fat Grams	Total Calories	% Fat Calories
white	1 oz	6.0	90	60%
yellow	1 oz	7.0	90	70%
provolone	1 oz	6.0	90	60%
reduced-sodium				
Muenster	1 oz	9.0	110	74%
■ (Athenos)				
Feta/crumbled				
basil & tomato	1 oz	6.0	80	68%
mild	1 oz	6.0	80	68%
traditional				
reduced-fat	1 oz	4.0	60	60%
regular	1 oz	6.0	80	68%
■ (Boar's Head)				
American				
white	1 oz	9.0	100	81%
yellow	1 oz	9.0	100	81%
blue cheese/creamy	1 oz	8.0	90	80%
butter kase	1 oz	9.0	100	81%
cheddar				
Canadian	1 oz	10.0	110	82%
horseradish	1 oz	9.0	110	74%
sharp				
white	1 oz	9.0	110	74%
yellow	1 oz	9.0	110	74%
Vermont				
white	1 oz	10.0	110	82%
yellow	1 oz	10.0	110	82%
Colby				
longhorn	1 oz	9.0	110	74%
Edam	1 oz	7.0	90	70%
feta	1 oz	4.0	60	60%
Gloucester				
double/yellow	1 oz	10.0	110	82%
Gouda	1 oz	9.0	110	74%
Havarti..all flavors	1 oz	10.0	110	74%
Monterey Jack..all flavors	1 oz	9.0	100	81%
mozzarella/low-moisture	1 oz	7.0	90	70%
Muenster..all styles	1 oz	8.0	100	72%
provolone..all styles	1 oz	8.0	100	72%
Swiss				
baby Swiss	1 oz	9.0	110	74%
Gold Label/imported	1 oz	8.0	110	65%
lacey	1 oz	6.0	90	60%
natural/no salt added	1 oz	8.0	110	65%
■ BONBEL (See (Laughing Cow) in this section)				
■ (Borden)/Processed				
American				
singles				
16 slices	1 oz	5.0	70	64%
24 slices	⅔ oz	4.5	60	68%

Food and Description	Amount	Fat Grams	Total Calories	% Fat Calories
Big Bread size	½ oz	6.0	80	68%
fat-free	1 slice	–	30	–
California				
cheddar..all styles	1 oz	9.0	110	65%
Monterey Jack	1 oz	8.0	100	72%
mozzarella/Lite Line	1 oz	2.0	50	36%
Swiss				
cheese food	⅔ oz	5.0	70	64%
fat-free	⅔ oz	–	25	–
Lite Line	1 oz	2.0	50	36%
sliced	1 oz	8.0	100	72%
■ (Cabot)				
cheddar				
aged w/horseradish				
brick	1 oz	9.0	110	74%
5-peppercorn/brick	1 oz	9.0	110	74%
light	1 oz	4.5	70	58%
mild/slices	1 oz	9.0	110	74%
sharp..all styles	1 oz	9.0	110	74%
tomato basil/brick	1 oz	9.0	110	74%
Monterey Jack/shredded	1 oz	9.0	110	74%
mozzarella Fancy blend/shredded	1 oz	7.0	100	63%
pepper Jack slices	1 oz	9.0	110	74%
Vermont				
extra sharp/brick	1 oz	9.0	110	74%
Hunter's seriously				
sharp cheddar/brick	1 oz	9.0	110	74%
light				
brick	1 oz	4.5	70	58%
slices	1 oz	4.5	70	58%
mild/brick	1 oz	9.0	110	74%
pepper Jack/brick	1 oz	9.0	110	74%
sharp				
brick	1 oz	9.0	110	74%
slices	1 oz	9.0	110	74%
■ (Chavrie)				
goat's milk cheese				
regular	1.1 oz	4.0	50	72%
w/basil				
& roasted garlic	1.1 oz	4.0	50	72%
■ (Churny)				
Maybud				
Edam/reduced-fat	1 oz	5.0	80	56%
farmers	1 oz	8.0	100	72%
Gouda/reduced-fat	1 oz	5.0	80	56%
Lite Line	1 oz	2.0	50	36%
regular..snack	1 oz	3.0	70	39%
■ (Cornville)				
Brie	1 oz	7.0	90	70%
Camembert	1 oz	7.0	90	70%

Food and Description	Amount	Fat Grams	Total Calories	% Fat Calories
■ (County Line)				
American/sliced				
16-count pkg	1 slice	5.0	70	64%
cheddar				
all styles	1 oz	10.0	120	75%
Colby				
jack	1 oz	9.0	110	74%
medium sharp	1 oz	10.0	120	75%
mild				
chunk	1 oz	10.0	120	75%
sliced	1 slice	9.0	110	74%
sharp	1 oz	10.0	120	75%
garden Jack	1 oz	9.0	110	74%
Monterey Jack	1 oz	9.0	110	74%
mozzarella				
part-skim/low-moisture				
finely shredded	¼ cup	5.0	80	56%
regular/chunk	1 oz	5.0	80	56%
string	1 oz	5.0	80	56%
Muenster	1 oz	9.0	110	74%
Swiss, Old World	1 oz	8.0	110	65%
taco/shredded	¼ cup	10.0	120	75%
■ CRACKER BARREL (See (Kraft) in this section)				
■ (Di Giorono)				
Parmesan				
chunk	2 tsp	2.0	25	72%
grated	2 tsp	2.0	20	90%
shredded	2 tsp	2.0	20	90%
Romano				
chunk	2 tsp	2.0	25	72%
grated	2 tsp	2.0	25	90%
shredded	2 tsp	2.0	20	90%
■ (Dorman's)				
natural				
blue				
Castello/70%	1 oz	12.0	135	80%
Danablu				
40%	1 oz	8.0	100	72%
60%	1 oz	10.0	110	82%
brick	1 oz	9.0	110	74%
Brie	1 oz	6.5	80	73%
Camembert/50%	1 oz	7.0	90	70%
cheddar				
reduced-fat/low sodium	1 oz	5.0	80	56%
regular	1 oz	9.0	110	74%
Colby	1 oz	9.0	110	74%
Edam	1 oz	8.0	100	72%
feta/45%	1 oz	7.0	90	70%
Gouda	1 oz	8.0	100	72%

Food and Description	Amount	Fat Grams	Total Calories	% Fat Calories
Havarti				
45%	1 oz	7.0	90	70%
60%	1 oz	11.0	120	83%
Monterey Jack				
reduced-fat/low-sodium	1 oz	5.0	80	56%
regular	1 oz	8.0	100	72%
mozzarella				
part-skim/low-sodium	1 oz	5.0	80	56%
reduced-fat/low-sodium	1 oz	4.0	80	45%
regular	1 oz	6.0	90	60%
Muenster				
low-sodium	1 oz	9.0	110	74%
reduced-fat/low-sodium	1 oz	5.0	80	56%
regular	1 oz	9.0	100	81%
Parmesan	1 oz	9.0	130	62%
provolone				
reduced-fat/low-sodium	1 oz	4.0	80	45%
regular	1 oz	7.0	100	63%
Romano	1 oz	7.0	100	63%
Swiss				
no salt added	1 oz	8.0	100	72%
reduced-fat/low-sodium	1 oz	5.0	90	50%
regular	1 oz	8.0	100	72%
tybo/45%	1 oz	7.5	100	68%
■ **(Dragone)**				
mozzarella				
part-skim/low-moisture	1 oz	5.0	80	56%
shredded/all-natural	¼ cup	6.0	80	45%
string				
part-skim	1 oz	6.0	80	45%
whole milk	1 oz	7.0	90	70%
Parmesan				
all styles	1 oz	7.0	110	57%
grated/shredded	¼ cup	7.0	110	57%
ricotta				
part skim	¼ cup	6.0	90	60%
whole milk	¼ cup	7.0	100	63%
■ **(Finlandia)**				
imported				
Gouda stick	1 oz	8.0	100	72%
Havarti stick	1 oz	8.0	100	72%
Muenster				
loaf	1 oz	8.0	100	72%
stick	1 oz	9.0	110	65%
Swiss				
Heavenly Light				
loaf	1 oz	4.0	80	45%
stick	1 oz	8.0	110	65%
high cut loaf	1 oz	8.0	110	65%
regular stick	1 oz	8.0	110	65%

Food and Description	Amount	Fat Grams	Total Calories	% Fat Calories
Sandwich Naturals/imported				
Gouda	1 oz	8.0	100	72%
Havarti	1 oz	9.0	110	65%
light Swiss	1 oz	4.0	80	45%
Muenster	1 oz	9.0	110	65%
Swiss	1 oz	8.0	110	65%
■ **(Friendship)**				
farmer	2 Tbs	2.5	50	45%
hoop	2 Tbs	2.0	20	90%
■ **(Frigo)**				
Cheese Heads/100% natural Mini Bars				
Colby Jack	¾ oz	7.0	80	90%
mild cheddar	¾ oz	7.0	80	90%
Cheese Heads/100% natural string cheese				
cheddar swirls	1 oz	6.0	80	45%
light natural	1 oz	3.0	60	45%
mozzarella & cheddar				
swirls/12-count	1 oz	5.0	80	56%
mozzarella				
part-skim/low-moisture	1 oz	5.0	80	56%
shredded/all-natural	¼ cup	6.0	80	45%
string				
part-skim	1 oz	6.0	80	45%
whole milk	1 oz	7.0	90	70%
Parmesan				
all styles	1 oz	7.0	110	57%
grated/shredded	¼ cup	7.0	100	63%
Parmesan & Romano				
all styles	1 oz	7.0	110	57%
grated/shredded	1 oz	9.0	130	62%
pizza/shredded	1 oz	3.0	65	42%
provolone/lite	1 oz	4.0	70	51%
ricotta				
low-salt	¼ cup	8.0	110	65%
part-skim	¼ cup	6.0	90	60%
whole milk	¼ cup	8.0	110	65%
Romano				
grated	1 oz	8.0	110	65%
grated/dry	1 oz	9.0	130	62%
shredded	¼ cup	7.0	100	63%
whole	1 oz	8.0	110	65%
■ **(Healthy Choice)**				
American				
white singles	¾ oz	1.0	40	23%
yellow singles	¾ oz	1.0	40	23%
94% fat-free				
cheddar/shredded	¼ cup	1.5	50	27%
Colby Jack	1 oz	1.5	50	27%
garlic & herbs/shredded	¼ cup	1.5	50	27%
Italian/shredded	¼ cup	1.5	50	27%

Food and Description	Amount	Fat Grams	Total Calories	% Fat Calories
jalapeño singles	¾ oz	1.0	40	23%
Mexican/shredded	¼ cup	1.5	50	27%
mozzarella	1 oz	1.5	50	27%
string	1 oz	1.5	50	27%
pizza..all styles	1 oz	1.5	50	27%
process cheese loaf	1" cube	–	35	–
Swiss singles	1 oz	1.0	40	23%
■ (Hickory Farms)				
Neufchatel				
chocolate	1 oz	8.0	110	65%
orange	1 oz	8.0	100	72%
peach	1 oz	8.0	90	80%
pineapple	1 oz	8.0	90	80%
rum date nut	1 oz	8.0	100	72%
strawberry	1 oz	8.0	90	80%
■ (Hoffman)..processed cheese food				
hot pepper	1 oz	7.0	90	70%
smoky sharp	1 oz	9.0	110	74%
super sharp	1 oz	9.0	110	74%
■ (Kaukauna)				
deli style				
cheese balls				
cheddar				
extra sharp				
w/almonds	1 oz	7.0	100	63%
garden vegetable w/almonds	1 oz	10.0	120	75%
horseradish w/almonds	1 oz	6.0	90	60%
port wine	1 oz	7.0	90	70%
sharp w/almonds/hazelnuts	1 oz	6.0	90	60%
smokey bacon w/almonds	1 oz	6.0	90	60%
cheese logs..cheddar				
double sharp w/almonds	1 oz	6.0	90	60%
garlic & herb w/almonds	1 oz	10.0	120	75%
port wine w/almonds	1 oz	6.0	90	60%
sharp w/almonds & hazelnuts	1 oz	6.0	90	60%
sharp hickory/smoke w/almonds	1 oz	6.0	90	60%
■ (Kraft)				
100% GRATED PARMESAN CHEESES				
grated				
Parmesan	2 tsp	1.5	20	68%
Parmesan & Romano	2 tsp	1.5	20	68%
Parmesan original	2 tsp	1.5	20	68%
Parmesan-style				
reduced-fat	2 tsp	1.0	20	45%
Romano	2 tsp	1.5	20	68%
shredded				
Parmesan	1 oz	8.0	110	65%
Parmesan-Romano				
& Asiago	1 oz	8.0	110	65%

Food and Description	Amount	Fat Grams	Total Calories	% Fat Calories
CRACKER BARREL—Natural Cheeses				
baby Swiss	1 oz	9.0	110	74%
cheddar				
extra sharp	1 oz	10.0	120	75%
cheese cuts	1 oz	10.0	120	75%
extra sharp white				
reduced-fat	1 oz	6.0	90	60%
sharp	1 oz	10.0	120	75%
sharp/slices	~1 oz	8.0	90	80%
sharp 2% milk reduced-fat	1 oz	6.0	90	60%
Vermont sharp				
cheese cuts	1 oz	10.0	120	75%
white	1 oz	9.0	110	74%
KRAFT DELI DELUXE CHEESES				
American slices				
16-count pkg	¾ oz	7.0	80	79%
24-count pkg	⅔ oz	6.0	70	77%
cheddar				
sharp/slices 10-count pkg	~1 oz	8.0	90	80%
Colby Jack slices 10-count pkg	~1 oz	7.0	90	70%
mozzarella/low-moisture				
slices/11-count pkg	¾ oz	5.0	60	75%
pepper Jack slices 10-count pkg	~1 oz	7.0	90	70%
Swiss slices				
11-count pkg	¾ oz	7.0	80	79%
16-count pkg	½ oz	5.0	70	64%
KRAFT EASY CHEESES				
American	~1 oz	6.0	90	60%
cheddar	~1 oz	6.0	90	60%
bacon	~1 oz	7.0	90	70%
sharp	~1 oz	6.0	90	60%
nacho cheese	~1 oz	7.0	90	70%
STRING CHEESES				
cheese sticks/Twist-ums				
mozzarella	1 oz	4.0	60	60%
mozarella & cheddar	1.13 oz	6.0	90	60%
NATURAL BRICK CHEESES				
cheddar				
& Monterey Jack				
cube cheese	1 oz	10.0	120	75%
marbled	1 oz	7.0	90	70%
shredded	1 oz	8.0	100	72%
bacon	1 oz	7.0	90	70%
extra sharp	1 oz	10.0	120	75%
medium				
8-oz brick	1 oz	9.0	110	74%
16-oz brick	1 oz	10.0	120	75%
mild				
2% milk reduced-fat	1 oz	6.0	80	68%
cube cheese	1 oz	11.0	130	76%

Food and Description	Amount	Fat Grams	Total Calories	% Fat Calories
longhorn	1 oz	9.0	110	74%
regular	1 oz	9.0	110	74%
shredded	1 oz	8.0	100	72%
finely	1 oz	9.0	110	74%
sharp				
2% milk reduced-fat	1 oz	6.0	80	68%
cube cheese	1 oz	11.0	130	76%
extra sharp	1 oz	10.0	120	75%
regular/16-oz brick	1 oz	10.0	120	75%
shredded	1 oz	9.0	110	74%
fat-free	1 oz	–	40	–
finely	1 oz	10.0	120	75%
Colby	1 oz	9.0	110	74%
2% milk reduced-fat	1 oz	6.0	80	68%
longhorn-style	1 oz	9.0	110	74%
midget	1 oz	9.0	110	74%
& Monterey Jack	1 oz	9.0	110	74%
cube cheese	1 oz	10.0	120	75%
marbled	1 oz	9.0	110	74%
Monterey Jack	1 oz	9.0	100	81%
2% milk reduced-fat	1 oz	6.0	80	68%
mozzarella..all styles	1 oz	5.0	80	56%
KRAFT NATURAL SHREDDED CHEESES				
Cheese Italian Style				
classic garlic				
w/seasonings	1 oz	10.0	120	75%
mozzarella & Parmesan				
finely shredded	1 oz	8.0	100	72%
Cheese Mexican Style/finely shredded				
cheddar Jack	1 oz	9.0	110	74%
w/jalapeño peppers	1 oz	9.0	110	74%
taco	1 oz	10.0	120	75%
classic melts				
cheddar & American	1 oz	10.0	120	75%
cheddar Jack & American	1 oz	10.0	120	75%
4-cheese	1 oz	10.0	120	75%
Italian-style 5-cheese	1 oz	6.0	90	60%
Mexican-style 4-cheese	1 oz	9.0	100	81%
mild cheddar 2% milk				
finely shredded				
8-oz bag	1 oz	6.0	80	68%
12-oz bag	1 oz	9.0	110	74%
Monterey Jack	1 oz	8.0	100	72%
mozzarella				
2% milk reduced-fat	1 oz	4.5	70	58%
fat-free	1 oz	–	45	–
low-moisture				
finely shredded	1 oz	4.5	70	58%
regular shredded	1 oz	5.0	80	56%

Food and Description	Amount	Fat Grams	Total Calories	% Fat Calories
pizza mozzarella				
& provolone	1 oz	7.0	90	70%
4-cheese	1 oz	7.0	90	70%
Swiss	1 oz	8.0	110	65%
KRAFT SINGLES				
American				
2% milk reduced-fat	1 slice	3.0	50	54%
regular/yellow	1 slice	4.5	60	68%
cheddar/sharp				
2% milk reduced-fat	1 slice	3.0	50	54%
manchego singles	1 slice	5.0	70	54%
mozzarella				
2% milk reduced-fat	1 slice	3.0	50	54%
regular 96-count box	1 slice	4.5	60	68%
pepper Jack				
2% milk reduced-fat	1 slice	3.0	50	54%
Swiss 2% milk reduced-fat	1 slice	3.0	50	54%
POLLY-O				
bite-size balls	1.5 oz	10.0	120	75%
cherry-size balls	1 oz	7.0	80	79%
shredded				
fat-free	¼ cup	–	45	–
lite	¼ cup	3.0	60	45%
part skim	¼ cup	5.0	80	56%
whole milk	¼ cup	7.0	90	70%
mozzarella w/Parmesan	¼ cup	8.0	100	72%
Parmesan/grated	2 tsp	1.5	20	27%
Parmesan & Romano				
grated	2 tsp	1.5	20	27%
ricotta				
fat-free	¼ cup	–	50	–
lite	¼ cup	3.0	70	39%
part-skim	¼ cup	6.0	90	60%
whole milk	¼ cup	8.0	110	65%
string cheese				
String-Ums & Polly-O				
mozzarella				
reduced-fat	1 oz	4.5	80	51%
regular	1 oz	6.0	80	68%
Twistarellas				
regular	1.13 oz	7.0	100	63%
	¾ oz	4.0	60	60%
super long	1.5 oz	9.0	120	60%
VELVEETA				
light loaf	1 oz	3.0	60	45%
Mexican loaf				
hot	1 oz	6.0	90	60%
mild				
loaf	1 oz	6.0	90	60%
shredded	¼ cup	9.0	130	60%

Food and Description	Amount	Fat Grams	Total Calories	% Fat Calories
original				
16-oz box/loaf	1 oz	6.0	90	60%
shredded	¼ cup	9.0	130	62%
slices/16-count pkg	¾ oz	4.5	60	68%
■ (Land O'Lakes)				
DELI CHEESES/Chunk				
Havarti	1 oz	8.0	110	65%
other				
cheddar white	1 oz	9.0	110	74%
Co-Jack semisoft	1 oz	9.0	110	74%
pepper Jack	1 oz	9.0	110	74%
NATURAL CHEESES				
American				
2# loaf	1 oz	9.0	110	74%
Golden Velvet	1 oz	6.0	80	68%
brick	1 oz	8.0	100	72%
chedarella	1 oz	8.0	100	72%
pre-sliced	1 slice	9.0	110	74%
semi-soft	1 oz	9.0	100	82%
pre-sliced	1 slice	9.0	110	74%
cheddar				
extra sharp	1 oz	9.0	110	74%
medium	1 oz	9.0	110	74%
mild	1 oz	9.0	110	74%
pre-sliced	1 oz	9.0	110	74%
sharp				
chunk	1 oz	9.0	110	74%
pre-sliced	1 slice	9.0	110	74%
white sharp	1 oz	9.0	110	74%
Co-Jack				
chunk	1 oz	9.0	110	74%
pre-sliced	1 slice	9.0	110	74%
Colby	1 oz	9.0	110	74%
pre-sliced	1 sice	9.0	110	74%
Havarti				
chunk	1 oz	8.0	110	65%
pre-sliced	1 slice	8.0	110	65%
Monterey Jack				
hot	1 oz	9.0	110	74%
regular	1 oz	9.0	110	74%
mozarella/pasteurized				
part-skim	1 oz	6.0	80	68%
pre-sliced	1 slice	6.0	80	68%
Muenster/pre-sliced	1 slice	8.0	100	72%
pepper Jack/pre-sliced	1 slice	9.0	110	74%
provolone w/smoke flavor				
pre-sliced	1 slice	8.0	100	72%
Snack'n Cheese to-Go				
chedarella	1 portion	7.0	80	79%

Food and Description	Amount	Fat Grams	Total Calories	% Fat Calories
cheddar				
medium	1 portion	7.0	80	79%
mild	1 portion	7.0	80	79%
Co-Jack	1 portion	7.0	80	79%
Monterey Jack	1 portion	7.0	80	79%
Swiss/pre-sliced	1 slice	8.0	110	65%
baby	1 oz	8.0	110	65%
pre-sliced/baby	1 slice	8.0	110	65%
PROCESSED CHEESES				
American				
pasteurized/pre-sliced				
sharp	1 slice	9.0	110	74%
white	1 slice	9.0	110	74%
yellow	1 slice	9.0	110	74%
singles ¾ oz				
individually				
wrapped	1 slice	5.0	70	64%
Jalapeño peppers				
pre-sliced	1 slice	7.0	90	70%
■ (Laughing Cow)				
NATURAL CHEESE				
Babybel/mini				
Bonbel	1 piece	6.0	70	77%
Gouda	1 piece	6.0	80	68%
mild cheddar	1 piece	5.0	70	64%
original				
light	1 piece	3.0	50	54%
regular	1 piece	6.0	70	77%
Cheezbits	6 pieces	6.0	70	77%
Gourmet Cheese				
& Baguettes	1 unit	4.5	75	54%
wedges				
creamy Swiss				
light creamy				
French onion	1 wedge	2.0	35	51%
garlic & herb	1 wedge	2.0	35	51%
Swiss original	1 wedge	2.0	35	51%
original creamy Swiss	1 wedge	4.0	50	72%
■ (Lifetime)				
fat-free..all styles	1 oz	–	40	–
■ LIGHT 'N' LIVELY (*See* COTTAGE CHEESE)				
■ (Litehouse)				
Idaho bleu cheese..crumbles	¼ cup	8.0	100	72%
■ (Miceli's)				
SPECIALTY & IMPORTED CHEESE				
cheddar/mild				
classic cut	1 oz	9.0	110	74%
mozzarella/fresh				
ciliegini				
classic cut	1 oz	5.0	80	56%

Food and Description	Amount	Fat Grams	Total Calories	% Fat Calories
fancy	1 oz	5.0	80	56%
ovoline	1 oz	5.0	70	64%
sliced	1 oz	5.0	80	56%
Parmesan				
grated	1 oz	1.5	20	68%
wedge	1 oz	7.0	100	63%
pizza				
classic cut/shredded	1 oz	6.0	80	68%
ricotta				
Chicago-style	2 oz	6.0	90	60%
fat-free	2 oz	–	45	–
light/low-fat	~2 oz	2.5	60	38%
part-skim	2 oz	5.0	80	56%
traditional	~2 oz	6.0	90	60%
■ (MONTRACHET) (See (Alouette) in this section)				
■ (Nikos)				
feta cheese-crumbled/tub				
plain	1 oz	6.0	80	68%
w/tomato & basil	1 oz	8.0	100	72%
■ (Polly-O) (See (Kraft) in this section)				
■ (Precious)				
mozzarella/part-skim	1 oz	6.0	80	68%
ricotta				
part-skim				
fat-free	¼ cup	–	40	–
low-fat	¼ cup	3.0	60	45%
original	¼ cup	6.0	100	54%
whole milk	¼ cup	8.0	110	65%
string/part-skim	1 oz	6.0	80	68%
■ (Quaker)				
pimiento loaf	2 Tbs	8.0	80	90%
relish loaf	2 Tbs	8.0	80	90%
scallion loaf	2 Tbs	9.0	90	90%
■ (Saladena) specialty & imported				
blue crumbles	1 oz	9.0	100	81%
feta	1 oz	7.0	90	70%
crumbles	1 oz	7.0	90	70%
Mediterranean	1 oz	6.0	90	60%
goat crumbles	1 oz	7.0	90	70%
Gorgonzola crumbles	1 oz	9.0	100	81%
Provençal	1 oz	6.0	80	68%
■ (Sargento)				
DELI-STYLE/Sliced Cheeses				
American Burger Cheese	1 slice	6.0	70	77%
cheddar				
medium	1 slice	6.0	80	68%
sharp	1 slice	6.0	80	68%
Colby	1 slice	7.0	80	79%
jarlsberg	1 slice	6.0	80	68%
Monterey Jack	1 slice	6.0	80	68%

Food and Description	Amount	Fat Grams	Total Calories	% Fat Calories
mozzarella	1 slice	4.0	60	60%
Muenster	1 slice	6.0	80	68%
provolone				
reduced-fat	1 slice	3.5	50	63%
regular	1 slice	5.0	70	64%
Swiss				
8-oz brick				
thick	1 slice	8.0	110	65%
thin	1 slice	5.0	70	64%
aged	1 slice	5.0	70	64%
reduced-fat	1 slice	4.0	60	60%
OTHER FINE CHEESES				
blue cheese/crumbled	¼ cup	8.0	100	72%
Parmesan/grated	2 tsp	1.5	25	54%
Parmesan & Romano	2 tsp	1.5	25	54%
ricotta				
fat-free	¼ cup	–	50	–
light	¼ cup	2.5	60	38%
part-skim	¼ cup	4.5	70	58%
whole-milk	¼ cup	6.0	90	60%
SHREDDED CHEESES				
Cheese blends				
4-cheese Mexican	¼ cup	9.0	110	74%
6-cheese Italian	¼ cup	7.0	90	70%
angel hair Parmesan, mozzarella				
& Romano	¼ cup	7.0	100	63%
cheddar Jack..all types	¼ cup	9.0	110	74%
Italian w/garlic	¼ cup	7.0	100	63%
mozzarella				
& provolone	¼ cup	7.0	90	70%
pepper Jack				
w/habañeros	¼ cup	7.0	90	70%
nacho & taco	¼ cup	9.0	110	74%
Parmesan & Romano	2 tsp	1.5	20	68%
pizza double cheese	¼ cup	6.0	90	60%
taco	¼ cup	9.0	110	74%
ChefStyle..cheddar				
all styles	¼ cup	9.0	110	74%
fancy				
Asiago/extra fine	2 tsp	1.5	20	68%
cheddar..all styles	¼ cup	9.0	110	74%
Colby Jack	¼ cup	9.0	110	74%
Monterey Jack	¼ cup	9.0	110	74%
mozzarella	¼ cup	6.0	80	68%
Parmesan	2 tsp	1.5	20	68%
Swiss	¼ cup	8.0	110	65%
reduced-fat				
4-cheese Italian	¼ cup	4.5	80	51%
4-cheese Mexican	¼ cup	6.0	80	68%

Food and Description	Amount	Fat Grams	Total Calories	% Fat Calories
cheddar/mild	¼ cup	6.0	80	68%
mozzarella	¼ cup	4.5	80	51%
SNACK CHEESES				
sticks				
cheddar				
mild				
6-count pkg	1 piece	8.0	100	72%
singles	1 piece	9.0	110	74%
Colby Jack				
6-count pkg	1 stick	7.0	80	79%
12-count pkg	1 piece	9.0	110	74%
single	1 piece	9.0	110	74%
Twirls/2-colored mozzarella				
6-pk pkg	1 piece	4.5	70	58%
12-pk pkg	1 piece	6.0	80	68%
singles	1 piece	6.0	80	68%
■ **(Stella)**				
BLENDS				
3-cheese				
European	¼ cup	8.0	100	72%
Italian	¼ cup	7.0	100	63%
Mediterranean	¼ cup	7.0	90	70%
Parmesan & Romano	¼ cup	6.0	100	60%
OTHER CHEESES				
Asiago/shredded	1 Tbs	2.5	30	75%
blue/crumbled	¼ cup	8.0	100	72%
feta/crumbled	¼ cup	4.5	70	58%
fontinella	1 oz	9.0	110	74%
Gorgonzola	¼ cup	8.0	100	72%
Romano	¼ cup	7.0	100	63%
Kasseri	1 oz	9.0	110	65%
Parmesan/shredded	¼ cup	7.0	100	63%
Swiss/natural	1 oz	8.0	100	72%
■ **(Treasure Cave)**				
blue cheese	¼ cup	8.0	100	72%
feta	¼ cup	4.5	60	68%
Gorgonzola	¼ cup	8.0	100	72%
Italian blend	¼ cup	7.0	110	57%
Parmesan	¼ cup	8.0	110	65%
Romano	¼ cup	7.0	110	57%
■ **(Weight Watchers)**				
fat-free				
American/white or yellow fat-free				
all styles	¾ oz	–	30	–
cheddar				
fat-free..all styles	¾ oz	–	30	–
low-fat..all styles	1 oz	5.0	80	56%
Parmesan/fat-free..grated	1 Tbs	–	15	–
Swiss/fat-free/sliced	¾ oz	–	30	–

Food and Description	Amount	Fat Grams	Total Calories	% Fat Calories
■ (WisPride)				
cheddar cheese ball				
sharp cheddar w/almonds				
& hazelnuts	1 oz	6.0	90	60%
Swiss w/almonds	1 oz	6.0	80	68%
CHEESE, COTTAGE (See COTTAGE CHEESE)				
CHEESE, CREAM (See CREAM CHEESE)				
CHEESE ALTERNATIVE/IMITATION				
■ (CEMAC) Nu Tofu				
fat-free..all styles				
regular...all styles	1 oz	4.0	70	51%
regular	1 oz	4.0	70	51%
■ (DORMAN'S) Lo-Chol				
cheddar	1 oz	7.0	100	63%
Colby	1 oz	7.0	100	63%
mozzarella	1 oz	6.0	90	60%
Muenster	1 oz	7.0	100	63%
Swiss	1 oz	7.0	100	63%
■ (FORMAGGI)				
American/sliced				
classic	1 oz	3.0	60	45%
white	1 slice	4.0	60	60%
yellow	1 slice	4.0	60	60%
zesty jalapeño	1 oz	3.0	60	45%
cheddar				
shredded	1 oz	3.0	60	45%
sliced	1 slice	4.0	60	60%
Parmesan/grated	2 tsp	1.0	15	60%
provolone/vintage	1 oz	3.0	60	45%
mozzarella/shredded	1 oz	3.0	60	45%
ricotta/fat-free	½ cup	–	40	–
Swiss/sliced	1 oz	3.0	60	45%
■ (FRIGO)				
cheddar	1 oz	7.0	90	70%
mozzarella	1 oz	7.0	90	70%
■ (Galaxy)				
soy cheese..all styles	1 oz	3.0	60	45%
■ (SMART BEAT) lactose-free				
American ⅔-oz slices	1 slice	–	25	–
cheddar ⅔-oz slices				
creamy	1 slice	2.0	40	45%
low-sodium	1 slice	–	25	–
mellow	1 slice	–	25	–
sharp	1 slice	–	25	–
■ (SOYA KAAS) tofu				
American cheddar/mild	1 oz	5.0	70	64%
garlic & herb	1 oz	5.0	70	64%
hickory smoked cheddar	1 oz	5.0	80	56%
mozzarella				
fat-free	1 oz	–	40	–
regular	1 oz	5.0	70	64%

Food and Description	Amount	Fat Grams	Total Calories	% Fat Calories
■ **(SOYCO) tofu**				
American/sliced				
mozzarella	1 slice	3.0	50	54%
Swiss				
regular	1 slice	3.0	50	54%
veggie	1 slice	2.0	40	45%
yellow				
regular	1 slice	3.0	50	54%
veggie	1 slice	2.0	40	45%
Caesar's Italian/grated	2 tsp	0.5	15	30%
Cajun/grated	2 tsp	0.5	15	30%
cheddar				
baked potato/grated	2 tsp	0.5	15	30%
fat-free	1 oz	–	30	–
low-fat	1 oz	3.0	60	45%
jalapeño				
fat-free	1 oz	–	30	–
low-fat	1 oz	3.0	60	45%
Monterey/low-fat	1 oz	3.0	60	45%
mozzarella				
fat-free	1 oz	–	30	–
low-fat	1 oz	3.0	60	45%
veggie/sliced	1 slice	2.0	40	45%
Parmesan/grated	2 tsp	0.5	15	30%
pepper Jack/veggie				
sliced	1 slice	2.0	40	45%
provolone/veggie/sliced	1 slice	2.0	40	45%
Romano/grated	2 tsp	0.5	15	30%
■ **(SOYMAGE) tofu**				
American/yellow/sliced	1 slice	–	20	–
cheddar	1 oz	–	40	–
grated cheese	2 tsp	0.5	15	30%
herb	1 oz	–	40	–
jalapeño	1 oz	–	40	–
mozzarella				
chunk	1 oz	–	40	–
sliced	1 slice	–	20	–
■ **(TOFUTTI) Better Than Cream Cheese**				
French onion	2 Tbs	8.0	80	90%
broccoli & cheddar	2 Tbs	8.0	80	90%
creamed spinach	2 Tbs	8.0	80	90%
garden vegetable	2 Tbs	8.0	80	90%
garlic & herb	2 Tbs	8.0	80	90%
herbs & chives	2 Tbs	8.0	80	90%
plain	2 Tbs	8.0	80	90%
smoked salmon	2 Tbs	8.0	80	90%
■ **(YVES) The Good Slice**				
all styles	1 slice	2.0	35	51%

CHEESE DIP (See DIP)

CHEESE DISH (See FROZEN ENTRÉE/DINNER; VEGETARIAN FOODS; WELSH RAREBIT)

Food and Description	Amount	Fat Grams	Total Calories	% Fat Calories
CHEESE SAUCE (*See* SAUCE)				
CHEESE SEASONING (*See* SEASONINGS)				
CHEESE SNACK (*See* SNACKS)				
CHEESE SOUP (*See* SOUP)				
CHEESE SPREAD (*See* CHEESE ALTERNATIVE/IMITATION; CREAM CHEESE)				
■ **(Alouette)**				
crème de Brie				
fines herbs	1 oz	8.0	220	33%
original	1 oz	8.0	220	33%
crème fraîche				
cooking & topping	1 oz	11.0	100	99%
gourmet layered/elegante				
roasted garlic & pesto	1 oz	10.0	100	90%
roasted sweet peppers				
& olive tapenade	1 oz	9.0	90	90%
sun-dried tomato/garlic	1 oz	9.0	100	72%
spreadable cheeses				
cucumber dill/light	1 oz	4.0	50	72%
garlic & herbs				
light	1 oz	4.0	50	72%
regular	1 oz	7.0	70	90%
peppercorn Parmesan	1 oz	7.0	80	79%
savory vegetable	1 oz	6.0	60	90%
spinach artichoke	1 oz	6.0	60	90%
sun-dried tomato	1 oz	7.0	70	90%
triple onion	1 oz	7.0	70	90%
■ **(Chavrie)** goat cheese spread				
basil & roasted garlic	2 Tbs	4.0	50	72%
original	2 Tbs	4.0	50	72%
Cheez Whiz (*See* (Kraft) in this section)				
■ **(Connoisseur)**				
aged English cheddar	2 Tbs	8.0	100	72%
Asiago	2 Tbs	7.0	90	70%
Brie	2 Tbs	7.0	90	70%
Gorgonzola	2 Tbs	7.0	90	70%
Swiss	2 Tbs	7.0	90	70%
■ **(Fleur de Lait)**				
light..all flavors	2 Tbs	4.5	60	68%
Neufchâtel spread				
Bermuda onion	2 Tbs	8.0	90	80%
date nut rum	2 Tbs	8.0	90	80%
garden vegetable	2 Tbs	8.0	80	90%
garlic & spice	2 Tbs	9.0	90	90%
herb & spice	2 Tbs	9.0	90	90%
lemon	2 Tbs	7.0	90	70%
lox/smoked salmon	2 Tbs	8.0	90	80%
mandarin orange	2 Tbs	7.0	90	70%
peach	2 Tbs	7.0	90	70%

Food and Description	Amount	Fat Grams	Total Calories	% Fat Calories
pineapple	2 Tbs	8.0	90	80%
strawberry	2 Tbs	8.0	90	80%
toasted onion	2 Tbs	9.0	90	90%
wild berry	2 Tbs	7.0	90	70%
■ (Heluva Good Cheese)				
cheese food/cold pack				
all flavors	2 Tbs	7.0	90	70%
■ (Kaukauna)				
DELI-STYLE				
cheese balls				
cheddar				
extra sharp				
w/almonds	1 oz	7.0	100	63%
garden vegetable				
w/almonds	1 oz	10.0	120	75%
horseradish				
w/almonds	1 oz	6.0	90	60%
port wine	1 oz	7.0	90	70%
sharp				
w/almonds				
& hazelnuts	1 oz	6.0	90	60%
smokey bacon				
w/almonds	1 oz	6.0	90	60%
cheese logs				
cheddar				
double sharp				
w/almonds	1 oz	6.0	90	60%
garlic & herb				
w/almonds	1 oz	10.0	120	75%
port wine				
w/almonds	1 oz	6.0	90	60%
sharp w/almonds				
& hazelnuts	1 oz	6.0	90	60%
sharp hickory smoke				
w/almonds	1 oz	6.0	90	60%
COLD PACK CUPS				
Lite 50..all flavors	2 Tbs	3.5	70	45%
original..all flavors	2 Tbs	7.0	90	70%
Stone Crock/sharp cheddar	2 Tbs	7.0	90	70%
■ (Kraft)				
Cheez Whiz				
jarred				
light	2 Tbs	3.0	80	34%
original	2 Tbs	7.0	90	70%
salsa con queso	2 Tbs	7.0	90	70%
squeezable/plain	2 Tbs	8.0	100	72%
Cracker Barrel whipped spreadables/cheddar & cream cheese				
all types	2 Tbs	8.0	80	90%

Food and Description	Amount	Fat Grams	Total Calories	% Fat Calories
Old English brand				
sharp spread	2 Tbs	8.0	90	80%
regular Kraft jarred spreads				
bacon	2 Tbs	8.0	90	80%
jalapeño pepper loaf	1 oz	6.0	80	68%
olive & pimiento	2 Tbs	6.0	70	77%
pimiento	2 Tbs	6.0	80	68%
pineapple	2 Tbs	5.0	70	64%
Roka/blue				
cheese spread	2 Tbs	7.0	80	79%
Velveeta spread/Mexican				
all types	1 oz	6.0	90	60%
■ (Land O'Lakes)				
Golden Velvet	1 oz	6.0	80	68%
■ (Laughing Cow) Spreadable cheeses				
Babybel/mini spreadable				
cheddar	1 oz	5.0	70	64%
original	1 oz	6.0	70	77%
original spreadable				
light	1 oz	2.0	30	60%
regular	1 oz	4.0	50	72%
■ (Merkts)				
all flavors	2 Tbs	8.0	100	72%
■ (Nabisco) Easy Cheese spread				
American	2 Tbs	6.0	90	60%
cheddar				
regular	2 Tbs	6.0	90	60%
sharp	2 Tbs	6.0	90	60%
cheddar 'n' bacon	2 Tbs	7.0	90	70%
nacho	2 Tbs	7.0	90	70%
■ (Owl's Nest)				
bacon	2 Tbs	9.0	110	65%
cheddary				
ranch	2 Tbs	8.0	100	72%
w/sharp cheddar cheese	2 Tbs	9.0	110	65%
garlic	2 Tbs	8.0	100	72%
horseradish				
w/sharp cheddar cheese	2 Tbs	9.0	100	81%
peppers galore	2 Tbs	9.0	100	81%
port wine	2 Tbs	8.0	100	72%
Swiss almond	2 Tbs	8.0	100	72%
Vermont/sharp white cheddar	2 Tbs	8.0	100	72%
Roka (*See* (Kraft) in this section)				
■ (Rondele)				
Deli-cups				
garden vegetable	2 Tbs	9.0	90	90%
garlic & herb				
light	2 Tbs	5.0	70	64%
original	2 Tbs	9.0	100	81%

Food and Description	Amount	Fat Grams	Total Calories	% Fat Calories
roasted garlic				
& artichoke	2 Tbs	10.0	100	90%
Vidalia onion	2 Tbs	9.0	100	90%
Gourmet Wheel				
4-pepper	2 Tbs	9.0	90	90%
Mediterranean	2 Tbs	9.0	100	81%
Snack Pack garlic				
& herb	2 Tbs	9.0	100	81%
Velveeta (*See* (Kraft) in this section)				
■ (Wispride)				
COLD PACK..Cheddar				
Lite 50..all flavors	2 Tbs	3.5	70	45%
regular..all flavors	2 Tbs	7.0	90	70%
DELI-STYLE				
cheese balls				
cheddar				
& cream w/almonds	1 oz	7.0	100	63%
extra sharp				
w/almonds	1 oz	7.0	100	63%
sharp cheddar				
w/almonds	1 oz	6.0	90	60%
w/almonds				
& hazelnuts	1 oz	6.0	90	60%
garden vegetable				
w/almonds	1 oz	10.0	120	75%
garlic & herb	1 oz	10.0	120	75%
horseradish				
w/almonds	1 oz	6.0	90	60%
port wine w/almonds	1 oz	6.0	90	60%
smokey bacon w/almonds	1 oz	6.0	90	60%
Swiss w/almonds	1 oz	6.0	80	68%
cheese logs..cheddar..w/almonds				
all types & flavors	1 oz	6.0	90	60%
CHEESE SUBSTITUTE (*See* CHEESE ALTERNATIVE/IMITATION)				
CHERIMOYA				
raw/whole/medium	2 lbs	2.0	515	3%
CHERRY				
canned or jarred				
(C&S) maraschino				
w/stems	1 large	–	10	–
(Del Monte)				
dark sweet				
in heavy syrup	½ cup	–	100	–
(Giant Foods)				
light sweet in				
heavy syrup	⅔ cup	–	110	–
Oregon/pitted				
in heavy syrup	½ cup	–	110	–

Food and Description	Amount	Fat Grams	Total Calories	% Fat Calories
tart red/pitted				
in water	⅔ cup	–	60	–
(Musselman's) red tart				
pitted	4.2 oz	–	50	–
(S&W)				
dark sweet				
in heavy syrup	½ cup	–	140	–
maraschino				
green or red	1 cherry	–	10	–
royal Anne				
light/sweet/pitted	½ cup	–	140	–
dried				
(Chukar)				
bing	2 oz	1.0	160	6%
Rainier	2 oz	1.0	160	6%
tart	2 oz	–	170	–
tart 'n' sweet	2 oz	–	180	–
(Sonoma)				
bing	¼ cup	–	140	–
sweet tart	¼ cup	–	140	–
(Traverse Bay) cherry snax				
chocolate-covered	1.3 oz	7.0	70	90%
yogurt-covered	1.2 oz	5.0	150	30%
red tart	1 oz	–	100	–
fresh				
sour red	1 cup	<1.0	51	9%
sweet	10 medium	0.7	49	13%
	1 cup	1.0	103	9%
(Dole)	1 cup	1.0	90	10%
frozen				
(Big Valley) dark sweet	½ cup	–	60	–
(Cascadian Farm)				
dark sweet	1 cup	1.0	72	13%
sweet				
sweetened	1 cup	<1.0	232	2%
unsweetened	3.5 oz	<1.0	60	8%
glacé				
(S&W)				
green cherries	5 pieces	–	80	–
red cherries	5 pieces	–	80	–
(Seneca)				
cherries/all colors	6 pieces	–	90	–
cherry pineapple mix	2 Tbs	–	100	–
CHERRY DRINK (*See also* FRUIT PUNCH; SOFT DRINK MIX)				
bottled				
(R. W. Knudsen)				
black	11 fl oz	–	180	–
celebratory/sparkling				
organic cherry	8 fl oz	–	110	–
cider	8 fl oz	–	120	–

Food and Description	Amount	Fat Grams	Total Calories	% Fat Calories
frozen				
(R. W. Knudsen)				
from concentrate	8 fl oz	–	130	–
(Welch's) Welchade	8 fl oz	–	130	–
CHERRY JUICE/JUICE BLEND/JUICE DRINK				
bottled, boxed, or canned				
(After the Fall)				
black cherry spritzer	12 fl oz	–	180	–
(Dole) mountain cherry	8 fl oz	–	120	–
(Hi-C) wild cherry	8 fl oz	–	120	–
(Libby's) Juicy Juice	8 fl oz	–	140	–
(Walnut Acres) juice	8 fl oz	–	140	–
(Welch's) 100% Juice/pourable				
cherry sensation	11.5 oz	–	130	–
(Tropicana Twister)				
cherry berry	8 fl oz	–	130	–
cherry raspberry	8 fl oz	–	130	–
frozen/prepared				
(Cascadian Farm) mountain				
concentrate	2 oz	–	120	–
from concentrate	8 fl oz	–	120	–
(Dole) mountain cherry	8 fl oz	–	140	–
CHERVIL				
dried	1 tsp	–	1	–
raw	4 oz	–	65	–
CHESTNUT				
Chinese				
boiled or steamed	1 oz	–	44	–
dried	1 oz	0.5	103	4%
roasted	1 oz	–	68	–
European				
boiled or steamed	1 oz	–	37	–
dried	1 oz	1.0	106	8%
roasted	1 oz	0.6	70	8%
Japanese				
boiled or steamed	1 oz	–	16	–
dried	1 oz	–	102	–
roasted	1 oz	–	57	–
CHESTNUT FLOUR (See FLOUR)				
CHICKEN (See LUNCHEON MEAT; VEGETARIAN FOODS)				
■ **CHICKEN & CHICKEN PARTS/FRESH**				
broiler/fryer				
dark meat				
meat & skin				
batter-dipped				
& fried	~9.5 oz	51.8	828	56%
flour-coated				
& fried	~6.5 oz	31.0	523	53%
roasted	~6 oz	26.0	423	55%
stewed	~6.5 oz	27.0	428	57%

Food and Description	Amount	Fat Grams	Total Calories	% Fat Calories
meat only				
fried	~5 oz	16.0	334	43%
roasted	~5 oz	13.6	286	43%
stewed	~5 oz	12.6	269	42%
giblets/organs				
giblets/chopped or diced				
flour-coated & fried	1 cup	19.5	402	44%
simmered	1 cup	6.9	228	27%
gizzard/simmered	1 oz	1.0	43	21%
	1 cup	5.0	222	20%
heart/simmered	3 oz	5.0	158	29%
	1 cup	11.5	268	39%
liver/simmered	~5 oz	7.6	219	31%
	1 cup	7.6	220	31%
half/meat & skin				
batter-dipped & fried	~1 lb	80.8	1347	54%
flour-coated & fried	~¾ lb	46.8	844	50%
roasted	~¾ lb	40.7	715	51%
stewed	~¾ lb	42.0	730	52%
light meat				
meat & skin				
batter-dipped & fried	~7 oz	29.0	520	50%
flour-coated & fried	~5 oz	15.7	320	44%
roasted	~5 oz	14.0	293	43%
stewed	~5 oz	15.0	302	45%
meat only				
fried	~5 oz	7.8	268	26%
roasted	~5 oz	6.0	242	22%
stewed	~5 oz	5.6	223	23%
parts				
backs				
meat & skin				
batter-dipped & fried	~4 oz	26.0	397	59%
flour-coated & fried	~2.5 oz	14.9	238	56%
roasted	~2 oz	11.0	159	62%
stewed	~2 oz	11.0	158	63%
meat only				
fried	~2 oz	8.9	167	48%
roasted	~1.5 oz	5.0	96	47%
stewed	~1.5 oz	4.7	88	48%
breast				
meat & skin				
batter-dipped & fried	~5 oz	18.5	364	46%
flour-coated & fried	~3.5 oz	8.7	218	36%
roasted	~3.5 oz	7.6	193	35%
stewed	~4 oz	8.0	202	36%
meat only				
fried	~3 oz	4.0	161	22%
roasted	~3 oz	3.0	142	19%
stewed	~3 oz	2.9	144	18%

Food and Description	Amount	Fat Grams	Total Calories	% Fat Calories
drumstick				
meat & skin				
batter-dipped & fried	~2.5 oz	11.0	193	51%
flour-coated & fried	~2 oz	6.7	120	50%
roasted	~2 oz	5.8	112	47%
stewed	~2 oz	6.0	116	47%
meat only				
fried	~1.5 oz	3.0	82	33%
roasted	~1.5 oz	2.0	76	24%
stewed	~1.5 oz	2.6	78	30%
leg				
meat & skin				
batter-dipped & fried	~5.5 oz	25.6	431	53%
flour-coated & fried	~4 oz	16.0	285	51%
roasted	~4 oz	15.0	265	51%
stewed	~4 oz	16.0	275	52%
meat only				
fried	~3 oz	8.8	195	40%
roasted	~3 oz	8.0	182	40%
stewed	~3.5 oz	8.0	187	39%
thigh				
meat & skin				
batter-dipped & fried	~3 oz	14.0	238	53%
flour-coated & fried	~2 oz	9.0	162	50%
roasted	~2 oz	9.6	153	56%
stewed	~2 oz	10.0	158	57%
meat only				
fried	~2 oz	5.0	113	40%
roasted	~2 oz	5.7	109	47%
stewed	~2 oz	5.0	107	42%
wing				
meat & skin				
batter-dipped & fried	~2 oz	10.7	159	61%
flour-coated & fried	~1 oz	7.0	103	61%
roasted	~1.5 oz	6.6	99	60%
stewed	~1.5 oz	6.7	100	60%
meat only				
fried	~1 oz	1.8	42	39%
roasted	~1 oz	1.7	43	36%
stewed	~1 oz	1.7	43	36%
whole/including meat, skin, giblets & neck				
batter-dipped & fried	~2¼ lb	180.0	2987	54%
flour-coated & fried	~1½ lb	108.0	1928	50%
roasted	~1½ lb	90.0	1598	51%
stewed	~1½ lb	92.9	1625	52%
■ **CHICKEN & CHICKEN PARTS/FRESH or FROZEN/BRAND NAME**				
(Butterball) fresh/raw				
best of the fryer	4 oz	11.0	180	55%

Food and Description	Amount	Fat Grams	Total Calories	% Fat Calories
breast fillet/boneless/skinless				
seasoned				
Italian-style	1 fillet	1.5	110	12%
lemon butter	1 fillet	1.5	110	12%
mesquite	1 fillet	1.5	110	12%
teriyaki	1 fillet	1.5	110	12%
thin	1 fillet	1.0	110	8%
drumsticks	4 oz	8.0	160	45%
thighs/family pack				
regular	1 4 oz	15.0	210	64%
skinless	1 4 oz	4.0	120	30%
whole chicken/seasoned				
BBQ	4 oz	15.0	220	61%
herb garlic	4 oz	15.0	220	61%
regular	4 oz	15.0	210	64%
wings				
drummettes	3 pieces	11.0	170	58%
regular				
family pack	4 oz	16.0	220	65%
regular	4 oz	16.0	220	65%
(Perdue) fresh				
breast				
skinless & boneless				
individually frozen	5.9 oz	1.5	160	8%
thin sliced/boneless				
skinless	2.8 oz	1.5	80	17%
breast tenderloins				
individually frozen	4 oz	1.5	110	12%
Fit 'n' Easy				
breast				
skinless & boneless	4 oz	1.0	110	8%
tenderloins	4 oz	1.0	120	8%
ground				
breast	4 oz	0.5	100	5%
regular	4 oz	12.0	180	60%
regular burger patties	4 oz	11.0	170	90%
Oven Stuffers				
roaster breast,				
skinless & boneless	4 oz	2.0	130	14%
Ovenables/boneless/seasoned				
Home-style	4 oz	1.0	100	9%
Italian-style	4 oz	4.5	130	31%
lemon pepper	4 oz	1.0	110	8%
teriyaki	4 oz	1.0	110	8%
roasting chicken/seasoned				
honey-flavored				
dark	4 oz	20.0	260	69%
white	4 oz	10.0	190	47%

Food and Description	Amount	Fat Grams	Total Calories	% Fat Calories
toasted garlic				
dark	4 oz	21.0	260	73%
white	4 oz	10.0	180	50%
thighs/skinless & boneless				
individually frozen	6.2 oz	16.0	260	55%
(Tyson)				
FRESH UNCOOKED				
breast				
boneless, skinless	4 oz	1.5	110	12%
skinless split	4 oz	1.5	110	12%
split w/ribs	4 oz	10.0	180	50%
Tasty Selections/boneless/skinless				
lemon herb	4 oz	1.0	100	9%
tenders	4 oz	0.5	100	5%
drumsticks	4 oz	9.0	160	51%
skinless	4 oz	3.5	120	26%
ground	4 oz	9.0	150	54%
leg				
quarters	4 oz	13.0	190	62%
whole	4 oz	17.0	230	67%
thigh	4 oz	16.0	220	65%
boneless/skinless				
cutlets	4 oz	4.0	110	33%
skinless	4 oz	4.0	110	33%
whole chicken				
cut up	4 oz	16.0	220	65%
family roaster	4 oz	15.0	210	64%
young chicken	4 oz	15.0	210	64%
wings	4 pieces	18.0	240	68%
INDIVIDUALLY FRESH FROZEN				
breasts				
boneless, skinless/half				
w/rib meat	4 oz	3.5	170	19%
half	4 oz	12.0	230	47%
Cornish game hen				
w/o giblets	4 oz	14.0	200	63%
drumsticks	2 pieces	7.0	140	45%
tenderloins, boneless				
skinless	2 pieces	0.5	80	6%
thighs	1 piece	34.0	380	81%
boneless/skinless	1 piece	11.0	170	58%
wings	4 pieces	18.0	240	68%

CHICKEN ENTRÉE/DINNER/CANNED, FULLY COOKED, or READY-TO-COOK (*See also* ASIAN FOOD; FROZEN ENTRÉE/DINNER; MEXICAN FOOD; PASTA ENTRÉE/DINNER; RICE DISH)

Food and Description	Amount	Fat Grams	Total Calories	% Fat Calories
(Banquet) *FROZEN*				
breast tenders				
buffalo-style				
seasoned	3 oz	18.0	270	60%
original	3 oz	19.0	280	61%

Food and Description	Amount	Fat Grams	Total Calories	% Fat Calories
nuggets/breaded				
fun race car shapes	3 oz	20.0	280	64%
original	3 oz	20.0	280	64%
patties/family pack	3 oz	21.0	290	65%
original	3 oz	20.0	280	64%
patties				
breaded	2.7 oz	19.0	260	66%
pieces/assorted pieces				
crispy, skinless	3.75 oz	16.0	260	55%
original crispy	3.87 oz	18.0	270	60%
popcorn chicken				
breast fritters	3 oz	9.0	190	43%
wings/breaded honey BBQ	4 oz	20.0	290	62%
(Betty Crocker) *BOX MIX*				
Chicken Helper/prepared as directed				
4-cheese	1 cup	12.0	310	35%
cheddar & broccoli	1 cup	10.0	310	29%
cheesy chicken				
enchilada	1 cup	9.0	350	23%
chicken fried rice	1 cup	8.0	260	28%
chicken				
& herb rice	1 cup	7.0	260	24%
chicken & mashed potatoes				
home-style	1 cup	10.0	250	36%
chicken & stuffing	1 cup	9.0	290	28%
chicken potato				
au gratin	1 cup	7.0	270	23%
creamy roasted garlic	1 cup	8.0	280	26%
fettuccini Alfredo	1 cup	8.0	300	24%
teriyaki	1 cup	6.0	300	18%
Parmesan pasta	1 cup	8.0	290	25%
Southwestern	⅔ cup	5.0	240	19%
Complete Meals/prepared as directed				
chicken & buttermilk				
biscuits	⅕ pkg	13.0	320	37%
home-style dumplings				
& chicken	⅕ pkg	9.0	250	32%
Oven Favorites/prepared as directed				
cheddar & mozzarella/served				
w/1 Tbs cheese sauce	½ cup	13.0	340	34%
creamy chicken & rice	1 cup	13.0	330	35%
home-style chicken				
& biscuit bake	⅔ cup	11.0	340	29%
stuffing & gravy	⅔ cup	11.0	280	35%
potatoes au gratin	⅕ pkg	12.0	300	36%
(Boar's Head) *COOKED/READY-TO-COOK*				
breasts				
aroastica-seasoned	1 oz	1.0	60	8%
BarBQ sauce–basted	2 oz	0.5	60	8%
blazing buffalo–style	2 oz	1.0	60	15%

Food and Description	Amount	Fat Grams	Total Calories	% Fat Calories
hickory-smoked	2 oz	0.5	60	8%
oven-roasted	2 oz	1.0	60	15%
(Butterball) *FROZEN*				
breasts				
crispy-baked				
Italian-style	1 piece	6.0	190	19%
lemon	1 piece	7.0	200	32%
original	1 piece	6.0	180	30%
Parmesan	1 piece	7.0	200	32%
Southwestern	1 piece	6.0	170	32%
Tenders				
baked breast	3 pieces	6.0	170	32%
grilled w/sauce				
hickory smoked	4 pieces	5.0	160	28%
Oriental	4 pieces	5.0	160	28%
(Dinty Moore) *CANNED/MICROWAVEABLE*				
canned stew				
chicken & dumplings	1 cup	8.0	230	31%
chicken stew	1 cup	11.0	220	45%
individual canned serving				
chicken & dumplings	1 cup	6.0	200	27%
microwavable				
American classics				
chicken & dumplings	1 bowl	9.0	280	29%
chicken & noodles	1 bowl	8.0	260	28%
chicken & rice	1 bowl	10.0	250	36%
chicken				
w/mashed potatoes	1 bowl	4.0	240	15%
microwave cup				
chicken & dumpling	1 cup	6.0	200	27%
chicken stew	1 cup	8.0	180	40%
noodles & chicken	1 cup	9.0	190	43%
(Green Giant) frozen				
CREATE A MEAL!/as packaged				
chicken Alfredo	2 cups	6.0	230	23%
garlic herb	2⅓ cups	9.0	230	35%
lemon pepper chicken	1½ cup	0.5	140	3%
stir-fry				
garlic	1⅔ cup	1.5	130	10%
lo mein	2⅓ cup	1.5	170	8%
teriyaki	1¾ cup	0.5	100	5%
Parmesan herb chix	1¾ cup	2.5	160	14%
sweet & sour	1½ cup	—	180	—
COMPLETE SKILLET MEAL/as packaged				
chicken				
Alfredo	¼ pkg	6.0	270	20%
cheesy pasta	¼ pkg	6.0	270	20%
creamy chix noodle	¼ pkg	5.0	290	16%
garlic chicken pasta	¼ pkg	7.0	260	24%
lo mein	¼ pkg	2.5	200	11%

Food and Description	Amount	Fat Grams	Total Calories	% Fat Calories
sweet & sour chix	¼ pkg	1.5	320	4%
teriyaki	¼ pkg	1.5	250	5%
(Hormel)				
CANNED				
America's Choice				
chunk chicken				
in broth	2 oz	1.0	50	28%
breast of chicken				
no salt	2 oz	1.0	50	18%
regular	2 oz	1.0	50	18%
chunk chicken	2 oz	2.5	60	38%
lemon	2 oz	1.0	50	18%
Southwest	2 oz	1.0	50	18%
tomato basil w/garlic	2 oz	1.0	50	18%
(Lloyd's) in BBQ sauce	¼ cup	3.0	90	30%
(Louis Rich)				
READY-TO-COOK/refrigerated				
breast cuts				
honey-roasted	3 oz	2.5	130	17%
oven-roasted	3 oz	2.5	130	17%
breast strips				
breaded/restaurant-style	3 oz	6.0	170	32%
grilled/large	3 oz	3.0	110	25%
Italian-style	3 oz	3.0	110	25%
Southwestern				
large size	3 oz	3.0	110	25%
regular size	3 oz	3.0	110	25%
(Perdue) *FULLY COOKED*				
breast				
cutlets				
home-style	1 pattie	2.5	120	19%
Italian-style/white	1 pattie	3.0	130	21%
original	3 oz	10.0	190	47%
tenderloins/white	3 oz	2.5	140	16%
Fit 'n' Easy/skinless & boneless				
breast tenderloins	3 oz	0.5	100	5%
fresh/cooked				
Cornish hen				
dark	3 oz	14.0	200	63%
white	3 oz	8.0	160	45%
drumsticks/roasted	1 piece	6.0	110	49%
ground	3 oz	11.0	170	58%
leg quarters	3 oz	17.0	220	70%
soup & stew baking chicken				
dark	3 oz	15.0	210	64%
white	3 oz	9.0	170	48%
thighs/roasted	1 thigh	19.0	240	71%
thin sliced/skinless				
& boneless	2 oz	1.0	80	11%

Food and Description	Amount	Fat Grams	Total Calories	% Fat Calories
whole chicken/cooked				
dark	3 oz	16.0	210	69%
white	3 oz	10.0	170	53%
whole chicken/cut-up				
country-style				
dark	3 oz	16.0	210	69%
white	3 oz	10.0	170	53%
whole chicken/quartered				
dark	3 oz	17.0	220	70%
white	3 oz	10.0	170	53%
whole chicken legs/roasted	1 leg	27.0	370	65%
wings/roasted	2 wings	15.0	210	64%
ground				
breast	3 oz	0.5	80	6%
burgers	3 oz	10.0	160	56%
individually frozen/fully cooked				
breast/skinless				
& boneless	4.2 oz	1.5	140	10%
hot & spicy wings	3 oz	12.0	180	60%
nuggets/breast	3.4 oz	16.0	250	58%
tenderloins/breast	3 oz	1.0	100	9%
thighs/boneless				
& skinless	1 thigh	9.0	180	45%
nuggets				
baseball-shaped	2.7 oz	10.0	190	47%
basketball-shaped	2.7 oz	10.0	190	47%
breast tenderloin	3 oz	10.0	200	45%
breast/white	2.7 oz	9.0	180	45%
chicken & cheese	2.7 oz	10.0	190	47%
football-shaped	2.7 oz	10.0	190	47%
fun shapes				
star & drumstick	4 pieces	9.0	170	48%
Oven Stuffer Roaster				
drumsticks	1 piece	11.0	190	52%
roaster				
dark	3 oz	15.0	210	64%
white	3 oz	9.0	170	48%
roaster breast/white	3 oz	1.5	120	11%
whole breast	3 oz	8.0	150	48%
Wingettes	3 pieces	15.0	220	61%
(Reser's) *FRESH*				
refrigerated chicken salad	½ cup	21.0	270	70%
(Schwan's) *FROZEN*/partially or fully cooked unless stated otherwise				
chicken bites	3 oz	7.0	160	39%
chicken breast				
fillet				
breaded	1 fillet	11.0	270	36%
broccoli & cheese	1 piece	15.0	240	56%
diced	3 oz	1.0	90	10%

Food and Description	Amount	Fat Grams	Total Calories	% Fat Calories
halves/roasted				
w/skin	1 piece	9.0	220	37%
lemon pepper	1 fillet	10.0	180	50%
Southern-style	1 fillet	13.0	230	51%
stuffed/seasoned	1 piece	15.0	240	56%
unbreaded	1 fillet	1.5	110	12%
Chicken Express/meal kit				
chicken & broccoli	1 bowl	18.0	500	32%
teriyaki	1 bowl	3.5	360	9%
w/fried rice	¼ bag	1.0	320	3%
Cordon Bleu	5 oz	15.0	290	47%
drumstick/roasted				
w/skin	1 piece	3.0	90	30%
Drummies	3 pieces	17.0	240	64%
meat for fajitas	½ cup	3.0	110	25%
nuggets, breaded	6 nuggets	15.0	230	59%
patties/breaded	1 patty	14.0	220	60%
strips/breaded				
tenderloin	3 pieces	1.0	180	5%
wings				
bar-b-que	4 pieces	11.0	170	58%
buffalo–style				
boneless	4 pieces	12.0	210	51%
hot	4 pieces	10.0	170	53%
teriyaki	4 pieces	14.0	250	50%
(Swanson)				
CHICKEN/Canned				
chicken à la king	5.25 oz	11.0	220	45%
chicken & dumplings	7.5 oz	11.0	220	45%
chicken stew	7.62 oz	7.0	160	39%
Mixin' Chicken in broth	¼ cup	8.0	110	65%
premium chunk				
chicken breast	2 oz	1.0	60	15%
CHICKEN/Frozen				
fried breast portion	4.5 oz	20.0	360	50%
nibbles	3.25 oz	19.0	300	57%
nuggets	3 oz	14.0	230	55%
pre-fried				
chicken parts	3.25 oz	16.0	270	53%
thighs & drumsticks	3.25 oz	18.0	290	56%
(Tyson)				
BOXED/BAGGED ITEMS/FULLY COOKED				
bites/box	13 pieces	10.0	180	50%
breast/diced				
bag	3 oz	1.0	90	10%
box	3 oz	3.5	120	26%
breast fillets/bag				
mesquite	1 piece	7.0	130	48%
regular	1 piece	16.0	290	50%
teriyaki	1 piece	6.0	170	32%

Food and Description	Amount	Fat Grams	Total Calories	% Fat Calories
breast strips				
fajita-style				
bag	3 oz	5.0	120	38%
box	3 oz	5.0	120	38%
grilled/box	3 oz	3.0	110	25%
Italian-style/box	3 oz	3.0	120	23%
lemon/box	3 oz	2.5	120	19%
regular/bagged or boxed	3 oz	3.5	120	26%
Southwest				
bag	3 oz	2.5	120	19%
box	3 oz	3.0	110	25%
meatballs/bag	3 oz	11.0	180	55%
nuggets				
bag	3 oz	1.0	90	10%
box	3 oz	1.0	90	10%
breast nuggets/box	5 pieces	16.0	280	51%
fun-shaped/box	5 pieces	14.0	240	53%
patties				
bagged	1 piece	11.0	180	55%
breast/box				
regular	1 piece	11.0	180	55%
Southwestern-style	1 piece	18.0	240	68%
popcorn chicken				
bites/bag	6 pieces	9.0	210	39%
regular/box	6 pieces	9.0	210	39%
strips/bag				
buffalo-style	2 pieces	10.0	230	39%
crispy	2 pieces	10.0	200	45%
tenderloins/breast/box	1 piece	7.0	150	42%
Southern-style	1 piece	7.0	150	42%
Spicy	1 piece	7.0	160	39%
tenders				
bag	5 pieces	14.0	240	53%
breast/box				
honey batter	3 pieces	13.0	200	59%
shaped/box	5 pieces	15.0	230	59%
wings				
BBQ-style/box	3 pieces	13.0	200	59%
buffalo/bag	4 pieces	15.0	220	61%
honey BBQ				
bag	4 pieces	14.0	220	57%
box	3 pieces	15.0	250	54%
hot and spicy/box	3 pieces	12.0	180	60%
hot and spicy/box	4 pieces	15.0	220	61%
Wings of Fire/box	3 pieces	16.0	260	55%
READY-TO-COOK				
chicken broccoli				
& cheese	1 piece	19.0	340	50%
chicken Kiev	1 piece	32.0	460	63%
Cordon Bleu	1 piece	17.0	350	44%

Food and Description	Amount	Fat Grams	Total Calories	% Fat Calories
REFRIGERATED ENTRÉES				
chicken medallions				
in marsala sauce	5 oz	4.0	130	28%
in sesame teriyaki sauce	5 oz	3.0	170	16%
in tomato & herb sauce	5 oz	3.5	120	26%
Premium Chunk Chicken Salad				
Kit	1 pkg	9.0	210	39%
(Weaver) *FROZEN/Boneless*				
breast strips				
buffalo	2 pieces	15.0	220	61%
crispy	2 pieces	14.0	220	57%
low-fat	3 pieces	1.5	120	11%
regular	3 pieces	14.0	230	55%
breast tenders				
honey batter	5 pieces	13.0	220	53%
regular	5 pieces	14.0	240	53%
croquettes				
w/¼ cup gravy	2 pieces	14.0	230	55%
w/o gravy	3 oz	20.0	340	53%
Mini-Drums/crispy	5 pieces	16.0	250	58%
nuggets	4 pieces	15.0	210	64%
patties				
breast	1 patty	10.0	170	52%
Italian	1 patty	14.0	210	60%
original	1 patty	11.0	180	55%
popcorn chicken/buffalo	1 serving	14.0	230	55%
wings				
buffalo-style hot	3 pieces	13.0	190	62%
honey BBQ	3 pieces	11.0	200	50%
CHICKEN SALAD (*See* CHICKEN ENTRÉE/DINNER)				
CHICKEN SEASONING (*See* SEASONINGS)				
CHICKEN SUBSTITUTES (*See* VEGETARIAN FOODS)				
CHICKPEA/GARBANZO BEAN				
canned				
(Arrowhead Mills) dry	¼ cup	2.0	170	11%
(Bush's Best)..16-oz can	4.5 oz	2.0	130	14%
(Eden) garbanzo	½ cup	1.5	120	11%
(Fermano's)	4.5 oz	2.0	110	16%
(Goya) Spanish-style	7.5 oz	2.0	150	12%
(Green Giant)	½ cup	1.5	110	12%
(Hain)	½ cup	2.5	120	19%
(Old El Paso)	½ cup	1.5	100	14%
(Progresso)				
chickpeas	½ cup	2.5	120	19%
garbanzo beans	½ cup	1.5	100	14%
(ShariAnn's) whole	½ cup	2.0	110	16%
(S&W)				
light/50% less salt	½ cup	1.5	80	17%
low-fat	½ cup	1.5	80	17%

Food and Description	Amount	Fat Grams	Total Calories	% Fat Calories
(Sun Vista)				
frijoles garbanzos	½ cup	1.5	110	12%
(Westbrae) Natural	½ cup	2.0	110	16%
dry				
boiled	½ cup	1.0	134	13%
raw	½ cup	6.0	364	15%
(Arrowhead Mills)	¼ cup	2.0	170	11%
(Best Yet)	¼ cup	2.0	110	16%
CHICORY/raw	8 oz	–	15	–
CHILI/CHILI BEANS				
CANNED				
(Armour)				
no beans	7.5 oz	14.0	280	45%
w/beans	7.5 oz	16.0	320	45%
(Austex)				
no beans	9.5 oz	41.0	530	70%
w/beans	8 oz	26.0	340	69%
(Bush's Best)..Chili Magic				
chili starter				
Louisiana hot	4.4 oz	1.5	110	12%
Texas medium	4.4 oz	2.0	120	15%
traditional mild	4.4 OZ	1.0	110	8%
(Castleberry's) w/beans	7.5 oz	21.0	350	54%
(Chili Man)				
no beans	7.5 oz	17.0	330	46%
w/beans	7.5 oz	27.0	380	64%
(Cincinnati Recipe) w/meat	4.3 oz	12.0	160	68%
(Dennison's)				
chili w/beans				
99% fat-free	7.5 oz	2.0	220	8%
99% fat-free				
turkey	7.5 oz	3.0	210	9%
con carne				
chunky	7.5 oz	12.0	320	34%
hot	7.5 oz	18.0	370	44%
hot & chunky	7.5 oz	13.0	320	37%
original	9 oz	17.0	370	41%
	7.5 oz	15.0	350	39%
cup	1 cup	12.0	300	36%
chili w/o beans	7.5 oz	18.0	330	49%
con carne w/mild				
green chilies	7.5 oz	17.0	370	41%
vegetarian				
99% fat-free	7.5 oz	1.0	180	5%
(Health Valley)				
99% fat-free				
medium turkey	1 cup	3.0	220	12%
other types..all flavors	1 cup	1.0	160	6%

Food and Description	Amount	Fat Grams	Total Calories	% Fat Calories
(Hormel)				
no beans	1 cup	9.0	210	39%
chunky	1 cup	6.0	210	26%
hot	1 cup	9.0	210	39%
hot & spicy	1 cup	10.0	230	39%
less salt	1 cup	9.0	210	39%
turkey	1 cup	3.0	190	14%
w/beans	1 cup	7.0	270	23%
chunky	1 cup	7.0	270	23%
home-style	1 cup	20.0	350	51%
hot	1 cup	7.0	270	23%
hot & spicy	1 cup	7.0	270	23%
less salt	1 cup	7.0	270	23%
turkey	1 cup	3.0	210	13%
vegetarian	1 cup	1.0	200	5%
(Kuner's) chili beans				
original in chili sauce	4.3 oz	2.0	120	15%
Southwestern black w/cumin & chili spices	4.3 oz	1.0	130	7%
(Pritikin) black bean				
spicy chili	1 cup	1.0	230	4%
(S&W)				
chili beans				
original				
w/zesty sauce	4.4 oz	1.0	110	8%
w/chipotle peppers	4.4 oz	–	90	–
chili makin's				
home-style	4.3oz	0.5	80	6%
original	4.3 oz	0.5	80	6%
(Skyline)				
original recipe	3 oz	9.0	150	54%
family size/tub	8.5 oz	14.0	270	47%
for chili dogs	1.7 oz	2.5	45	50%
(Stagg)				
Chicken Grande	1 cup	12.0	250	43%
Chili Laredo	1 cup	15.0	320	42%
Chunkero	1 cup	17.0	310	49%
classic	1 cup	17.0	330	46%
Country Brand	1 cup	17.0	330	46%
Dynamite Hot	1 cup	17.0	340	45%
Fiesta Grill	1 cup	9.0	240	34%
Ranch House	1 cup	11.0	270	37%
Rio Blanco	1 cup	12.0	250	43%
Silverado/beef	1 cup	3.0	230	12%
Steak House	1 cup	22.0	340	58%
Turkey Ranchero	1 cup	3.0	240	11%
Private Reserve	1 cup	17.0	330	46%
Vegetable Garden	1 cup	1.0	200	5%

Food and Description	Amount	Fat Grams	Total Calories	% Fat Calories
FROZEN				
(Skyline)				
calzones				
chili	½ box	15.0	330	41%
chili & hot dog	½ box	17.0	350	44%
chili/original	½ box	22.0	320	62%
chili & spaghetti	½ box	12.0	330	33%
coney bites w/chili	⅓ box	17.0	240	64%
JARRED				
(Bush's Best)				
home-style chili				
no beans..original	7.5 oz	14.0	240	53%
w/beans..all styles	7.5 oz	10.0	260	35%
MICROWAVEABLE				
(Health Valley) low-fat vegetarian chili cups				
all styles	⅓ cup	1.0	120	8%
(Hormel) Microcup Meals				
chili				
no beans	1 cup	8.0	190	38%
w/beans	1 cup	6.0	220	25%
chili mac	1 cup	9.0	200	41%
hot w/beans	1 cup	6.0	220	25%
(Stagg) Chili Smart Pak/shelf stable				
no beans				
Country Brand mild w/sweet bell peppers	7.15 oz	17.0	330	46%
Rio Blanco chicken w/white sauce	7.15 oz	12.0	250	43%
Steak House	7.15 oz	22.0	330	60%
w/beans				
Chunkero mild	7.15 oz	17.0	320	48%
classic	7.15 oz	17.0	310	49%
Dynamite Hot w/habanero peppers	7.15 oz	17.0	340	45%
Fiesta Grill w/fire-roasted tomatoes	7.15 oz	11.0	260	38%
Laredo w/green chilies & jalapeños	7.15 oz	16.0	310	46%
Ranch House chicken	7.15 oz	9.0	270	30%
Silverado beef	7.15 oz	7.0	250	25%
Turkey Ranchero	7.15 oz	7.0	250	25%
Vegetable Garden 4-bean	7.15 oz	1.0	200	5%
(The Allens)				
Mexican chili beans frijols enchilados	4.4 oz	1.0	130	7%
(Trappey's)				
red kidney beans w/chili gravy	4.4 oz	1.0	110	8%

Food and Description	Amount	Fat Grams	Total Calories	% Fat Calories
CHILI SAUCE (See SAUCE)				
CHINESE FOOD (See ASIAN FOOD, also FROZEN ENTRÉE/DINNER)				
CHINESE PARSLEY (See CILANTRO)				
CHIVES				
freeze-dried	1 Tbs	–	1	–
raw	1 Tbs	–	1	–
	¼ cup	–	2	–
CHOCOLATE (See BAKING BITS, CHIPS, CHUNKS & PIECES; CANDY)				
CHOCOLATE/HOT (See COCOA; MILK MIXES)				
CHOCOLATE SYRUP (See ICE CREAM TOPPING; MILK MIX)				
CHUB (See CISCO)				
CHUTNEY				
(Patak's) Original				
hot mango spice	1 Tbs	–	60	–
(Major Grey's)				
apple curry	1 Tbs	–	25	–
apricot chardonnay	1 Tbs	–	25	–
cranberry	1 Tbs	–	40	–
mango				
hot	1 Tbs	–	60	–
mild	1 Tbs	–	60	–
peach Zinfandel	1 Tbs	–	25	–
pear cardamom	1 Tbs	–	25	–
CIDER				
BOTTLED OR BOXED				
(Alpenglow) apple/sparkling	8 fl oz	–	120	–
(Indian Summer)				
all styles and flavors	8 fl oz	–	120	–
(Knudsen) Thirst Quencher				
cherry	8 fl oz	–	130	–
cider & spice	8 fl oz	–	120	–
(Lucky Leaf) apple	8 fl oz	–	150	–
(Martinelli's) apple				
sparkling cider	8 fl oz	–	140	–
(Musselman's)				
apple/100%				
from concentrate	8 fl oz	–	120	–
sparkling	8 fl oz	–	150	–
(Odwalla) Essentials				
harvest apple	8 fl oz	–	130	–
(TreeTop) apple	8 fl oz	–	120	–
(Zeigler) chilled				
all styles & flavors	8 fl oz	–	120	–
MIX				
(Alpine) apple cider drink/prepared				
original	8 fl oz	–	80	–
spiced	8 fl oz	–	80	–
sugar-free	8 fl oz	–	15	–

Food and Description	Amount	Fat Grams	Total Calories	% Fat Calories
CILANTRO/CHINESE PARSLEY/CORIANDER LEAF				
dried	1 tsp	–	2	–
	1 Tbs	–	5	–
fresh	1 tsp	–	2	–
	1 Tbs	–	5	–
CINNAMON/ground	1 tsp	–	10	–
CISCO/CHUB				
meat only				
raw	3 oz	1.5	85	16%
smoked	2 oz	6.5	100	59%
CITRON/candied (*See* individual fruits listings)				
CITRUS JUICE/JUICE DRINK (*See also* FRUIT PUNCH)				
BOTTLED, BOXED, OR CANNED				
(Season's Best)				
citrus medley	8 fl oz	–	120	–
FROZEN OR REFRIGERATED..prepared				
(Hanson's)				
citrus orange	8 fl oz	–	130	–
citrus punch	8 fl oz	–	130	–
(Tropicana) citrus punch	8 fl oz	–	140	–
CLAM (*See also* SEAFOOD ENTRÉE/DINNER)				
CANNED				
(3 Diamonds) whole	2 oz	0.5	45	10%
(Bumble Bee)				
baby/fancy whole	3.33 oz	1.0	50	18%
(Chicken of the Sea)				
baby whole	2.22 oz	–	35	–
chopped	¼ cup	–	30	–
minced	¼ cup	–	30	–
smoked baby	1 can	14.0	200	63%
whole	2 oz	–	30	–
(Crown Prince)				
baby				
boiled	⅓ cup	1.5	50	27%
natural	⅓ cup	1.0	50	18%
(Doxsee) solids & liquid				
chopped	1.85 oz	–	25	–
minced	1.85 oz	–	25	–
(Empress) baby/whole	4 oz	1.0	60	15%
(Geisha)				
baby				
fancy smoked/boxed				
in cottonseed	1.875 oz	9.0	130	62%
whole	3.33 oz	0.5	50	9%
chopped	2.16 oz	–	30	–
minced	2.16 oz	–	30	–
(Gorton's)				
chopped	¼ cup	–	20	–

Food and Description	Amount	Fat Grams	Total Calories	% Fat Calories
(Progresso) minced	¼ cup	–	25	–
(Snow's)				
chopped in clam juice	1.85 oz	–	25	–
FRESH				
breaded & fried	3 oz	9.0	171	47%
	20 small	21.0	380	50%
raw	3 oz	0.8	63	11%
steamed	3 oz	1.7	126	12%
	20 small	1.8	133	12%
FROZEN				
(Gorton's)..fried/crunchy	2.87 oz	14.0	240	53%
(Matlaw's)				
casino	1.3 oz	3.0	60	45%
stuffed				
box	3.7 oz	8.0	180	40%
tray	2.7 oz	6.0	130	42%
(Mrs. Paul's)..fried	½ box	12.0	250	43%
(Sea Pak Shrimp Co)..strips	5 oz	23.0	410	50%
(Van De Kamp's) fried	18 pieces	12.0	250	43%
CLAM CHOWDER (*See* SOUP)				
CLAM JUICE				
(Mott's)				
Clamato				
bloody Caesar	8 fl oz	–	50	–
picante	8 fl oz	–	60	–
regular	8 fl oz	–	60	–
CLAM SAUCE (*See* SAUCE)				
CLOVES/ground	1 tsp	–	7	–
CLUB SODA (*See* COCKTAIL MIXER; SOFT DRINK)				
COBBLER (*See* PIE & COBBLER)				
COCKTAIL SAUCE (*See* SAUCE)				
COCKTAIL/COCKTAIL MIXERS (*See also* LIQUEUR; LIQUOR, DISTILLED; WINE)				
generic				
Alexander	2.5 fl oz	1.8	179	9%
Bacardi	2.5 fl oz	–	118	–
Black Russian	3 fl oz	–	255	–
Bloody Mary	5 fl oz	–	116	–
bourbon & soda	4 fl oz	–	105	–
brandy	1 fl oz	–	75	–
daiquiri	2 fl oz	–	111	–
Gibson	2.5 fl oz	–	158	–
gimlet	2.5 fl oz	–	132	–
gin rickey	7 fl oz	–	114	–
gin & tonic	7.5 fl oz	–	171	–
Gold Cadillac	4.5 fl oz	3.6	394	8%
grasshopper	2.25 fl oz	3.6	164	20%
highball	8 fl oz	–	165	–
mai tai	4.5 fl oz	–	310	–
Manhattan	2.5 fl oz	–	128	–
margarita	~3 fl oz	–	170	–

Food and Description	Amount	Fat Grams	Total Calories	% Fat Calories
martini	2.5 fl oz	–	156	–
mint julep	10 fl oz	–	215	–
old-fashioned	4 fl oz	–	180	–
piña colada/canned	4.5 fl oz	11.0	347	29%
rum/hot buttered	~9 fl oz	11.9	317	34%
screwdriver	7 fl oz	–	174	–
Singapore sling	8 fl oz	–	228	–
sloe gin fizz	8 fl oz	–	121	–
stinger	3 fl oz	–	282	–
tequila sunrise	5.5 fl oz	–	189	–
Tom Collins	7.5 fl oz	–	121	–
	10 fl oz	–	180	–
whiskey sour	3 fl oz	–	123	–
White Russian	3.5 fl oz	1.0	268	3%
COCKTAIL MIXER (*See also* SOFT DRINK; WATER; individual fruit juice listings)				
(Bacardi) frozen/prepared				
fruit mixers w/o alcohol				
margarita	8 fl oz	–	90	–
piña colada	8 fl oz	4.0	170	21%
rum runner	8 fl oz	–	120	–
strawberry daiquiri	8 fl oz	–	120	–
(Baja Bob's) bottle mix				
Bloody Mary				
lean & mean	4 oz	–	20	–
margarita..all types	4 oz	–	10	–
piña colada	4 oz	1.0	30	30%
Collins	8 fl oz	–	100	–
ginger ale				
cherry				
diet	8 fl oz	–	–	–
regular	8 fl oz	–	90	–
	12 fl oz	–	120	–
cranberry				
diet	8 fl oz	–	–	–
regular	8 fl oz	–	90	–
golden				
diet	8 fl oz	–	–	–
regular	8 fl oz	–	90	–
plain				
diet	8 fl oz	–	–	–
regular	8 fl oz	–	100	–
half-and-half	8 fl oz	–	100	–
hi-spot	8 fl oz	–	110	–
island lime	8 fl oz	–	120	–
Jamaica cola	8 fl oz	–	100	–
lemon sour	8 fl oz	–	100	–
seltzer/sparkling water	8 fl oz	–	–	–
sour mixer	8 fl oz	–	80	–
sunripe orange	8 fl oz	–	110	–
tonic water..all types	8 fl oz	–	–	–

Food and Description	Amount	Fat Grams	Total Calories	% Fat Calories
vanilla cream brown	8 fl oz	–	110	–
Vichy water	8 fl oz	–	–	–
(Coco Lopez) w/o alcohol				
cream of coconut				
makes 8 fl oz	2 Tbs	5.0	110	41%
piña colada				
canned	3 fl oz	2.0	140	13%
jarred	4 fl oz	4.0	160	23%
(Holland House)				
Bloody Mary/bottled				
regular	4.5 fl oz	–	20	–
smooth 'n' spicy	4 fl oz	–	15	–
daiquiri				
raspberry/bottled	4 fl oz	–	140	–
regular/dry mix	1 pkg	–	65	–
strawberry/bottled	4 fl oz	–	180	–
mai tai/dry mix	1 pkg	–	64	–
margarita				
regular				
bottled	4 oz	–	100	–
dry mix	1 pkg	–	57	–
strawberry/bottled	4 fl oz	–	180	–
old-fashioned/bottled	1 fl oz	–	33	–
piña colada				
dry mix	1 pkg	–	82	–
sweet & sour	4 fl oz	–	130	–
Tom Collins				
dry mix	1 pkg	–	65	–
whiskey sour				
bottled	4 fl oz	–	130	–
dry mix	1 pkg	–	64	–
(Jero) bottle mixes				
Bloody Mary				
regular	1 serving	–	170	–
spicy jalapeño	1 serving	–	45	–
cherry bar mix	1 serving	–	45	–
grenadine	1 serving	–	90	–
Manhattan	1 serving	–	60	–
margarita	1 serving	–	190	–
old-fashioned	1 serving	–	130	–
piña colada	1 serving	2.0	290	62%
strawberry				
daiquiri	1 serving	–	310	–
margarita	1 serving	–	310	–
sweet & sour	1 serving	–	150	–
triple sec	1 serving	–	40	–
(Major Peters') bottle mixes				
Bloody Mary..all styles	1 serving	–	45	–
grenadine	1 serving	–	80	–

Food and Description	Amount	Fat Grams	Total Calories	% Fat Calories
lime juice				
sweetened West India				
from concentrate	1 serving	–	10	–
mai tai	1 serving	–	200	–
margarita	1 serving	–	200	–
old-fashioned	1 serving	–	150	–
piña colada				
⅕ bottle	1 serving	–	260	–
⅙ bottle	1 serving	–	320	–
strawberry				
daiquiri	1 serving	–	200	–
margarita	1 serving	–	200	–
sweet & sour	1 serving	–	200	–
triple sec	1 serving	–	35	–
(Mr. & Mrs. T) bottled				
Bloody Mary				
regular	4.5 fl oz	–	20	–
rich & spicy	4.5 fl oz	–	30	–
margarita				
regular	3 fl oz	–	80	–
strawberry	3.5 fl oz	–	100	–
piña colada	4 fl oz	<1.0	150	3%
sweet & sour	3 fl oz	–	70	–
(Rose's) grenadine syrup	1 fl oz	–	65	–
(Schweppe's)				
bitter lemon	8 fl oz	–	110	–
club soda				
regular	8 fl oz	–	–	–
sodium-free	8 fl oz	–	–	–
Collins mixer	8 fl oz	–	90	–
ginger ale				
diet	8 fl oz	–	–	–
dry grape	8 fl oz	–	90	–
regular	8 fl oz	–	80	–
lemon sour	8 fl oz	–	100	–
seltzer/sparkling water	8 fl oz	–	–	–
tonic water				
citrus	8 fl oz	–	80	–
cranberry	8 fl oz	–	80	–
plain				
diet	8 fl oz	–	–	–
regular	8 fl oz	–	90	–
(Tabasco) Bloody Mary	8 fl oz	–	60	–
COCOA (*See also* MILK MIX)				
(Baker's)	3.5 oz	13.0	220	53%
(Ghirardelli)				
sweet ground chocolate				
& cocoa	1 Tbs	1.5	20	68%
unsweetened	1 Tbs	1.5	20	68%

Food and Description	Amount	Fat Grams	Total Calories	% Fat Calories
(Hershey)				
European	1 Tbs	0.5	20	23%
	½ cup	3.0	90	30%
Original	1 Tbs	0.5	20	23%
	⅓ cup	3.0	110	25%
(Nestlé)	1 Tbs	0.5	15	30%
COCONUT				
(Baker's) Angel Flake				
canned	2 Tbs	6.0	70	77%
packaged	2 Tbs	5.0	70	64%
premium shred	2 Tbs	5.0	70	64%
sweetened	2 Tbs	5.0	70	64%
(Durkee) flaked	2 Tbs	6.0	80	68%
(Fisher)..Chef's Naturals	2 Tbs	5.0	70	64%
(Griffin's)	2 Tbs	4.0	70	51%
(Let's Do Organic)				
flakes	2 Tbs	10.0	100	90%
shredded				
light	2 Tbs	6.0	60	90%
regular	2 Tbs	10.0	100	90%
COCONUT CREAM				
canned/sweetened				
(Coco Lopez)	2 Tbs	5.0	110	41%
raw	1 Tbs	5.0	50	18%
	1 cup	83.0	795	94%
COCONUT MILK				
CANNED				
(A Taste of Thai) unsweetened				
light	⅓ cup	4.0	45	80%
original	⅓ cup	15.0	140	96%
(Native Forest)				
classic	¼ cup	10.0	100	90%
light	¼ cup	5.0	50	90%
GENERIC	1 Tbs	3.0	30	90%
	1 cup	48.0	445	97%
frozen	1 Tbs	3.0	30	90%
	1 cup	50.0	486	93%
raw	1 Tbs	3.6	35	92%
	1 cup	57.0	552	93%
COCONUT WATER	1 Tbs	–	3	–
	1 cup	0.5	46	10%
COD (*See also* COD ROE; SEAFOOD ENTRÉE/DINNER)				
Atlantic & Pacific				
breaded & fried	3 oz	9.0	175	46%
canned	3 oz	0.7	89	7%
cooked—dry heat	3 oz	0.7	89	7%
dried	3 oz	2.0	246	7%
raw	3 oz	0.6	70	7%
COD ROE	3 oz	1.7	111	14%

Food and Description	Amount	Fat Grams	Total Calories	% Fat Calories
COFFEE/COFFEE-LIKE BEVERAGE				
FLAVORED				
bottled/carton				
(Folger's) Jakada/Coffee Latte				
French roast	10.5 oz	3.5	170	19%
mocha	10.5 oz	3.5	190	17%
vanilla	10.5 oz	3.5	170	19%
(Maxwell House) iced cappuccino				
Coffee Cappio	8 fl oz	2.5	130	17%
Mocha Cappio	8 fl oz	2.5	140	16%
Vanilla Cappio	8 fl oz	2.5	140	16%
(Nescafé Frothe)				
chocolate mocha	8.47 oz	–	80	–
Divinely Mocha	8.47 oz	3.0	90	30%
Enchanting Vanilla	8.47 oz	3.0	90	30%
(Silk) by White Wave				
soylatte coffee				
carton	1 cup	3.5	170	19%
soylatte/bottle	11 oz	5.0	220	20%
(Starbucks) Frappuccino	9.5 fl oz	3.0	190	14%
INSTANT				
(Flavia)				
French vanilla	1 cup	–	2	–
hazelnut	1 cup	–	3	–
Irish crème	1 cup	–	3	–
(General Foods) International Coffee/Cappuccino/prepared				
Café Francais	1 cup	3.5	60	53%
Café Mocha/decaf	1 cup	2.0	60	30%
Café Vienna				
decaf/sugar-free				
/fat-free	1 cup	1.5	30	45%
regular	1 cup	2.5	70	32%
Cappuccino Coolers				
chocolate	1 cup	–	60	–
French vanilla	1 cup	–	60	–
Coffee Drink Mix				
crème caramel	1 cup	2.0	70	26%
French vanilla café				
decaffeinated	1 cup	2.5	60	38%
fat-free	1 cup	–	25	–
fat-free/sugar-free	1 cup	–	5	–
regular	1 cup	2.5	60	38%
sugar-free	1 cup	–	25	–
hazelnut	1 cup	2.0	60	30%
Irish cream café	1 cup	1.5	60	23%
Italian cappuccino	1 cup	2.0	60	30%
Kahlúa café	1 cup	2.0	60	30%
orange cappuccino				
regular	1 cup	2.0	60	30%

Food and Description	Amount	Fat Grams	Total Calories	% Fat Calories
sugar-free	1 cup	1.5	30	45%
Suisse Mocha				
decaffeinated	1 cup	2.0	60	30%
fat-free	1 cup	–	25	–
fat-free/sugar-free	1 cup	–	5	–
regular	1 cup	2.0	60	30%
sugar-free	1 cup	–	25	–
Swiss white chocolate	1 cup	3.0	70	39%
Viennese chocolate				
café	1 cup	1.5	50	27%
(Hills Bros) prepared				
Bavarian mint mocha				
regular	6 fl oz	1.0	50	18%
sugar-free	6 fl oz	1.0	35	26%
Café Vienna	6 fl oz	2.0	60	30%
double mocha	1 serving	3.5	120	26%
Dutch chocolate	6 fl oz	2.0	60	30%
English toffee	1 serving	4.5	120	34%
French vanilla				
decaf	1 serving	4.5	120	34%
regular	1 serving	4.5	120	34%
hazelnut	1 serving	4.5	120	34%
Orange Capri	6 fl oz	2.0	60	30%
Swiss Mocha				
regular	6 fl oz	2.0	60	30%
sugar-free	6 fl oz	2.0	40	45%
white chocolate				
caramel	1 serving	4.5	120	34%
(Land O' Lakes) Cappuccino Classics/mix				
amaretto	1 pkt	3.0	130	21%
chocolate supreme	1 pkt	5.0	150	30%
French vanilla	1 pkt	3.0	130	21%
Suisse mocha	1 pkt	3.5	140	23%
Suprema	1 pkt	3.0	140	19%
(Maxwell House) cappuccino/prepared				
amaretto	1 cup	1.0	90	10%
Irish cream	1 cup	1.0	90	10%
mocha				
decaffeinated	1 cup	2.5	100	23%
regular	1 cup	2.5	100	23%
sugar-free	1 cup	3.0	60	45%
vanilla				
decaffeinated	1 cup	1.0	90	10%
regular	1 cup	1.0	90	10%
sugar-free	1 cup	3.0	60	45%
(MJB) prepared				
banana nut mocha				
sugar-free	6 fl oz	2.0	40	45%
café mocha	6 fl oz	1.0	50	18%

Food and Description	Amount	Fat Grams	Total Calories	% Fat Calories
cherry mocha	6 fl oz	1.0	50	18%
fudge mocha..sugar-free	6 fl oz	2.0	40	45%
mint mocha				
regular	6 fl oz	1.0	50	18%
sugar-free	6 fl oz	1.0	35	26%
vanilla mocha..sugar-free	6 fl oz	2.0	40	45%
NON-FLAVORED/prepared/unless otherwise noted				
(Brim)				
decaf	6 fl oz	–	2	–
regular	6 fl oz	–	4	–
(Folger's) ground				
decaffeinated	1 Tbs	–	17	–
regular	1 Tbs	–	16	–
(Kava) mix only	1 tsp	–	2	–
(Maxwell House) decaf	6 fl oz	–	2	–
(Mountain Blend) instant	6 fl oz	–	5	–
(Sanka) decaf	6 fl oz	–	2	–
(Yuban)	6 fl oz	–	2	–
espresso	2 fl oz	–	1	–
regular				
(Nescafé) instant/prepared				
Brava	6 fl oz	–	4	–
classic	6 fl oz	–	4	–
decaf	6 fl oz	–	4	–
(Pero) hot beverage drink w/malt & barley/no caffeine/prepared	6 fl oz	–	4	–
(Postum) coffee-flavored grain beverage prepared w/water	8 fl oz	–	10	–
(Sanka) instant	6 fl oz	–	2	–
(Taster's Choice)				
decaffeinated	6 fl oz	–	4	–
regular	6 fl oz	–	4	–
(Worthington) Natural Touch Kaffree Roma/mix only	1 tsp	–	10	–
(Yuban)	6 fl oz	–	4	–
COFFEE CREAMER (*See* CREAM; CREAMER, NONDAIRY)				
COLD CUTS (*See* LUNCHEON MEAT)				
COLESLAW (*See* individual restaurant listings)				
COLLARDS				
canned				
(Glory Foods) seasoned	½ cup	1.0	50	18%
(Luck's) chopped greens				
seasoned w/pork	½ cup	3.0	60	45%
(The Allen's)				
seasoned Southern style	½ cup	0.5	35	13%
Verduras collards				
Picadas/chopped	½ cup	0.5	30	15%
(The Allen's Sunshine)				
seasoned Southern style	½ cup	0.5	35	13%

Food and Description	Amount	Fat Grams	Total Calories	% Fat Calories
fresh				
cooked	½ cup	–	13	–
raw/chopped	½ cup	–	18	–
frozen/chopped				
(Best Yet)	3.3 oz	–	30	–
(McKenzie's)	3.2 oz	–	30	–
(Pictsweet)	3.3 oz	–	25	–

CONDIMENTS (*See* ASIAN FOOD; MEXICAN FOOD; SAUCE; SEASONINGS; individual listings)

COOKIE (*See also* BROWNIE/BROWNIE-LIKE BARS; CRACKER; CAKE, SNACKS)

■ **(Archway)**

Food and Description	Amount	Fat Grams	Total Calories	% Fat Calories
ABC sugar cookies	12 cookies	4.5	130	31%
almond crescent	2 cookies	3.5	100	32%
apple bar/fat-free	1 bar	–	60	–
apple raisin	1 cookie	4.0	110	33%
apple-filled oatmeal	1 cookie	3.0	90	30%
apricot-filled oatmeal	1 cookie	3.0	90	30%
Aunt Mary's sugar cookies	1 cookie	4.0	130	28%
Bells & Stars	3 cookies	7.0	150	42%
carrot cake	1 cookie	5.0	120	38%
cashew nougat	3 cookies	11.0	170	58%
cherry-filled	1 cookie	3.0	90	30%
chocolate/fat-free	1 cookie	–	90	–
chocolate brownie cookie	1 cookie	5.0	140	32%
chocolate chip				
bag	5 cookies	7.0	160	39%
brownie	1 cookie	5.0	140	32%
drop	1 cookie	3.5	90	35%
ice box	1 cookie	5.0	110	41%
semi-sweet	1 cookie	6.0	140	39%
sugar-free	1 cookie	5.0	110	41%
walnut	1 cookie	7.0	140	45%
coconut macaroon				
original	1 cookie	6.0	100	54%
striped	1 cookie	5.0	100	45%
Cookie Jar Hermits	1 cookie	2.5	90	25%
dark molasses	1 cookie	3.5	120	26%
date-filled oatmeal	1 cookie	3.0	90	30%
devil's food/fat-free	1 cookie	–	60	–
Dutch apple	1 cookie	4.5	110	37%
Dutch cocoa	1 cookie	3.5	100	32%
frosty				
lemon	1 cookie	4.0	100	36%
orange	1 cookie	4.5	110	37%
fruit & honey bar	1 bar	6.0	190	28%
fruitcake cookies	3 cookies	5.0	140	32%
gingerbread cookies	3 cookies	5.0	140	32%
gingersnap				
iced	4 cookies	4.0	120	30%
original	5 cookies	5.0	150	30%

Food and Description	Amount	Fat Grams	Total Calories	% Fat Calories
reduced-fat	5 cookies	3.5	140	23%
iced molasses	1 cookie	3.5	120	26%
iced oatmeal				
10-oz pkg	1 cookie	4.5	120	34%
14-oz pkg	4 cookies	4.0	120	38%
Jar Hermits	1 cookie	4.5	180	23%
lemon				
drop	1 cookie	3.5	90	35%
snaps	5 cookies	7.0	150	42%
sugar-free	1 cookie	5.0	110	41%
malted nutty nougat	3 cookies	10.0	160	56%
molasses				
old-fashioned	1 cookie	3.0	100	27%
nutty nougat	3 cookies	12.0	170	64%
oatmeal				
chocolate chip	1 cookie	4.5	120	34%
date-filled	1 cookie	3.0	100	27%
pecan	1 cookie	7.0	140	45%
raisin	1 cookie	3.5	120	26%
raisin bran				
fat-free	1 cookie	–	110	–
original/packaged	1 cookie	3.5	110	29%
raspberry/fat-free	1 cookie	–	100	–
sugar-free	1 cookie	5.0	110	41%
party treats	3 cookies	7.0	140	45%
peanut butter				
chocolate	1 cookie	7.0	150	42%
home-style	1 cookie	7.0	140	45%
old-fashioned	1 cookie	5.0	100	45%
sugar-free	1 cookie	6.0	110	49%
pecan crunch	1 cookie	8.0	150	48%
pecan ice box	1 cookie	6.0	110	49%
pfeffernusse	2 cookies	1.0	100	9%
raspberry-filled	1 cookie	3.0	90	30%
rocky road				
original	1 cookie	6.0	130	42%
sugar-free	1 cookie	5.0	100	45%
Ruth's golden oatmeal	1 cookie	5.0	120	38%
shortbread/fat-free	1 cookie	5.0	110	41%
strawberry-filled	1 cookie	3.0	90	30%
sugar	1 cookie	3.0	100	27%
sugar drop cookies	1 cookie	2.5	80	28%
trees	3 cookies	8.0	150	48%
vanilla wafer	5 cookies	4.0	130	28%
wedding cake	3 cookies	8.0	160	45%
windmill/old-fashioned	1 cookie	3.5	90	35%
■ (Austin)				
peanut butter chocolate stix	1 bar	8.0	130	55%
Seanimals	10 cookies	5.0	140	32%

Food and Description	Amount	Fat Grams	Total Calories	% Fat Calories
vanilla cream	1.8 oz	11.0	260	38%
zoo animal cracker	17 cookies	2.0	120	15%
■ (Bakery Wagon)				
cobbler/fat-free				
apple	1 cookie	–	70	–
boysenberry	1 cookie	–	70	–
cranberry apple	1 cookie	–	70	–
mixed fruit	1 cookie	–	70	–
peach/apricot	1 cookie	–	70	–
raspberry	1 cookie	–	70	–
strawberry	1 cookie	–	70	–
cookie/low-fat				
apple-filled oat	1 cookie	1.5	90	15%
date-filled oat	1 cookie	1.5	90	15%
iced molasses				
mini	3 cookies	2.0	130	14%
regular	1 cookie	2.0	90	20%
raspberry-filled oat	1 cookie	1.5	90	15%
soft oatmeal				
iced	1 cookie	1.5	100	5%
plain	1 cookie	1.5	90	15%
gingersnap	5 cookies	7.0	160	37%
■ (Barbara's Bakery)				
animal cookies/vanilla	8 cookies	4.5	120	34%
crisp cookies				
chocolate chip	1 cookie	5.0	80	56%
double Dutch chocolate	1 cookie	4.0	80	45%
old-fashioned oatmeal	1 cookie	3.0	60	45%
traditional shortbread	1 cookie	4.0	80	45%
fig bars				
fat-free				
apple cinnamon	1 bar	–	60	–
raspberry	1 bar	–	60	–
wheat-free	1 bar	–	60	=
whole wheat fig	1 bar	–	60	–
low-fat traditional				
blueberry	1 bar	0.5	60	8%
fig/traditional	1 bar	0.5	15%	
Snackimals				
chocolate chip	10 cookies	4.0	120	30%
oatmeal/wheat-free	10 cookies	4.0	110	33%
vanilla	10 cookies	4.0	120	33%
■ (Betty Crocker)				
mix/prepared				
bar & cookie mixes				
chocolate peanut butter	1 bar	7.0	150	42%
Sunkist lemon bar	1 bar	4.5	140	29%

Food and Description	Amount	Fat Grams	Total Calories	% Fat Calories
cookie mixes				
chocolate				
chip	2 cookies	8.0	160	45%
chunk	2 cookies	6.0	150	36%
double chocolate				
chunk	2 cookies	6.0	150	34%
peanut butter chip	2 cookies	7.0	150	42%
double chocolate chunk	2 cookies	6.0	150	34%
oatmeal	2 cookies	6.0	150	36%
oatmeal chocolate chip	2 cookies	7.0	150	42%
peanut butter	2 cookies	8.0	160	45%
rainbow	2 cookies			
sugar cookie	3 cookies	8.0	160	45%
gingerbread cake				
cookie mix				
mix only	⅓ pkg	6.0	220	25%
prepared	1 cookie	6.0	230	23%
■ (Break Cake)				
brownie creme/2-oz cookie	1 cookie	8.0	240	30%
chips & creme	1 cookie	6.0	140	39%
chocolate chip	1 oz	6.0	140	39%
chocolate sugar wafer	4 cookies	9.0	200	41%
coconut macaroon				
2-oz cookie	2 cookies	14.0	270	47%
devil's food creme	1 cookie	5.0	130	35%
gingersnap	5 cookies	5.0	130	42%
hermit/2-oz cookie	1 cookie	7.0	230	27%
marshmallow pie				
banana	1.2 oz	5.0	150	30%
chocolate	1.2 oz	5.0	150	30%
devil's food	1.2 oz	4.0	140	26%
double-decker chocolate	3 oz	11.0	360	28%
oatmeal	5 cookies	6.0	140	39%
peanut butter	1 cookie	7.0	140	45%
peanut butter wafer	1 cookie	9.0	180	45%
raisin creme	1 cookie	5.0	140	32%
shortbread	5 cookies	6.0	140	39%
strawberry wafer	4 cookies	11.0	220	45%
striper wafer	1 cookie	10.0	190	47%
vanilla sugar wafer	4 wafers	11.0	220	45%
■ (Brown & Haley) box mix/mix only				
Almond Roca buttercrunch	1 oz	2.0	110	16%
■ CAMEO (See (Nabisco) in this section)				
■ (Carr's)				
biscuits for tea				
dark chocolate	2 biscuits	6.0	130	41%
milk chocolate	2 biscuits	6.0	130	41%
plain	2 biscuits	6.0	140	39%

Food and Description	Amount	Fat Grams	Total Calories	% Fat Calories
Chococcines	2 cookies	9.0	150	54%
Imperials				
dark chocolate	2 cookies	7.0	150	42%
milk chocolate	2 cookies	7.0	140	45%
& crème	2 cookies	7.0	130	48%
ginger lemon cremes	2 cookies	7.0	140	45%
Hob-Nobs	2 cookies	6.0	140	39%
Petits Bijoux	4 cookies	5.0	140	32%
Sweet Grahams	2 pieces	6.0	140	39%

■ **CHIPS AHOY** (*See* (Nabisco) in this section)
■ **CHIPS DELUXE** (*See* (Keebler) in this section)
■ **(Dare)**
Breaktime

chocolate chip	1 cookie	1.7	37	41%
coconut	1 cookie	1.4	35	36%
ginger	1 cookie	1.1	34	29%
oatmeal	1 cookie	1.3	35	33%

Dare

blueberry cheesecake	1 cookie	4.6	90	46%
butter creme	1 cookie	3.9	85	41%
café mocha	1 cookie	3.5	78	40%
carrot cake	1 cookie	5.0	92	49%
chocolate chip	1 cookie	3.8	76	45%
chocolate fudge	1 cookie	4.8	97	45%
cinnamon Danish	1 cookie	1.4	44	29%
coconut creme	1 cookie	5.2	99	47%
French creme	1 cookie	5.3	80	60%
golden caramel	1 cookie	3.3	73	41%
Harvest of the Rain Forest	1 cookie	4.0	69	52%
lemon creme	1 cookie	4.5	95	43%
maple leaf creme	1 cookie	3.8	85	40%
milk chocolate fudge	1 cookie	4.8	97	45%

Sun Maid

chocolate & raisins	1 cookie	3.0	56	48%
raisin	1 cookie	2.5	52	43%

Simple Pleasures

almond cookie	1 cookie	1.3	35	33%
chocolate thins	1 cookie	1.3	35	33%
digestive	1 cookie	2.1	46	41%
oatmeal	1 cookie	3.4	74	41%
snaps				
cinnamon	1 cookie	0.7	31	20%
spice	1 cookie	1.0	33	27%
social tea	1 cookie	0.6	29	18%
lemon	1 cookie	0.6	29	18%
sugar	1 cookie	0.7	47	13%

■ **(Delicious)**

almond windmill	3 cookies	5.0	130	35%
animal crackers	9 cookies	5.0	130	35%

Food and Description	Amount	Fat Grams	Total Calories	% Fat Calories
butter thins	10 cookies	5.0	110	41%
Chiquita				
Bananarama	2 cookies	4.0	120	30%
chocolate chip	2 cookies	8.0	140	51%
chocolate chip				
thins	10 cookies	5.0	110	41%
coconut bar	3 cookies	7.0	140	45%
fig bar	1 cookie	1.0	70	13%
	2 cookies	2.0	130	14%
gingersnap	4 cookies	3.0	130	21%
Heath English				
toffee crunch	3 cookies	10.0	170	53%
honey graham				
cinnamon	2 whole	5.0	130	35%
plain	2 whole	3.5	120	26%
iced oatmeal	2 cookies	6.0	130	42%
jelly top	47 pieces	8.0	260	28%
Ileath				
English toffee	3 cookies	10.0	170	53%
striped toffee delights	2 cookies	8.0	140	51%
macaroon	2 cookies	6.0	130	42%
maple leaf creme	2 cookies	5.0	120	38%
Nestlé				
Butterfinger	3 cookies	6.0	130	42%
Raisinets oatmeal	3 cookies	4.5	140	29%
oatmeal				
iced	2 cookies	5.0	120	38%
plain	2 cookies	5.0	130	35%
w/Raisinets	3 cookies	4.5	140	29%
sandwich cookies				
assorted	3 cookies	6.0	150	36%
assorted creme	3 cookies	6.0	150	36%
banana creme	3 cookies	6.0	150	36%
chocolate creme	3 cookies	6.0	150	36%
duplex	3 cookies	5.0	140	32%
duplex creme	3 cookies	6.0	150	36%
lemon	3 cookies	5.0	140	32%
lemon creme	3 cookies	6.0	150	36%
peanut butter creme	3 cookies	6.0	150	36%
	2 cookies	5.0	150	30%
strawberry creme	3 cookies	6.0	150	36%
vanilla	3 cookies	5.0	140	32%
vanilla creme	3 cookies	6.0	150	36%
	2 cookies	5.0	150	30%
shortbread	4 cookies	6.0	140	39%
Skippy peanut butter	3 cookies	10.0	150	60%
sugar cookie	2 cookies	5.0	130	35%
sugar wafer				
assorted				
regular	4 wafers	6.0	140	39%

Food and Description	Amount	Fat Grams	Total Calories	% Fat Calories
sugar-free	3 wafers	10.0	150	60%
chocolate				
regular	3 wafers	9.0	150	54%
sugar-free	6 wafers	11.0	170	58%
chocolate/strawberry	1 cookie	2.0	35	26%
lemon	1 cookie	2.0	35	26%
mini creme	1 cookie	1.5	25	54%
strawberry				
regular	3 wafers	9.0	150	54%
sugar-free	6 wafers	11.0	170	58%
strawberry/vanilla	1 cookie	2.0	35	26%
vanilla				
regular	3 wafers	9.0	150	54%
sugar-free	6 wafers	11.0	170	58%
vanilla wafers				
fat-free	8 cookies	–	110	–
original	8 cookies	4.5	130	31%
■ (Drake's)				
chocolate chip	2 cookies	7.0	140	45%
chocolate, chocolate chip	2 cookies	5.0	130	35%
coconut	2 cookies	6.0	140	39%
coconut macaroon	1 cookie	7.0	135	47%
lemon	2 cookies	5.0	130	35%
oatmeal	2 cookies	5.0	130	35%
■ (Duncan Hines)..box mix/prepared				
box mix				
chocolate chip	2 cookies	8.0	170	42%
fudge brownie cookie	2 cookies	7.0	140	45%
golden sugar	2 cookies	7.0	150	42%
peanut butter	2 cookies	8.0	140	51%
■ ELFIN DELIGHTS (See (Keebler) in this section)				
■ (Entenmann's) Soft Baked				
Carb Counting/chewy				
chocolate chip	1 oz	7.0	130	48%
Chewy Snack Barz				
brownie chip/8-count	1 bar	7.0	170	37%
rainbow chip/8-count	1 bar	8.0	180	40%
original recipe/8-count				
chocolate chip	1 bar	9.0	180	45%
chocolate brownie..fat-free	2 cookies	–	80	–
chocolate chip/pouch				
cookie bites	1.5 oz	11.0	220	45%
devil's food/low-fat cookie cake	1 cookie	0.5	60	8%
Happy Valentine's Day	~1 oz	7.0	130	48%
butter	2 cookies	7.0	130	48%
holiday butter	2 cookies	7.0	130	48%
oatmeal				
chocolate chip/fat-free	2 cookies	–	100	–
raisin/1.5-oz pouch	1 pouch	8.0	190	38%
oatmeal raisin/fat-free	2 cookies	–	100	–

Food and Description	Amount	Fat Grams	Total Calories	% Fat Calories
soft-baked				
chocolate chip				
original	1 oz	7.0	150	42%
	¾ oz	5.0	100	45%
milk chocolate chip	3 cookies	7.0	150	42%
original recipe				
chocolate chip	3 cookies	7.0	150	42%
cookie bites 1.5-oz pouch	1 pouch	11.0	210	47%
■ (Estee)				
chocolate chip				
original	4 cookies	7.0	150	42%
sugar-free	3 cookies	3.5	110	29%
chocolate sandwich	3 cookies	6.0	160	34%
chocolate walnut				
sugar-free	3 cookies	3.5	110	29%
coconut				
original	4 cookies	6.0	140	39%
sugar-free	3 cookies	3.5	110	29%
fig bar/low-fat	2 bars	1.0	100	9%
fudge	4 cookies	7.0	150	42%
lemon				
sugar-free	3 cookies	3.0	110	25%
thins	4 cookies	6.0	140	39%
oatmeal raisin	4 cookies	5.0	130	35%
original sandwich	3 cookies	6.0	160	34%
peanut butter sandwich	3 cookies	7.0	160	39%
shortbread	4 cookies	4.0	130	28%
Smart Treats	3 cookies	3.0	110	25%
■ (Famous Amos)				
chocolate chip	4 cookies	7.0	150	42%
individual pkg	1 pkg	9.0	200	41%
chocolate chip & pecan	4 cookies	8.0	150	48%
chocolate crème sandwich	3 cookies	6.0	150	18%
low-fat/iced/individual pkg				
gingersnaps	1 pkg	3.0	200	9%
lemonsnaps	1 pkg	2.5	200	11%
oatmeal				
chocolate chip				
& walnut	4 cookies	7.0	150	42%
raisin	4 cookies	5.0	140	32%
■ (Featherweight)				
chocolate chip	4 cookies	5.0	140	32%
creme wafer				
chocolate	7 cookies	8.0	160	45%
vanilla	7 cookies	7.0	160	39%
double chocolate chip	4 cookies	5.0	140	32%
lemon	4 cookies	5.0	140	32%
oatmeal raisin	4 cookies	5.0	140	32%
peanut butter	4 cookies	5.0	140	32%
vanilla	4 cookies	5.0	140	32%

Food and Description	Amount	Fat Grams	Total Calories	% Fat Calories
■ (Fifty/50)				
LOW-FAT/Fructose-sweetened				
apple cinnamon				
cookie bar	1 bar	1.5	120	11%
fudge brownie bar	1 bar	1.5	110	12%
sandwich				
chocolate	3 cookies	7.0	160	39%
duplex	3 cookies	7.0	160	39%
vanilla	3 cookies	7.0	170	37%
SUGAR-FREE/Fructose-sweetened				
butter	4 cookies	8.0	160	45%
chocolate chip	4 cookies	10.0	170	53%
coconut	4 cookies	10.0	160	56%
fudge brownie	4 cookies	8.0	160	45%
oatmeal/hearty	4 cookies	6.0	140	39%
peanut butter wafers	4 cookies	7.0	160	39%
chocolate	6 wafers	9.0	150	54%
chocolate raspberry	6 wafers	9.0	150	54%
strawberry vanilla	6 wafers	9.0	150	54%
vanilla	6 wafers	9.0	150	54%
SUGAR-FREE/Sweetened w/Maltitol				
chocolate chip	4 cookies	7.0	140	45%
lemon crème	3 cookies	7.0	150	42%
oatmeal	4 cookies	6.0	140	39%
shortbread	8 cookies	8.0	160	45%
■ (Grandma's)				
Homestyle/big cookies				
chocolate chip	1 cookie	9.0	200	41%
fudge chocolate chip	1 cookie	7.0	190	33%
molasses	1 cookie	4.0	160	23%
oatmeal raisin	1 cookie	6.0	180	30%
peanut butter	1 cookie	10.0	200	45%
Rich & Chewy				
chocolate chip/soft	1 pkg	12.0	270	40%
Sandwich Creme				
mini				
fudge	9 cookies	7.0	150	42%
peanut butter	9 cookies	7.0	150	42%
vanilla	9 cookies	7.0	150	42%
regular-size				
peanut butter	5 cookies	10.0	210	43%
vanilla	5 cookies	10.0	210	43%
■ (Hain)				
animal graham				
chocolate	15 cookies	3.0	120	23%
original	15 cookies	3.0	80	34%
graham cracker				
chocolate	2 cookies	3.0	120	23%
cinnamon	2 cookies	3.0	80	34%
honey	2 cookies	3.0	80	34%

Food and Description	Amount	Fat Grams	Total Calories	% Fat Calories
■ **(Health Valley)**				
Café Creations				
chocolate chip	1 cookie	5.0	100	45%
chocolate, chocolate				
chip	1 cookie	5.0	100	45%
raisin oatmeal	1 cookie	3.5	90	35%
Carb Fit..all types	2 cookies	8.0	110	65%
chocolate				
chip oatmeal	1 cookie	4.0	100	36%
chunk	1 cookie	7.0	120	53%
Cookie Cremes sandwich cookies				
all flavors	2 cookies	5.0	120	38%
double chocolate chunk	1 cookie	7.0	120	53%
fat-free cookies				
apple spice	3 cookies	–	100	–
apricot delight	3 cookies	–	100	–
raisin oatmeal	3 cookies	–	100	–
Fat-Free Healthy Chips				
all styles	3 cookies	–	100	–
low-fat biscotti style	2 cookies	3.0	120	23%
mini chocolate, chocolate chip	1 cookie	4.0	100	36%
oatmeal				
peanut	1 cookie	4.0	100	36%
raisin	1 cookie	3.5	90	35%
white chocolate chunk	1 cookie	7.0	140	45%
■ **HONEY MAID** (*See* (Nabisco) in this section)				
■ **(Keebler)**				
Chips Deluxe				
Carb Sensible Cookies				
chocolate chip	1 cookie	4.0	70	51%
w/pecans	1 cookie	5.0	70	64%
chocolate, chocolate				
chip peanut butter	1 cookie	4.0	70	51%
regular cookies				
chocolate chip				
mini	4 cookies	8.0	150	48%
original	1 cookie	4.5	80	51%
chocolate lover's	1 cookie	4.5	80	51%
coconut	1 cookie	4.5	80	51%
crunchy walnut	1 cookie	6.0	90	60%
rainbow				
mini	4 cookies	8.0	150	48%
regular	1 cookie	4.0	80	45%
soft & chewy	1 cookie	3.0	70	39%
w/peanut butter cups	1 cookie	4.5	90	45%
E. L. Fudge sandwich cookies				
butter fudge sandwich	2 cookies	5.0	130	35%
w/fudge crème filling	2 cookies	5.0	120	38%
Butterfinger-blasted	2 cookies	9.0	180	45%
fudge w/fudge crème filling	2 cookies	6.0	120	45%

Food and Description	Amount	Fat Grams	Total Calories	% Fat Calories
mini fudge w/crème filling	7 cookies	6.0	130	42%
peanut butter double stuffed	2 cookies	9.0	180	45%
Fudge Shoppe cookies				
Deluxe grahams	3 cookies	7.0	140	45%
Fudge Lover's fudge sticks	3 pieces	10.0	160	56%
Fudge Sticks	3 pieces	8.0	150	48%
Fudge Stripes				
original	3 cookies	7.0	150	42%
reduced-fat	3 cookies	7.0	150	42%
Grasshopper	4 cookies	7.0	150	42%
Grahams				
chocolate	8 crackers	4.0	140	26%
cinnamon crisp				
low-fat	8 crackers	1.5	110	12%
regular	8 crackers	3.0	130	21%
honey graham				
low-fat	9 crackers	1.5	120	11%
regular	8 crackers	4.0	140	26%
original	8 crackers	3.5	130	24%
KEEBLER				
"ON THE GO" cookie snacks				
animal/frosted	6 pieces	6.0	130	42%
E. L. Fudge				
mini	1 pkg	12.0	260	42%
mini butter sandwich				
w/fudge creme	1 pkg	12.0	280	39%
Fudge Stripe/minis	1 pkg	13.0	270	43%
sandies w/pecans	1 pkg	17.0	300	51%
Original cookies				
animal cookies	10 pieces	4.0	130	28%
frosted	8 pieces	7.0	150	42%
iced	6 pieces	5.0	140	32%
country-style oatmeal	2 cookies	6.0	130	34%
Danish wedding	4 cookies	6.0	130	34%
gingersnaps	5 cookies	6.0	150	36%
vanilla wafers				
mini	18 cookies	6.0	140	39%
original	8 cookies	6.0	150	36%
Sandies				
caramel pecan	1 cookie	5.0	80	56%
chocolate chip & pecan	1 cookie	5.0	80	56%
cinnamon	1 cookie	5.0	80	56%
Fruit Delights				
apple cobbler	1 cookie	3.5	80	39%
strawberry				
cheesecake cookie	1 cookie	3.5	80	39%
original				
w/almonds	1 cookie	5.0	90	50%
w/pecans	1 cookie	5.0	80	56%
pecan	1 cookie	5.0	90	50%
mini	4 cookies	10.0	160	56%

Food and Description	Amount	Fat Grams	Total Calories	% Fat Calories
Simply Shortbread	1 cookie	4.5	80	51%
25% reduced-fat w/pecans	1 cookie	3.5	80	39%
Soft Batch cookies				
chocolate chip	1 cookie	3.5	80	45%
Sugar Wafers				
peanut butter	4 wafers	9.0	160	51%
vanilla	3 wafers	6.0	130	42%
Vienna Fingers				
fudge thins	4 cookies	7.0	160	39%
mint fudge thins	4 cookies	7.0	160	39%
original	2 cookies	6.0	150	36%
reduced-fat (25%)	2 cookies	4.5	140	29%
■ (Krinos)				
Viennese Wafers				
coffee	4 wafers	9.0	170	48%
hazelnut	4 wafers	7.0	170	37%
peanut butter	4 wafers	7.0	170	37%
sesame cream	4 wafers	8.0	170	42%
vanilla	4 wafers	7.0	170	37%
■ (Lance)				
Choc-O-Lunch 1.5-oz package	1 pkg	8.0	200	36%
chocolate chip mini cookies				
1-oz package	½ pkg	4.0	130	28%
Lem-O-Lunch	5 cookies	9.0	210	39%
oatmeal crèmes	1 cookie	9.0	240	34%
On a Nekot cookie				
peanut butter	6 cookies	12.0	250	43%
S'Mores	6 cookies	13.0	250	43%
peanut butter wafers	1 pkg	12.0	220	49%
strawberry cookies	5 cookies	9.0	210	39%
sugar wafers	4 cookies	8.0	150	48%
Van-O-Lunch	6 cookies	8.0	210	34%
vanilla	4 wafers	8.0	150	48%
variety pack cookies 1.75-oz pkg	1 pkg	13.0	250	47%
■ (Little Debbie)				
BARS				
caramel cookie bar	1 bar	8.0	160	45%
holiday crispy bar	1 bar	6.0	190	28%
marshmallow crispy bars	1 bar	3.5	140	23%
Big Packs	1 bar	4.5	190	21%
nutty bar wafer bar				
Big Packs	1 pkg	20.0	330	55%
boxed	1 pkg	17.0	290	53%
individual pkg	2 oz	18.0	310	52%
	1.5 oz	13.0	230	51%
peanut butter bar				
boxed	1 pkg	15.0	280	48%
individual pkg	1 pkg	14.0	250	50%

Food and Description	Amount	Fat Grams	Total Calories	% Fat Calories
COOKIES				
apple flips	1 pkg	6.0	150	36%
chocolate chip cookie				
individual pkg	1 cookie	9.0	180	45%
	1.35 oz	9.0	190	43%
coconut round	1 pkg	7.0	150	42%
cookie wreaths	1 pkg	5.0	100	45%
Easter puffs	1 pkg	6.0	150	36%
Figaroos				
fat-free/individual pkg	1 pkg	–	180	–
regular	1 pkg	3.5	150	21%
fudge delights	1 cookie	2.0	110	16%
fudge round				
boxed	1 pkg	6.0	150	36%
individual pkg	2.5 oz	12.0	310	35%
	3 oz	14.0	380	33%
German chocolate				
cookie ring	1 cookie	8.0	140	51%
ginger	1 pkg	3.0	90	30%
lemon creme wafer	1 pkg	5.0	100	45%
oatmeal delights	1 cookie	2.0	110	16%
oatmeal raisin				
individual pkg	1 cookie	6.0	160	34%
PB&J oatmeal pie	1 pkg	5.0	140	32%
peanut cluster	1 pkg	11.0	190	52%
Pumpkin Delight	1 pkg	5.0	150	30%
Star Crunch Cosmic Snack				
individual pkg	1 pkg	12.0	290	37%
	1 oz	5.0	140	32%
CRÈME PIES				
chocolate chip	1 cookie	6.0	150	36%
jelly	1 cookie	7.0	150	42%
oatmeal				
original				
boxed	1 pkg	7.0	170	29%
individual pkg	2.5 oz	12.0	310	35%
	3 oz	14.0	370	34%
reduced-fat	1 pkg	2.5	130	17%
raisin				
boxed	1 pkg	5.0	140	32%
individual pkg	1 pkg	11.0	280	35%
MARSHMALLOW PIES				
banana				
boxed	1 pkg	8.0	240	30%
individual pkg	2.5 oz	11.0	320	31%
	1.5 oz	6.0	180	30%
chocolate				
boxed	1 pkg	5.0	160	28%
individual pkg	1.5 oz	7.0	180	35%
marshmallow supremes	1 pkg	5.0	140	32%

Food and Description	Amount	Fat Grams	Total Calories	% Fat Calories
■ (Lil Dutch Maid)				
almond windmill	2 cookies	3.0	110	25%
Chip Delight	4 cookies	7.0	150	42%
chocolate cream	3 cookies	6.0	150	36%
coconut macaroon	2 cookies	5.0	130	35%
duplex cream	3 cookies	6.0	150	36%
oatmeal	4 cookies	4.5	140	30%
vanilla cream	3 cookies	6.0	150	36%
vanilla wafers	9 cookies	9.0	170	48%
■ (LU)				
Aloha	1 cookie	5.0	75	60%
barre chocolat	1 cookie	3.0	65	42%
chips chocolat				
fudge	1 cookie	4.0	75	48%
regular	1 cookie	5.0	85	53%
chocolatiers	3 cookies	11.0	170	58%
craquelin	1 cookie	3.0	55	49%
crokine	2 cookies	–	20	–
Euphrates	2 cookies	2.0	40	45%
fondant	4 cookies	8.0	170	37%
gaufrettes	2 cookies	4.0	85	42%
Marie LU				
mini	12 cookies	5.0	130	35%
original	3 cookies	6.0	170	32%
whole wheat	3 cookies	4.0	140	26%
milk lunch	4 cookies	4.0	140	26%
palmito	1 cookie	3.0	50	54%
petit-beurre	4 cookies	4.0	150	26%
Petite Écolier/little schoolboy				
dark chocolate	2 cookies	7.0	130	48%
milk chocolate	2 cookies	7.0	130	48%
Pimm's				
orange	2 cookies	4.0	100	35%
raspberry	2 cookies	3.0	100	27%
truffe	4 cookies	11.0	180	55%
■ (Manischewitz)				
chocolate chip	3 cookies	7.0	150	42%
macaroon				
almond	2 cookies	5.0	100	45%
banana split	2 cookies	4.0	110	33%
cappuccino chip	2 cookies	5.0	100	45%
chocolate				
almond	2 cookies	5.0	110	41%
chip	2 cookies	5.0	100	45%
chunk cherry	2 cookies	4.0	110	33%
plain	2 cookies	4.0	90	40%
coconut	2 cookies	6.0	100	54%
cookies 'n' cream	2 cookies	5.0	100	45%
fudgey nut brownie	2 cookies	5.0	100	45%
honey nut	2 cookies	5.0	100	45%

Food and Description	Amount	Fat Grams	Total Calories	% Fat Calories
rocky road	2 cookies	5.0	100	45%
toffee crunch	2 cookies	5.0	100	45%
■ (Mother's)				
ABC				
cinnamon grahams	12 cookies	5.0	140	32%
sugar cookies	12 cookies	4.5	130	31%
almond shortbread	3 cookies	12.0	190	57%
Animal Parade	9 pieces	6.0	135	40%
butter-flavored	5 cookies	6.0	140	39%
Candy Blasters	2 cookies	6.0	120	45%
candy chip	4 cookies	7.0	150	42%
checkerboard wafer	4 wafers	9.0	150	54%
chocolate chip				
angel	3 cookies	11.0	190	52%
bag	5 cookies	5.0	140	32%
Hawaiian	2 cookies	11.0	180	55%
package	2 cookies	8.0	160	45%
parade	4 cookies	5.0	130	35%
small	5 cookies	7.0	160	39%
chocolate cream	2 cookies	8.0	190	38%
chocolate marble cream	2 cookies	8.0	190	38%
circus animal	6 cookies	7.0	140	45%
classic assortment	2 cookies	7.0	140	45%
cocadas coconut	5 cookies	8.0	160	45%
coffee cream sandwich	2 cookies	7.0	180	35%
cookie parade	4 cookies	7.0	140	45%
dinosaur grahams	2 cookies	4.0	140	26%
double-fudge sandwich	2 cookies	9.0	180	45%
duplex sandwich				
reduced-fat	3 cookies	5.0	160	28%
English tea sandwich	2 cookies	7.0	180	35%
fig bar				
regular				
fat-free	1 bar	–	70	–
regular	1 bar	1.5	80	17%
whole wheat				
fat-free	1 bar	–	70	–
regular	1 bar	3.0	80	34%
Flaky Flix				
fudge wafer	2 cookies	7.0	140	45%
vanilla wafer	2 cookies	8.0	140	51%
fudge circus animal	6 cookies	7.0	140	45%
fudge graham	2 cookies	8.0	150	48%
Gaucho peanut butter				
sandwich	2 cookies	8.0	190	38%
gingerbread man	6 cookies	6.0	140	39%
holiday				
candy ship	4 cookies	7.0	150	42%
frosted	4 cookies	6.0	130	42%
striped shortbread	2 cookies	8.0	140	51%

Food and Description	Amount	Fat Grams	Total Calories	% Fat Calories
sugar	2 cookies	7.0	150	42%
sugar cut-out	9 cookies	4.5	130	31%
iced/old-fashioned				
chocolate	2 cookies	7.0	160	37%
lemonade	2 cookies	8.0	160	45%
iced oatmeal				
bag	4 cookies	4.0	120	30%
package	2 cookies	4.0	130	28%
iced raisin	2 cookies	8.0	170	42%
macaroons/old-fashioned	2 cookies	11.0	170	58%
Marias	3 cookies	4.5	170	24%
Marie Lu	3 cookies	4.5	160	25%
mint square	2 cookies	8.0	150	48%
oatmeal	2 cookies	5.0	130	35%
butterscotch	2 cookies	5.0	120	38%
chocolate chip	2 cookies	5.0	120	38%
crème sandwich	2 cookies	9.0	190	43%
old-fashioned				
oatmeal & raisin	2 cookies	6.0	140	39%
original	2 cookies	5.0	110	41%
raisin	5 cookies	7.0	150	42%
walnut chocolate chip	2 cookies	7.0	140	45%
peanut butter				
old-fashioned	2 cookies	9.0	150	54%
square	2 cookies	8.0	160	45%
Rainbow wafer	4 wafers	8.0	140	51%
Striped shortbread	3 cookies	8.0	170	42%
sugar	2 cookies	6.0	140	39%
sugar-free				
checkerboard wafers	6 wafers	9.0	140	58%
chocolate chip	4 cookies	7.0	140	45%
chocolate crème	3 cookies	7.0	150	42%
lemon-flavored crème	3 cookies	7.0	150	42%
oatmeal	4 cookies	6.0	140	39%
peanut butter	4 cookies	9.0	160	45%
pecan shortbread	4 cookies	11.0	170	58%
shortbread	8 cookies	8.0	160	45%
vanilla crème	3 cookies	7.0	150	42%
sugared lemon-flavor				
old-fashioned	2 cookies	8.0	150	48%
taffy sandwich	2 cookies	8.0	190	38%
Triplet assortment	2 cookies	7.0	150	42%
vanilla				
123 artificially				
flavored	12 cookies	4.5	130	31%
crème sandwiches	2 cookies	7.0	180	35%
wafer	8 cookies	5.0	140	32%
Zoo Pals	14 cookies	5.0	140	32%

Food and Description	Amount	Fat Grams	Total Calories	% Fat Calories
■ **(Mrs. Fields)**				
BITE-SIZE NIBBLER COOKIES				
butter	2 cookies	4.5	110	37%
chewy chocolate fudge	2 cookies	4.5	120	34%
cinnamon sugar	2 cookies	4.5	120	34%
Debra's Special Nibbler	2 cookies	4.5	100	41%
milk chocolate				
w/walnuts	2 cookies	6.0	120	45%
w/o nuts	2 cookies	5.0	110	41%
M&M Nibbler	2 cookies	5.0	110	41%
peanut butter	2 cookies	6.0	110	49%
semi-sweet chocolate	2 cookies	5.0	100	41%
triple chocolate	2 cookies	6.0	110	49%
white chunk macadamia	2 cookies	7.0	120	53%
REGULAR-SIZE COOKIES				
butter toffee	1 cookie	13.0	290	40%
cinnamon sugar	1 cookie	12.0	300	36%
coconut & macadamias	1 cookie	13.0	280	42%
Debra's Special	1 cookie	12.0	280	39%
milk chocolate				
macadamia	1 cookie	18.0	320	51%
& walnuts	1 cookie	17.0	320	48%
w/o nuts	1 cookie	13.0	280	42%
oatmeal				
chocolate chip	1 cookie	13.0	280	42%
raisins & walnuts	1 cookie	12.0	280	39%
peanut butter	1 cookie	16.0	310	46%
milk chocolate	1 cookie	17.0	300	51%
semi-sweet chocolate	1 cookie	14.0	280	45%
w/walnuts	1 cookie	16.0	310	46%
Snickerdoodle Jumbo	1 cookie	29.0	640	41%
white chocolate				
macadamia	1 cookie	17.0	310	49%
■ **(Murray)**				
REGULAR COOKIES				
chocolate chip	2 cookies	7.0	150	42%
coconut	2 cookies	8.0	150	48%
coconut macaroon	3 cookies	6.0	120	45%
lemon cremes				
sandwich	3 cookies	5.0	140	32%
oatmeal/old-fashioned				
iced	2 cookies	6.0	140	39%
Southern Kitchen	2 cookies	6.0	140	39%
sugar wafers/duplex	5 cookies	7.0	140	45%
windmill	3 cookies	5.0	140	32%
cremes	3 cookies	5.0	140	32%
SUGAR-FREE COOKIES				
chocolate chip	3 cookies	8.0	150	48%
& pecan	3 cookies	10.0	160	56%
cremes	3 cookies	6.0	120	45%

Food and Description	Amount	Fat Grams	Total Calories	% Fat Calories
chocolate	3 cookies	7.0	120	53%
double fudge	3 cookies	7.0	140	45%
fudge-dipped				
shortbread	5 cookies	7.0	130	48%
wafers	4 cookies	10.0	140	64%
gingersnap	7 cookies	4.5	130	31%
lemon				
low-fat/iced	7 cookies	1.5	120	9%
sandwich	3 cookies	6.0	120	45%
sugar wafers	4 cookies	10.0	130	69%
oatmeal	5 cookies	7.0	150	42%
peanut butter	3 cookies	9.0	150	54%
shortbread	8 cookies	6.0	120	45%
pecan	3 cookies	11.0	170	58%
vanilla sugar wafers	4 cookies	10.0	130	69%
■ (Nabisco)				
CHIPS AHOY/Chocolate Chip Cookies				
Candy Blasts	½ oz	4.0	80	45%
caramel/6-count	1 cookie	9.0	180	45%
chunky	1 cookie	4.0	80	45%
white fudge	½ oz	4.0	80	45%
chocolate				
chewy	1.2 oz	7.0	150	42%
12-count	1.58 oz	10.0	210	43%
chewy real				
chocolate chips	1.2 oz	8.0	170	42%
chip/4 cookies	1.4 oz	9.0	200	41%
Cremewiches				
chocolate				
w/chocolate crème	1 oz	7.0	150	42%
w/peanut butter	1 oz	8.0	150	48%
w/vanilla crème	1 oz	7.0	150	42%
mini chocolate chip				
2-GO! 1.25 oz bag	1 bag	10.0	210	43%
1.5 oz	1 pkg	10.0	210	43%
bite-size	1.3 oz	9.0	170	48%
GO-Pack	1 oz	7.0	150	42%
Go-Tubes	1 oz	7.0	150	42%
Packs 2 GO!/12-count	1.4 oz	9.0	200	41%
real chocolate chip	3 cookies	8.0	160	45%
1.4 oz package	1 pkg	9.0	200	41%
reduced-fat	1 cookie	5.0	140	32%
HONEY MAID GRAHAMS				
apple cinnamon sticks	1 oz	3.0	130	21%
chocolate	8 cookies	3.0	120	23%
sticks	1 oz	3.0	130	21%
cinnamon	8 cookies	3.0	140	19%
low-fat	8 cookies	1.5	120	11%
sticks	1 oz	2.5	120	17%
GO-Pack	1 oz	3.0	130	21%

Food and Description	Amount	Fat Grams	Total Calories	% Fat Calories
honey/original	8 cookies	2.5	120	17%
	1 oz	3.0	140	19%
low-fat	8 cookies	1.5	120	11%
sticks	1 oz	3.0	130	21%
oatmeal crunch	1 oz	3.0	130	21%
NABISCO FAMILY FAVORITES				
Barnum's Animals				
box/2.125 oz	½ box	4.0	130	28%
Snak Sacks/bag	1 oz	4.0	130	28%
Biscos sugar wafer	8 cookies	6.0	140	39%
Cameo creme sandwich	2 cookies	5.0	130	35%
Famous wafers/chocolate	~1 oz	5.0	140	32%
gingersnap				
old-fashioned	4 cookies	2.5	120	19%
grahams				
fudge-covered grahams	1 serving	7.0	140	45%
original	8 cookies	3.0	130	21%
Imperio/combination				
Combinato	1.25 oz	7.0	170	37%
Lorna Doone shortbread	4 cookies	7.0	140	45%
Mallomars/pure chocolate	2 cookies	5.0	120	38%
Marshmallow fudge twirls	1 piece	6.0	130	42%
Morelianas/orange Naranja	1 oz	5.0	130	35%
national arrowroot				
biscuit	1 cookie	0.5	20	23%
oatmeal				
iced	1 cookie	3.0	80	34%
regular	1 cookie	3.0	80	34%
Pecanz/pecan shortbread	½ oz	5.0	90	50%
Social Tea biscuits	6 cookies	4.0	120	30%
zwieback	1 piece	1.0	35	26%
NEWTONS				
cobblers				
apple	2 cookies	–	90	–
caramel apple				
snackable dessert	2 cookies	2.5	130	17%
cinnamon	2 cookies	–	90	–
Cherries 'n' Cheesecake				
snackable dessert	1.3 oz	2.5	120	19%
fig				
2-count	2 oz	4.0	200	18%
fat-free	2 cookies	–	90	–
Packs 2-GO!/12-pack	1 oz	–	100	–
regular	2 cookies	2.5	110	20%
	2 oz pkg	4.5	210	19%
peach apricot	2 cookies	–	70	–
raspberry	2 cookies	–	90	–
& yogurt	2 cookies	2.5	130	17%
strawberry	2 cookies	–	90	–
& yogurt	2 cookies	3.0	130	21%

Food and Description	Amount	Fat Grams	Total Calories	% Fat Calories
kiwi	1 oz	1.5	100	14%
Snackable Dessert				
Shortcake	1.3 oz	3.0	130	21%
NILLA VANILLA WAFER				
chocolate reduced-fat	1 oz	2.0	110	16%
original	1 oz	6.0	140	39%
reduced-fat	1 oz	2.0	120	15%
NUTTER BUTTER				
4-count pack	1 pkg	11.0	260	38%
Bites/99 Cents package	⅓ pkg	6.0	150	36%
Bites/1.25-oz package	1 pkg	7.0	170	37%
Bites/Snak Saks	1 oz	6.0	140	39%
Bites-to-Go pak	1 oz	6.0	140	39%
peanut butter sandwich	2 cookies	6.0	130	42%
1.9-oz package	1 pkg	11.0	260	38%
peanut butter				
creme patty	5 cookies	10.0	170	53%
OREO				
chocolate	1.32 oz	7.0	160	39%
creme/4-count	1.12 oz	7.0	150	42%
football	1.2 oz	7.0	160	39%
fudge-covered	~1 oz	5.0	90	50%
fudge mint–covered	1 oz	4.5	90	45%
reduced-fat	1.2 oz	3.5	140	23%
Cookie Barz				
6-count	1 bar	10.0	180	50%
8-count	1 bar	8.0	150	48%
20-count	1 bar	10.0	180	50%
individual	1.23 oz	10.0	180	50%
Double Delight Chocolate				
coffee 'n' crème	1 oz	7.0	150	42%
mint 'n' crème	1 oz	7.0	140	45%
Double Stuff Chocolate	1 oz	7.0	140	45%
1.5-oz package	1 pkg	10.0	210	43%
mini				
chocolate	1.25 oz	7.0	170	37%
12-count	1 pkg	9.0	200	41%
bite size/3-oz pkg	⅓ pkg	6.0	140	39%
crème	1.25 oz	7.0	170	37%
12-count	1 pkg	9.0	200	41%
fun-size				
Easter	1 oz	6.0	130	42%
Halloween	1 oz	6.0	130	42%
Go-Pak Cup/bite-size	¼ cup	6.0	140	38%
Go-Pak/chocolate	1 pkg	10.0	210	43%
Oreo & mini Chips Ahoy				
20 pack	1 pkg	7.0	170	37%
Oreo, Nutter Butter &				
Chips Ahoy				
12-count	1 pkg	7.0	170	37%

Food and Description	Amount	Fat Grams	Total Calories	% Fat Calories
red & white crème	1 oz	6.0	140	38%
Snak Saks				
chocolate	1 pkg	6.0	140	38%
peanut butter				
& chocolate crème	1 oz	7.0	140	45%
Spring w/purple crème	1 oz	7.0	150	42%
Uh-Oh w/chocolate crème	1.2 oz	7.0	170	37%
White fudge covered	¾ oz	6.0	110	49%
Winter 4 Fun shapes				
w/red crème	1 oz	7.0	140	45%
SNACKWELL'S				
BITE-SIZE				
chocolate chip	~1 oz	4.0	130	28%
double chocolate chip	~1 oz	4.0	130	28%
peanut butter chip	~1 oz	4.0	120	30%
CARBWELL				
fudge brownie cookie	1 serving	3.5	90	35%
fudge-striped				
shortbread	1 serving	9.0	150	54%
fudge-covered grahams	1 serving	9.0	150	54%
FAT-FREE				
devil's food cookie cakes	1 cookie	–	50	–
ORIGINAL				
chocolate sandwich	1 oz	3.0	110	25%
coconut creme	2 cookies	4.0	110	33%
golden devil's food	1 cookie	0.5	50	9%
mint creme	2 cookies	3.5	110	29%
oatmeal raisin	2 cookies	3.0	110	25%
peanut butter/bite-size	13 cookies	4.0	120	30%
SUGAR-FREE				
chocolate chip	1 oz	8.0	150	48%
chocolate sandwich	1 oz	6.0	130	42%
crème sandwich	1 oz	6.0	130	42%
fudge-striped shortbread	~1 oz	9.0	150	54%
lemon crème sandwich	1 oz	6.0	130	42%
oatmeal	~1 oz	2.5	90	25%
shortbread	1 oz	5.0	130	35%
TEDDY GRAHAMS				
Graham Snacks				
Bob the Builder	1 oz	4.0	120	30%
cinnamon	1 oz	4.0	120	30%
chocolate	1 oz	4.5	130	31%
honey & cinnamon sticks	1.25 oz	5.0	150	30%
cinnamon	1 oz	4.0	130	28%
99 cents/cinnamon	1 oz	4.0	130	28%
1.25-oz package	1 pkg	5.0	160	28%
Clifford the Big				
Red Dog	1 oz	4.0	130	28%
honey/chocolate	1.25 oz	4.5	150	27%
honey	1 oz	4.0	130	28%

Food and Description	Amount	Fat Grams	Total Calories	% Fat Calories
1.25-oz package	1 pkg	4.5	150	27%
Dora the Explorer	1 oz	4.0	130	28%
fun-size				
holiday	1 oz	3.5	120	26%
Halloween	1 oz	3.5	120	26%
Mint/Snack Saks	1 oz	4.0	130	28%
Mini chocolate chip				
Snack Saks	1 oz	4.5	140	29%
■ (Nestlé) Toll House				
refrigerated/ready-to-bake				
Break & Bake				
chocolate chip	1 cookie	5.0	110	41%
chocolate chip				
& caramel	1 cookie	4.5	100	41%
& fudge	1 cookie	5.0	110	41%
& peanut butter	1 cookie	5.0	100	45%
chocolate chunk	1 cookie	5.0	110	41%
peanut butter	1 cookie	7.0	150	42%
sugar	1 cookie	5.0	110	41%
Ultimates				
chip & chunks	1 cookie	11.0	200	50%
chocolate chip lovers	1 cookie	10.0	200	45%
macadamia white fudge	1 cookie	11.0	200	49%
peanut butter chips				
& chunks	1 cookie	10.0	190	47%
walnut chocolate	1 cookie	6.0	110	49%
rolled cookies				
chocolate chip				
original	1 cookie	6.0	140	38%
reduced-fat	1 cookie	3.5	130	24%
sugar	1 cookie	5.0	120	38%
■ (New Morning)				
grahams				
cinnamon	2 sheets	3.0	130	21%
honey	2 sheets	3.0	130	21%
GrahamWiches				
chocolate &				
peanut butter crème	2 cookies	5.0	120	38%
peanut butter crème	2 cookies	5.0	130	35%
vanilla crème	2 cookies	5.0	130	35%
Mini Bites				
chocolate grahams	22 pieces	3.0	110	25%
honey graham	22 pieces	3.0	110	25%
■ (Nonni's)				
biscotti				
chocolate	1 piece	6.0	130	42%
cioccolate	1 piece	6.0	130	42%
twin pack	1 piece	6.0	130	42%
decaf	1 piece	5.0	130	35%
Decadence	1 piece	5.0	130	35%

Food and Description	Amount	Fat Grams	Total Calories	% Fat Calories
original	1 piece	4.0	100	36%
twin pack	1 piece	4.0	100	36%
Paradise	1 piece	6.0	130	42%
value pack	1 piece	4.0	100	36%
Cio	1 piece	6.0	130	42%
Noci Cio	1 piece	6.0	150	36%
■ **OREO** (*See* (Nabisco) in this section)				
■ **(Otis Spunkmeyer)**				
frozen cookie dough = baked cookies				
Café Collection Cookies/thaw & serve 5 oz				
Serving size = 2-oz cookie/servings per cookie/2.5				
chocolate chunk	1 serving	11.0	250	40%
oatmeal raisin	1 serving	8.0	230	31%
white chocolate				
macadamia nut	1 serving	13.0	270	51%
Supreme Indulgence Super Premium/2-oz size				
chocolate chunk	1 cookie	12.0	250	43%
oatmeal raisin	1 cookie	9.0	230	35%
peanut butter				
chocolate chip	1 cookie	13.0	260	45%
white chunk				
macadamia nut	1 cookie	15.0	270	50%
Sweet Discovery/1.3-oz medium-size				
butter sugar	1 cookie	8.0	160	45%
buttercrunch toffee	1 cookie	8.0	170	42%
Café Vienna	1 cookie	8.0	170	42%
Carnival	1 cookie	7.0	160	39%
chocolate chip				
double	1 cookie	9.0	180	45%
chocolate w/Reese's				
Pieces candy	1 cookie	8.0	170	42%
milk chocolate chunk	1 cookie	8.0	170	42%
regular	1 cookie	8.0	170	42%
w/pecans	1 cookie	9.0	170	48%
w/walnuts	1 cookie	9.0	180	45%
oatmeal				
cranberry	1 cookie	6.0	150	36%
raisin	1 cookie	6.0	160	34%
peanut butter	1 cookie	10.0	180	50%
chocolate chunk	1 cookie	10.0	180	50%
Rocky Road	1 cookie	8.0	160	45%
triple chocolate	1 cookie	8.0	170	42%
turtle	1 cookie	9.0	170	48%
white chocolate				
macadamia nut	1 cookie	10.0	180	50%
Sweet Discovery/4-oz/old-fashioned size				
butter sugar	½ cookie	12.0	250	43%
Buttercrunch Toffee	½ cookie	12.0	250	43%
Carnival	½ cookie	11.0	250	45%
chocolate chip				
double chocolate	½ cookie	14.0	270	47%

Food and Description	Amount	Fat Grams	Total Calories	% Fat Calories
milk chocolate chunk	½ cookie	13.0	250	47%
regular	½ cookie	11.0	250	40%
oatmeal raisin	½ cookie	10.0	230	39%
peanut butter				
chocolate chunk	½ cookie	11.0	240	41%
regular	½ cookie	15.0	270	50%
turtle	½ cookie	13.0	250	47%
white chocolate				
macadamia nut	½ cookie	15.0	280	48%
Sweet Discovery/4-oz cookies				
chocolate chip	1 cookie	17.0	370	41%
oatmeal raisin	1 cookie	15.0	350	39%
peanut butter	1 cookie	21.0	390	48%
white chocolate				
macadamia nut	1 cookie	20.0	390	46%
Sweet Discovery/Bite Size cookies				
butter sugar	1 cookie	4.0	90	40%
chocolate chip	1 cookie	4.5	100	41%
double	1 cookie	5.0	100	45%
oatmeal raisin	1 cookie	3.5	90	35%
peanut butter	1 cookie	5.0	100	45%
white chocolate				
macadamia nut	1 cookie	5.0	100	45%
Sweet Discovery/"Spunkies"				
chocolate chip	4 cookies	6.0	130	42%
peanut butter	4 cookies	7.0	140	45%
Traditional Recipe/1.5-oz cookies				
Carnival	1 cookie	8.0	180	40%
chocolate chip				
double chocolate	1 cookie	9.0	180	45%
regular	1 cookie	8.0	180	40%
oatmeal raisin	1 cookie	8.0	180	40%
peanut butter	1 cookie	11.0	190	52%
Ranger	1 cookie	9.0	190	43%
sugar	1 cookie	8.0	180	40%
white chocolate				
macadamia nut	1 cookie	9.0	190	43%
Traditional Recipe/2.5-oz cookies				
Carnival	1 cookie	14.0	310	41%
chocolate chip	1 cookie	14.0	310	41%
double chocolate	1 cookie	15.0	310	44%
oatmeal raisin	1 cookie	13.0	300	39%
peanut butter	1 cookie	18.0	320	51%
Ranger	1 cookie	16.0	310	46%
sugar	1 cookie	14.0	310	41%
■ (Pamela's)				
BISCOTTI				
almond anise	2 pieces	6.0	170	32%
chocolate walnut	2 pieces	6.0	170	32%
lemon almond	2 pieces	7.0	170	37%

Food and Description	Amount	Fat Grams	Total Calories	% Fat Calories
CARB-CONSCIOUS				
chocolate chip				
walnut	1 cookie	3.5	60	53%
coconut	1 cookie	4.5	60	68%
peanut butter	1 cookie	3.5	50	63%
ORGANIC COOKIES				
chocolate chunk pecan				
shortbread	2 cookies	11.0	190	52%
dark chocolate,				
chocolate chunk	2 cookies	8.0	160	45%
espresso chocolate				
chunk	2 cookies	8.0	160	45%
oatmeal				
raisin walnut	2 cookies	9.0	170	48%
spicy ginger	2 cookies	7.0	160	39%
TRADITIONAL COOKIES (wheat and gluten-free)				
butter shortbread	1 cookie	6.0	120	45%
carob hazelnut	1 cookie	7.0	120	53%
chocolate chip				
chunky	1 cookie	6.0	120	45%
walnut	1 cookie	8.0	130	55%
ginger w/sliced				
almonds	1 cookie	5.0	110	41%
peanut butter	1 cookie	5.0	90	50%
shortbread				
lemon	1 cookie	6.0	120	30%
pecan shortbread	1 cookie	8.0	130	55%
swirl	1 cookie	7.0	120	53%
■ (Peak Frean's)				
arrowroot	4 biscuits	4.5	150	27%
coffee creme	2 biscuits	6.0	140	39%
crème/assorted	1 oz	6.0	140	39%
fruit creme	2 biscuits	5.0	130	35%
ginger crisp	~1 oz	4.5	150	27%
Nice biscuits	4 biscuits	6.0	160	34%
Petit Beurre	1 oz	4.0	130	28%
shortcake	3 cookies	7.0	140	45%
■ (Pepperidge Farm)				
Chocolate Chunk/Crispy Cookies				
Chesapeake/dark chocolate				
pecan	1 cookie	8.0	140	51%
Nantucket/dark chocolate				
chunk	1 cookie	7.0	140	45%
Sanibel/milk chocolate				
almond	1 cookie	8.0	140	51%
Sausalito/milk chocolate				
macadamia	1 cookie	8.0	140	51%
Sedona/dark chocolate toffee				
& pecans	1 cookie	7.0	130	48%
Tahoe/white chocolate				
macadamia	1 cookie	6.0	130	42%

Food and Description	Amount	Fat Grams	Total Calories	% Fat Calories
Distinctive cookies				
Bordeaux				
milk chocolate	3 cookies	9.0	160	51%
original	4 cookies	5.0	130	35%
Brussels				
individual pkg	2 cookies	4.0	100	36%
mint	3 cookies	10.0	190	47%
regular pkg	3 cookies	7.0	150	42%
Brussels mint	3 cookies	10.0	190	47%
Chantilly/raspberry	3 cookies	3.0	120	23%
Chessmen				
butter pecan	3 cookies	6.0	130	42%
butterscotch	3 cookies	5.0	120	38%
individual pkg	3 cookies	4.0	100	36%
regular pkg	3 cookies	5.0	120	38%
Geneva	3 cookies	9.0	160	51%
Lido	1 cookie	5.0	90	50%
double chocolate	2 cookies	8.0	140	51%
milk chocolate	3 cookies	10.0	180	50%
Salzburg	2 cookies	6.0	150	36%
Verona				
apricot/raspberry	3 cookies	6.0	140	39%
strawberry	3 cookies	5.0	140	32%
Old-Fashioned home-style cookies				
ginger man	4 cookies	4.0	130	28%
lemon nut	3 cookies	9.0	170	48%
sugar	3 cookies	6.0	140	39%
Soft-baked cookies				
Augusta	1 cookie	7.0	130	48%
milk chocolate caramel chewy	1 cookie	6.0	140	39%
Nantucket/dark chocolate				
chunk	1 cookie	7.0	140	45%
Santa Cruz/oatmeal raisin	1 cookie	5.0	140	32%
Sausalito/milk chocolate				
macadamia	1 cookie	8.0	140	51%
Pirouette				
chocolate hazelnut	2 cookies	6.0	140	42%
chocolate mint	2 cookies	6.0	140	42%
French vanilla	2 cookies	6.0	140	42%
■ (Pillsbury)				
Cookie Mix/Snack Batch				
chocolate chip/mix only	~1 oz	2.0	100	18%
Ready to Bake/refrigerated cookie dough				
chocolate chip	1 cookie	6.0	120	45%
w/walnuts	1 cookie	7.0	120	45%
sugar	1 cookie	6.0	120	45%
Refrigerated Cookie Dough				
chocolate chip				
double & chunk	1 cookie	7.0	140	45%
home-baked classics	1 cookie	8.0	160	45%

Food and Description	Amount	Fat Grams	Total Calories	% Fat Calories
reduced-fat	1 cookie	3.0	110	25%
roll	1 cookie	7.0	140	45%
tub	1 cookie	7.0	140	45%
w/walnuts	1 cookie	7.0	130	48%
chocolate chunk	1 cookie	7.0	140	45%
M&M's	2 cookies	6.0	150	36%
holiday	1 cookie	6.0	150	36%
oatmeal chocolate chip	1 cookie	6.0	120	45%
peanut butter	1 cookie	6.0	130	42%
holiday	1 cookie	6.0	130	42%
shaped				
Christmas tree	2 slices	8.0	160	45%
flag	2 slices	8.0	160	45%
ghost	2 slices	8.0	160	45%
gingerbread	2 slices	7.0	140	45%
holiday	2 slices	7.0	140	45%
Linus/Great Pumpkin	2 slices	8.0	160	45%
Peter Cottontail	2 slices	8.0	160	45%
Rudolph	2 slices	8.0	160	45%
shamrock	2 slices	8.0	160	45%
Snoopy valentine	2 slices	8.0	160	45%
Valentines	2 slices	8.0	160	45%
sugar	2 cookies	5.0	130	35%
holiday	2 cookies	5.0	130	35%
white chocolate chunk	2 cookies	6.0	30	42%
■ (Rippin' Good)				
Carousel	6 cookies	6.0	140	39%
chocolate chip creme	2 cookies	6.0	160	34%
cookie jar	3 cookies	6.0	150	36%
creme wafers/assorted	3 cookies	7.0	140	45%
duplex creme	2 cookies	4.0	100	36%
fudge stripe oatmeal	2 cookies	8.0	140	51%
gingersnap	5 cookies	4.0	130	26%
granola & peanut butter sandwich	2 cookies	6.0	140	39%
iced oatmeal	2 cookies	2.0	90	30%
iced spice	3 cookies	3.0	130	21%
lemon crisp	3 cookies	8.0	160	45%
macaroon cremes	2 cookies	8.0	160	45%
marshmallow blossoms	2 cookies	2.0	90	30%
marshmallow daisies	2 cookies	2.0	90	30%
marshmallow fudge stripes	2 cookies	4.0	100	36%
peanut butter	2 cookies	4.0	100	36%
Rippie Cremes vanilla sandwich	3 cookies	6.0	160	34%
spice wafer	3 cookies	4.0	140	26%
striped dainties	1 cookie	3.0	50	54%

■ **SIMPLE PLEASURES** (*See* (Dare) in this section)

Food and Description	Amount	Fat Grams	Total Calories	% Fat Calories
■ **SNACKWELL'S** (*See* (Nabisco) in this section)				
■ **(Spaans Cookie Co.)**				
FAT-FREE COOKIES				
Oat bran 'n' raisin	2 cookies	–	80	–
LOW-FAT COOKIES				
banana	2 cookies	3.0	100	27%
chocolate chip	2 cookies	3.0	110	25%
fudge 'n' chips	2 cookies	3.0	100	27%
oat bran 'n' chips	2 cookies	3.0	100	27%
REGULAR COOKIES				
butter melt	2 cookies	6.0	130	42%
chocolate chip				
plain	2 cookies	6.0	120	45%
w/walnuts	1 cookie	7.0	130	48%
cinnamon bears	1 cookie	4.0	100	36%
cocoa bears	1 cookie	4.0	100	36%
coconut krispies	2 cookies	5.0	120	38%
date oatmeal	2 cookies	4.5	120	34%
fruit 'n' honey	2 cookies	3.5	110	29%
fudge 'n' chips				
w/walnuts	2 cookies	6.0	120	45%
fudge brownie	2 cookies	4.5	120	34%
harvest	2 cookies	6.0	130	42%
holiday	2 cookies	7.0	130	48%
oat bran 'n' raisin	1 cookie	4.5	110	37%
peanut butter	2 cookies	7.0	130	48%
shortbread	2 cookies	5.0	120	38%
soft oatmeal	2 cookies	3.5	110	29%
Speculaas/windmills	2 cookies	6.0	130	42%
sugar bear	1 cookie	4.0	100	36%
toasted almond	2 cookies	7.0	130	48%
SUGAR-FREE COOKIES				
cherry crisps	3 cookies	5.0	110	41%
chocolate chip swirls	3 cookies	5.0	110	41%
crunchy vanilla	3 cookies	5.0	120	38%
Dutch chocolate	3 cookies	5.0	110	41%
lemon coconut	3 cookies	6.0	120	30%
peanut butter	3 cookies	6.0	120	30%
spiced windmill	3 cookies	5.0	110	41%
■ **(Stella D'Oro)**				
Biscotti				
almond	~½ oz	4.5	100	41%
chocolate almond	~½ oz	4.0	90	41%
chocolate chunk	~½ oz	4.0	90	40%
French vanilla	~½ oz	3.5	90	35%
Breakfast Treats				
chocolate	¾ oz	3.0	90	30%
original	¾ oz	3.0	90	30%
mini	1 oz	3.5	120	26%
Viennese cinnamon	¾ oz	2.5	90	25%

Food and Description	Amount	Fat Grams	Total Calories	% Fat Calories
Coffee Treats/toast				
almond	1 oz	4.5	110	20%
angel wings	~1 oz	12.0	170	64%
anisette	1 oz	1.0	130	7%
low-fat	1.3 oz	1.0	130	7%
mini	1 oz	1.0	130	7%
sponge				
low-fat	~1 oz	1.0	90	10%
original	~1 oz	1.0	90	10%
banana walnut	~1 oz	2.0	100	18%
blueberry	~1 oz	1.0	100	9%
cinnamon raisin	~1 oz	1.0	100	9%
Roman egg biscuits	1 oz	4.0	130	28%
Cookies				
almond				
delight	1 oz	8.0	160	45%
toast	1 oz	2.5	110	20%
Anginetti	1 oz	3.5	130	24%
egg jumbo	~1 oz	1.5	120	11%
Lady Stella assortment	1 oz	4.5	130	31%
Margherite				
combination	1 oz	5.0	130	35%
mini	1.2 oz	5.0	150	30%
original	1 oz	4.5	130	31%
Swiss fudge	~1 oz	9.0	170	48%
■ (Tastykake)				
chocolate chip	3 cookies	6.0	130	42%
oatmeal raisin	3 cookies	6.0	130	42%
sugar	3 cookies	6.0	120	45%
■ (Tofutti) non-dairy				
chocolate chip	1 cookie	6.0	139	39%
fig bars	1 cookie	2.0	100	18%
oatmeal raisin	1 cookie	4.0	118	31%
peanut butter	1 cookie	7.0	137	46%
■ TOLL HOUSE (*See* (Nestlé) in this section)				
■ (Twix)				
cookie bars				
caramel	2 bars	14.0	280	45%
peanut butter	2 bars	17.0	280	55%
■ (Umeya)..fortune cookie	4 cookies	0.5	110	4%
■ (Voortman)				
Almonette	1 cookie	6.0	100	54%
chocolate chip	1 cookie	4.5	100	41%
chunky	1 cookie	11.0	230	43%
jumbo	1 cookie	11.0	230	43%
sugar-free	1 cookie	6.0	100	54%
chocolate wafer	3 cookies	9.0	160	51%
sugar-free	3 cookies	11.0	160	62%
coconut delight	1 cookie	5.0	90	50%
Dutch creme	1 cookie	4.5	110	37%

Food and Description	Amount	Fat Grams	Total Calories	% Fat Calories
fudge swirl	1 cookie	5.0	90	50%
Gingerboy	1 cookie	4.0	90	40%
maple cream sandwich	1 cookie	5.0	110	41%
oatmeal				
apple	1 cookie	3.0	80	34%
fudge-striped	1 cookie	6.0	130	42%
raisin/jumbo	1 cookie	10.0	270	33%
Peanut Delight	1 cookie	7.0	120	53%
jumbo	1 cookie	14.0	240	53%
shortbread	1 cookie	6.0	110	49%
sugar-free	1 cookie	7.0	120	53%
swirl	2 cookies	6.0	110	49%
sugar	1 cookie	4.0	90	40%
vanilla wafer	3 cookies	9.0	170	43%
windmill	1 cookie	4.0	100	36%
■ (Weight Watchers)				
apple raisin bar	1 cookie	2.0	70	26%
chocolate sandwich	2 cookies	4.0	140	26%
oatmeal raisin	2 cookies	2.0	120	15%
vanilla sandwich	2 cookies	3.0	140	19%
■ (Westbrae)				
COOKIE JAR CLASSICS				
Dutch apple cinnamon	1 cookie	4.0	110	32%
honey almond	1 cookie	4.0	110	32%
raspberry vanilla	1 cookie	4.0	110	32%
REGULAR COOKIES				
crispy chocolate chip	1 cookie	4.0	110	32%
soft chocolate chip				
coconut	1 cookie	4.5	110	37%
pecan	1 cookie	4.5	110	37%
walnut	1 cookie	5.0	110	41%
soft chocolate chocolate chip	1 cookie	3.0	90	30%
RICE MALT COOKIES				
gingersnap	3 cookies	5.0	130	35%
oatmeal	3 cookies	6.0	140	39%
COOKIE CRUMBS (See also CRACKER CRUMBS/MEAL)				
(Nabisco)				
Oreo				
cookie crumbs	2 Tbs	4.0	90	40%
crunchies	~½ oz	2.5	50	45%
COOKING SPRAY				
(Crisco)				
natural blend oil	⅓-sec spray	14.0	120	100%
natural butter				
no-stick	⅓-sec spray	–	–	–
original w/canola oil	⅓-sec spray	14.0	120	100%
pure all-natural oil				
100% extra-virgin	⅓-sec spray	14.0	120	100%
(Mazola)				
butter/fat-free	2-sec spray	–	–	–

Food and Description	Amount	Fat Grams	Total Calories	% Fat Calories
original canola (Pam)	2-sec spray	–	–	–
butter flavor	⅓-sec spray	<1	–	–
Pam for baking	⅓-sec spray	<1	–	–
olive oil	⅓-sec spray	<1	–	–
original (Weight Watchers)	⅓-sec spray	<1	–	–
butter	⅓-sec spray	–	–	–
cooking	⅓-sec spray	–	–	–
CORIANDER LEAF (*See* CILANTRO)				
CORIANDER SEED				
whole	1 tsp	<1.0	5	53%
	1 Tbs	0.9	15	53%
	1 oz	5.0	85	53%
CORN				
CANNED/JARRED				
(Blue Boy)				
cream-style sweet	½ cup	–	25	–
whole-kernel sweet	½ cup	–	90	–
(Bristol) baby				
corn on cob	4 ears	–	12	–
(Del Monte)				
cream-style				
golden				
no salt added	½ cup	0.5	90	5%
regular	½ cup	0.5	90	5%
supersweet	½ cup	0.5	60	8%
traditional				
home-style	½ cup	1.0	100	9%
white	½ cup	1.0	100	9%
whole kernel				
fiesta	½ cup	1.0	50	18%
gold & white	⅓ cup	0.5	80	6%
golden				
regular	½ cup	1.0	90	10%
supersweet				
no salt added	½ cup	1.0	60	15%
no sugar added	½ cup	1.0	60	15%
sweet/summer crisp	½ cup	1.0	70	13%
white	½ cup	1.0	60	15%
(Fancifood) baby corn	6 pieces	–	25	–
(Green Giant)				
cream-style	½ cup	0.5	100	5%
Mexicorn	⅓ cup	–	60	–
Niblets				
white shoepeg	⅓ cup	0.5	80	6%
yellow				
extra-sweet				
plain	⅓ cup	0.5	80	6%
regular	⅓ cup	0.5	50	9%

Food and Description	Amount	Fat Grams	Total Calories	% Fat Calories
50% less sodium	⅓ cup	–	60	–
no salt or				
sugar added	⅓ cup	–	60	–
regular	⅓ cup	–	70	–
shoepeg corn	⅓ cup	0.5	80	6%
super sweet yellow				
and white corn	⅓ cup	–	50	–
whole kernel/sweet				
50% less sodium	½ cup	0.5	80	6%
regular	½ cup	0.5	80	6%
(Kame) Baby cocktail corn	½ cup	–	20	–
(Libby's)				
sweet				
cream-style	½ cup	–	90	–
vacuum packed	⅓ cup	1.0	70	27%
whole kernel	½ cup	1.0	90	10%
(S&W)				
cream-style				
traditional				
home-style	½ cup	0.5	60	8%
w/starch	½ cup	1.0	100	9%
whole kernel				
regular	½ cup	1.0	90	10%
sweet 'n' crisp	⅓ cup	1.5	70	19%
young/sweet/tender	½ cup	1.0	90	10%
(Stokely)				
cream-style..all types	½ cup	1.0	100	9%
whole kernel				
crisp 'n' sweet	½ cup	1.5	80	17%
gold & white				
naturally sweet	½ cup	1.0	80	11%
golden	½ cup	1.5	60	23%
white	½ cup	1.0	190	10%
(WestBrae)				
golden	½ cup	1.0	90	10%
white	½ cup	1.0	100	9%
FRESH/sweet/white or yellow				
kernels/cooked	½ cup	1.0	89	10%
whole ear	1 medium	1.0	89	10%
FROZEN				
(Birds Eye)				
corn on the cob				
big ears	1 ear	1.0	160	6%
corn blend				
gold & white	½ cup	1.0	60	5%
little ears	2 ears	1.0	120	8%
sweet corn on cob	2 ears	1.0	110	8%
kernels				
baby gold & white	½ cup	1.0	80	11%
baby white	⅔ cup	0.5	60	8%

Food and Description	Amount	Fat Grams	Total Calories	% Fat Calories
baby whole	½ cup	0.5	100	5%
cut kernels	⅓ cup	0.5	70	6%
sweet young & tender (C&W)	½ cup	1.0	80	11%
early harvest petite..all styles (Cascadian Farm)	⅔ cup	1.0	80	11%
golden sweet				
w/butter sauce	½ cup	3.0	100	27%
sweet corn	½ cup	1.0	90	10%
(Green Giant)				
corn on the cob				
extra sweet	1 ear	–	120	–
Nibblers/6-ear pkg	1 ear	0.5	70	6%
Niblets/4-ear pkg	1 ear	1.0	150	6%
cream-style sweet	½ cup	0.5	90	5%
kernels				
Niblets				
boil-in-bag				
corn & butter	⅔ cup	2.5	110	20%
no sauce	⅔ cup	0.5	80	6%
extra sweet	⅔ cup	1.0	70	13%
family-size				
in butter sauce	¾ cup	1.5	100	14%
regular	⅔ cup	0.5	80	6%
regular/white				
extra sweet	⅔ cup	0.5	50	9%
shoepeg white/boil-in-bag				
no sauce	½ cup	0.5	70	6%
white corn				
& butter	⅔ cup	2.0	110	16%
Southwest/boil-in-bag corn				
& roasted red peppers	½ cup	0.5	80	6%
(McKenzie's)				
golden cream	½ cup	–	100	–
Southern				
white corn Silver				
Queen–style	½ cup	1.0	80	11%
white creamed Silver				
Queen–style	½ cup	–	100	–
(Ore-Ida) corn on the cob				
mini gold	1 ear	1.0	80	11%
regular	1 ear	1.5	140	10%
(Pictsweet)				
corn on the cob				
3" ear	1 ear	<1.0	50	8%
6" ear	1 ear	1.0	110	8%
kernels/cut	½ cup	1.0	80	11%

CORN CAKE (*See* RICE CAKES)
CORN CHIPS (*See* TORTILLA CHIPS)
CORN CHOWDER (*See* SOUP)

Food and Description	Amount	Fat Grams	Total Calories	% Fat Calories
CORN DISH (*See also* FROZEN ENTRÉE/DINNER; VEGETABLES, MIXED)				
CANNED/JARRED				
(Aunt Nellie's) corn relish	1 Tbs	–	20	–
(Del Monte) Savory Sensations				
corn 'n' butter	½ cup	2.5	90	25%
Santa Fe corn				
in hearty sauce	½ cup	1.0	70	13%
(Green Giant) corn relish	1 Tbs	–	20	–
FROZEN				
(Green Giant)				
Niblets in butter				
sauce	⅔ cup	1.5	110	12%
white shoepeg in				
butter sauce	¾ cup	2.0	110	16%
(Mrs. Paul's)				
corn fritter	1 fritter	6.0	130	42%
CORN DOG (*See also* FRANKFURTER)				
(State Fair) w/Ball Park				
breakfast				
bite				
blueberry	3 pieces	11.0	210	47%
chicken	3 pieces	13.0	220	53%
original	3 pieces	14.0	230	55%
stick/individually wrapped				
blueberry	2.85 oz	13.0	240	49%
chicken	2.9 oz	8.0	210	34%
original	2.85 oz	12.0	230	47%
cheeseburger flavor				
stickwich	4 oz	15.0	270	50%
cheese corn dog	3.25 oz	19.0	250	68%
chicken				
jumbo	4 oz	10.0	260	35%
Classic				
all-meat	2.67 oz	10.0	210	43%
jumbo	4 oz	17.0	340	45%
large	3.2 oz	13.0	270	43%
beef	2.67 oz	12.0	180	60%
jumbo	4.0 oz	19.0	300	57%
Fiesta jalapeño cheese	3.2 oz	11.0	220	45%
low-fat/5-count	1	2.5	150	15%
meat	2.7 oz	10.0	220	41%
w/sleeve	4.0 oz	25.0	330	68%
turkey				
classic	2.67 oz	7.0	190	33%
jumbo	4 oz	12.0	280	39%
large	3.2 oz	10.0	220	41%
light	4 oz	6.0	210	26%
mini	4 oz	17.0	310	49%
w/sleeve	4 oz	12.0	280	39%

Food and Description	Amount	Fat Grams	Total Calories	% Fat Calories
CORNFLAKE CRUMBS				
(Kellogg's)	2 Tbs	–	40	–
CORN GRITS (See also CEREAL)				
(Albers)				
quick hominy/dry				
white	¼ cup	0.5	140	3%
yellow	¼ cup	0.5	140	3%
(Arrowhead Mills)				
corn grits/dry				
white	¼ cup	–	150	–
yellow	¼ cup	–	130	–
(Aunt Jemima)				
quick/dry	1 pkt	0.5	130	3%
regular/old-fashioned	1 pkt	0.5	140	3%
(Jim Dandy) enriched/dry				
quick	1.6 oz	0.5	160	3%
regular	~1.5 oz	0.5	160	3%
(Quaker)				
instant/dry				
4-cheddar cheese blend	1 pkt	2.5	100	23%
American cheese	1 pkt	1.5	100	14%
country bacon	1 pkt	0.5	100	5%
ham 'n' cheese	1 pkt	1.5	100	14%
original	1 pkt	–	100	–
quick/dry				
golden grits	¼ cup	0.5	120	4%
regular	¼ cup	0.5	130	3%
real				
butter flavor	1 pkt	1.5	100	14%
cheddar cheese	1 pkt	1.5	100	14%
red eye & country				
gravy	1 pkt	0.5	100	5%
regular old-fashioned				
white hominy	¼ cup	0.5	140	4%
(Spice Hunter) microwavable cups				
butter & cheddar	1 cup	3.0	180	15%
ham & cheddar	1 cup	3.0	180	15%
CORN NUT (See SNACKS)				
CORN PONE (See BREAD)				
CORN STARCH				
(Argo)	1 Tbs	–	30	–
(Cream) 100% pure	1 Tbs	–	30	–
(Maizena)				
caramel flavor	1 Tbs	–	35	–
regular flavor	1 Tbs	–	30	–
strawberry flavor	1 Tbs	–	35	–
vanilla flavor	1 Tbs	–	35	–
CORN SYRUP (See PANCAKE & WAFFLE SYRUP)				

Food and Description	Amount	Fat Grams	Total Calories	% Fat Calories
CORNBREAD (*See* BREAD)				
CORNED BEEF (*See* BEEF; LUNCHEON MEAT)				
CORNED BEEF HASH (*See* BEEF DISH/ENTRÉE)				
CORNISH GAME HEN (*See also* CHICKEN)				
fresh & frozen				
(Perdue) whole				
dark meat	3 oz	15.0	210	64%
white meat	3 oz	10.0	170	53%
(Tyson) w/giblets	4 oz	12.0	180	60%
fully cooked				
(Perdue) oven-roasted				
dark meat	3 oz	9.0	140	58%
white meat	3 oz	7.0	130	48%
CORNMEAL/Dry				
(Albers) yellow or white	3 Tbs	–	110	–
(Arrowhead Mills)				
blue	¼ cup	1.5	130	10%
yellow	¼ cup	1.0	120	8%
(Aunt Jemima) self-rising				
white/enriched				
bolted	3 Tbs	0.5	90	5%
de-germed	3 Tbs	0.5	90	5%
(Martha White) enriched				
yellow/plain	3 Tbs	1.0	120	8%
(Quaker)				
masa harina	¼ cup	1.5	110	12%
preparada para				
tortillas	⅓ cup	4.5	160	25%
white/enriched	3 Tbs	0.5	90	5%
yellow/enriched	3 Tbs	0.5	90	5%
CORNMEAL MIX (*See also* BAKE & FRY MIX)				
(Aunt Jemima) self-rising				
buttermilk white	3 Tbs	0.5	80	6%
white/bolted	3 Tbs	0.5	80	6%
yellow	3 Tbs	4.5	140	29%
(Martha White) dry				
self-rising/enriched				
white	3 Tbs	1.0	110	8%
yellow	3 Tbs	1.0	110	8%
(Miracle Maize) mix only				
country-style	3 Tbs	0.5	130	3%
sweet	3 Tbs	0.5	100	5%
COTTAGE CHEESE (*See also* CHEESE)				
(Borden)				
creamed				
2% fat	½ cup	2.0	90	20%
4% fat	½ cup	5.0	120	38%
dry curd/5% fat	½ cup	1.0	80	11%

Food and Description	Amount	Fat Grams	Total Calories	% Fat Calories
(Breakstone)				
creamed				
2% fat				
large curd	½ cup	2.5	90	25%
small curd	½ cup	2.5	90	25%
snack size	4 oz	2.0	90	20%
4% fat				
large curd	½ cup	5.0	120	38%
small curd	½ cup	5.0	120	38%
snack size	4 oz	5.0	110	41%
dry curd/<0.5% fat	¼ cup	–	45	–
ricotta	¼ cup	–	45	–
(Crowley) creamed				
1% fat				
calcium-fortified	½ cup	1.0	90	10%
plain	½ cup	1.0	90	10%
w/pineapple	½ cup	1.0	110	8%
2% fat	½ cup	2.5	105	21%
4% fat				
plain	½ cup	5.0	120	38%
w/peaches	½ cup	3.0	140	19%
w/pineapple	½ cup	4.0	140	26%
(Friendship) creamed				
1% fat				
plain	½ cup	1.0	90	10%
lactose reduced	½ cup	1.0	90	10%
no salt added	½ cup	1.0	90	10%
w/pineapple	½ cup	1.0	110	8%
2% fat/large				
curd pot-style	½ cup	2.5	90	25%
4% fat				
large curd	½ cup	5.0	120	38%
small curd	½ cup	5.0	120	38%
w/pineapple	½ cup	4.0	140	25%
non-fat	½ cup	–	80	–
(Hood)				
1% low-fat				
black pepper & herbs	½ cup	1.0	80	11%
chive & toasted onion	½ cup	0.5	80	6%
no salt added	½ cup	1.0	80	11%
pineapple cherry	½ cup	1.0	110	8%
plain	½ cup	1.0	80	11%
w/peaches	½ cup	1.0	110	8%
w/strawberries	½ cup	1.0	120	8%
4% fat				
chive				
country-style	½ cup	4.5	110	37%
large curd	½ cup	4.5	110	37%
pineapple	½ cup	3.5	130	24%

Food and Description	Amount	Fat Grams	Total Calories	% Fat Calories
fat-free				
pineapple	½ cup	–	100	–
plain	½ cup	–	80	–
(Kemps)				
creamed				
1% fat/light	4 oz	1.5	90	15%
2% fat/low-fat	4 oz	2.5	90	25%
4% fat	4 oz	5.0	110	41%
fat-free	4 oz	–	80	–
dry curd	4 oz	1.0	80	11%
large curd	4 oz	5.0	110	41%
(Knudsen) creamed				
1.5% fat "On the Go"				
peach	½ cup	1.5	110	12%
pineapple	½ cup	2.0	120	15%
strawberry	½ cup	1.5	110	12%
tropical fruit	½ cup	2.0	110	18%
2% low-fat				
single serve/4-count	1 cup	2.0	90	20%
small curd	½ cup	2.5	100	23%
4% fat				
large curd	½ cup	5.0	130	35%
small curd	½ cup	5.0	120	38%
Nonfat/free				
On the Go!	4 oz	–	70	–
regular	½ cup	–	80	–
(Land O'Lakes) creamed				
1% fat	½ cup	1.0	90	10%
2% fat	½ cup	2.0	100	18%
4% fat	½ cup	5.0	120	38%
(Light 'n' Lively) creamed				
1% fat				
plain	½ cup	1.0	80	11%
w/garden salad	½ cup	1.5	80	17%
w/peach & pineapple	½ cup	1.0	110	8%
low-fat snack size	½ cup	1.0	80	11%
non-fat	½ cup	–	80	–
(Pet)				
2% Go lightly low-fat	½ cup	1.0	90	10%
4% small curd	½ cup	5.0	120	38%
(Sealtest) creamed				
1% fat	½ cup	1.3	99	12%
2% fat/small curd	½ cup	2.5	107	21%
4% fat				
large curd	½ cup	4.5	114	35%
small curd	½ cup	4.5	114	35%
(Weight Watchers) creamed				
1% fat	½ cup	1.0	90	10%
2% fat	½ cup	2.0	90	20%

Food and Description	Amount	Fat Grams	Total Calories	% Fat Calories
COUSCOUS (*See also* PASTA, SOUP/DEHYDRATED)				
(Casbah) mix only				
almond chicken				
vegetarian	1 pkg	2.0	160	11%
asparagus au gratin				
organic	1 pkg	2.0	150	12%
cheddar broccoli	1 pkg	2.0	130	14%
Hearty Harvest	1 pkg	1.0	180	5%
(Marrakesh Express) dry mix				
mango salsa	2 oz	–	190	–
Parmesan cheese	2 oz	1.0	200	5%
plain	2 scoops	–	220	–
roasted chicken				
w/vegetables	2 oz	–	190	–
sun-dried tomato				
& herb	2 oz	–	190	–
wild mushroom	2 oz	0.5	190	2%
(Melting Pot) dry mix				
mango salsa	2 oz	–	190	–
Parmesan cheese	2 oz	1.0	200	5%
plain	2 scoops	–	220	–
roasted chicken				
w/vegetables	2 oz	–	190	–
sun-dried tomato				
& herb	2 oz	–	190	–
wild mushroom	2 oz	0.5	190	2%
(Near East) mix/prepared				
couscous				
broccoli	1 cup	2.5	210	11%
herbed chicken	1 cup	3.5	220	14%
Mediterranean curry	1 cup	3.5	220	14%
original/plain	1 cup	2.0	230	8%
Parmesan	1 cup	3.0	220	12%
roasted garlic				
& olive oil	1 cup	4.5	230	18%
toasted pine nut	1 cup	6.0	230	23%
tomato lentil	1 cup	3.5	220	14%
wild mushroom herb	1 cup	4.0	230	16%
Couscous Moroccan				
pasta	1¼ cups	6.0	260	21%
COWPEA (*See* BLACK-EYED PEA)				
CRAB (*See also* CRAB, IMITATION; CRAB DISH; SEAFOOD ENTRÉE/DINNER)				
CANNED/meat only				
(3 Diamonds)				
fancy w/leg meat	3 oz	–	40	–
fancy white	3 oz	–	45	–
lump	2 oz	–	45	–
(Bumble Bee) Orleans				
fancy lump crabmeat				
premium select	2 oz	1.0	40	23%

Food and Description	Amount	Fat Grams	Total Calories	% Fat Calories
fancy lump/premium				
select	2 oz	1.0	40	23%
(Chicken of the Sea) drained				
crabmeat	2 oz	–	40	–
fancy	2 oz	–	40	–
jumbo lump	2 oz	0.5	35	13%
lump	2 oz	0.5	35	13%
pink	2 oz	–	30	–
white	2 oz	–	30	–
(Crown Prince) drained	½ cup	–	50	–
(Geisha)				
lump	2 oz	0.5	45	10%
snow	2 oz	–	35	–
white	2 oz	0.5	50	9%
(Phillips)				
backfin/pasteurized				
hand-picked	2 oz	–	45	–
(S&W) Dungeness	⅓ cup	1.0	80	11%
FRESH/refrigerated meat only				
Brand-specific				
(Phillips) tub				
backfin				
pasteurized	2 oz	–	45	–
claw/pasteurized	2 oz	–	45	–
Non-Brand				
Alaska/Alaskan king				
cooked—moist heat	3 oz	1.0	82	11%
	1 leg	2.0	129	14%
blue				
cooked—moist heat	3 oz	1.5	90	15%
raw	3 oz	1.0	75	12%
Dungeness				
cooked—moist heat	3 oz	1.0	95	9%
raw	3 oz	1.0	75	12%
queen/raw	3 oz	1.0	76	12%
raw	3 oz	1.0	71	13%
	1 leg	1.0	145	6%
soft shell				
cooked—moist heat	3 oz	1.5	90	15%
fried	1 medium	13.0	213	55%
FROZEN				
(Phillips)				
cocktail crab claws				
restaurant-style	2 oz	–	45	–
CRAB, IMITATION				
(Icicle Seafood)	⅔ cup	–	90	–
(Louis Kemp)				
Crab Delights/fat-free				
chunks	3.2 oz	–	80	–
flake-style	3.2 oz	–	80	–

Food and Description	Amount	Fat Grams	Total Calories	% Fat Calories
shreds	3.2 oz	–	80	–
leg-style	3.2 oz	–	80	–
CRAB DISH (See also SEAFOOD ENTRÉE/DINNER)				
CANNED/PACKAGED				
Bumble Bee seafood salad				
ready-to-eat/2.8 oz	1 pkg	17.0	200	77%
FROZEN				
(Mrs. Paul's)				
deviled crab cake	1 cake	8.0	190	38%
(Nancy's) seafood				
crab cakes				
6-oz package	1 pkg	20.0	350	51%
MIX				
(Zatarain's) crab cake mix				
New Orleans–style				
mix only	1.15 oz	0.5	100	5%
CRAB SOUP (See SOUP)				
CRABAPPLE				
canned				
(Lucky Leaf) spiced	½ cup	–	110	–
fresh/raw/w/skin				
sliced	½ cup	–	40	–
whole	3 oz	–	60	–
CRACKER (See also COOKIE; SNACKS)				
■ (Adrienne's)				
Appeleazers				
double cheddar	1 oz	5.0	130	35%
garlic & herb	1 oz	4.0	130	28%
original	1 oz	4.0	130	28%
Courtney's English Water Crackers				
classic	4 crackers	1.0	60	15%
cracked pepper	4 crackers	1.0	60	15%
savory herb	4 crackers	1.0	60	15%
sun-dried tomato	4 crackers	1.0	60	15%
Darcia's Crostini				
aged cheddar	8 pieces	3.5	90	35%
cheddar	8 pieces	3.5	90	35%
fennel	8 pieces	3.5	90	35%
onion	8 pieces	3.5	90	35%
original	8 pieces	3.5	90	35%
rosemary	8 pieces	3.5	90	35%
Gourmet Lavosh Hawaii flatbread				
bite-size	1 oz	3.0	120	23%
caraway & rye	1 oz	3.0	115	23%
Classic Island	1 oz	3.0	120	23%
mini-bite snack	1 oz	3.0	120	23%
peppercorn	1 oz	3.0	115	23%
portion-control pkgs	1 oz	3.0	120	23%
rosemary garlic	1 oz	3.0	125	22%

Food and Description	Amount	Fat Grams	Total Calories	% Fat Calories
slightly onion	1 oz	3.0	120	23%
10-grain	1 oz	3.0	110	25%
■ (Ak-Mak)				
100% whole wheat cracker bread	5 crackers	2.0	116	16%
Armenian				
regular	1 sheet	2.0	100	18%
round				
no seeds	1 cracker	1.0	100	9%
seeded	1 cracker	2.0	100	18%
whole wheat	1 cracker	2.0	116	16%
whole wheat	1 sheet	2.0	116	16%
■ (Austin)				
snack pack/individual packages				
cheddar on wheat				
sandwich crackers				
reduced fat	1 pkt	7.0	170	37%
regular	1 pkg	10.0	200	45%
cheese Dolphins & Friends	1 pkg	10.0	200	45%
cheese & peanut butter				
reduced-fat	1 pkg	7.0	170	37%
cheese on cheese				
sandwich crackers	1 pkg	10.0	200	45%
grilled cheese sandwich				
cookies	1 pkg	10.0	200	45%
PB&J sandwich crackers	1 pkg	10.0	200	45%
peanut butter on cheese sandwich				
crackers	1 pkg	10.0	200	45%
toast sandwich				
reduced-fat	1 pkg	7.0	170	37%
regular	1 pkg	10.0	200	45%
■ (Barbara's Bakery)				
Cheese Bites	22 crackers	3.0	120	23%
Go-Go Grahams/organic				
chocolate	8 crackers	3.5	130	24%
cinnamon	8 crackers	3.5	130	24%
honey	8 crackers	3.5	130	24%
lemon-ginger	8 crackers	3.5	130	24%
Rite Lite Rounds				
original	5 crackers	2.0	60	30%
savory poppy seed	5 crackers	2.0	60	30%
tamari sesame	5 crackers	2.0	70	26%
Wafer Crisps				
French onion	3 wafers	1.0	60	30%
roasted garlic & herb	3 wafers	1.0	60	30%
sun-dried tomato & basil	3 wafers	1.0	60	30%
toasted sesame	3 wafers	1.0	60	30%

Food and Description	Amount	Fat Grams	Total Calories	% Fat Calories
Wheatines/all natural				
cracked pepper	4 crackers	1.0	50	18%
original	4 crackers	1.0	50	18%
■ **(Bisca)**				
Organic Water Crackers				
cracked pepper	4 crackers	1.0	60	15%
garlic & herb	4 crackers	1.0	60	15%
original	4 crackers	1.0	60	15%
mini	8 crackers	1.0	60	15%
sesame mini	8 crackers	1.5	70	19%
■ **(Blue Diamond)**				
Nut-Thins				
almond	~16 crackers	3.5	120	26%
hazelnut	~16 crackers	3.0	120	23%
pecan	~16 crackers	3.5	120	26%
Smokehouse	~16 crackers	3.5	120	26%
■ **BRETON** (*See* (Dare) in this section)				
■ **(Burns & Ricker)**				
Crispini				
fat-free	½ cup	–	110	–
seeds & spice	5 pieces	3.0	110	25%
sesame	5 pieces	3.0	110	25%
sesame garlic	5 pieces	3.0	110	25%
S.F. stone-ground wheat	5 pieces	<0.5	110	4%
Pita Crisps/~5 per oz				
pesto	1 oz	5.0	130	35%
tomato & onion	1 oz	6.0	130	42%
Tuscany Toast				
pesto	10 pieces	5.0	120	38%
tomato & onion	10 pieces	6.0	130	42%
■ **(Campbell's)**				
soup & oyster	32 pieces	3.0	70	39%
■ **(Carr's)**				
Assortments				
biscuits for cheese	3 biscuits	2.5	83	27%
distinctive flavor assortment	3 crackers	2.5	70	32%
Cocktail Crackers				
Cocktail Cheddars	22 pieces	8.0	150	48%
Cocktail Croissant original golden	22 crackers	3.0	140	19%
sesame & spring vegetable	22 crackers	3.5	140	23%
Entertainers				
cheddar crackers	3 crackers	4.0	80	45%
croissant crackers	3 crackers	3.0	70	39%
poppy & sesame crackers	4 crackers	5.0	80	56%
Wheatolo English biscuits	1 biscuit	3.0	70	39%
whole wheat crackers	2 crackers	3.5	80	39%

Food and Description	Amount	Fat Grams	Total Calories	% Fat Calories
Monterey crackers				
hearty wheat	3 crackers	1.5	50	27%
roasted vegetable	3 crackers	1.5	50	27%
savory wheat	3 crackers	2.0	60	30%
sesame onion	3 crackers	2.5	60	38%
rosemary crackers	7 crackers	5.0	130	35%
table water crackers				
plain	5 crackers	1.5	70	19%
w/cracked pepper	5 crackers	1.5	70	19%
w/roasted garlic & herbs	5 crackers	1.5	70	19%
w/toasted sesame seeds	5 crackers	1.5	70	19%
■ **COMBOS** (See (M&M * Mars) in this section)				
■ **CRISPINI** (See (Burns & Ricker) in this section)				
■ **(Dare)**				
BREMER				
crackers				
caraway	1 oz	2.5	130	17%
soup & chili	½ oz	1.5	60	23%
wafers				
cracked wheat/box	½ oz	1.5	66	20%
low-sodium/box	½ oz	1.5	70	19%
original/can	½ oz	1.5	70	19%
sesame	½ oz	1.8	68	24%
BRETON				
mini crackers				
cheddar	~¾ oz	3.7	87	38%
French onion	~½ oz	5.0	100	45%
garden vegetable	¾ oz	3.8	87	39%
original	1 oz	3.5	70	45%
wheat	~½ oz	4.2	89	42%
regular crackers				
Cabaret crisp & cream	~½ oz	3.5	70	45%
multigrain thin wheat	~½ oz	3.5	70	45%
original thin wheat	~½ oz	3.0	60	45%
reduced fat & sodium thin wheat	~½ oz	1.5	60	23%
sesame thin wheat	~½ oz	3.0	60	45%
Vinta	~½ oz	3.0	70	39%
Vivant zesty vegetable	~½ oz	2.5	60	38%
■ **(Delicious)**				
cheddar cheese				
low-fat	22 crackers	1.5	110	12%
original	24 crackers	4.5	140	29%
snack	28 crackers	7.0	150	42%
chicken-flavored snack	10 crackers	9.0	160	51%
cracked pepper/fat-free	17 crackers	–	110	–

Food and Description	Amount	Fat Grams	Total Calories	% Fat Calories
crispy bacon	11 crackers	7.0	150	42%
garden vegetable				
low-fat	14 crackers	1.5	120	11%
original	13 crackers	7.0	150	42%
graham crackers				
chocolate	2 crackers	3.0	130	21%
cinnamon	2 crackers	3.5	130	24%
honey	2 crackers	3.0	130	21%
hearty wheat snack	13 crackers	6.0	140	39%
Saltines				
original	5 crackers	1.5	60	27%
unsalted tops	5 crackers	1.5	60	27%
savory ranch	10 crackers	8.0	160	45%
sesame wheat	13 crackers	7.0	150	42%
snack crackers	9 crackers	8.0	150	48%
soup & chili crackers	37 crackers	1.5	60	23%
sour cream & chive snack	9 crackers	9.0	160	51%
tangy onion snack	11 crackers	6.0	140	39%
■ (Devonsheer)				
melba rounds				
organic				
garlic	5 pieces	1.0	60	15%
plain				
regular	5 pieces	–	50	–
unsalted	5 pieces	–	50	–
sesame				
regular	5 pieces	2.0	60	30%
unsalted	5 pieces	2.0	60	30%
other				
12-grain	5 pieces	–	50	–
honey bran	5 pieces	–	50	–
onion	5 pieces	–	50	–
savory herb	5 pieces	0.5	50	9%
vegetable	5 pieces	–	50	–
melba toast				
12-grain	3 pieces	–	50	–
garlic	3 pieces	–	50	–
plain				
regular	3 pieces	–	50	–
unsalted	3 pieces	–	50	–
rye	3 pieces	–	50	–
sesame				
regular	3 pieces	1.0	50	18%
unsalted	3 pieces	1.0	50	18%
vegetable	3 pieces	–	50	–
wheat				
regular	3 pieces	–	50	–
unsalted	3 pieces	–	50	–

Food and Description	Amount	Fat Grams	Total Calories	% Fat Calories
■ (Eden)				
rice crackers				
brown rice	1 oz	2.0	120	15%
nori maki	15 crackers	–	110	–
■ (Edward & Sons)				
Brown Rice Snaps				
toasted onion	8 crackers	–	60	–
vegetable	8 crackers	0.5	60	8%
■ (Estee) sugar-free				
Classic				
cracked pepper	18 crackers	2.0	120	15%
golden	10 crackers	2.0	130	14%
wheat	17 crackers	1.5	100	14%
grahams				
chocolate	2 crackers	2.0	110	
cinnamon	2 crackers	2.0	90	20%
old-fashioned	2 crackers	2.0	90	20%
■ (Finn)				
crispbread/dark				
plain	2 pieces	–	40	–
w/caraway seeds	2 pieces	–	40	–
■ (Frito-Lay)				
Cheetos				
bacon cheddar	1 pkg	9.0	190	43%
cheddar cheese	1 pkg	11.0	210	47%
golden toast & cheddar	1 pkg	14.0	240	53%
Doritos				
jalapeño & cheddar	1 pkg	13.0	230	51%
nacho cheesier	1 pkg	14.0	240	53%
Peanut Pan				
cheese peanut butter	1 pkg	10.0	210	43%
toast peanut butter	1 pkg	11.0	210	47%
■ (Goodman's) matzo crackers				
Passover				
egg	1 matzo	1.0	130	7%
plain	1 matzo	–	130	–
■ (Hain)				
Bites				
cheddar				
golden	22 pieces	1.5	120	11%
white	22 pieces	1.5	120	11%
other crackers				
original				
no salt added	11 pieces	–	110	–
Regular	11 pieces	–	110	–
Saltines				
no salt added	5 pieces	–	60	–
regular	5 pieces	–	60	–

Food and Description	Amount	Fat Grams	Total Calories	% Fat Calories
sesame				
no salt added	11 pieces	6.0	140	39%
regular	11 pieces	6.0	140	39%
soup/oyster	35 pieces	–	60	–
vegetable				
no salt added	11 pieces	6.0	140	39%
regular	11 pieces	6.0	140	39%
whole wheat				
Hain rich				
no salt added	11 pieces	6.0	130	42%
regular	11 pieces	6.0	130	42%
regular whole wheat				
no salt added	11 pieces	2.5	70	32%
original	11 pieces	2.5	70	32%
■ (Health Valley)				
LOW-FAT				
bruschetta vegetable				
no salt added	6 crackers	1.0	60	15%
regular	6 crackers	1.0	60	15%
cracked pepper	5 crackers	1.0	60	15%
French onion	10 crackers	1.0	60	15%
garden herb	6 crackers	1.0	60	15%
sesame	5 crackers	1.0	60	15%
stoned wheat	5 crackers	1.0	60	15%
whole wheat	6 crackers	1.5	60	23%
ORIGINAL				
amaranth graham	6 crackers	3.0	120	23%
oat bran graham	6 crackers	3.0	120	23%
rice bran	6 crackers	3.0	110	25%
OTHER				
corn bread crackers				
bell pepper	4 crackers	1.5	60	23%
butter	4 crackers	1.5	60	23%
honey	4 crackers	1.5	60	23%
■ (Ideal)				
crispbread				
extra thins	3 slices	–	48	–
fiber thins	2 slices	–	40	–
oat bran thins	2 slices	–	50	–
flatbread				
fiber w/sesame seeds	2 slices	–	40	–
whole grain/no salt	2 slices	–	43	–
■ (J. J. Flats)				
breadflats				
flavorall	1 piece	2.5	60	38%
garlic	1 piece	2.0	60	30%
onion	1 piece	2.0	60	30%
plain	1 piece	2.0	60	30%
poppy	1 piece	2.0	60	30%
multigrain	1 piece	1.5	60	23%

Food and Description	Amount	Fat Grams	Total Calories	% Fat Calories
sesame	1 piece	1.0	50	18%
■ (Kashi)				
Tasty Little Crackers				
7-grain	15 crackers	3.0	130	21%
Country Cheddar	18 crackers	3.0	130	21%
honey sesame	15 crackers	3.0	130	21%
natural ranch	18 crackers	3.0	130	21%
■ (Kame)				
rice crunch crackers				
plain	16 pieces	1.0	110	8%
sesame	16 pieces	1.5	110	12%
unsalted	16 pieces	1.0	100	9%
■ (Kavli)				
Norwegian crispbread				
crispy thin	2 slices	<1.0	15	10%
hearty thick	1 slice	<1.0	35	10%
rye bran	2 slices	–	30	–
■ (Keebler)				
CRACKER SANDWICHES				
cheese & peanut butter	1 pkg	9.0	190	43%
club & cheddar	1 pkg	14.0	260	48%
original	1 pkg	9.0	180	45%
toast & peanut butter	1 pkg	10.0	200	45%
wheat & cheddar	1 pkg	10.0	200	45%
KRISPY CRACKERS				
Saltines				
fat-free	5 crackers	–	60	–
mild cheddar	5 crackers	–	60	–
original	5 crackers	1.5	60	19%
unsalted tops	5 crackers	1.5	60	19%
whole wheat	5 crackers	1.5	60	–
soup & oyster	17 crackers	1.5	70	19%
MUNCH'EMS/Baked				
cheddar	39 crackers	6.0	140	39%
original/seasoned	41 crackers	5.0	140	32%
ranch	40 crackers	5.0	140	32%
sour cream & onion	39 crackers	5.0	140	32%
OTHER CRACKERS				
Club Crackers				
33% reduced fat	4 crackers	3.0	70	75%
50% reduced sodium	5 crackers	2.0	70	26%
original	4 crackers	3.0	70	39%
export soda crackers	3 crackers	1.5	60	23%
Rumbly Grahams				
chocolate chip	23 pieces	4.5	140	29%
cinnamon	20 pieces	5.0	140	32%
honey	20 pieces	5.0	140	32%
Scooby-Doo				
cheese crackers	49 crackers	7.0	150	42%
Pizza-roni crackers	46 crackers	7.0	150	42%

Food and Description	Amount	Fat Grams	Total Calories	% Fat Calories
Toasteds				
buttercrisp	5 crackers	3.5	80	39%
onion	5 crackers	3.0	80	34%
sesame	5 crackers	4.0	80	45%
wheat	5 crackers	3.5	80	39%
Touch of Cheddar	4 crackers	2.5	70	32%
Wheatables				
honey wheat	17 crackers	6.0	140	39%
original				
reduced-fat	19 crackers	4.0	140	26%
regular	16 crackers	6.0	140	39%
7-grain	17 crackers	6.0	140	39%
Zesta Saltines				
Export Sodas	3 crackers	1.5	60	23%
fat-free	5 crackers	–	60	–
original	5 crackers	1.5	60	23%
reduced-sodium	5 crackers	1.5	60	23%
soup & oyster	45 crackers	3.0	70	39%
unsalted tops	5 crackers	1.5	60	23%
SUNSHINE				
Cheez-It				
Big 14 ounce	12 crackers	8.0	160	68%
cheddar Jack	26 crackers	8.0	160	68%
chili cheese	25 crackers	8.0	160	68%
hot & spicy	26 crackers	8.0	150	48%
juniors	44 crackers	7.0	140	45%
original	26 crackers	8.0	160	45%
Parmesan garlic	26 crackers	7.0	150	42%
party mix	½ cup	4.5	130	31%
reduced-fat	30 crackers	4.5	140	29%
white cheddar	26 crackers	7.0	150	42%
Twisterz				
cheddar & more				
cheddar	17 crackers	6.0	140	39%
hot wings &				
cheesy blue	17 crackers	6.0	140	39%
HiHo				
original	5 crackers	4.5	80	51%
reduced-fat	5 crackers	2.0	70	26%
TOWN HOUSE				
bistro crackers				
corn bread	2 crackers	3.0	80	34%
multigrain	2 crackers	3.0	80	34%
rye	2 crackers	3.5	80	39%
regular				
original	5 crackers	4.5	80	51%
reduced				
fat/50%	6 crackers	2.0	70	39%

Food and Description	Amount	Fat Grams	Total Calories	% Fat Calories
sodium	5 crackers	4.5	80	51%
wheat	5 crackers	4.5	80	51%
■ (Lance)				
Captain's Wafers				
cream cheese & chives	6 crackers	10.0	200	45%
grilled cheese	6 crackers	10.0	200	45%
peanut butter w/honey	6 crackers	9.0	190	43%
smokehouse cheddar	6 crackers	6.0	180	30%
cheese on wheat crackers	6 crackers	11.0	200	50%
malt/peanut butter on				
crispy malt crackers	6 crackers	10.0	190	47%
Nipchee/cheddar cheese				
on cheese crackers	6 crackers	12.0	200	54%
peanut butter on wheat	6 crackers	11.0	200	50%
Toastchee				
original				
peanut butter & cheese				
sandwich cracker	6 crackers	12.0	220	49%
reduced-fat	6 crackers	7.0	180	35%
toasty/peanut butter				
on a buttery cracker	6 crackers	11.0	190	52%
Variety Pack				
Captain's Choice	6 crackers	10.0	200	45%
Old Favorites	6 crackers	11.0	200	50%
■ (Little Debbie)				
cheddar on				
cheese crackers				
~1 oz package	1 pkg	7.0	130	48%
1.39 oz package	1 pkg	10.0	190	47%
peanut butter cheese				
crackers				
~1-oz package	1 pkg	7.0	130	48%
1.39-oz package	1 pkg	10.0	190	47%
peanut butter toasty				
crackers				
~1-oz package	1 pkg	6.0	130	42%
1.39-oz package	1 pkg	10.0	190	47%
■ (M&M * Mars)				
Combos				
snack crackers				
cheddar cheese				
family bag	1 oz	6.0	140	39%
individual package	1.7 oz pkg	11.0	240	41%
pepperoni pizza				
family bag	1 oz	6.0	140	39%
individual package	1.7 oz pkg	11.0	240	41%
■ (Manischewitz)				
matzo				
apple cinnamon	1 matzo	–	110	–

Food and Description	Amount	Fat Grams	Total Calories	% Fat Calories
egg & onion	1 matzo	1.0	100	9%
everything				
matzo	1 matzo	0.5	110	4%
matzo crackers	12 pieces	0.5	110	4%
no salt	1 matzo	–	110	–
saltine				
original	1 matzo	2.0	110	16%
unsalted	1 matzo	–	110	–
savory garlic	1 matzo	–	100	–
thin				
original	1 matzo	–	100	–
tea	1 matzo	–	100	–
unsalted				
matzo	1 matzo	–	90	–
matzo crackers	12 pieces	0.5	110	4%
whole wheat	1 oz	0.5	110	4%
Tam Tams				
everything	10 pieces	5.0	130	35%
garlic	10 pieces	4.0	130	28%
no salt	10 pieces	4.0	130	28%
onion	10 pieces	5.0	140	32%
original	10 pieces	4.0	130	28%
■ MUNCH'EMS (See (Keebler) in this section)				
■ (Nabisco)				
NABISCO				
Barnum's animal crackers				
box	1 oz	4.0	130	26%
Snak Saks	1 oz	4.0	130	26%
Cheese Nips				
cheddar	1 oz	6.0	150	36%
$.99 pkg	1 oz	6.0	150	36%
4-cheese				
$.99/1.25-oz pkg	1 pkg	7.0	150	42%
mini	1 oz	6.0	150	36%
Nickelodeon Rocket				
Power	1 oz	7.0	140	45%
Packs 2 go!				
1.65-oz package	1 pkg	10.0	230	39%
reduced-fat	1 oz	3.5	130	24%
salsa & cheddar				
doubles	1 oz	7.0	150	42%
Thin Crisps/100-calorie				
packs/6-count	~1 oz pkg	3.0	100	27%
Flavor Crisps				
bacon-baked snack	1 oz	8.0	160	45%
Better Cheddars/baked				
Chicken in a Biskit	1 oz	10.0	170	53%
original	1 oz	8.0	150	48%
reduced-fat	1 oz	6.0	140	39%

Food and Description	Amount	Fat Grams	Total Calories	% Fat Calories
Sociables/baked				
savory	1 oz	3.5	70	45%
Swiss cheese/baked	1 oz	7.0	140	45%
Twigs sesame & cheese				
snack sticks	1 oz	7.0	150	42%
vegetable thins/baked	1 oz	9.0	160	51%
graham crackers	1 oz	3.0	130	21%
Harvest Crisps				
wheat thins				
garden vegetable	1 oz	3.5	130	24%
5-grain	1 oz	3.5	140	23%
Honey Maid Graham Crackers				
apple cinnamon				
sticks	~1 oz	3.0	130	21%
chocolate	1 oz	3.0	130	21%
sticks	1 oz	3.0	130	21%
cinnamon	1 oz	2.5	130	17%
Go-Pak	⅓ pkg	3.0	130	21%
low-fat	~1 oz	1.5	120	11%
sticks	1 oz	2.5	120	19%
honey	1.22 oz	3.0	140	19%
low-fat	~1 oz	1.5	120	9%
sticks	~1 oz	2.5	130	17%
oatmeal crunch	1 oz	3.0	130	21%
Nut Thins				
almond	1 oz	4.5	140	29%
hazelnut	1 oz	4.0	120	30%
pecan	1 oz	5.0	130	35%
Premium Saltines				
fat-free	½ oz	–	60	–
gold	½ oz	3.0	70	39%
low-sodium	½ oz	1.5	60	23%
multigrain	½ oz	1.5	60	23%
original	½ oz	1.5	60	23%
soup & oyster	½ oz	1.5	60	23%
unsalted tops	½ oz	2.0	70	26%
Social tea biscuits	1 oz	4.0	120	30%
Toast Crackers				
w/cheddar cheese	1.4 oz pkg	11.00	200	50%
8-count	1.38 oz pkg	12.0	200	54%
w/peanut butter	1.38 oz pkg	10.0	190	47%
Wheatsworth stone-ground				
wheat cracker	~½ oz	3.5	80	39%
RED OVAL FARMS				
stoned wheat				
Wheat thins				
lower sodium	~1 oz	1.5	60	23%
mini	~1 oz	3.0	130	21%
regular	½ oz	1.5	60	23%

Food and Description	Amount	Fat Grams	Total Calories	% Fat Calories
RITZ				
Bits				
Cracker sandwiches				
cheese	1 oz	9.0	150	54%
$.99	1 oz	10.0	160	56%
Go-Pak	½ pkg	9.0	160	51%
Packs 2 Go!	1.5 oz pkg	14.0	230	55%
chips				
oven-toasted/crunch				
cheddar	1 oz	6.0	150	36%
original	1 oz	5.0	140	32%
sour cream				
& onion	1 oz	6.0	150	36%
crisp crackers				
crispy baked	1 oz	5.0	140	32%
graham cracker				
fun-size holiday	1 oz	7.0	140	45%
Go-Pak	½ pkg	8.0	160	45%
jalapeño cheddar	1 oz	6.0	140	39%
peanut butter	1.25 oz pkg	9.0	180	45%
1.5-oz pkg		14.0	230	55%
$.99	1 oz	8.0	150	48%
1.5-oz package	1 pkg	11.0	210	47%
12-count				
1.25-oz package	1 pkg	9.0	180	45%
Packs 2 Go!				
1.5-oz package	1 pkg	11.0	210	47%
peanut butter fudge	1 oz	8.0	150	48%
s'mores	1 oz	6.0	150	36%
1.25-oz package	1 pkg	7.0	170	37%
fun-size				
Halloween	1 oz	6.0	140	39%
Other Ritz Crackers				
assortment/cheese, cracked				
pepper & wheat	~½ oz	4.0	80	45%
baseball shape	~½ oz	4.0	80	45%
bite-size/original	1.3 oz pkg	9.0	190	43%
cracked pepper wheat				
assortment	~½ oz	4.0	80	45%
football shape	~½ oz	4.0	80	45%
garlic butter/4-count	~½ oz	4.0	80	45%
low-sodium	~½ oz	4.0	80	45%
original	~½ oz	4.0	80	23%
reduced-fat/4-count	~½ oz	2.0	70	26%
peanut butter	1.4 oz	9.0	190	43%
	1.75 oz bag	13.0	260	45%
reduced-fat	½ oz	2.0	70	26%
Snack/cheddar baked				
Mix	1.5 pkg	9.0	200	41%
Mixers/Snak Saks	1.14 oz	7.0	150	42%

Food and Description	Amount	Fat Grams	Total Calories	% Fat Calories
star-studded shape	~½ oz	4.0	80	45%
sticks	1 oz	7.0	150	42%
w/peanut butter				
1.38-oz package	1 pkg	9.0	190	43%
w/real cheese/8-count				
1.38-oz package	1 pkg	12.0	200	54%
w/whole wheat	~½ oz	2.5	70	32%
SNACKWELL'S				
fat-free/cracked pepper	½ oz	–	60	–
reduced-fat				
cracked pepper	½ oz	1.5	60	23%
French onion	1 oz	3.0	130	21%
wheat	½ oz	1.5	70	19%
zesty cheese	1 oz	3.0	130	21%
TRISCUIT				
cheddar	1 oz	4.5	120	34%
garden herb	1 oz	4.0	120	30%
low-sodium	1 oz	5.0	130	35%
original	1 oz	5.0	130	35%
reduced-fat	1 oz	3.0	120	23%
roasted garlic	1 oz	4.5	120	34%
Thin Crisps				
French onion	1 oz	4.5	130	10%
original	1 oz	4.5	130	10%
whole wheat	1 oz	5.0	130	35%
whole wheat				
deli-style rye	1 oz	1.5	120	11%
original	1 oz	4.5	120	34%
WHEAT THINS				
big	1 oz	6.0	140	39%
honey	1 oz	6.0	150	36%
low-salt	1 oz	6.0	150	36%
multigrain	1 oz	4.5	140	29%
original	1 oz	6.0	150	36%
ranch	1 oz	6.0	140	39%
reduced-fat	1 oz	4.0	130	28%
snack				
baked original	1 oz	6.0	150	36%
minis				
100-calorie packs	1 pack	3.0	100	27%
zwieback toast	2 pieces	1.0	35	26%
■ **(New Morning)**				
grahams				
cinnamon	2 sheets	3.0	130	21%
honey	2 sheets	3.0	130	21%
GrahamWiches				
chocolate &				
peanut butter crème	2 cookies	5.0	120	38%
peanut butter crème	2 cookies	5.0	130	35%
vanilla crème	2 cookies	5.0	130	35%

Food and Description	Amount	Fat Grams	Total Calories	% Fat Calories
Mini Bites				
chocolate grahams	22 pieces	3.0	110	25%
■ (Old London)				
FLATBREAD CRACKERS				
everything	2 pieces	2.5	60	38%
sesame	2 pieces	2.0	60	30%
MELBA SNACK				
bacon	5 pieces	1.5	60	23%
garlic	5 pieces	1.0	60	15%
Mexicali corn	5 pieces	1.5	60	23%
nacho	5 pieces	2.0	70	26%
onion	5 pieces	1.5	60	23%
rye	5 pieces	1.5	60	23%
sesame	5 pieces	3.0	60	45%
white	5 pieces	1.0	60	15%
whole wheat	5 pieces	1.0	60	15%
MELBA TOAST				
garlic	3 pieces	–	50	–
onion	3 pieces	–	45	–
rye	3 pieces	–	45	–
sesame				
regular	3 pieces	1.0	50	18%
unsalted	3 pieces	1.5	50	27%
wheat	3 pieces	–	50	–
white	3 pieces	–	50	–
whole grain				
regular	3 pieces	–	45	–
unsalted	3 pieces	–	45	–
■ (O.T.C.)				
chowder & oyster	3 pieces	2.0	70	26%
wine	11 pieces	3.0	130	21%
■ (Pepperidge Farm)				
ENTERTAINING CRACKERS				
butter thins	4 crackers	3.0	70	39%
country cheese	2 crackers	4.0	80	45%
hearty wheat	3 crackers	3.5	80	39%
quartet assortment	3 crackers	2.5	70	32%
trio collection	4 crackers	2.5	70	32%
GOLDFISH CRACKERS				
cheddar cheese–blasted				
burstin' BBQ	51 pieces	6.0	140	39%
extra cheddar	51 pieces	6.0	140	39%
nothing but nacho	51 pieces	4.5	140	29%
X-plosive pizza	51 pieces	6.0	140	39%
cinnamon	1 oz	6.0	150	36%
crisps				
cheddar Jack	1 oz	7.0	150	42%
cheesy sour				
cream onion	1 oz	7.0	150	42%
4-cheese	1 oz	7.0	150	42%

Food and Description	Amount	Fat Grams	Total Calories	% Fat Calories
honey	1 oz	6.0	150	36%
Liberty w/real cheese	1 oz	6.0	140	39%
low-salt	55 pieces	6.0	140	39%
reduced-sodium	60 pieces	6.0	150	36%
regular	55 pieces	6.0	140	39%
sandwich snackers				
cheddar w/peanut				
butter filling	1 oz	6.0	140	39%
original				
w/cheese filling	1 oz	7.0	150	42%
w/peanut butter				
filling	1 oz	6.0	140	39%
white cheddar	1 oz	7.0	150	42%
SNACK STICKS				
pretzel	12 sticks	–	120	–
pumpernickel	12 sticks	1.5	120	11%
3-cheese	12 sticks	6.0	150	36%
wheat	12 sticks	3.5	130	24%
WATER BISCUITS				
cracked pepper	5 crackers	1.0	60	15%
traditional	5 crackers	1.0	60	15%
■ (Pritikin)				
brown rice crackers				
low-sodium				
onion & garlic	7 crackers	–	60	–
unsalted				
plain	7 crackers	–	60	–
w/sesame seeds	7 crackers	–	60	–
whole wheat/unsalted	8 crackers	–	50	–
RED OVAL FARMS (*See* (Nabisco) in this section)				
RITZ (*See* (Nabisco) in this section)				
■ (Ry-Krisp)				
fat-free	2 crackers	–	60	–
fiber plus	1 slice	1.0	35	26%
golden rye	1 slice	–	30	–
hearty rye	1 slice	–	50	–
light rye	2 slices	–	50	–
natural	2 crackers	–	40	–
seasoned	2 crackers	1.0	45	20%
sesame	2 crackers	2.0	50	36%
■ (Ryvita)				
breaks	1 slice	–	48	–
crispbread				
Allinson Organic				
whole meal	1 slice	–	17	–
dark	1 slice	–	38	–
dark rye				
plain	1 slice	–	28	–
multigrain	1 slice	0.5	37	12%
original wheat	1 slice	–	18	–

Food and Description	Amount	Fat Grams	Total Calories	% Fat Calories
crackerbread				
high fiber	1 slice	–	16	–
original	1 slice	–	19	–
whole meal	1 slice	–	18	–
■ (Sesmark)				
rice thins				
brown	15 pieces	1.5	120	11%
cheddar	15 pieces	2.5	130	12%
original sesame	15 pieces	2.5	130	12%
teriyaki-flavored	13 pieces	2.5	130	17%
savory rice minis				
chili cheese	35 pieces	2.0	120	15%
lightly salted	40 pieces	1.5`	120	11%
nacho corn	35 pieces	2.0	120	15%
sesame garlic	37 pieces	2.5	120	19%
savory thins				
cracked wheat	15 pieces	1.5	100	14%
original	15 pieces	2.5	120	19%
teriyaki	13 pieces	3.0	130	21%
toasted onion & garlic	15 pieces	1.5	110	12%
sesame thins				
cheddar	9 pieces	9.0	150	54%
garlic	9 pieces	9.0	150	54%
original	9 pieces	9.0	150	54%
unsalted	11 pieces	10.0	160	56%
■ SNACKWELL'S (*See* (Nabisco) in this section)				
■ SUNSHINE (*See* (Keebler) in this section)				
■ TRISCUIT (*See* (Nabisco) in this section)				
■ TWIX (*See* CANDY)				
■ (Valley Lahvosh)				
cracker bread				
hearts	9 crackers	1.0	110	8%
rounds				
2" dia	7 crackers	1.0	110	8%
3" dia	4 crackers	1.0	110	8%
5" dia	1 cracker	0.5	70	6%
15" dia	1.8 oz	2.0	190	9%
wheat rounds				
3" dia	4 crackers	1.0	110	8%
5" dia	1 cracker	0.5	60	8%
15" dia	1.8 oz	2.0	190	9%
sweetheart crispies	7 crackers	2.0	120	15%
■ (Wasa)				
crispbread				
fiber rye	1 slice	1.0	30	30%
hearty rye	1 slice	–	40	–
multigrain	1 slice	–	45	–
organic rye	1 slice	–	35	–
sesame				
No'e'	1 slice	1.0	30	30%

Food and Description	Amount	Fat Grams	Total Calories	% Fat Calories
Runda	1 slice	1.5	55	9%
rye				
light	1 slice	–	25	–
original	1 slice	–	35	–
sodium-free	1 slice	–	30	–
wheat doré	1 slice	1.0	50	18%
■ (Westbrae)				
natural wafers				
5-piece	7 crackers	–	50	–
no salt	7 crackers	0.5	50	11%
onion garlic				
brown rice	7 crackers	–	50	–
sesame	7 crackers	–	50	–
tamari	7 crackers	–	50	–
CRACKER CRUMBS/MEAL (*See also* MATZO MEAL & MIX)				
(Golden Dipt)				
cracker meal/no salt				
extra fine	¼ cup	1.0	145	6%
fine	¼ cup	1.0	145	6%
medium	¼ cup	1.0	145	6%
Modern Maid				
matzo meal	¼ cup	1.0	145	6%
(Manischewitz) matzo	¼ cup	0.5	130	3%
(Nabisco)				
Cracker meal/baking				
topping	¼ cup	–	110	–
CRANBERRY				
dried				
(Ann's House of Nuts)	⅓ cup	–	130	–
(Ocean Spray)				
Craisins				
cherry	⅓ cup	–	130	–
orange	⅓ cup	–	130	–
regular	⅓ cup	–	130	–
(Sanoma)	⅓ cup	–	120	–
(Sun-Maid)	⅓ cup	–	140	–
(Traverse Bay)				
cranberries	⅓ cup	0.5	140	3%
cranberries/berry & cherry				
w/cherries				
and blueberries	⅓ cup	1.0	150	6%
fresh				
chopped	½ cup	–	27	–
	1 cup	–	54	–
(Dole)	½ cup	–	23	–
(Ocean Spray)	2 oz	–	30	–
	1 cup	–	50	–
whole/w/o stems	½ cup	–	23	–
	1 cup	–	46	–

Food and Description	Amount	Fat Grams	Total Calories	% Fat Calories
CRANBERRY BEAN				
fresh				
boiled	½ cup	<1.0	120	4%
canned	½ cup	<1.0	110	4%
raw	½ cup	1.0	330	3%
CRANBERRY JUICE/JUICE BLEND/JUICE BLEND DRINK				
BOTTLED/BOXED/CANNED				
(Dole)				
cranberry				
cocktail	8 fl oz	–	140	–
	10 fl oz	–	160	–
	11.5 fl oz	–	200	–
crangrape	8 fl oz	–	170	–
(Knudsen)				
cranberry nectar	8 fl oz	–	140	–
Just juice	8 fl oz	–	60	–
Sparkling cranberry	8 fl oz	–	130	–
(Langer's)				
cranberry cocktail	8 fl oz	–	140	–
cranberry drink/diet	8 fl oz	–	30	–
cranberry drink blend				
apple/Fuji	8 fl oz	–	160	–
Caribbean	8 fl oz	–	135	–
grape	8 fl oz	–	165	–
orange	8 fl oz	–	130	–
raspberry				
diet	8 fl oz	–	30	–
regular	8 fl oz	–	150	–
cranberry juice	8 fl oz	–	140	–
cranberry juice blend				
grape	8 fl oz	–	150	–
raspberry	8 fl oz	–	145	–
(Martinelli's)..sparkling apple-cranberry				
	8 fl oz	–	110	–
(Ocean Spray)				
CRAVIN' LESS SUGAR JUICE DRINK				
cranberry				
wild berry	8 fl oz	–	80	–
JUICE & TEA				
cranberry	8 fl oz	–	100	–
white cranberry				
peach	8 fl oz	–	100	–
LIGHT STYLE				
juice cocktail				
cranberry	8 fl oz	–	40	–
white cranberry	8 fl oz	–	40	–
juice drink				
crangrape	8 fl oz	–	40	–
cranraspberry	8 fl oz	–	40	–

Food and Description	Amount	Fat Grams	Total Calories	% Fat Calories
PREMIUM 100% JUICE BLENDS				
cranberry				
& Concord grape	8 fl oz	–	150	–
& Georgia peach	8 fl oz	–	140	–
& mixed berry	8 fl oz	–	150	–
& Pacific				
raspberry	8 fl oz	–	140	–
& Red Delicious				
apple	8 fl oz	–	130	–
cranberry blend	8 fl oz	–	140	–
REDUCED-CALORIE				
cranapple	8 fl oz	–	50	–
cranberry juice				
cocktail	8 fl oz	–	50	–
cranraspberry	8 fl oz	–	50	–
REGULAR JUICE COCKTAIL				
cranberry	8 fl oz	–	130	–
apple	8 fl oz	–	160	–
grape	8 fl oz	–	160	–
raspberry	8 fl oz	–	140	–
strawberry	8 fl oz	–	140	–
w/calcium	8 fl oz	–	150	–
REGULAR JUICE DRINK				
cranapple	8 fl oz	–	160	–
crancherry	8 fl oz	–	150	–
crangrape	8 fl oz	–	160	–
cranmango	8 fl oz	–	130	–
cranraspberry	8 fl oz	–	140	–
cranstrawberry	8 fl oz	–	140	–
crantangerine	8 fl oz	–	130	–
SPRITZER				
cranberry	11.75 oz	–	160	–
(Old Orchard)				
low-carb				
apple cranberry	8 fl oz	–	26	–
cranberry	8 fl oz	–	29	–
cranberry raspberry	8 fl oz	–	23	–
white cranberry	8 fl oz	–	39	–
(Snapple)				
cranberry apple				
bottle	12 fl oz	–	200	–
can	11.5 oz	–	190	–
cranberry raspberry				
diet	8 fl oz	–	10	–
regular	8 fl oz	–	120	–
cranberry raspberry				
diet	8 fl oz	–	10	–
tea	8 fl oz	–	10	–
winter whipper	10 fl oz	–	150	–
cranberry twist	8 fl oz	–	100	–

Food and Description	Amount	Fat Grams	Total Calories	% Fat Calories
(Tropicana)				
cranberry apple	10 fl oz	–	170	–
cranberry cocktail	8 fl oz	–	140	–
cranberry grape	8 fl oz	–	170	–
Twister/Orange				
Cranberry Clash	8 fl oz	–	130	–
	10 fl oz	–	160	–
light	8 fl oz	–	45	–
	10 fl oz	–	60	–
regular	8 fl oz	–	120	–
	10 fl oz	–	160	–
(Walnut Acres) Organic				
all styles	8 fl oz	–	110	–
(Welch's) cranberry				
cocktail drink	5.5 fl oz	–	100	–
	10 fl oz	–	140	–
juice cocktail	5.5 fl oz	–	100	–
	8 fl oz	–	–	
	10 fl oz	–	140	–
juice cocktail drink				
cranberry	11.5 fl oz	–	200	–
	8.45 fl oz	–	180	–
cranberry grape	8 fl oz	–	170	–
JuiceMakers				
cranberry apple				
juice cocktail	8 fl oz	–	120	–
Sparkling Juice				
Celebration	8 fl oz	–	160	–
FROZEN/prepared, unless noted otherwise				
(Old Orchard)				
apple cranberry	8 fl oz	–	120	–
cranberry blend	8 fl oz	–	120	–
cranberry raspberry	8 fl oz	–	130	–
(Seneca) juice cocktail				
cranberry	8 fl oz	–	130	–
cranberry apple	8 fl oz	–	140	–
(Welch's)				
juice 100% blend/11.5-oz can				
concentrate	2 oz	–	150	–
juice cocktail				
cranberry apple	8 fl oz	–	160	–
cranberry cherry	8 fl oz	–	150	–
cranberry cocktail				
light	8 fl oz	–	50	–
regular	8 fl oz	–	140	–
cranberry orange	8 fl oz	–	140	–
cranberry raspberry	8 fl oz	–	150	–
light	8 fl oz	–	50	–
regular	8 fl oz	–	150	–

Food and Description	Amount	Fat Grams	Total Calories	% Fat Calories
CRANBERRY SAUCE/canned				
(Ocean Spray) canned				
cranberries	2 oz	–	30	–
Cran-Fruit cranberry crushed fruit				
orange	¼ cup	–	120	–
raspberry	¼ cup	–	120	–
strawberry	¼ cup	–	120	–
jellied	¼ cup	–	110	–
whole berry	¼ cup	–	110	–
(S&W)				
all styles	¼ cup	–	100	–
CRANBERRY-ORANGE RELISH				
canned	½ cup	–	246	–
uncooked	½ cup	–	245	–
CRAYFISH/mixed species				
cooked—moist heat	3 oz	1.0	97	9%
raw	3 medium	<1.0	24	19%
	3 oz	0.9	76	11%
CREAM (*See also* CREAMER, NONDAIRY; SOUR CREAM; SOUR CREAM SUBSTITUTE; WHIPPED TOPPING)				
(Alouette)				
crème fraîche				
cooking & topping				
cream	1 oz	11.0	100	100%
(Creamland) half-and-half				
ultra-pasteurized	2 Tbs	3.0	35	77%
(Devon Cream Company)				
clotted cream	2 Tbs	15.0	140	96%
w/brandy	2 Tbs	14.0	140	90%
w/Drambuie	2 Tbs	13.0	130	90%
w/Grand Marnier	2 Tbs	14.0	130	97%
w/strawberries	2 Tbs	9.0	100	81%
double Devon cream	2 Tbs	13.0	130	90%
(Hood)				
half-and-half	2 Tbs	3.5	40	79%
heavy	1 Tbs	5.0	50	90%
light	1 Tbs	3.0	30	90%
(Land O'Lakes)				
half-and-half	2 Tbs	3.5	35	9%
fat-free	2 Tbs	–	20	–
light	1 Tbs	1.0	20	45%
gourmet	2 Tbs	3.5	40	79%
heavy gourmet				
whipping	1 Tbs	5.0	50	90%
(Rockview Farms) whipping cream				
heavy grade A	1 Tbs	5.0	50	90%
(Sunshine Dairy) whipping				
heavy grade A	1 Tbs	5.0	50	90%

Food and Description	Amount	Fat Grams	Total Calories	% Fat Calories
(Umpqua) whipping				
old-fashioned heavy	1 Tbs	6.0	60	90%
CREAM CHEESE (See also CHEESE ALTERNATIVE/IMITATION; CHEESE SPREAD)				
(Breakstone) Temp-Tee				
whipped	3 Tbs	8.0	80	90%
(Connoisseur)				
apple cinnamon	1 oz	7.0	110	57%
cranberry	1 oz	8.0	100	72%
mango peach	1 oz	7.0	110	57%
(Darigold)	2 Tbs	10.0	100	90%
(Dorman's)				
70% fat	2 Tbs	10.0	100	90%
65% fat	2 Tbs	8.0	90	80%
(Fleur de Lait) Premium light				
all flavors	2 Tbs	4.5	60	68%
(Formagg)				
fat-free	2 Tbs	–	25	–
original	2 Tbs	7.0	80	79%
(Fresh Cut)				
all flavors	2 Tbs	9.0	90	90%
(Friendship)				
New York–style				
reduced-fat	2 Tbs	3.0	50	54%
soft	2 Tbs	10.0	100	90%
(Healthy Choice) fat-free				
herbs & garlic	2 Tbs	–	25	–
plain	2 Tbs	–	25	–
strawberry	2 Tbs	–	35	–
(Heluva Good Cheese)	2 Tbs	10.0	100	90%
(Keller's)				
boxed/brick	1 oz	9.0	100	81%
(Kraft)				
Philadelphia brand				
brick				
fat-free	1 oz	–	30	–
Neufchâtel ⅓ less fat	1 oz	6.0	70	77%
original	1 oz	10.0	100	90%
regular/soft				
fat-free/plain	2 Tbs	–	30	–
light	2 Tbs	5.0	70	64%
original	2 Tbs	10.0	100	90%
whipped				
regular	2 Tbs	7.0	70	90%
w/chives	2 Tbs	6.0	70	77%
w/mixed berries	2 Tbs	6.0	70	77%
Philly's flavors/soft				
blueberry	2 Tbs	8.0	100	63%
garden vegetable				
fat-free	2 Tbs	–	30	–
regular	2 Tbs	9.0	90	90%

Food and Description	Amount	Fat Grams	Total Calories	% Fat Calories
honey nut	2 Tbs	10.0	110	82%
pineapple	2 Tbs	9.0	100	81%
raspberry	2 Tbs	8.0	100	63%
strawberry				
fat-free	2 Tbs	–	30	–
light	2 Tbs	7.0	70	90%
regular	2 Tbs	8.0	90	80%
(Weight Watchers) light	2 Tbs	3.0	40	68%
(Wispride)..cream cheese spread				
all flavors	2 Tbs	8.0	90	80%
(Wolferman's)				
cream cheese spread & toppings				
garlic herb	½ tsp	–	–	–
raspberry	2 tsp	–	25	–
spinach artichoke	½ tsp	–	–	–
strawberry	2 tsp	–	25	–
CREAM OF TARTAR	1 tsp	–	7	–
	1 Tbs	–	23	–
CREAMER, NONDAIRY (*See also* CREAM)				
LIQUID				
(International Delight)				
amaretto				
fat-free	1 Tbs	–	30	–
original	1 Tbs	2.0	45	40%
reduced-calorie	1 Tbs	2.0	30	60%
chocolate cream	1 Tbs	1.5	40	34%
cinnamon hazelnut				
fat-free	1 Tbs	–	30	–
regular	1 Tbs	1.5	40	34%
French vanilla				
original	1 Tbs	2.0	45	40%
royal				
fat-free	1 Tbs	–	30	–
original	1 Tbs	2.0	45	40%
hazelnut				
original	1 Tbs	2.0	45	40%
reduced-calorie	1 Tbs	2.0	30	60%
Irish cream				
fat-free	1 Tbs	–	30	–
original	1 Tbs	1.5	45	30%
Southern pecan	1 Tbs	1.5	40	34%
vanilla hazelnut				
fat-free	1 Tbs	–	45	–
toffee caramel	1 Tbs	1.5	40	34%
(Mocha Mix)				
original	1 Tbs	1.5	20	68%
(Morningstar)				
French vanilla	1 Tbs	2.0	45	40%
hazelnut	1 Tbs	1.5	40	34%
Irish cream	1 Tbs	1.5	40	34%

Food and Description	Amount	Fat Grams	Total Calories	% Fat Calories
(Nestlé)				
Coffee-mate				
amaretto	1 Tbs	2.0	40	45%
cafe mocha				
fat-free	1 Tbs	–	25	–
regular	1 Tbs	2.0	40	45%
chocolate raspberry	1 Tbs	2.0	40	45%
cinnamon vanilla	1 Tbs	2.0	40	45%
crème	1 Tbs	2.0	40	45%
French vanilla	1 Tbs	2.0	40	45%
fat-free	1 Tbs	–	25	–
hazelnut				
fat-free	1 Tbs	–	25	–
regular	1 Tbs	2.0	40	45%
Irish cream				
fat-free	1 Tbs	–	25	–
regular	1 Tbs	2.0	40	45%
original				
fat-free	1 Tbs	–	10	–
low-fat	1 Tbs	0.5	10	45%
regular	1 Tbs	1.0	20	45%
Coffee-mate half-and-half				
hazelnut	1 Tbs	4.0	70	51%
original	1 Tbs	3.5	40	79%
vanilla	1 Tbs	4.0	60	60%
(Real) half-and-half				
almond roca	2 Tbs	1.0	80	11%
French vanilla	2 Tbs	2.0	80	23%
Irish cream	2 Tbs	3.5	80	39%
(Rich's) frozen				
Coffee Rich				
light	1 Tbs	1.0	10	90%
original	1 Tbs	1.5	25	54%
Farm Rich				
fat-free	1 Tbs	–	10	–
light	1 Tbs	1.0	10	90%
original	1 Tbs	1.5	20	68%
Poly Rich	1 Tbs	1.0	20	68%
POWDERED				
(Dean Foods) Cremora				
fat-free	1 tsp	–	10	–
lite	1 tsp	–	10	–
original	1 tsp	0.5	15	30%
Royale	1 tsp	1.0	15	60%
(Nestlé)				
Coffee-mate				
cinnamon vanilla creme	4 tsp	2.5	60	38%
French vanilla	4 tsp	2.5	60	38%
fat-free	4 tsp	–	50	–
hazelnut	4 tsp	3.0	60	45%

Food and Description	Amount	Fat Grams	Total Calories	% Fat Calories
fat-free	4 tsp	–	50	–
original				
fat-free	1 tsp	–	10	–
light	1 tsp	–	10	–
regular	1 tsp	0.5	10	45%
half-and-half				
hazelnut	2 Tbs	4.0	60	40%
original	2 Tbs	3.5	40	79%
vanilla	2 Tbs	4.0	60	40%
Latte Creations				
classic	2 Tbs	6.0	100	54%
mocha	2 Tbs	4.0	90	40%
vanilla	2 Tbs	4.0	90	40%
CREPE				
FROZEN				
(Chef Francois)	1 crepe	3.0	80	34%
MIX				
(Krusteaz) prepared	2 crepes	3.0	100	27%
READY-TO-SERVE				
(Freida's)				
French bistro-style	1 crepe	0.5	30	15%
(French-style)				
7" crepes	1 crepe	0.5	30	15%
(Table de France)				
9" dia	1 crepe	1.0	45	20%
CRISPBREAD (*See* CRACKER)				
CROAKER				
breaded & fried	3 oz	10.0	188	48%
raw	3 oz	2.7	89	27%
CROISSANT				
FROZEN				
(Chef Pierre) prebaked/all-butter				
1-oz croissant	1 croissant	5.0	110	41%
2-oz croissant	1 croissant	9.0	210	39%
3-oz croissant	1 croissant	22.0	360	55%
(Sara Lee) all-butter/petite	2 croissants	11.0	230	43%
READY-TO-SERVE				
(Awrey's)				
butter	1 oz	6.0	110	49%
	2 oz	13.0	220	53%
sliced	3 oz	19.0	330	52%
unsliced	3 oz	19.0	330	52%
sandwich				
sliced	1.5 oz	8.0	160	45%
	2.5 oz	14.0	270	47%
tip-to-tip				
croissant/sliced	2 oz	12.0	220	49%
(Pepperidge Farm) all-butter				
petite/all-butter	1 croissant	6.0	120	45%
sandwich	1 croissant	7.0	170	37%

Food and Description	Amount	Fat Grams	Total Calories	% Fat Calories
(Sara Lee)				
FOOD SERVICE				
100% vegetable				
shortening				
sliced	2 oz	11.0	220	45%
	3 oz	15.0	320	42%
unsliced	.9 oz	5.0	100	45%
butter				
sliced	2 oz	12.0	220	49%
	3 oz	18.0	330	48%
unsliced	1.25 oz	5.0	110	41%
	2 oz	9.0	210	38%
	3 oz	22.0	360	55%
natural butter-flavored				
sliced	2 oz	14.0	240	53%
	2.5 oz	13.0	270	43%
	3 oz	21.0	360	53%
unsliced	1.125 oz	11.0	240	41%
	1.5 oz	8.0	160	45%
	2 oz	11.0	220	45%
1½-oz croissant	1 croissant	8.0	170	43%
2-oz croissant	1 croissant	10.0	220	41%
3-oz sandwich				
croissant	1 croissant	15.0	320	42%
sandwich croissant				
sliced	1 croissant	11.0	220	45%
*RETAIL/*frozen				
French-style				
petite	2 croissants	11.0	230	43%
plain	1 croissant	8.0	170	42%
CROUTONS				
(Arnold) crispy				
classic				
Italian	5 croutons	1.5	30	45%
seasoned	5 croutons	1.0	30	30%
home-style/larger				
garlic herb	5 croutons	1.0	30	30%
(Brownberry) (*See* (Arnold) in this section)				
(Cardini)				
Caesar	2 Tbs	1.5	35	39%
garlic & butter	2 Tbs	1.5	35	39%
Italian	2 Tbs	1.5	30	45%
(Chatham Village)				
Caesar	2 Tbs	1.5	35	39%
cheese & garlic	2 Tbs	2.5	40	56%
garden herb	2 Tbs	1.5	35	39%
garlic & butter	2 Tbs	1.5	35	39%
garlic & onion				
fat-free	2 Tbs	–	25	–

Food and Description	Amount	Fat Grams	Total Calories	% Fat Calories
(Devonsheer)				
Italian	2 Tbs	0.5	30	15%
onion & garlic	2 Tbs	0.5	30	15%
(Edward & Sons) organic/vegan				
Italian herbs	2 Tbs	0.5	28	16%
lightly salted	2 Tbs	0.5	30	15%
onion garlic	2 Tbs	0.5	30	15%
(Fresh Gourmet) premium				
FAT-FREE				
garlic Caesar	5 croutons	–	20	–
Parmesan ranch	5 croutons	–	15	–
REGULAR				
butter & garlic	5 croutons	1.0	25	36%
cheese & garlic	5 croutons	1.0	25	36%
classic Caesar	5 croutons	1.0	25	36%
country ranch	5 croutons	1.0	25	36%
garden herb	5 croutons	1.0	25	36%
Italian-seasoned	5 croutons	1.5	25	54%
(Mrs. Cubberson's) restaurant-style				
Caesar salad	5 croutons	1.0	30	30%
cheese & garlic	5 croutons	1.0	30	30%
fat-free	5 croutons	–	30	–
onion & garlic	5 croutons	1.0	30	30%
ranch	5 croutons	1.0	30	30%
seasoned	5 croutons	1.0	30	30%
(Old London)				
RESTAURANT-STYLE				
garlic	2 Tbs	1.0	30	30%
Italian	2 Tbs	1.0	30	30%
sourdough	2 Tbs	1.0	30	30%
TOASTETTES/round croutons				
Caesar	10 croutons	1.0	25	36%
cheese garlic	10 croutons	1.0	25	36%
buttermilk ranch	10 croutons	1.0	25	36%
herb-seasoned	10 croutons	1.0	25	36%
toasted onion	10 croutons	1.0	25	36%
(Pepperidge Farm)				
CLASSIC CUT				
fat-free				
Caesar/fat-free	6 croutons	–	30	–
spicy Italian	6 croutons	–	30	–
regular				
cheese garlic	11 croutons	1.0	35	26%
onion garlic	11 croutons	1.0	30	30%
seasoned	11 croutons	1.0	30	30%
GENEROUS CUT				
buttermilk ranch	6 croutons	1.0	30	30%
classic Caesar	6 croutons	1.5	35	39%
cracked pepper				
& Parmesan	6 croutons	1.0	35	26%

Food and Description	Amount	Fat Grams	Total Calories	% Fat Calories
sourdough cheese	6 croutons	1.0	30	30%
zesty Italian	6 croutons	1.5	35	39%
CROWDER PEA/bag or canned				
(Lowe's) 16-oz bag	3 oz	1.0	120	8%
(Luck's) seasoned w/pork	7.5 oz	7.0	200	32%
(The Allens)				
crowder peas	4.4 oz	1.0	110	8%
(The Allen's East Texas Fair)				
crowder peas	4.4 oz	1.0	110	8%
CRUMPET				
(Wolferman's)				
blueberry	1 crumpet	–	90	–
cinnamon sugar	1 crumpet	–	90	–
classic	1 crumpet	-	90	–
raspberry	1 crumpet	1.0	90	10%
CUCUMBER (See also PICKLE)				
raw				
sliced	½ cup	–	7	–
whole	1 medium	–	29	–
CUCUMBER DISH (See also PICKLE; PICKLE RELISH)				
(Rosoff's) cucumber salad	1 oz	–	12	–
(Schorr's) cucumber garden salad	1 oz	–	12	–
CUMIN SEED/whole	1 tsp	0.5	8	56%
CURD TOPPING				
(Wolferman's)				
Elizabethan curd				
lemon	1 Tbs	2.0	60	30%
raspberry	1 Tbs	2.0	60	30%
CURRANT				
BLACK				
dried	½ cup	–	204	–
raw	½ cup	–	36	–
	½ lb	–	140	–
RED OR WHITE/raw	½ cup	–	31	–
	½ lb	–	125	–
ZANTE/dried				
(Del Monte) dried	½ cup	–	200	–
(S&W) canned	¼ cup	–	130	–
(Sun-Maid) zante	¼ cup	–	130	–
CURRY (See also SAUCE)				
(A Taste of Thai)..curry bases				
green	1 tsp	1.5	15	90%
Panang	1 tsp	2.0	25	72%
red	1 tsp	1.5	20	68%
yellow	1 tsp	3.0	30	90%
CURRY POWDER/ground	1 tsp	–	6	–
CUSK				
raw	3 oz	1.0	74	12%
steamed	1 oz	<1.0	30	15%
	1 lb	3.0	481	6%

Food and Description	Amount	Fat Grams	Total Calories	% Fat Calories
CUSTARD (*See* also PIE & COBBLER; PUDDING & MOUSSE)				
homemade/USDA Standard Home Recipe				
baked	1 cup	14.6	305	43%
boiled	½ cup	7.0	164	38%
zabaglione	¼ cup	4.0	80	45%
mix				
(Con-Gelli) dry mix only				
caramel custard	1 serving	–	60	–
CUTTLEFISH				
cooked—moist heat	3 oz	1.0	135	6%
raw	3 oz	0.6	67	8%

D

Food and Description	Amount	Fat Grams	Total Calories	% Fat Calories
DANDELION GREENS/fresh				
cooked	½ cup	–	17	–
raw/chopped	½ cup	–	13	–
DANISH (*See* PASTRY)				
DATE				
(Amport) diced	¼ cup	–	130	–
(Del Monte)				
chopped	¼ cup	–	120	–
pitted/medium	5-6 dates	–	120	–
(Dole)				
chopped	1 oz	–	120	–
dried/ground	1 oz	–	110	–
pitted/medium	5-6 dates	–	120	–
(Frieda's) Medjool	2-3 dates	–	120	–
(Sun Giant)				
chopped	1 cup	1.0	490	2%
whole/pitted	10 medium	1.0	220	4%
(Sun-Maid) chopped				
California				
chopped	1.3 oz	–	120	–
natural California				
pitted	1.3 oz	–	120	–
DATE FILLING (Solo)	2 Tbs	1.0	100	9%
DEER (*See* VENISON)				
DESSERT TOPPING (*See* CREAM; ICE CREAM TOPPING; WHIPPED TOPPING)				

Food and Description	Amount	Fat Grams	Total Calories	% Fat Calories

DIETING AID (*See* BREAKFAST DRINK; GRANOLA/GRANOLA-TYPE BAR; NUTRITIONAL LIQUID SUPPLEMENT)

DILL LEAVES/fresh	1 cup	–	5	–
DILL SAUCE (*See* SAUCE)				
DILL SEED				
dried	1 tsp	–	3	–
whole	1 tsp	–	6	–

DINNER (*See* ASIAN FOOD; BEEF DISH/ENTRÉE; EGG DISH/MEAL; FAST FOOD; FROZEN ENTRÉE/DINNER; MEXICAN FOOD; PASTA ENTRÉE/DINNER; PIZZA; PORK ENTRÉE; RICE DISH; SEAFOOD ENTRÉE/DINNER; VEGETARIAN FOODS; individual listings)

DIP (*See also* SALAD DRESSING; SAUCE; SEASONINGS)

■ FROZEN

(Calavo) Mexican-style avocado				
guacamole	2 Tbs	4.5	50	81%
(Heinz) T.G.I. Friday's				
spinach cheese &				
artichoke	2 Tbs	3.5	45	70%

■ MIX
(Note: Unless otherwise stated, data are for dry mix only)

(Frito-Lay)				
Ruffles dip mixes				
French onion				
naturally & artificially flavored				
mix	1/16 pkt	–	5	–
prepared	2 Tbs	6.0	70	77%
ranch				
mix only	1/16 pkt	–	5	–
prepared	2 Tbs	6.0	70	77%
(Hidden Valley)				
Fiesta				
prepared	2 Tbs	6.0	70	77%
French onion				
prepared	2 Tbs	6.0	70	77%
garden vegetable				
prepared	2 Tbs	6.0	70	77%
original ranch				
fat-free	2 Tbs	–	35	–
prepared	2 Tbs	3.0	40	68%
regular recipe w/sour				
cream party dip				
prepared	2 Tbs	6.0	70	77%
(Knorr)				
DIP MIX				
cracked pepper ranch	½ tsp	–	5	–
garden dill	½ tsp	–	5	–
onion chive	½ tsp	–	5	–
RECIPE CLASSICS/ soup, dip & recipe mix				
French onion	⅓ box	1.0	35	26%

Food and Description	Amount	Fat Grams	Total Calories	% Fat Calories
roasted garlic herb	⅓ box	1.5	80	17%
vegetable	¼ box	0.5	30	15%
(Lipton)				
DIP MIX				
onion	1/16 pkg	–	5	–
*RECIPE SECRETS/*soup & dip mix				
beefy onion	⅛ pkg	0.5	25	18%
onion mushroom	⅕ pkg	0.5	30	15%
ranch	⅙ pkg	–	30	–
savory herb w/garlic	⅛ pkg	–	30	–
vegetable	⅕ pkg	–	30	–
(McCormick/Schilling)				
Dip Classics				
country herb	1 tsp	–	10	–
French onion	¾ tsp	–	5	–
garlic & pepper	¾ tsp	–	5	–
ranch	¾ tsp	–	5	–
spinach	½ tsp	–	10	–
spring onion	½ tsp	–	5	–
vegetable	½ tsp	–	5	–
■ **READY-TO-SERVE**				
(Athenos) hummus				
3 pepper/spicy	2 Tbs	3.5	60	53%
artichoke & garlic	2 Tbs	2.5	45	50%
black olive	2 Tbs	3.0	50	54%
cucumber dill	2 Tbs	4.0	60	60%
Greek-style	2 Tbs	3.5	60	53%
original	2 Tbs	3.5	60	53%
pesto	2 Tbs	3.5	50	63%
roasted				
eggplant	2 Tbs	2.5	45	50%
garlic	2 Tbs	3.5	50	63%
red pepper	2 Tbs	3.5	60	53%
scallion	2 Tbs	3.5	50	63%
(Armour)				
bacon cheddar cheese	2 Tbs	2.5	40	56%
bean	2 Tbs	1.0	40	23%
cheddar/jalapeño	2 Tbs	2.5	35	64%
cheese/chili	2 Tbs	1.5	30	45%
nacho bean	2 Tbs	1.0	40	23%
(Calavo) guacamole				
medium	2 Tbs	4.0	50	72%
mild	2 Tbs	4.0	50	81%
original avocado	2 Tbs	3.0	45	60%
spicy	2 Tbs	4.5	50	81%
(Dean's)				
bacon & horseradish	2 Tbs	5.0	60	75%
creamy dill	2 Tbs	4.5	50	81%
creamy taco	2 Tbs	4.5	50	81%

Food and Description	Amount	Fat Grams	Total Calories	% Fat Calories
French onion				
fat-free	2 Tbs	–	25	–
light	2 Tbs	2.0	35	51%
original	2 Tbs	5.0	60	75%
w/bacon	2 Tbs	5.0	60	75%
green onion	2 Tbs	4.5	60	68%
guacamole				
regular	2 Tbs	8.0	80	90%
zesty	2 Tbs	9.0	90	90%
ranch	2 Tbs	5.0	60	75%
veggie	2 Tbs	5.0	60	75%
(Frito-Lay)				
DIP KITS				
Doritos				
nacho cheesier				
& spicy queso	½ pkg	10.0	190	47%
& zesty picante	½ pkg	8.0	170	42%
Fritos				
chili cheese				
& scoops	1 kit	33.0	510	58%
fiesta cheese dip				
& scoops	1 kit	28.0	450	56%
Ruffles & French				
onion–flavored dip	1 kit	34.0	460	67%
Tostitos & cheese dip	1 kit	25.0	430	52%
Wavy Lay's & ranch–				
flavored dip	1 kit	34.0	470	65%
PARTY BOWL DIPS				
Southwestern salsa	2 Tbs	–	10	–
spicy queso	2 Tbs	2.5	40	56%
thick 'n' chunky salsa	2 Tbs	–	15	–
zesty bean & cheese	2 Tbs	2.0	40	45%
REGULAR FRITOS TUB DIPS				
bean				
hot	2 Tbs	1.0	40	23%
original	2 Tbs	1.0	40	23%
black bean	2 Tbs	–	30	–
cheddar cheese/mild	2 Tbs	4.0	60	60%
chili cheese	2 Tbs	3.0	45	60%
French onion	2 Tbs	5.0	60	75%
jalapeño cheese	2 Tbs	4.0	50	72%
RUFFLES DIPS				
French onion	2 Tbs	5.0	50	90%
ranch	2 Tbs	5.0	60	75%
TOSTITOS DIPS				
all-natural salsa				
hot	2 Tbs	–	15	–
medium	2 Tbs	–	15	–
mild	2 Tbs	–	15	–

Food and Description	Amount	Fat Grams	Total Calories	% Fat Calories
fire-roasted tomato				
salsa	2 Tbs	–	15	–
queso supreme	2 Tbs	2.5	45	50%
restaurant-style				
medium salsa				
con queso	2 Tbs	2.5	40	56%
salsa	2 Tbs	–	15	–
roasted garlic-flavored				
salsa	2 Tbs	–	15	–
(Guiltless Gourmet) spicy				
black bean				
mild	2 Tbs	–	30	–
spicy	2 Tbs	–	30	–
salsa dip				
roasted red pepper	2 Tbs	–	15	–
Southwestern grill	1 Tbs	–	15	–
(Heluva Good Cheese)				
bacon horseradish	2 tbs	5.0	60	75%
clam	2 Tbs	5.0	50	90%
French onion				
light	2 Tbs	2.0	35	51%
original	2 Tbs	5.0	60	75%
home-style onion	2 tbs	5.0	60	75%
jalapeño cheddar/light	2 tbs	2.0	40	45%
ranch	2 Tbs	5.0	60	75%
(Kaukauna)				
chili & cheese				
con queso deli/				
Mexican/medium	2 Tbs	5.0	70	64%
French onion	2 Tbs	3.0	50	54%
Nacho cheese/medium	2 Tbs	6.0	80	68%
salsa & cheese				
con queso deli/				
Mexican/medium	2 Tbs	4.5	70	58%
veggie ranch	2 Tbs	3.0	50	54%
(Kemp's)				
farmer's market dill	2 Tbs	15.0	140	96%
French onion	2 Tbs	4.5	60	68%
(Kraft)				
CHEEZ WHIZ				
Cheezin 'n' squeezing	2 Tbs	8.0	100	72%
light	2 Tbs	3.5	80	39%
original	2 Tbs	7.0	90	70%
salsa con queso	2 Tbs	7.0	90	70%
HANDI-SNACKS				
cheese dip				
& breadsticks	⅓ pkg	4.5	110	37%
& crackers	⅓ pkg	6.0	100	54%
& Mr. Salty				

Food and Description	Amount	Fat Grams	Total Calories	% Fat Calories
pretzels	⅛ pkg	3.5	100	32%
& Ritz crackers	⅛ pkg	6.0	100	54%
OTHER				
avocado/guacamole	2 Tbs	4.5	60	68%
bacon cheddar	2 Tbs	5.0	60	75%
cheese/premium				
jalapeño	2 Tbs	5.0	60	75%
nacho	2 Tbs	5.0	60	75%
French onion				
fat-free	2 Tbs	–	25	–
regular	2 Tbs	4.5	60	68%
green onion	2 Tbs	4.5	60	68%
ranch/creamy				
fat-free	2 Tbs	–	25	–
regular	2 Tbs	4.5	60	68%
(LiteHouse)				
FRUIT DIPS				
caramel				
fat-free	2 Tbs	–	110	–
Hershey's	2 Tbs	3.0	120	23%
low-fat	2 Tbs	–	110	–
toffee	2 Tbs	1.5	120	11%
caramel apple				
fat-free	2 Tbs	–	110	–
premium	2 Tbs	4.5	120	34%
chocolate/fat-free	2 Tbs	–	70	–
cinnamon vanilla	2 Tbs	6.0	90	60%
strawberry crème	2 Tbs	6.0	90	60%
vanilla crème	2 Tbs	6.0	90	60%
GLAZE DIPS				
apple cinnamon	3 Tbs	–	70	–
blueberry	3 Tbs	–	70	–
peach	3 Tbs	–	70	–
strawberry				
regular	3 Tbs	–	100	–
sugar-free	3 Tbs	–	35	–
VEGGIE DIPS				
avocado	2 Tbs	15.0	140	96%
dilly	2 Tbs	16.0	150	96%
jalapeño cheddar	2 Tbs	16.0	150	96%
onion	2 Tbs	11.0	110	90%
ranch	2 Tbs	13.0	120	98%
salsa	2 Tbs	6.0	60	90%
(Marie's)				
blue cheese	2 Tbs	8.0	80	90%
dill	2 Tbs	8.0	80	90%
French onion	2 Tbs	8.0	80	90%

Food and Description	Amount	Fat Grams	Total Calories	% Fat Calories
ranch				
home-style	2 Tbs	8.0	80	90%
light	2 Tbs	3.0	45	60%
spinach	2 Tbs	8.0	85	85%
(Marzetti)				
FOR FRUIT				
caramel apple				
fat-free	2 Tbs	–	120	–
	2 oz	–	160	–
light	2 Tbs	1.5	110	12%
old-fashioned	1 oz	6.0	150	36%
	1.5 oz	8.0	210	34%
chocolate	1.36 oz	2.0	110	16%
cream cheese	2 Tbs	3.0	70	39%
peanut butter caramel	2 Tbs	7.0	130	48%
FOR VEGETABLES				
bacon ranch	2 Tbs	12.0	120	90%
blue cheese	3 oz	44.0	420	94%
	2 Tbs	15.0	149	96%
celery & carrot	1.5 oz	24.0	220	98%
cheese veggie topping	2 Tbs	7.0	90	70%
dill				
fat-free veggie	2 Tbs	–	30	–
light	2 Tbs	6.0	60	90%
regular	2 Tbs	14.0	140	90%
French onion				
light	2 Tbs	6.0	70	77%
regular	2 Tbs	13.0	130	90%
guacamole	2 Tbs	12.0	120	90%
ranch				
fat-free	2 Tbs	–	35	–
garlic	2 Tbs	14.0	140	90%
light	2 Tbs	6.0	80	68%
organic	2 Tbs	14.0	130	97%
veggie				
fat-free	2 Tbs	–	35	–
light	2 Tbs	6.0	70	77%
singles	2 Tbs	13.0	130	90%
sour cream & onion				
fat-free	2 Tbs	–	35	–
Southwestern				
fat-free	2 Tbs	–	30	–
original	2 Tbs	14.0	140	90%
GLAZE DIP				
for strawberries				
regular	1.6 oz	–	60	–
sugar-free	1.6 oz	–	10	–
(Old El Paso)				
black bean	2 Tbs	–	25	–

Food and Description	Amount	Fat Grams	Total Calories	% Fat Calories
cheese 'n' salsa				
medium	2 Tbs	3.0	40	68%
mild	2 Tbs	3.0	40	68%
jalapeño	2 Tbs	1.0	30	30%
(Phillip's) seafood dip				
crab & spinach				
original	2 Tbs	5.0	60	75%
restaurant recipe	2 Tbs	5.0	60	75%
(Reeser's) Fresh dips				
artichoke jalapeño	2 Tbs	7.0	80	79%
French onion/toasted	2 Tbs	5.0	60	75%
ranch	2 Tbs	11.0	110	90%
spinach dip/creamy	2 Tbs	9.0	90	90%
(Rod's)				
DIP				
French onion				
regular	2 Tbs	6.0	70	77%
w/bacon	2 Tbs	6.0	70	77%
green onion	2 Tbs	6.0	70	77%
ranch	2 Tbs	6.0	70	77%
DIP & DRESSING				
avocado	2 Tbs	11.0	110	90%
French onion/fat-free	2 Tbs	–	25	–
guacamole				
regular	2 Tbs	11.0	110	90%
zesty	2 Tbs	8.0	80	90%
ranch				
regular	2 Tbs	11.0	110	90%
fat-free	2 Tbs	–	25	–
w/bacon	2 Tbs	11.0	110	90%
(Skyline Chili)..chili dip				
chili & cream cheese	2 Tbs	9.0	120	68%
w/mild cheddar cheese	2 Tbs	9.0	120	68%
(Snyder's)				
Eat Smart/tres bean				
w/jalapeño & lime	2 Tbs	–	25	–
flame-roasted				
salsa con queso	2 Tbs	2.0	35	51%
mild cheddar cheese	2 Tbs	9.0	100	81%
mustard/tangy honey	2 Tbs	1.0	70	13%
(T. Marzetti's)				
FRUIT DIPS				
apple dip				
caramel				
fat-free	2 Tbs	–	120	–
light	2 Tbs	1.5	110	12%
peanut butter	2 Tbs	7.0	130	48%
apple dip caramel				
fat-free	2 oz	–	160	–

Food and Description	Amount	Fat Grams	Total Calories	% Fat Calories
old-fashioned				
cup	2 oz	8.0	210	34%
tub	1.5 oz	6.0	150	36%
chocolate-flavored				
fat-free	2 Tbs	–	100	–
regular	2 Tbs	2.0	110	16%
cream cheese	2 Tbs	3.0	70	39%
VEGGIE DIPS				
blue cheese	2 Tbs	19.0	180	95%
dill	2 Tbs	14.0	140	90%
ranch				
bacon	2 Tbs	12.0	120	90%
fat-free	2 Tbs	–	35	–
light	2 Tbs	6.0	70	77%
organic	2 Tbs	14.0	130	97%
original	2 Tbs	14.0	140	90%
Southwestern ranch	2 Tbs	12.0	120	90%
spinach	2 Tbs	14.0	140	90%
(Tribe of Two Sheiks) hummus				
classic	2 Tbs	3.0	50	54%
dill	2 Tbs	3.0	50	54%
forty-spice	2 Tbs	3.0	50	54%
jalapeño	2 Tbs	3.0	50	54%
roasted garlic	2 Tbs	3.0	50	54%
scallion	2 Tbs	3.0	50	54%
DISTILLED LIQUOR (See LIQUOR, DISTILLED)				
DOCK				
cooked-drained	3 oz	0.5	17	26%
raw/chopped	3 oz	0.5	15	30%
DOGFISH (See also SHARK)				
raw	3 oz	8.0	135	53%
DOLPHIN FISH (See also MAHIMAHI)				
raw	3 oz	0.6	73	7%
DONUT (See also BAGELS; COOKIES; PASTRY)				
(Awrey's)				
dunkers				
almond	2 donuts	11.0	240	41%
glazed				
regular	2 donuts	11.0	240	41%
rings	1 donut	16.0	270	53%
sour cream	1 donut	19.0	380	45%
plain	2 donuts	18.0	330	49%
powdered sugar				
jelly Bismark	1 donut	14.0	270	47%
(Dolly Madison)				
chocolate				
gems	4 gems	15.0	260	52%
iced/old-fashioned	1 donut	14.0	300	42%
cinnamon sticks	1 stick	9.0	170	48%

Food and Description	Amount	Fat Grams	Total Calories	% Fat Calories
cinnamon sugar				
gems	6 gems	17.0	360	43%
sticks	2 sticks	12.0	230	47%
crunch				
gems	6 gems	18.0	390	42%
regular	1 donut	6.0	140	39%
dunking sticks	2 sticks	19.0	360	48%
frosted	1 donut	6.0	130	42%
glazed/old-fashioned	1 donut	14.0	300	42%
iced/jumbo	1 donut	12.0	230	47%
plain				
jumbo	1 donut	11.0	190	52%
regular	2 donuts	10.0	170	53%
powdered sugar/gems	6 gems	17.0	360	43%
sugar				
jumbo	1 donut	12.0	230	47%
regular	1 donut	6.0	130	42%
white iced				
old-fashioned	1 donut	14.0	230	55%
yeast glazed	1 donut	8.0	180	40%
(Entenmann's)				
DONUT HOLES/glazed				
Little Bites	4 pieces	11.0	220	45%
DONUTS				
classic				
frosted				
devil's food	1 donut	20.0	320	56%
rich frosted/8-count	1 donut	19.0	280	61%
ultimate chocolate				
lovers/8-count	1 donut	19.0	310	55%
Donut Shoppe				
popems				
cinnamon	4 pieces	13.0	250	47%
glazed	4 pieces	10.0	210	43%
holiday	4 pieces	10.0	220	41%
rich-frosted				
holiday	4 pieces	22.0	310	64%
popettes				
softee powdered	4 pieces	13.0	240	49%
holiday donuts	1 donut	21.0	330	57%
(Freihofer's)				
Donut holes				
powdered mini	1 donut	6.0	120	45%
Donuts				
super softee	1 donut	12.0	210	51%
éclair/fine baked	1 éclair	8.0	200	36%
(Hostess)				
DONETTES/bite-size donuts				
crumb	3 donettes	10.0	230	39%

Food and Description	Amount	Fat Grams	Total Calories	% Fat Calories
frosted	3 donettes	12.0	200	54%
powdered	3 donettes	9.0	180	45%
DONETS				
blueberry	1 donut	13.0	210	56%
frosted	1 donut	11.0	180	55%
glazed/old-fashioned	1 donut	13.0	260	45%
plain	1 donut	7.0	140	45%
powdered	1 donut	8.0	150	48%
raspberry O's	1 donut	10.0	230	39%
(Krispy Kreme)				
apple fritter	1 fritter	21.0	380	50%
cake				
cinnamon sugar	1 donut	14.0	280	45%
pumpkin spice	1 donut	18.0	340	48%
traditional	1 donut	13.0	230	51%
caramel kreme crunch	1 donut	19.0	350	49%
chocolate				
iced crème-filled	1 donut	21.0	350	54%
iced cruller	1 donut	15.0	290	47%
iced custard-filled	1 donut	17.0	300	51%
malted kreme	1 donut	21.0	390	48%
cinnamon twist	1 twist	9.0	230	35%
coffee & kreme	1 donut	20.0	360	50%
dulce de leche	1 donut	4.5	290	14%
glazed				
blueberry-filled	1 donut	16.0	290	50%
chocolate iced	1 donut	12.0	250	43%
w/sprinkles	1 donut	12.0	260	42%
cruller	1 donut	14.0	240	53%
custard-filled	1 donut	16.0	290	50%
lemon-filled	1 donut	16.0	290	50%
original	1 donut	12.0	200	54%
raspberry-filled	1 donut	16.0	300	48%
sour cream	1 donut	18.0	340	48%
strawberry-filled	1 donut	16.0	290	50%
twist	1 twist	9.0	210	39%
vanilla-iced	1 donut	12.0	240	45%
honey & oat	1 donut	18.0	340	48%
key lime pie	1 donut	18.0	330	49%
maple iced	1 donut	12.0	240	45%
New York cheesecake	1 donut	19.0	330	52%
powdered				
cream-filled	1 donut	21.0	340	56%
raspberry	1 donut	16.0	300	48%
vanilla-iced				
cream-filled	1 donut	20.0	340	53%
custard-filled	1 donut	16.0	290	50%
raspberry-filled	1 donut	16.0	350	41%
w/sprinkles	1 donut	13.0	270	43%

Food and Description	Amount	Fat Grams	Total Calories	% Fat Calories
(Little Debbie)				
donut sticks				
box	1 pkg	14.0	230	55%
individual	1 pkg	13.0	220	53%
mini donuts				
frosted	1 pkg	22.0	360	55%
glazed	1 pkg	12.0	280	39%
powdered/packaged	1.78 oz	10.0	210	43%
	2.5 oz	16.0	310	46%
(Rich's) frozen				
éclairs				
Bavarian crème	1 éclair	12.0	220	49%
mini	2.3 oz	13.0	250	47%
cappuccino	1 éclair	12.0	220	49%
(Sara Lee)				
CAKE				
assorted/variety pack	1 donut	14.0	280	45%
glazed				
old-fashioned				
sour cream	1 donut	9.0	250	32%
vanilla cake	1 donut	9.0	340	24%
iced chocolate chip	1 donut	13.0	280	42%
powdered sugar	1 donut	13.0	290	40%
YEAST-RAISED				
apple fritter	1 fritter	19.0	360	48%
golden glazed	1 donut	11.0	270	37%
sugar-coated				
raspberry-filled	1 donut	9.0	250	32%
sweet centers/variety	1 center	10.0	260	35%
(TastyKake)				
apple fritter	1.5 oz	9.0	170	48%
Krispy Stix	1.5 oz	6.0	180	30%
mini donuts				
bubble gum	6 donuts	10.0	250	36%
cinnamon	6 donuts	11.0	210	47%
plain glazed	6 donuts	12.0	270	40%
powdered sugar	6 donuts	14.0	290	43%
rich frosted	6 donuts	23.0	380	54%
regular				
cinnamon	1 donut	11.0	210	47%
coated	1 donut	13.0	220	53%
plain	1 donut	12.0	210	51%
premium frosted	1 donut	15.0	250	54%
sugar	1 donut	11.0	200	50%
(Winchell's)				
CAKE DONUTS				
buttermilk bar/glazed	1 donut	16.0	260	55%
cinnamon crumb	1 donut	18.0	240	68%
iced				
French	1 donut	13.0	220	53%
old-fashioned	1 donut	19.0	260	66%

Food and Description	Amount	Fat Grams	Total Calories	% Fat Calories
plain	1 donut	15.0	230	59%
glazed old-fashioned	1 donut	18.0	250	65%
plain	1 donut	14.0	215	59%
DONUT HOLES				
iced	4 pieces	15.0	230	59%
plain	4 pieces	14.0	215	59%
RAISED DONUTS				
apple fritter	1 fritter	41.0	670	55%
bear claw	1 donut	30.0	560	48%
chocolate Bavarian	1 donut	18.0	325	50%
jelly				
glazed	1 donut	17.0	320	48%
sugar	1 donut	17.0	315	49%
rounds				
chocolate	1 donut	16.0	240	60%
glazed	1 donut	15.0	230	59%
sugar	1 donut	15.0	225	60%
twists				
chocolate	1 twist	16.0	240	60%
glazed	1 twist	15.0	230	59%
sugar	1 twist	15.0	225	60%
DRESSING (*See* MAYONNAISE/MAYONNAISE-TYPE DRESSING; SALAD DRESSING; STUFFING/DRESSING)				
DRUM/freshwater				
baked	3 oz	5.0	130	35%
raw	3 oz	4.0	100	36%
DUCK				
domesticated				
raw				
liver	1.5 oz	2.0	60	30%
roasted				
meat & skin	~¾ lb	108.0	1287	76%
meat only	8 oz	25.0	456	49%
wild/raw	3 oz	9.0	170	48%
breast meat only	3 oz	3.5	105	30%
meat & skin	9.5 oz	41.0	570	65%
DUMPLING (*See also* FROZEN ENTRÉE/DINNER; PASTA; PASTRY)				
dry/pasta				
(Creamette)				
yolk-free dumplings	2 oz	1.0	210	4%
(Skinner) dumplings	2 oz	1.0	210	4%
dry/potato				
(Monterey Pasta Co.)				
gnocchi/Italian potato dumpling	3.7 oz	2.5	90	25%
frozen				
(Chef Pierre)				
apple dumplings				
w/cinnamon sauce	1 dumpling	21.0	480	39%
(Mary B's)				
open kettle dumplings	⅓ pkg	4.0	160	23%

E

Food and Description	Amount	Fat Grams	Total Calories	% Fat Calories
ÉCLAIR (*See* DONUT; PASTRY)				
EEL				
cooked—dry heat	3 oz	12.7	200	57%
raw	3 oz	10.0	156	58%
smoked	~2 oz	16.0	188	77%
EGG (*See also* EGG SUBSTITUTE; VEGETARIAN FOODS)				
GENERIC				
chicken				
boiled, hard or soft	1 medium	4.0	70	51%
	1 large	5.6	79	64%
fried in butter	1 large	7.0	95	66%
pickled	1 large	5.0	80	56%
poached	1 large	5.6	79	64%
raw				
white only	1 medium	–	14	–
	1 large	–	16	–
	1 cup	–	120	–
whole	1 medium	4.0	70	51%
	1 large	5.6	79	64%
yolk only	1 medium	4.0	56	64%
	1 large	5.6	63	64%
duck/raw	1 egg	9.6	130	67%
goose/raw	1 egg	19.0	276	62%
quail/raw	1 egg	1.0	14	64%
turkey/raw	1 egg	9.0	135	60%
INDIVIDUAL BRANDS				
(Eggland's Best)				
large	1 egg	4.0	40	90%
(Land O'Lakes)				
cage-free all-natural	1 egg	4.5	70	58%
extra-large	1 egg	5.0	80	56%
large	1 egg	4.5	70	58%
(Papetti) refrigerated				
all whites	~1 oz	–	25	–
quick eggs	2 oz	–	30	–
(Sauder) Free range				
extra-large	1 egg	5.0	80	56%
(Wilcox)				
100% organic				
brown/large	1 egg	4.5	70	58%

Food and Description	Amount	Fat Grams	Total Calories	% Fat Calories
Dino super jumbo	1 egg	7.0	100	63%
Omega 3–fortified brown egg	1 egg	4.5	70	58%

EGG DISH/MEAL (*See also* BREAKFAST SANDWICH; EGG; EGG SUBSTITUTE; FROZEN ENTRÉE/DINNER; individual FAST FOOD listings; VEGETARIAN FOODS)

FROZEN OR REFRIGERATED

(Chef's Omelet)				
ham & cheese	½ pkg	12.0	180	60%
sausage & cheese	½ pkg	18.0	240	68%
3–cheese	½ pkg	16.0	230	63%
Western-style	½ pkg	9.0	150	54%
(Nancy's) quiche/microwavable				
petite appetizers				
assortment				
box of 48				
classic French	6 quiches	24.0	400	54%
Florentine	6 quiches	21.0	370	51%
Florentine puffs	12 pieces	21.0	400	47%
Santa Fe quiche				
tartlets	12 tarts	40.0	650	55%
single servings				
broccoli cheddar	1 quiche	26.0	430	54%
cheese trio				
bistro favorite	1 quiche	28.0	450	56%
classic French	1 quiche	33.0	470	63%
Florentine	1 quiche	26.0	440	53%
Lorraine	1 quiche	29.0	490	53%
(Schwan's)				
Pour-a-Quiche				
broccoli & cheddar	4.3 oz	16.0	200	72%
original	4.3 oz	14.0	180	70%
(Swanson)				
egg, cheese & bacon on a biscuit	1 sdw	22.0	310	64%
sausage, egg & cheese on a croissant	1 sdw	33.0	470	63%
(Weight Watchers) Handy Omelet				
English muffin sandwich	1 sdw	5.0	210	21%

JARRED

(Penrose) Pickled				
5.5-oz jar	1 egg	3.0	45	60%
36-oz jar	1 egg	3.0	50	54%

PRECOOKED

(Mountain House) Pouch				
eggs w/bacon	1 pouch	18.0	320	51%
eggs w/ham & peppers	1 pouch	21.0	350	54%
scrambled eggs	1 pouch	18.0	310	52%

EGG NOG (*See also* MILK; MILK MIX)

(Borden) Premium/can	4 oz	9.0	160	51%

Food and Description	Amount	Fat Grams	Total Calories	% Fat Calories
(Dairyland)				
classic	4 oz	5.0	155	29%
light	4 oz	3.2	108	21%
original	4 oz	2.0	118	15%
(Eagle Family) Premium	4 oz	9.0	160	51%
REFRIGERATED				
(Farm Rich) non-dairy	8 fl oz	18.0	380	43%
(HP Hood) Southern Comfort				
fat-free/sugar-free	8 oz	–	110	–
golden	4 oz	8.0	180	40%
light	4 oz	4.0	140	26%
traditional				
non-alcohol	4 oz	8.0	190	38%
vanilla	4 oz	8.0	180	40%
vanilla spice	4 oz	9.0	210	39%
(Kemp's)				
Holly Nog	4 fl oz	2.0	110	16%
light	4 fl oz	3.0	120	23%
original	4 fl oz	9.0	175	46%
premium	4 fl oz	9.0	180	45%
(Land O'Lakes)				
light	4 fl oz	3.0	130	21%
original	4 fl oz	8.0	170	42%
(Sinton's)				
Colorado	4 oz	8.0	170	42%
old-fashioned	4 oz	8.0	170	42%

EGG ROLL (*See* ASIAN FOOD; FROZEN ENTRÉE/DINNER; SEAFOOD ENTRÉE/DINNER)
EGG SALAD (*See* EGG DISH/MEAL)
EGG SUBSTITUTE

Food and Description	Amount	Fat Grams	Total Calories	% Fat Calories
(Con Agra) Egg Beaters				
frozen				
fat-free	¼ cup	–	30	–
refrigerated				
all types	¼ cup	–	30	–
(Just Whites)				
dried egg whites	2 tsp	–	14	–
(Morningstar Farms) frozen				
Better'n Eggs	¼ cup	–	20	–
Scramblers	¼ cup	–	35	–
(Nulaid) no cholesterol/no fat				
cheese	¼ cup	–	40	–
original	¼ cup	–	30	–
(Papetti Foods)				
Better'n Eggs	2 oz	–	30	–
The Right Egg	2 oz	–	30	–
(Second Nature)				
no cholesterol	2 fl oz	2.0	60	30%
no fat	2 fl oz	–	35	–
w/garden vegetables	2.5 fl oz	–	40	–
(Simply Eggs)	1.75 fl oz	1.0	35	26%

Food and Description	Amount	Fat Grams	Total Calories	% Fat Calories
(Tofutti) Egg Watchers	¼ cup	–	30	–
(Wonderslim) fat & egg				
substitute	¼ cup	–	35	–
EGGPLANT/fresh				
boiled/drained	½ cup	–	13	–
jarred				
(Food Club) roasted	1 oz	3.0	35	77%
(Patak's Original)				
relish/brinjal eggplant				
sweet & spicy/				
medium	½ oz	4.0	70	51%
(Peloponnese) baba ghanoush				
eggplant & tahini				
spread	1 oz	3.0	40	68%
raw				
(Frieda's)	⅔ cup	–	20	–
EGGPLANT DISH (See FROZEN ENTRÉE/DINNER)				
ELDERBERRY/raw	1 cup	0.8	105	7%
	½ lb	1.0	154	6%
ELK/meat only				
raw	1 oz	0.4	31	17%
	1 pound	6.6	504	12%
roasted	3 oz	1.6	124	12%
ENCHILADA (See FROZEN ENTRÉE/DINNER; MEXICAN FOOD)				
ENCHILADA SAUCE (See MEXICAN FOOD; SAUCE)				
ENDIVE/raw	½ cup	–	4	–
ENGLISH MUFFIN (See MUFFIN)				
ESCARGOT (See SNAIL/ESGARGOT)				
ESCAROLE/raw	4 oz	–	20	–
ESCAROLE SOUP (See SOUP)				
EXTRACTS & FLAVORINGS				
(Durkee)				
almond extract	1 tsp	–	13	–
anise extract	1 tsp	–	16	–
banana flavor	1 tsp	–	15	–
black walnut flavor	1 tsp	–	4	–
brandy flavor	1 tsp	–	15	–
butter flavor	1 tsp	–	3	–
cherry extract	1 tsp	–	3	–
chocolate flavor	1 tsp	–	7	–
coconut flavor	1 tsp	–	8	–
crème de menthe extract	1 tsp	–	9	–
lemon extract	1 tsp	–	17	–
maple extract	1 tsp	–	6	–
orange extract	1 tsp	–	14	–
peppermint extract	1 tsp	–	15	–
pineapple flavor	1 tsp	–	6	–
raspberry extract	1 tsp	–	10	–
rum flavor	1 tsp	–	14	–
strawberry extract	1 tsp	–	12	–

Food and Description	Amount	Fat Grams	Total Calories	% Fat Calories
vanilla butter & nut extract	1 tsp	–	5	–
vanilla extract	1 tsp	–	8	–
vanilla flavor	1 tsp	–	3	–
(McCormick/Schilling)				
black walnut extract				
cold	1 tsp	–	12	–
heated	1 tsp	–	<1	–
brandy imitation				
extract	1 tsp	–	20	–
chocolate extract				
cold	1 tsp	–	8	–
heated	1 tsp	–	2	–
coconut imitation extract	1 tsp	–	7	–
lemon extract				
cold	1 tsp	–	35	–
heated	1 tsp	–	<1	–
orange extract	1 tsp	–	23	–
pineapple imitation				
extract	1 tsp	–	12	–
root beer concentrate	1 tsp	–	13	–
rum imitation extract	1 tsp	–	19	–
sherry extract	1 tsp	–	14	–
vanilla				
cold	1 tsp	–	12	–
heated	1 tsp	–	<1	–

F

Food and Description	Amount	Fat Grams	Total Calories	% Fat Calories
FAJITA (See MEXICAN FOOD; FROZEN ENTRÉE/DINNER)				
FALAFEL				
mix				
(Casbah) prepared	5 balls	3.0	160	17%
(Fantastic Foods) Fantastic Falafel				
mix only	½ cup	4.0	250	14%
prepared	1 cup	4.0	250	14%
(Near East) vegetarian				
chickpea/fava bean mix				
prepared	1 cup	15.0	230	59%

Food and Description	Amount	Fat Grams	Total Calories	% Fat Calories
pita stuffers dry mix				
w/garbanzo beans	1.25 oz	2.0	120	15%
FAST FOOD (*See* listings in separate section at end of book)				
FAT (*See also* BEEF TALLOW; BUTTER; COOKING SPRAY; LARD; MARGARINE, MARGARINE SPREAD & SPRAY; OIL; PORK FAT; SHORTENING, VEGETABLE)				
bacon fat	1 Tbs	14.0	126	100%
beef fat/separable/raw	1 Tbs	12.0	108	100%
chicken fat	1 Tbs	12.0	115	100%
duck fat	1 Tbs	12.0	115	100%
pork backfat/raw	2 oz	50.0	464	100%
FAT SUBSTITUTE (*See also* OIL; SHORTENING, VEGETABLE)				
(Wonderslim) fat & egg substitute	¼ cup	–	35	–
FAVA BEAN/canned				
(Progresso)	½ cup	0.5	110	4%
FENNEL LEAVES/raw	2 oz	–	15	–
FENNEL SEED	1 tsp	–	7	–
FENUGREEK SEED	1 tsp	–	12	–
FIELD PEA				
(Allen's)				
field peas	½ cup	1.0	120	8%
tiny	½ cup	1.0	120	8%
(Bush's Best)				
field peas w/snaps	½ cup	0.5	110	4%
(Glory Foods)				
field peas	½ cup	–	80	–
w/snaps	½ cup	–	70	–
(Trappey's)				
flavored w/slab bacon	½ cup	0.5	100	5%
tender	½ cup	1.0	90	10%
w/snaps	½ cup	1.0	110	8%
FIG				
CANNED				
(Oregon Fruit)				
Kadota/whole				
in heavy syrup	½ cup	1.0	130	7%
DRIED				
(Blue Ribbon Orchard Choice)				
Calimyrna	½ cup	–	120	–
Mission				
figlets	1.4 oz	–	120	–
figs	½ cup	–	120	–
(Krinos) Katanata	3 figs	–	100	–
(Mariani) Calimyrna	½ cup	2.0	250	7%
(Sun-Maid)				
Calimyrna	¼ cup	–	120	–
Mission	¼ cup	–	120	–
FRESH	1 medium	–	37	–
	1 large	–	47	–
FILBERT/HAZELNUT (*See also* HAZELNUT BUTTER/SPREAD)				
(Diamond)				
in the shell	1 oz	19.0	190	90%

Food and Description	Amount	Fat Grams	Total Calories	% Fat Calories
shelled	1 oz	19.0	190	90%
(Planters) chopped	2 oz	35.0	350	90%
FISH (See GEFILTE FISH; SEAFOOD ENTRÉE/DINNER; individual listings)				
FISH CHOWDER (See SOUP)				
FISH SEASONING (See SEASONINGS)				
FIVE SPICE SEASONING (See SEASONINGS)				
FLAN (See CUSTARD)				
FLATBREAD (See CRACKER)				
FLATFISH (See also FLOUNDER)				
cooked	3 oz	1.0	100	9%
raw	3 oz	1.0	80	11%
FLAVORINGS (See EXTRACTS & FLAVORINGS)				
FLAXSEED				
(Arrowhead Mills)	3 Tbs	10.0	140	64%
FLOUNDER (See also SEAFOOD ENTRÉE/DINNER)				
baked				
w/butter	3 oz	7.0	171	37%
w/o butter	3 oz	1.0	80	11%
FLOUR				
acorn	1 oz	9.0	142	57%
all-purpose				
(Gold Medal)				
unbleached	¼ cup	–	100	–
(Martha White)				
bleached/enriched	¼ cup	–	100	–
(Robin Hood)	¼ cup	0.4	120	3%
unbleached	¼ cup	0.4	120	3%
whole wheat	¼ cup	0.6	120	5%
amaranth				
(Arrowhead Mills)	⅓ cup	2.5	120	19%
arrowroot	1 Tbs	–	29	–
barley				
(Arrowhead Mills)	⅓ cup	1.0	95	9%
blended				
(Arrowhead Mills)				
Perfect Harvest				
whole grains	¼ cup	1.5	130	10%
blending				
(Robin Hood) best for				
bread	¼ cup	0.4	120	3%
(Gold Medal)..all types	¼ cup	–	100	–
(Hodgson Mill) best for bread	¼ cup	–	100	–
(Pillsbury)	¼ cup	–	100	–
(Red Band) better for bread	¼ cup	–	100	–
buckwheat				
(Arrowhead Mills)	⅓ cup	1.5	115	12%
(Hodgson Mill)	⅓ cup	1.0	160	6%
cake or pastry				
(Arrowhead Mills)				
soft pastry	¼ cup	0.5	100	5%

Food and Description	Amount	Fat Grams	Total Calories	% Fat Calories
(Softasilk)				
velvet cake	¼ cup	–	100	–
(Presto) self-rising	¼ cup	–	90	–
(Robin Hood)	¼ cup	0.4	125	3%
(Swan's Down) cake	¼ cup	–	100	–
carob				
(St. John's Bread)	1 cup	3.0	420	6%
corn	1 oz	0.7	102	6%
	1 cup	3.0	430	6%
cottonseed				
low-fat	1 oz	–	95	–
partially defatted	1 oz	–	40	–
	1 cup	6.0	335	16%
gluten				
(La Pina) Supreme				
Hygluten	¼ cup	–	100	–
kamut				
(Arrowhead Mills)	⅓ cup	1.0	130	7%
(Eden) Organic	¼ cup	1.5	200	7%
millet				
(Arrowhead Mills)	⅓ cup	1.5	130	10%
multigrain				
(Arrowhead Mills)				
multi-blend	¼ cup	0.5	120	4%
oat				
(Arrowhead Mills)	⅓ cup	3.0	120	23%
(Hodgson Mill)				
oat bran blend	¼ cup	1.0	110	8%
pastry				
(Arrowhead Mills)	¼ cup	0.5	110	4%
peanut				
defatted	1 oz	–	92	–
	1 cup	–	200	–
low-fat	1 oz	6.0	120	45%
	1 cup	13.0	260	45%
potato	1 cup	1.5	632	2%
quinoa				
(Quinoa) gluten-free,				
whole-grain	¼ cup	2.0	130	14%
rice				
(Arrowhead Mills)				
brown	¼ cup	1.0	130	7%
white	¼ cup	–	120	–
(Lundberg Family Farms)				
Nutra-farmed				
brown rice	¼ cup	1.5	120	11%
organic	¼ cup	1.5	110	12%
(Tres Estrellas)	¼ cup	1.0	150	6%
rye				
(Arrowhead Mills)	¼ cup	0.5	110	4%

Food and Description	Amount	Fat Grams	Total Calories	% Fat Calories
(Hodgson Mill)	¼ cup	1.0	90	10%
(Krusteaz) medium	⅓ cup	0.5	110	4%
(Pillsbury)				
medium	¼ cup	–	100	–
(Robin Hood)	¼ cup	0.5	122	4%
self-rising				
(Martha White)				
bleached/enriched	¼ cup	0.5	110	4%
sesame				
high-fat	4 oz	42.0	595	64%
low-fat	1 cup	–	95	–
	4 oz	2.0	380	5%
partially defatted	4 oz	14.0	440	29%
soy				
(Arrowhead Mills)	¼ cup	4.5	100	41%
spelt				
(Arrowhead Mills)	⅓ cup	1.0	130	7%
sunflower seed	1 Tbs	<1.0	16	4%
	1 cup	1.3	261	4%
tortilla				
(La Pina)				
flour for tortillas	¼ cup	–	100	–
triticale	1 oz	0.5	95	5%
	1 cup	2.5	440	5%
white				
(Arrowhead Mills)				
unbleached	¼ cup	0.5	120	4%
(Gold Medal)				
all-purpose	¼ cup	–	100	–
organic	¼ cup	–	100	–
self-rising	¼ cup	–	100	–
unbleached	¼ cup	–	100	–
Wondra	¼ cup	–	100	
(Hodgson Mill)				
regular	¼ cup	–	100	–
seasoned	¼ cup	–	90	–
(Pillsbury)				
all-purpose				
bleached	¼ cup	–	100	–
unbleached	¼ cup	–	100	–
self-rising				
bleached	¼ cup	–	100	–
unbleached	¼ cup	–	100	–
Shake & Blend	¼ cup	–	100	–
(Quaker) Aunt Jemima				
self-rising				
enriched	3 Tbs	–	90	–
(Robin Hood)				
all-purpose	¼ cup	–	100	–
home-style	¼ cup	0.3	120	2%

Food and Description	Amount	Fat Grams	Total Calories	% Fat Calories
whole wheat				
(Alma)				
coarse wheat	¼ cup	–	100	–
fine wheat	¼ cup	–	100	–
(Arrowhead Mills)				
stone-ground	¼ cup	1.0	130	7%
(Gold Medal)				
whole wheat	¼ cup	0.5	90	5%
(Hodgson Mill)				
50/50	¼ cup	1.0	100	9%
whole wheat	¼ cup	1.0	100	9%
(Pillsbury)	¼ cup	1.0	120	8%
(Robin Hood)				
60% whole wheat	¼ cup	0.5	120	4%
whole wheat	¼ cup	0.6	120	5%
FRANKFURTER (*See also* CORN DOG; FRANKFURTER, VEGETARIAN; SAUSAGE; VEGETARIAN FOODS; individual FAST FOOD listings)				
(Armour)				
jumbo	2 oz	17.0	200	77%
(Ball Park)				
RETAIL				
Ball Park Franks				
beef franks	2 oz	16.0	180	80%
franks	2 oz	16.0	180	80%
Better for You				
fat-free				
beef franks	1.78 oz	–	55	–
franks	1.78 oz	–	50	–
light				
beef franks	1.78 oz	7.0	100	63%
franks	1.78 oz	7.0	100	63%
smoked white turkey				
bun-size	1.78 oz	–	45	–
bun-size				
beef	2 oz	16.0	180	80%
regular	2 oz	16.0	180	80%
Grillmaster				
beef	2.9 oz	12.0	240	45%
Cajun	2.9 oz	24.0	260	83%
garlic	2.9 oz	24.0	260	83%
smokey	2.9 oz	24.0	260	83%
singles				
beef franks	1.6 oz	13.0	150	78%
cheese	1.6 oz	13.0	150	78%
franks	1.6 oz	13.0	150	78%
Smokies	2 oz	17.0	180	85%
(Boar's Head)				
frankfurters				
beef				
cocktail	5 franks	15.0	170	79%

Food and Description	Amount	Fat Grams	Total Calories	% Fat Calories
light				
natural casing	1.6 oz	6.0	90	60%
skinless	1.6 oz	6.0	90	60%
natural casing	2 oz	14.0	160	79%
skinless	1.6 oz	11.0	120	83%
pork & beef				
natural casing	2 oz	14.0	150	84%
skinless	2 oz	14.0	150	84%
(Eckrich) jumbo				
cheese	1 frank	17.0	180	85%
regular	1 frank	17.0	190	80%
turkey, chicken				
& pork	1.6 oz	12.0	140	77%
jumbo	2 oz	14.0	170	74%
(Farmer John)				
Dodger Dogs/extra-long				
meat wiener	2.7 oz	21.0	190	99%
Frankfooter/extra-long				
beef frank	2.7 oz	20.0	230	78%
franks				
beef	1.6 oz	12.0	140	77%
Picante Dog				
spice meat wiener	1.6 oz	12.0	130	83%
wieners				
pork & beef	1.6 oz	11.0	130	76%
(Healthy Choice)				
beef hot dogs				
bun-size				
low-fat	1 frank	2.5	70	32%
meat	1 frank	2.5	70	32%
turkey..pork & beef				
frank..low-fat	1 frank	2.5	70%	32%
(Hebrew National)				
franks				
¼ pound dinner	4 oz	32.0	350	82%
97% fat-free	1 frank	1.5	45	30%
beef				
7-count	1.75 oz	14.0	150	84%
dinner/4-count	4 oz	32.0	350	82%
reduced-fat	1.7 oz	10.0	120	75%
cocktail franks				
4-count	4 links	16.0	180	80%
6-count	1 link	15.0	160	84%
Franks in a Blanket	5 pieces	24.0	290	74%
(Hillshire Farm)				
bun-size				
all-beef super dogs	4 oz	34.0	350	87%
beef	2 oz	17.0	180	85%
cheese	2 oz	17.0	180	85%

Food and Description	Amount	Fat Grams	Total Calories	% Fat Calories
regular	2 oz	17.0	180	85%
light & mild/jumbo	1 frank	8.0	110	65%
Lit'l Beef franks	2 oz	15.0	170	79%
Lit'l Smokies				
beef	6 pieces	15.0	170	79%
meat	6 pieces	16.0	180	80%
wieners				
bun-size	2 oz	17.0	180	85%
foot-long	3.25 oz	26.0	280	84%
light & mild	1 wiener	8.0	90	80%
Lit'l wieners	6 pieces	16.0	170	85%
natural casing	2 oz	17.0	180	85%
(Hormel)				
cocktail franks				
Smokies	6 smokies	15.0	170	79%
beef	6 smokies	16.0	180	80%
w/cheese	6 smokies	14.0	170	74%
	1 oz link	7.0	80	79%
corn dogs	2.75 oz	11.0	220	45%
hot dogs				
fat-free	1 frank	–	45	–
hot dogs/beef/fat-free	1 frank	–	45	–
franks				
beef	2 oz	15.0	170	79%
fat-free	1 frank	–	45	–
(Jennie-O) Turkey Store				
corn dogs	1 dog	10.0	230	39%
turkey franks				
w/natural smoke flavor	1.2 oz	5.0	70	64%
	1.59 oz	8.0	90	80%
	1.98 oz	11.0	130	76%
(Johnsonville)				
cocktail links/fully cooked				
beef links	6 links	16.0	180	80%
Little Smokies	6 links	16.0	180	80%
wieners	1.75 oz	14.0	150	84%
(Kahn's)				
franks				
beef				
bun-size	1 frank	16.0	180	80%
jumbo	2 oz	17.0	180	85%
regular	1 frank	14.0	150	84%
beef 'n cheddar	1 frank	16.0	180	80%
fat-free/jumbo	1 frank	–	40	–
pork & beef				
bun-size	1 frank	17.0	190	81%
jumbo	2 oz	16.0	170	85%
smoky				
Big Red	1 frank	14.0	170	74%

Food and Description	Amount	Fat Grams	Total Calories	% Fat Calories
(Old Wisconsin) wieners				
premium smoked	1.7 oz	14.0	160	79%
	2 oz	17.0	180	85%
(Oscar Mayer)				
corn dogs..5-count	3.25 oz	15.0	260	52%
Hot & Spicy hot dogs	2.7 oz	19.0	210	81%
Little Smokies				
cheese	2 oz	16.0	180	80%
regular	2 oz	15.0	170	79%
Lunchables				
All Star				
hot dogs	1 box	19.0	450	38%
hot dogs w/cola	1 box	19.0	480	36%
original smoked				
hot dogs	2.7 oz	23.0	240	86%
premium				
beef franks	2.7 oz	23.0	240	86%
turkey franks				
bun-length	1 frank	10.0	120	75%
cheese	1 frank	8.0	100	72%
regular	1 frank	8.0	100	72%
XXL Hot Dogs				
deli-style beef				
franks	2.7 oz	22.0	230	86%
(Shelton's)				
turkey franks	1.2 oz	4.5	60	68%
(Wambler Longacre)				
chicken	1.6 oz	9.0	110	74%
	2 oz	11.0	130	76%
turkey	1.6 oz	9.0	110	74%
	2 oz	11.0	130	76%
(Wranglers)				
beef	1 frank	15.0	170	79%
cheese	1 frank	15.0	170	79%
jalapeño	1 frank	15.0	170	79%
smoked	1 frank	15.0	170	79%

FRANKFURTER, VEGETARIAN (*See* VEGETARIAN FOODS)
FRENCH FRIES (*See* FROZEN ENTRÉE/DINNER; POTATO; individual FAST FOOD listings)
FRENCH ONION SOUP (*See* SOUP)
FRENCH TOAST
bread

Food and Description	Amount	Fat Grams	Total Calories	% Fat Calories
(Arnold) cinnamon				
French toast	1 slice	3.0	100	27%
(Pepperidge Farm)				
swirl bread				
brown sugar				
& cinnamon	1 slice	3.5	140	23%
French vanilla	1 slice	3.5	140	23%
maple syrup & cinnamon	1 slice	2.0	130	14%

frozen
(Aunt Jemima)

Food and Description	Amount	Fat Grams	Total Calories	% Fat Calories
SLICES				
cinnamon				
12.5-oz box/6-count	2 slices	6.0	220	25%
home-style	2 slices	6.0	240	23%
STICKS				
cinnamon/4.2 oz	¼ box	14.0	380	33%
12-count box	4 sticks	13.0	350	33%
cinnamon sticks				
w/syrup cups	6.6 oz	13.0	540	22%
(Bob Evans)				
Stuffed French Toast				
w/apples & cream cheese	1 box	17.0	460	33%
w/berries & cream cheese	1 box	17.0	360	33%
(Eggo)				
French Toaster Sticks				
chocolate chip	2 slices	6.0	210	26%
cinnamon	2 slices	6.0	220	25%
original	2 slices	6.0	220	25%
(Farm Rich) sticks				
blueberry	⅓ box	12.0	290	37%
cinnamon sprinkle	⅙ box	15.0	330	41%
original	⅓ box	12.0	300	36%
(Swanson)				
Great Starts				
French toast & sausage	1 meal	24.0	410	53%
FRITTER (*See* APPLE FRITTERS; CORN DISH; DONUT; PASTRY)				
FROG/legs				
floured & fried	1 oz	4.8	70	61%
	3 oz	17.0	250	61%
raw	3 oz	<1.0	63	7%
FROSTING (*See* CAKE FROSTING/ICING)				
FROZEN ENTRÉE/DINNER (*See also* ASIAN FOOD; BEEF DISH/ENTRÉE; CHICKEN ENTRÉE/DINNER; MEXICAN FOOD; PASTA ENTRÉE/DINNER; PIZZA; POTATO DISH/ENTRÉE; RICE DISH; VEGETARIAN FOODS)				
■ (Advance)				
ADVANCE FAST FIXIN'				
BBQ ribs	3 oz	8.0	120	60%
beef				
fingers				
12-oz tray	3 oz	18.0	260	62%
meatballs				
12-oz tray	3 oz	19.0	250	68%
28-oz tray	3 oz	17.0	260	59%
Italian	3 oz	13.0	200	59%
patties/breaded	3 oz	18.0	260	62%
chicken				
breaded/12-count	1 piece	12.0	200	54%
breast				
nuggets	3 oz	12.0	200	54%

Food and Description	Amount	Fat Grams	Total Calories	% Fat Calories
patties	3 oz	12.0	200	54%
strips	3 oz	12.0	200	54%
nuggets/cheese	3 oz	10.0	200	45%
popcorn chicken	3.3 oz	10.0	190	47%
chuckwagon patties				
beef & turkey	3 oz	18.0	260	62%
EASY BEGINNINGS				
sliced chicken breast				
fajita fillet-style	2.5 oz	3.0	100	27%
garlic & herb-style	2.5 oz	2.0	100	18%
RESTAURANT-STYLE				
beef				
burgers	3 oz	18.0	230	70%
country-fried steak	4.55 oz	20.0	350	51%
fajitas				
beef	3 oz	4.5	140	29%
chicken				
breast	2.4 oz	3.0	100	27%
thigh	3 oz	8.0	140	51%
Philly beef steak	3.5 oz	3.5	80	39%
Salisbury steaks w/gravy	5.33 oz	23.0	330	63%
steak fingers	3.25 oz	10.0	230	39%
chicken				
breast tenders	2 oz	3.0	100	27%
breasts				
chicken-fried	4.55 oz	15.0	330	41%
fire-roasted	5 oz	3.0	180	15%
tenders				
BBQ-style	4.8 oz	11.0	180	55%
buffalo-style				
20-oz bag	2 oz	11.0	210	47%
24-oz bag	4.8 oz	10.0	160	56%
■ (Banquet)				
BONE-IN CHICKEN				
fried chicken pieces				
country-fried..8 pieces	3 oz	18.0	280	58%
honey BBQ..skinless..8 pieces	3 oz	13.0	220	53%
hot & spicy..8 pieces	3 oz	18.0	280	58%
original..8 pieces	3 oz	14.0	250	50%
original..12 pieces	3 oz	18.0	280	58%
skinless..8 pieces	3 oz	13.0	240	49%
Southern-fried..8 pieces	3 oz	18.0	280	58%
wings				
hot & spicy	3 oz	17.0	240	64%
honey BBQ	3 oz	15.0	220	61%
BONELESS CHICKEN & MISC.				
nuggets				
breast	7 nuggets	20.0	280	64%
fun..our original	4 nuggets	24.0	300	72%
fun-shaped	4 nuggets	20.0	280	64%

Food and Description	Amount	Fat Grams	Total Calories	% Fat Calories
mozzarella	6 nuggets	18.0	280	58%
original	5 nuggets	21.0	290	65%
plain	7 nuggets	20.0	280	64%
Southern-fried	6 nuggets	17.0	260	59%
patties				
breast				
grilled	1 patty	4.5	110	37%
honey BBQ	1 patty	9.0	150	54%
fat-free	1 patty	–	100	–
original	1 patty	17.0	240	64%
Southern-fried	1 patty	16.0	230	63%
popcorn chicken	11 pieces	9.0	190	43%
tenders				
fat-free	3 tenders	–	120	–
original	5 tenders	16.0	250	58%
Southern-fried	5 tenders	16.0	260	55%
COUNTRY SKILLET				
chicken				
bites	5 bites	16.0	270	53%
nuggets				
original	5 nuggets	16.0	270	53%
Southern-fried	5 nuggets	18.0	270	60%
patties	1 patty	11.0	190	52%
tenders	3 tenders	14.0	240	53%
FAMILY SERVE ENTRÉES				
beef stew	1 cup	7.0	170	37%
broccoli..chicken..cheese				
w/rice	1 cup	9.0	220	37%
chicken				
& broccoli Alfredo	1 cup	19.0	350	49%
& dumplings	1 cup	14.0	270	47%
gravy				
& charbroiled beef	1 patty	15.0	210	64%
& meat loaf	1 serving	11.0	170	64%
& Salisbury steak	1 serving	18.0	230	70%
& sliced beef	1 serving	7.0	120	53%
& sliced turkey	1 serving	9.0	130	62%
lasagna w/meat sauce	1 cup	9.0	230	35%
macaroni & cheese	1 cup	5.0	200	23%
noodles & beef	1 cup	6.0	150	36%
FRENCH BREAD PIZZA				
cheese	1 pizza	11.0	330	30%
deluxe	1 pizza	12.0	330	33%
pepperoni	1 pizza	15.0	380	36%
HEARTY ONES				
chicken-fried steak	1 meal	50.0	820	55%
chicken-fried steak meal	1 meal	40.0	630	57%
fried chicken	1 meal	55.0	910	54%
pork rib	1 meal	40.0	720	50%
potpies				

Food and Description	Amount	Fat Grams	Total Calories	% Fat Calories
chicken	½ pie	32.0	510	56%
turkey	½ pie	32.0	510	56%
Swiss steak	1 meal	54.0	740	66%
turkey	1 meal	32.0	620	46%
KID CUISINE				
beef patty w/cheese	1 meal	18.0	440	37%
cheese pizza	1 meal	11.0	430	23%
chicken nugget meal	1 meal	19.0	460	37%
chicken nuggets	1 meal	24.0	500	43%
corn dog meal	1 meal	18.0	490	33%
fish sticks	1 meal	12.0	330	33%
fried chicken	1 meal	38.0	600	57%
hamburger pizza	1 meal	11.0	400	25%
macaroni & cheese	1 meal	11.0	370	27%
taco roll-ups	1 meal	18.0	420	39%
MEALS				
BBQ beef patty	1 meal	19.0	380	45%
BBQ chicken meal	1 meal	13.0	330	35%
BBQ pork rib meal	1 meal	20.0	400	45%
beef enchilada	1 meal	12.0	370	29%
beef patty meal	1 meal	20.0	310	58%
cheese enchilada	1 meal	10.0	350	26%
chicken & pasta marinara meal	1 meal	17.0	390	39%
chicken enchilada meal	1 meal	10.0	350	26%
chicken fingers w/brownie	1 meal	30.0	570	47%
chicken-fried steak	1 meal	23.0	420	49%
chicken nugget meal	1 meal	21.0	410	46%
fish stick	1 meal	20.0	470	38%
fried chicken	1 meal	20.0	310	58%
fried chicken meal	1 meal	27.0	470	52%
fried rice w/chicken	1 meal	9.0	330	25%
home-style noodles w/chicken	1 meal	19.0	400	43%
honey-roasted turkey meal	1 meal	6.0	230	23%
lasagna w/meat sauce	1 meal	9.0	320	25%
macaroni & cheese	1 meal	14.0	420	30%
Mexican	1 meal	20.0	450	40%
Mexican-style enchilada				
combo meal	1 meal	12.0	370	29%
meat loaf meal	1 meal	11.0	240	41%
pepperoni pizza meal	1 meal	23.0	480	43%
pork cutlet	1 meal	25.0	430	52%
Salisbury steak meal	1 meal	24.0	380	57%
sliced beef meal	1 meal	10.0	270	33%
Swedish meatballs	1 meal	19.0	400	43%
turkey meal	1 meal	11.0	270	37%
veal Parmesan w/pasta	1 meal	16.0	330	44%
Yankee pot roast meal	1 meal	8.0	210	34%
POTPIES				
beef	1 pie	25.0	430	52%
chicken	1 pie	23.0	400	52%

Food and Description	Amount	Fat Grams	Total Calories	% Fat Calories
chicken & broccoli	1 pie	20.0	350	51%
macaroni & cheese	1 pie	5.0	210	21%
turkey	1 pie	21.0	390	48%
vegetable cheese	1 pie	17.0	340	45%
■ (Birds Eye)				
EASY RECIPE CREATIONS/gourmet meal starter/as packaged				
basil herb primavera	2 cups	11.0	260	38%
Oriental lo mein	2⅓ cups	2.5	200	11%
roasted garlic Parmesan	1⅔ cups	10.0	240	38%
sesame ginger teriyaki	2¼ cups	1.5	140	10%
spicy Szechuan				
w/cashews	1¾ cups	4.5	180	23%
sweet & sour				
w/pineapple tidbits	1⅔ cups	0.5	200	2%
tortellini parmigiana	2¼ cups	12.0	240	45%
HEARTY SPOONFULS				
cheesy cream of broccoli	1 bowl	10.0	230	39%
chicken, rice & vegetables	1 bowl	2.0	160	11%
home-style chicken noodle	1 bowl	1.5	140	10%
Italian minestrone	1 bowl	4.0	240	15%
SIMPLY GRILLIN'/ side dishes				
garden herb	¼ box	6.0	140	39%
potatoes & onions	¼ box	7.0	180	35%
roasted corn & potatoes	⅕ box	5.0	140	32%
roasted garlic	⅕ box	4.5	120	34%
*Voila! All-in-One Meal/*as packaged (unless otherwise noted)				
beef				
steak/beef sirloin & garlic potatoes	5.7 oz	7.0	190	33%
teriyaki	7 oz	4.0	160	23%
chicken				
Alfredo/prepared	1 cup	8.0	240	30%
down-home chicken				
and vegetables	8.4 oz	5.0	180	25%
fajita	8.4 oz	6.0	150	36%
garden herb	6.3 oz	11.0	280	35%
garlic	7.3 oz	9.0	240	34%
pesto primavera	6.3 oz	7.0	210	30%
roasted garlic chicken				
& vegetables	8.8 oz	2.5	120	18%
stir-fry	7.3 oz	3.0	160	17%
teriyaki	7 oz	2.5	150	15%
3-cheese	7.3 oz	8.0	210	34%
Tuscano/chicken & sausage	8.4 oz	8.0	170	42%
shrimp/garlic	6.3 oz	8.0	220	33%
■ (Bob Evans Farms)				
chicken & noodles	1 pouch	12.0	220	49%
chicken potpie	1 pie	28.0	510	49%

Food and Description	Amount	Fat Grams	Total Calories	% Fat Calories
country gravy & sausage w/potatoes				
brunch bowl	1 bowl	19.0	380	45%
home fries/diced	2.85 oz	–	80	–
macaroni & cheese				
special recipe	10 oz	16.0	330	44%
pulled pork w/wildfire				
BBQ sauce	2 oz	6.0	150	36%
Snackwiches				
bacon/egg/cheese burrito	3 burritos	18.0	330	49%
sausage cheeseburgers/large	1 burger	16.0	270	53%
sausage & cheese burrito	3 burritos	11.0	330	30%
sausage gravy & biscuits	½ box	23.0	390	53%

■ **(Boston Market)**

BEEF

fillet of beef w/peppercorn				
mustard sauce	1 meal	16.0	360	40%
meat loaf w/gravy	1 meal	25.0	400	56%
pot roast w/vegetables				
& mashed potatoes	1 meal	18.0	420	39%
Salisbury steak w/mushroom				
gravy & macaroni	1 meal	42.0	750	50%
Swedish meatballs in a				
creamy sauce w/noodles	½ box	26.0	440	53%

CHICKEN

country-fried w/mashed potatoes				
& gravy	1 meal	35.0	620	51%
glazed rotisserie white meat w/mashed				
potatoes, gravy & green beans	1 meal	19.0	440	39%
home-style chicken w/noodles in				
creamy sauce w/carrots	1 meal	20.0	580	31%
primavera w/penne pasta				
& vegetables	1 meal	19.0	520	33%
white meat w/teriyaki sauce	1 meal	11.0	460	22%

POTPIES

chicken	½ box	38.0	570	60%
chicken/broccoli/cheese	½ box	42.0	630	60%
turkey	½ box	36.0	540	60%

SIDES

chili bowl	1 bowl	13.0	3340	34%
mini loaves	1 loaf	6.0	210	26%
potatoes				
mashed	½ box	9.0	180	45%
new	½ box	6.0	130	42%
soup bowl	1 bowl	4.5	200	20%

TURKEY

breast medallions w/dressing				
& gravy	1 meal	18.0	490	33%
oven-roasted breast w/mashed				
potatoes & gravy	1 meal	19.0	400	43%

Food and Description	Amount	Fat Grams	Total Calories	% Fat Calories
■ **(Chef America)** stuffed sandwiches, etc.				
Croissant pockets/singles				
chicken Alfredo	1 sandwich	15.0	320	42%
chicken, broccoli & cheddar	1 sandwich	15.0	310	44%
chicken Parmesan	1 sandwich	20.0	370	49%
egg, sausage & cheese	1 sandwich	20.0	360	50%
5-cheese pizza	1 sandwich	20.0	390	46%
ham & cheddar	1 sandwich	16.0	340	42%
meatballs & mozzarella	1 sandwich	15.0	330	41%
pepperoni pizza	1 sandwich	20.0	390	46%
Philly steak & cheese	1 sandwich	19.0	360	48%
turkey, bacon club	1 sandwich	15.0	320	42%
Hot Pockets/singles				
bacon, egg & cheese	1 sandwich	7.0	170	37%
barbecue sauce				
w/beef	1 sandwich	12.0	340	32%
beef & cheddar	1 sandwich	17.0	360	3%
beef taco	1 sandwich	13.0	320	37%
cheeseburger	1 sandwich	14.0	340	37%
chicken & cheddar w/broccoli	1 sandwich	11.0	300	33%
chicken fajita	1 sandwich	11.0	290	34%
chicken melt				
w/bacon	1 sandwich	17.0	350	44%
4-cheese pizza	1 sandwich	20.0	390	46%
4-meat & 4-				
cheese pizza	1 sandwich	19.0	360	48%
fruit pastries w/icing				
apple	1 piece	9.0	240	34%
cream cheese & strawberry	1 piece	10.0	240	38%
strawberry	1 piece	8.0	240	30%
ham, egg & cheese	1 sandwich	7.0	150	42%
ham 'n' cheese	1 sandwich	13.0	310	38%
Italian-style meat trio	1 sandwich	16.0	350	41%
jalapeño steak & cheese	1 sandwich	14.0	320	39%
meatballs w/mozzarella	1 sandwich	14.0	330	38%
pepperoni pizza	1 sandwich	15.0	350	39%
pepperoni & sausage	1 sandwich	20.0	380	47%
Philly steak & cheese	1 sandwich	18.0	370	44%
pizza minis				
double cheese	5 pieces	11.0	240	41%
pepperoni	5 pieces	12.0	240	45%
sausage & pepperoni	5 pieces	10.0	230	39%
sausage, egg & cheese	1 sandwich	7.0	170	37%
sausage pizza	1 sandwich	19.0	360	48%
steak fajita	1 sandwich	11.0	280	35%
3-cheese & chicken				
quesadilla	1 sandwich	13.0	320	37%
turkey & ham w/cheese	1 sandwich	13.0	300	39%
Hot Pockets/value packs				
bacon, egg & cheese				
12-count	1 piece	16.0	310	46%

Food and Description	Amount	Fat Grams	Total Calories	% Fat Calories
ham 'n' cheese				
3-pack	1 piece	13.0	310	38%
12-count	1 piece	13.0	310	38%
meatballs & mozzarella				
12-count	1 piece	14.0	330	37%
pepperoni pizza				
3-pack	1 piece	17.0	360	43%
12-count	1 piece	17.0	360	43%
Lean Pockets/singles				
bacon, egg & cheese	1 sandwich	4.5	150	27%
barbecue sauce w/beef	1 sandwich	7.0	290	22%
cheeseburger	1 sandwich	7.0	280	23%
chicken broccoli				
& cheddar	1 sandwich	7.0	260	24%
chicken fajita	1 sandwich	7.0	260	24%
chicken Parmesan	1 sandwich	7.0	280	23%
ham & cheddar	1 sandwich	7.0	280	23%
ham & cheese				
Ultra 12 grams net carbs	1 sandwich	6.0	210	26%
meatballs & mozzarella				
original	1 sandwich	7.0	290	22%
Ultra 12 grams net carbs	1 sandwich	6.0	200	27%
pepperoni pizza deluxe	1 sandwich	7.0	280	23%
Philly steak & cheese	1 sandwich	7.0	280	23%
sausage, egg & cheese	1 sandwich	4.5	140	29%
sausage & pepperoni pizza	1 sandwich	7.0	280	23%
steak fajita	1 sandwich	7.0	260	24%
supreme pizza				
Ultra 12 grams net carbs	1 sandwich	6.0	200	27%
3-cheese & chicken				
quesadilla	1 sandwich	7.0	280	23%
turkey & ham w/cheddar	1 sandwich	7.0	280	23%
turkey, broccoli & cheese	1 sandwich	7.0	270	23%
Lean Pockets/value packs				
meatballs & mozzarella				
12-count	1 piece	7.0	290	22%
pepperoni pizza				
12-count	1 piece	7.0	280	23%
Philly steak & cheese				
12-count	1 piece	7.0	280	23%
Pot Pie Express/singles				
chicken	1 pie	17.0	350	44%
chicken & broccoli	1 pie	17.0	350	44%
turkey	1 pie	17.0	350	44%
Pot Pie Express/value packs				
chicken/12-count	1 pie	18.0	340	48%
Toaster Breaks				
melts				
ham & cheese	1 melt	8.0	180	40%
Philly steak & cheese	1 melt	10.0	190	47%

Food and Description	Amount	Fat Grams	Total Calories	% Fat Calories
pizza				
double cheese	1 serving	9.0	190	43%
pepperoni	1 serving	10.0	200	45%
sausage & pepperoni	1 serving	8.0	180	40%
■ (Chef's Choice)				
BEEF				
stir-fry	1⅔ cups	3.0	180	15%
steak ranchero	1⅔ cups	7.0	300	21%
BOWLS				
beef				
garlic beef & broccoli	1 bowl	17.0	360	43%
hearty beef stew	1 bowl	10.0	270	33%
chicken				
cacciatore	1 bowl	12.0	310	35%
fajita	1 bowl	14.0	330	38%
primavera	1 bowl	17.0	330	46%
Toscana	1 bowl	17.0	370	41%
low-carb/11-oz bowls				
beef				
garlic beef & broccoli	1 bowl	17.0	360	43%
chicken				
cacciatore	1 bowl	12.0	310	35%
primavera	1 bowl	17.0	330	46%
Toscana	1 bowl	17.0	370	41%
pork				
Mexican-style	1 bowl	19.0	370	46%
shrimp				
stir-fry	1 bowl	3.0	130	21%
CHICKEN				
Alfredo	1¼ cups	12.0	330	33%
fried rice	1⅓ cups	3.0	270	10%
garlic primavera	1½ cups	3.5	230	14%
marinara	1⅔ cups	6.0	250	22%
Santa Fe	1⅔ cups	4.5	270	15%
stir-fry	1⅔ cups	2.5	220	10%
SHRIMP				
shrimp Alfredo	1¼ cups	10.0	280	32%
fried rice	1½ cups	2.0	230	8%
linguini	1⅓ cups	1.0	190	5%
stir-fry	1⅔ cups	1.0	160	6%
SUN-UP SKILLET BREAKFAST				
ham breakfast	8 oz	10.0	290	31%
■ (Dining In)				
chicken breasts/fire-roasted	¼ pkg	3.0	180	15%
chicken parmigiana				
w/spaghetti & tomato sauce	⅓ pkg	13.0	310	38%
home-style favorites				
meat loaf w/red sauce	4.85 oz	12.0	230	47%
meat lasagna				
w/four cheeses	⅓ pkg	15.0	310	44%

Food and Description	Amount	Fat Grams	Total Calories	% Fat Calories
popcorn chicken breaded patties	3 oz	10.0	190	47%
Salisbury steak w/mashed potatoes	¼ pkg	29.0	450	58%
seafood favorites				
catfish w/shrimp & 7-vegetable medley	1 pkg	6.0	120	45%
stuffed green peppers w/homemade tomato sauce	¼ pkg	13.0	200	59%
■ (Ethnic Gourmet)				
CHINESE				
chicken				
kung pao	1 bowll	10.0	420	21%
Szechuan vegetarian	1 bowl	6.0	380	14%
shrimp fried rice	1 bowl	17.0	460	33%
tofu/kung pao wrap	1 wrap	17.0	410	37%
INDIAN-STYLE				
chicken				
biryani	1 bowl	12.0	410	26%
korma	1 meal	10.0	360	25%
tandoori w/spinach	1 meal	10.0	330	27%
tikka masala	1 meal	11.0	350	28%
JAPANESE-STYLE				
teriyaki				
chicken	1 bowl	3.0	340	8%
vegetarian	1 bowl	2.5	330	7%
KOREAN-STYLE				
beef bulgogi (beef & vegetables)	1 meal	12.0	350	31%
SINGAPOREAN-STYLE				
Singapore noodles	1 bowl	8.0	290	25%
THAI-STYLE				
chicken massaman	1 meal	9.0	330	25%
chicken pad Thai	1 meal	8.0	430	16%
lemongrass & basil chicken	1 meal	12.0	400	27%
pad Thai w/shrimp	1 bowl	7.0	350	17%
VIETNAMESE-STYLE				
Thit Ga Kho Tieu (chicken & vegetables)	1 meal	2.5	330	7%
■ (Farm Rich)				
Cheese Dippers/breaded sticks				
Italian 4-cheese	¼ pkg	11.0	180	55%
mozzarella	¼ pkg	10.0	180	50%
Fiesta Dippers				
cheddar cheese stuffed jalapeños	¼ pkg	7.0	170	37%
cream cheese stuffed jalapeños	¼ pkg	7.0	130	48%
Pizza Dippers/pizza crusts				
double cheese stuffed	¼ box	7.0	170	37%
Pizza Snacks/4-cheese	¼ box	6.0	130	42%
Pizzatas Pizza Snacks				
3-meat supreme	¼ box	7.0	150	42%

Food and Description	Amount	Fat Grams	Total Calories	% Fat Calories
grilled American cheese	¼ box	8.0	160	45%
pepperoni	¼ box	7.0	150	42%
■ (Freezer Queen)				
COOK-IN-POUCH				
chicken à la king	1 pouch	1.5	60	23%
creamed chipped beef	1 pouch	5.0	100	45%
gravy				
& Salisbury steak	1 pouch	10.0	150	60%
& sliced beef	1 pouch	1.0	60	15%
& sliced turkey	1 pouch	2.0	70	26%
DELUXE FAMILY ENTRÉES				
beef & peppers w/rice	1 pkg	11.0	200	50%
cheesy chicken & broccoli				
w/rice	~⅓ pkg	8.0	260	28%
chicken & biscuits	⅓ pkg	4.5	180	23%
lasagna in meat sauce	8 oz	5.0	180	25%
pork ribs in BBQ sauce				
boneless	⅙ pkg	11.0	200	50%
turkey & dressing				
w/gravy	8 oz	5.0	180	25%
FAMILY BUFFET				
chicken nuggets	1 serving	15.0	250	54%
gravy & sliced beef	⅙ pkg	4.5	110	37%
w/mashed potatoes	¼ pkg	5.0	220	20%
white turkey				
w/mashed potatoes	¼ pkg	8.0	290	25%
meat loaf slices & home-style				
gravy w/mashed potatoes	¼ pkg	26.0	450	52%
Salisbury steak & gravy				
w/macaroni & cheese	¼ pkg	20.0	430	42%
FAMILY ENTRÉES				
beef				
charbroiled patties				
& mushroom gravy	1 patty	12.0	180	60%
gravy & Salisbury steak	1 steak	14.0	230	55%
king-size beef patties				
in onion gravy	¼ pkg	16.0	240	60%
noodles w/beef	8 oz	5.0	140	32%
broccoli				
in cheese sauce	4 oz	1.5	80	17%
pasta, cauliflower &				
carrots w/sauce	4 oz	0.5	120	4%
chicken				
croquettes/gravy				
& breaded	1 piece	4.5	130	31%
nuggets	3 oz	13.0	230	51%
macaroni & cheese	⅓ pkg	7.0	260	24%
meat loaf slices				
w/home-style gravy	1 slice	10.0	150	60%
turkey				
croquettes/gravy				

Food and Description	Amount	Fat Grams	Total Calories	% Fat Calories
& breaded	1 piece	8.0	160	45%
sliced turkey w/gravy	⅓ pkg	2.0	70	26%
MEALS				
beef				
& peppers				
w/sauce & rice	1 meal	4.5	330	12%
charbroiled patty w/gravy				
mashed potatoes, peas				
& carrots	1 meal	16.0	280	51%
sliced w/gravy, mashed				
potatoes & peas	1 meal	7.0	200	32%
chicken				
nuggets w/apple dessert				
& potato puffs	1 meal	19.0	340	50%
patty w/mashed potatoes & corn	1 meal	18.0	360	45%
sweet & sour w/rice	1 meal	2.5	300	8%
fish sticks w/macaroni				
& cheese & peas	1 meal	11.0	290	34%
lasagna w/meat sauce	1 meal	13.0	380	31%
meatloaf w/gravy, mashed				
potatoes & peas	1 meal	13.0	250	47%
pork/boneless rib-shaped patty				
w/BBQ sauce & veg	1 meal	18.0	340	48%
pot roast w/gravy, vegetables				
& green beans	1 meal	7.0	220	29%
Salisbury steak & gravy				
w/whipped potatoes	1 meal	14.0	280	45%
turkey & gravy w/dressing				
& mashed potatoes	1 meal	9.0	260	31%
veal parmigiana w/pasta in				
tomato sauce & peas	1 meal	7.0	200	32%
■ (Golden) Blintzes				
apple raisin	1 blintz	2.0	80	23%
blueberry	1 blintz	1.0	90	10%
cheese	1 blintz	2.0	80	23%
cherry	1 blintz	1.0	95	9%
potato	1 blintz	4.0	90	40%
■ (Green Giant)				
CREATE A MEAL!/prepared				
beefy noodle	1¼ cups	14.0	350	36%
cheesy pasta & vegetables	1¼ cups	21.0	420	45%
chicken Alfredo	1¼ cups	13.0	400	29%
garlic herb chicken	1¼ cups	15.0	380	36%
home-style stew	1 cup	16.0	340	42%
lemon pepper chicken	1⅔ cups	8.0	310	23%
lo mein	1¾ cups	7.0	320	20%
skillet lasagna	1¼ cups	13.0	340	34%
stir-fry				
garlic & ginger	1½ cups	7.0	270	23%
teriyaki	1¼ cups	6.0	230	23%

Food and Description	Amount	Fat Grams	Total Calories	% Fat Calories
sweet & sour	1¼ cups	7.0	340	19%
Szechuan	1¼ cups	14.0	310	41%
SKILLET MEALS/as packaged				
beef stew	¼ pkg	3.5	180	18%
chicken Alfredo	¼ pkg	6.0	270	20%
chicken lo mein	¼ pkg	2.5	200	11%
chicken teriyaki	¼ pkg	3.5	180	18%
chicken & cheesy pasta	¼ pkg	7.0	260	24%
creamy chicken noodle	¼ pkg	5.0	290	16%
garlic chicken pasta	¼ pkg	7.0	260	24%
steak teriyaki	¼ pkg	1.5	250	5%
sweet & sour chicken	¼ pkg	1.5	320	4%
■ **(Healthy Choice)**				
DINNER MEALS				
beef pot roast	1 meal	9.0	320	25%
beef Stroganoff	1 meal	9.0	320	25%
beef tips portabello	1 meal	8.0	280	26%
blackened chicken	1 meal	6.0	300	18%
boneless beef ribs				
w/classic BBQ sauce	1 meal	9.0	360	20%
charbroiled beef patty	1 meal	9.0	310	26%
chicken broccoli Alfredo	1 meal	7.0	300	21%
chicken enchiladas	1 meal	7.0	360	18%
chicken parmigiana	1 meal	9.0	320	25%
chicken teriyaki	1 meal	6.0	270	20%
country breaded chicken	1 meal	9.0	370	22%
country herb chicken	1 meal	6.0	280	19%
grilled turkey breast	1 meal	5.0	250	18%
herb-baked fish	1 meal	9.0	360	23%
honey-glazed chicken	1 meal	6.0	320	17%
lemon pepper fish	1 meal	5.0	280	16%
mesquite chicken BBQ	1 meal	5.0	300	15%
Oriental-style chicken &				
veg. stir-fry	1 meal	6.0	360	15%
oven-roasted beef	1 meal	7.0	280	23%
roasted chicken breast	1 meal	8.0	280	26%
Salisbury steak	1 meal	9.0	360	23%
stuffed pasta shells	1 meal	6.0	290	19%
sweet & sour chicken	1 meal	7.0	340	19%
traditional meat loaf	1 meal	9.0	340	24%
traditional Salisbury steak	1 meal	7.0	330	19%
traditional turkey breast	1 meal	5.0	330	14%
ENTRÉES & QUICK MEALS				
beef teriyaki	1 meal	7.0	310	20%
breaded chicken breast strips				
w/mac & cheese	1 meal	5.0	290	16%
cheddar broccoli potatoes	1 meal	7.0	270	23%
cheesy rice & chicken	1 meal	5.0	250	18%
chicken breast & vegetables	1 meal	7.0	260	24%
chicken carbonara	1 meal	7.0	290	22%

Food and Description	Amount	Fat Grams	Total Calories	% Fat Calories
chicken enchilada	1 meal	7.0	300	21%
chicken fettuccini Alfredo	1 meal	7.0	290	22%
chicken picatta	1 meal	5.0	260	17%
country-glazed chicken	1 meal	5.0	230	20%
fettuccini Alfredo	1 meal	7.0	280	23%
garlic chicken Sonoma	1 meal	4.0	230	16%
grilled chicken breast				
& pasta	1 meal	7.0	250	25%
w/mashed potatoes	1 meal	5.0	190	24%
home-style chicken & pasta	1 meal	6.0	250	22%
lasagna bake	1 meal	7.0	270	23%
macaroni & cheese	1 meal	7.0	290	22%
mandarin chicken	1 meal	3.5	250	13%
manicotti w/3 cheeses	1 meal	5.0	280	16%
Oriental-style chicken	1 meal	5.0	240	19%
rigatoni w/broccoli				
& cheese	1 meal	7.0	270	23%
roast turkey breast	1 meal	6.0	220	25%
Salisbury steak & red-				
skin mashed potatoes	1 meal	6.0	200	27%
sesame chicken	1 meal	6.0	260	21%
slow-roasted turkey breast				
& mashed potatoes	1 meal	7.0	210	30%
spaghetti & sauce				
w/seasoned beef	1 meal	6.0	310	17%
tuna casserole	1 meal	7.0	270	23%
FLAVOR ADVENTURES				
beef				
Merlot	1 meal	8.0	240	30%
Oriental-style	1 meal	9.0	310	26%
steak/grilled				
in roasted garlic sauce	1 meal	7.0	220	29%
whiskey	1 meal	6.0	280	19%
chicken				
country herb-roasted	1 meal	5.0	240	19%
grilled basil	1 meal	9.0	330	25%
grilled Caesar	1 meal	8.0	300	24%
grilled marinara				
margerita	1 meal	8.0	340	21%
princess	1 meal	7.0	310	20%
roasted chardonnay	1 meal	8.0	290	25%
Tuscany	1 meal	9.0	340	24%
MIXED GRILLS				
chicken				
honey BBQ dip sauce	1 meal	7.0	380	17%
honey mustard dip sauce	1 meal	7.0	360	18%
roasted garlic & red				
peppers dip sauce	1 meal	10.0	320	28%
teriyaki dip sauce	1 meal	7.0	340	19%
tomato garlic dip sauce	1 meal	7.0	370	17%

Food and Description	Amount	Fat Grams	Total Calories	% Fat Calories
steak				
BBQ sauce	1 meal	8.0	420	17%
w/teriyaki dip sauce	1 meal	9.0	350	23%
w/zesty steak sauce	1 meal	8.0	350	21%
■ (Hormel)				
QUICK MEAL				
BBQ beef sandwich	1 sandwich	17.0	370	41%
BBQ pork sandwich	1 sandwich	16.0	360	40%
rib-shaped sandwich	1 sandwich	24.0	430	50%
cheesy dog	1 "dog"	17.0	310	49%
cheeseburger	1 burger	20.0	400	45%
bacon	1 burger	23.0	440	47%
chicken sandwich	1 sandwich	13.0	285	41%
corn dog				
mini	10 mini's	15.0	240	56%
regular	1 "dog"	12.0	240	45%
fish fillet sandwich	1 sandwich	16.0	400	36%
grilled chicken sandwich	1 sandwich	12.0	320	34%
ham & Swiss	1 sandwich	8.0	330	22%
hamburger	1 burger	17.0	370	41%
jumbo dog	1 "dog"	21.0	350	54%
pepperoni bagel	1 bagel	15.0	350	39%
sausage & egg biscuit	1 biscuit	24.0	390	55%
sausage, egg				
& cheese muffin	1 muffin	8.0	260	38%
■ HOT POCKETS (*See* (Chef America) in this section)				
■ (Italian Village)				
cavatelli/low-salt	3.5 oz	1.0	250	4%
gnocchi/potato	4.6 oz	1.0	260	3%
manicotti/cheese	3.3 oz	10.0	190	47%
ravioli				
beef square	4 oz	3.5	220	14%
bite-size/cheese	4 oz	2.5	220	11%
cheese				
garlic lover's square	4 oz	4.0	200	18%
large round	4.8 oz	6.0	240	23%
mini round	4 oz	4.0	220	16%
square	3.7 oz	2.5	190	12%
villa prima				
florentine	4.5 oz	4.0	210	17%
4-cheese	4.5 oz	9.0	260	31%
garlic basil	4 oz	2.5	170	13%
portabello mushroom	4 oz	2.5	170	13%
tortellini				
cheese	3.5 oz	3.0	230	12%
meat	3.5 oz	4.0	250	14%
■ (Kid Cuisine) (*See* Banquet, within this category)				
■ (Lean Cuisine)				
CAFÉ CLASSICS/ Bowls				
chicken				

Food and Description	Amount	Fat Grams	Total Calories	% Fat Calories
& vegetables	1 bowl	6.0	310	17%
fried rice	1 bowl	8.0	410	18%
grilled Caesar	1 bowl	5.0	240	19%
teriyaki	1 bowl	2.5	340	6%
teriyaki steak	1 bowl	7.0	340	19%
3-cheese				
stuffed rigatoni	1 bowl	6.0	280	19%
CAFÉ CLASSICS/Meals				
beef				
orange	1 meal	7.0	300	21%
Oriental	1 meal	3.0	210	9%
oven-roasted	1 meal	3.5	210	15%
peppercorn	1 meal	7.0	220	29%
portabello	1 meal	7.0	220	29%
pot roast	1 meal	6.0	200	27%
Southern beef tips	1 meal	5.0	250	18%
bow-tie pasta & chicken	1 meal	4.0	220	16%
chicken				
a l'orange	1 meal	1.5	230	6%
& vegetables	1 meal	5.0	250	18%
baked	1 meal	4.5	230	18%
carbonara	1 meal	7.0	270	23%
fiesta grilled	1 meal	6.0	260	21%
glazed	1 meal	5.0	230	20%
grilled	1 meal	5.0	160	28%
herb-roasted	1 meal	3.5	190	17%
honey mustard	1 meal	4.0	260	14%
honey-roasted	1 meal	6.0	270	20%
in peanut sauce	1 meal	7.0	280	23%
in wine sauce	1 meal	5.0	220	20%
marsala	1 meal	4.0	140	26%
Mediterranean	1 meal	4.0	260	14%
Parmesan	1 meal	5.0	270	16%
piccata	1 meal	6.0	270	20%
roasted garlic	1 meal	5.0	230	20%
sesame	1 meal	8.0	320	23%
sweet & sour	1 meal	2.5	290	8%
teriyaki	1 meal	3.5	280	11%
w/almonds	1 meal	4.0	260	14%
w/basil cream sauce	1 meal	7.0	260	24%
fish..baked	1 meal	6.0	290	19%
honey-roasted pork	1 meal	4.0	230	16%
lasagna..cheese w/chicken	1 meal	8.0	280	26%
meat loaf & whipped potatoes	1 meal	8.0	270	27%
shrimp & angel-hair pasta	1 meal	5.0	240	19%
turkey				
glazed tenderloins	1 meal	6.0	270	20%
roasted breast	1 meal	2.5	270	8%
DINNERTIME SELECTIONS				
beef				

Food and Description	Amount	Fat Grams	Total Calories	% Fat Calories
Salisbury steak	1 meal	9.0	320	25%
steak tips Dijon	1 meal	7.0	310	20%
chicken				
fettuccini	1 meal	8.0	380	19%
Florentine	1 meal	6.0	370	15%
glazed	1 meal	6.0	310	17%
grilled w/penne pasta	1 meal	6.0	340	16%
Oriental glazed	1 meal	2.0	330	5%
roasted	1 meal	4.5	320	13%
Tucson	1 meal	6.0	270	20%
rigatoni				
jumbo	1 meal	10.0	390	23%
turkey breast...roasted	1 meal	7.0	340	19%
EVERYDAY FAVORITES				
Alfredo pasta w/chicken				
& broccoli	1 meal	6.0	270	20%
angel-hair pasta	1 meal	4.0	260	14%
cheddar potato, deluxe	1 meal	6.0	250	22%
cheese				
cannelloni	1 meal	4.5	240	17%
ravioli	1 meal	7.0	260	24%
chicken				
chow mein	1 meal	3.5	230	14%
enchilada suiza	1 meal	5.0	290	16%
fettuccini	1 meal	6.0	270	20%
honey Dijon grilled	1 meal	8.0	230	31%
lasagna				
5-cheese	1 meal	7.0	310	20%
Florentine	1 meal	6.0	270	19%
w/meat sauce	1 meal	7.0	280	23%
mandarin	1 meal	3.5	270	12%
pie	1 pie	8.0	300	24%
roasted	1 meal	7.0	260	24%
fettuccini				
Alfredo	1 meal	7.0	280	23%
primavera	1 meal	7.0	270	23%
home-style turkey	1 meal	5.0	240	19%
Hunan beef & broccoli	1 meal	4.0	230	16%
lasagna				
cheese Florentine bake	1 meal	7.0	270	23%
classic 5-cheese	1 meal	7.0	310	20%
w/meat sauce	1 meal	7.0	310	20%
macaroni & beef	1 meal	6.0	270	20%
macaroni & cheese	1 meal	7.0	300	21%
Oriental-style dumplings	1 meal	6.0	300	18%
penne pasta	1 meal	3.5	270	12%
❋ pot stickers/Oriental-style	1 pkg	6.0	320	17%
potato				
cheddar deluxe	1 meal	7.0	260	24%
roasted w/broccoli	1 meal	5.0	240	19%

Food and Description	Amount	Fat Grams	Total Calories	% Fat Calories
Santa Fe rice & beans	1 meal	5.0	300	28%
spaghetti				
w/meatballs	1 meal	5.0	260	17%
w/meat sauce	1 meal	5.0	240	19%
steak tips portabello	1 meal	4.0	130	28%
stuffed cabbage	1 meal	5.0	190	24%
Swedish meatballs	1 meal	7.0	290	22%
teriyaki stir-fry	1 meal	4.5	300	14%
3-bean chili w/rice	1 meal	7.0	270	23%
turkey..roasted w/vegetables	1 meal	2.0	120	15%
vegetable eggroll	1 meal	6.0	330	16%
vegetable lasagna	1 meal	7.0	260	24%

■ **LEAN POCKETS** (*See* (Chef America) in this section)
■ **(Life Choice)**

Beef pot roast	1 pkg	13.0	310	38%
cheesy broccoli scramble	1 pkg	34.0	480	64%
cheesy chicken Florentine	1 pkg	16.0	360	40%
chicken Parmesan	1 pkg	13.0	330	35%
hearty meat loaf	1 pkg	16.0	370	40%
herb-roasted chicken	1 pkg	19.0	390	44%
home-style baked chicken	1 pkg	6.0	210	26%
Italian sausage scramble	1 pkg	32.0	480	60%
open-roasted turkey	1 pkg	6.0	250	21%
roasted turkey breast	1 pkg	4.5	260	16%
Salisbury steak	1 pkg	7.0	280	23%
sausage, beef & bacon				
scramble	1 pkg	30.0	470	57%
slow-roasted beef tips	1 pkg	13.0	310	38%
3-meat Alfredo	1 pkg	32.0	500	58%

■ **(Marie Callender's)**
FAMILY SERVE ENTRÉES

country-fried chicken & gravy				
w/mashed potatoes	1 serving	27.0	460	53%
escalloped noodles & chicken	1 cup	20.0	360	50%
fettuccini Alfredo				
w/chicken & broccoli	1 serving	26.0	390	60%
lasagna	1 cup	17.0	310	49%
lasagna w/meat sauce	1 cup	16.0	310	46%
meat loaf w/mashed potatoes	1 serving	16.0	250	58%
Salisbury steak				
w/macaroni & cheese	1 serving	25.0	470	48%
turkey w/mashed potatoes	1 serving	16.0	310	46%

DINNERS

beef Stroganoff	1 meal	14.0	410	31%
beef tips..sliced in gravy	1 meal	19.0	410	42%
chicken-fried steak	1 meal	41.0	640	58%
chicken				
Cordon Bleu	1 meal	23.0	490	42%
honey-roasted	1 meal	21.0	470	40%
Parmigiana	1 meal	33.0	580	51%
Southwestern	1 meal	10.0	360	25%

Food and Description	Amount	Fat Grams	Total Calories	% Fat Calories
country-fried chicken	1 meal	34.0	660	46%
fish w/mac & cheese dinner	1 meal	16.0	400	36%
grilled chicken				
& mashed potatoes	1 meal	25.0	470	48%
ham steak	1 meal	13.0	410	29%
herb-roasted chicken				
& mashed potatoes	1 meal	35.0	580	54%
meat loaf w/mashed potatoes	1 meal	30.0	510	53%
pork chop dinner	1 meal	36.0	630	51%
pot roast	1 meal	15.0	400	34%
roast beef	1 meal	19.0	380	45%
Salisbury steak	1 meal	22.0	440	45%
sweet & sour chicken	1 meal	15.0	580	23%
turkey w/gravy & dressing	1 meal	11.0	360	28%
ONE-DISH CLASSICS				
cheese ravioli..marinara				
sauce	1 meal	20.0	610	30%
cheesy chicken breast & rice	1 meal	20.0	470	38%
chicken				
breast & rice w/cream sauce	1 meal	27.0	560	43%
carbonara	1 meal	19.0	520	33%
chunky w/noodles	1 meal	36.0	650	50%
teriyaki	1 meal	3.5	420	8%
chili..w/cornbread	1 meal	21.0	480	39%
country-style beef stew				
w/cornbread	1 meal	9.0	430	19%
fettuccini				
Alfredo	1 meal	55.0	900	55%
primavera	1 meal	27.0	550	44%
w/broccoli & chicken	1 meal	43.0	730	53%
grilled chicken beast w/pasta	1 meal	21.0	570	33%
home-style				
chicken & potato casserole	1 meal	14.0	400	32%
tuna and noodles	1 meal	35.0	610	52%
lasagna bake w/meat sauce	1 meal	15.0	470	29%
macaroni & chese	1 cup	13.0	340	34%
meat lasagna	1 cup	12.0	270	40%
spaghetti & meat sauce	1 meal	25.0	690	33%
stuffed pasta medley	1 meal	19.0	470	36%
Swedish meatballs	1 meal	25.0	560	40%
turkey breast medallions				
w/pasta	1 meal	32.0	630	46%
POTPIES				
beef				
9.5 oz	1 pie	42.0	650	58%
16.5 oz	1 cup	32.0	510	56%
chicken				
9.5 oz	1 pie	43.0	660	59%
16.5 oz	1 cup	35.0	540	58%
chicken & broccoli				
9.5 oz	1 pie	43.0	670	58%
16.5 oz	1 cup	45.0	630	64%

Food and Description	Amount	Fat Grams	Total Calories	% Fat Calories
chicken au gratin				
9.5 oz	1 pie	46.0	690	60%
16.5 oz	1 cup	37.0	560	59%
turkey				
9.5 oz	1 pie	43.0	660	59%
16.5 oz	1 cup	35.0	540	58%
■ (Michael Angelo's)				
chicken				
Capri	1 meal	15.0	640	21%
Parmesan	1 meal	16.0	730	20%
eggplant Parmesan	1 meal	19.0	280	61%
fettuccini Alfredo w/baked				
chicken breast	1 meal	18.0	740	22%
Italian-style sausage				
w/classic tomato sauce	1 meal	11.0	160	62%
lasagna				
vegetable	8 oz	7.0	230	27%
w/meat sauce	9 oz	10.0	290	31%
Tre Bella Raviolo w/spinach				
pesto, pepperoni	1 meal	19.0	280	61%
■ (Michelina's)				
AUTHENTICO				
black bean chili w/rice	1 pkg	5.0	400	11%
chicken				
& vegetable stir-fry	1 pkg	4.0	200	18%
fried	1 pkg	18.0	310	52%
glazed w/rice	1 pkg	3.5	250	13%
honey BBQ w/rice	1 pkg	3.0	290	9%
littles	1 pkg	14.0	300	42%
pesto w/penne	1 pkg	6.0	250	22%
pop'n chicken	1 pkg	17.0	350	44%
primavera w/spirals	1 pkg	6.0	250	22%
corn dawgs	1 dawg	16.0	320	45%
fettuccini Alfredo	1 pkg	16.0	370	38%
w/chicken & broccoli	1 pkg	11.0	300	33%
fettuccini primavera				
w/chicken	1 pkg	9.0	270	30%
lasagna				
Alfredo	1 pkg	16.0	340	42%
4-cheese	1 pkg	7.0	280	23%
4-cheese layered	1 pkg	11.0	260	37%
w/meat sauce	1 pkg	7.0	280	23%
linguini w/clams	1 pkg	3.5	290	11%
macaroni				
& beef	1 pkg	5.0	250	18%
& cheese	1 pkg	4.0	240	15%
& cheese w/ham	1 pkg	13.0	310	38%
& sharp cheddar cheese	1 pkg	15.0	400	34%
meatballs & mashed				
potatoes	1 pkg	14.0	270	47%

Food and Description	Amount	Fat Grams	Total Calories	% Fat Calories
meat loaf	1 pkg	16.0	270	53%
noodles				
Romanoff w/meatballs	1 pkg	7.0	300	9%
Stroganoff	1 pkg	14.0	320	39%
w/chicken, peas				
& carrots	1 pkg	10.0	260	35%
penne w/chicken	1 pkg	3.5	330	10%
pepper steak w/rice	1 pkg	4.0	250	14%
ravioli/cheese	1 pkg	18.0	390	42%
rigatoni/stuffed cheese	1 pkg	8.0	300	24%
roast turkey	1 pkg	9.0	250	28%
roasted sirloin supreme	1 pkg	5.0	230	20%
Salisbury steak	1 pkg	16.0	290	50%
spaghetti				
& meatballs	1 pkg	8.0	300	24%
w/meat sauce	1 pkg	4.0	250	14%
Swedish meatballs	1 pkg	17.0	390	39%
teriyaki chicken w/rice	1 pkg	2.5	280	8%
vegetable chicken stir-fry	1 pkg	5.0	200	23%
HOME-STYLE BOWLS				
beef & vegetable stew	1 bowl	6.0	230	23%
chicken				
& noodles	1 bowl	6.0	300	18%
Alfredo w/broccoli	1 bowl	21.0	490	38%
grilled chicken Caesar	1 bowl	4.5	310	13%
rigatoni/cheese-stuffed	1 bowl	9.0	360	23%
shrimp alfredo	1 bowl	16.0	370	39%
shrimp & vegetables alfredo	1 bowl	9.0	370	22%
LEAN GOURMET				
beef pepper steak w/rice	1 pkg	4.5	260	16%
beef Stroganoff	1 pkg	5.0	250	18%
cheese manicotti				
w/marinara sauce	1 pkg	5.0	290	16%
chicken				
Alfredo Florentine	1 pkg	5.0	250	18%
French recipe	1 pkg	4.5	180	23%
glazed	1 pkg	3.5	260	12%
fettuccini Alfredo	1 pkg	6.0	270	20%
lasagna				
5-cheese	1 pkg	5.0	220	20%
layered w/meat sauce	1 pkg	7.0	250	25%
macaroni & cheese	1 pkg	5.0	300	15%
meat loaf	1 pkg	8.0	210	34%
pasta in wine &				
mushroom sauce	1 pkg	6.0	290	19%
rigatoni/cheese-stuffed	1 pkg	7.0	260	24%
roasted sirloin supeme	1 pkg	5.0	230	20%
Salisbury steak	1 pkg	7.0	200	32%
Santa Fe–style				
rice & beans	1 pkg	9.0	350	23%

Food and Description	Amount	Fat Grams	Total Calories	% Fat Calories
shrimp w/pasta				
& vegetables	1 pkg	6.0	260	21%
spaghetti & meat sauce	1 pkg	5.0	280	16%
Swedish meatballs	1 pkg	7.0	290	22%
SIGNATURE MEALS				
beef pot roast	1 pkg	7.0	260	24%
chicken				
Alfredo w/broccoli	1 pkg	19.0	400	43%
breaded parmigiano	1 pkg	15.0	410	33%
marsala	1 pkg	13.0	270	43%
Salisbury steak & gravy	1 pkg	19.0	410	42%
shrimp Alfredo	1 pkg	13.0	290	49%
YU SING BOWLS (See ASIAN FOOD)				
ZAP'EMS				
chili-mac	1 pkg	21.0	420	45%
lasagna				
mozzarella	1 pkg	8.0	260	28%
primavera	1 pkg	10.0	260	35%
macaroni				
& beef	1 pkg	7.0	240	26%
& cheese	1 pkg	11.0	320	31%
noodles & chicken	1 pkg	10.0	280	32%
pasta primavera	1 pkg	4.0	220	16%
pizza				
cheese	1 pizza	21.0	420	45%
pepperoni	1 pizza	8.0	440	16%
snack	1 pkg	27.0	470	52%
rockin' taco	1 pkg	18.0	350	46%
shells & cheese	1 pkg	11.0	350	28%
spaghetti				
& meatballs	1 pkg	7.0	260	24%
marinara	1 pkg	2.0	230	8%
w/tomato & basil sauce	1 pkg	3.0	240	11%
vegetable stir-fry	1 pkg	4.5	240	16%
wheels & cheese	1 pkg	12.0	350	31%
■ (Morton)				
MEALS				
breaded chicken patty	1 meal	17.0	290	53%
chicken nuggets	1 meal	19.0	340	50%
macaroni & cheese	1 cup	8.0	240	30%
meat loaf w/tomato sauce	1 meal	13.0	250	47%
Mexican meal	1 meal	9.0	270	30%
Salisbury steak	1 meal	20.0	310	58%
turkey w/gravy & dressing	1 meal	10.0	240	38%
Western meal	1 meal	18.0	310	52%
POTPIES				
vegetable pie				
w/beef	1 pie	21.0	340	56%
w/chicken	1 pie	18.0	320	51%
w/turkey	1 pie	18.0	310	52%

Food and Description	Amount	Fat Grams	Total Calories	% Fat Calories
■ (Mrs. Paul's) Bowls				
shrimp				
Alfredo	1 bowl	9.0	300	27%
& tortellini	1 bowl	4.0	340	11%
fried rice	1 bowl	2.0	290	6%
garlic butter	1 bowl	3.5	290	11%
stir-fry	1 bowl	1.0	330	3%
sweet & sour	1 bowl	1.0	310	3%
Thai-style peanut	1 bowl	6.0	330	16%
■ (On-Cor)				
BOWLS (Family)				
rice				
chicken & vegetable	⅕ pkg	1.5	190	7%
sweet & sour chicken	⅕ pkg	1.5	190	7%
teriyaki chicken	⅕ pkg	1.5	190	7%
CLASSICS				
chicken parmigiana	⅙ pkg	11.0	260	38%
lasagna w/meat sauce	⅕ pkg	8.0	230	31%
macaroni & beef	⅕ pkg	13.0	260	45%
stuffed green peppers	¼ pkg	15.0	240	56%
Swedish meatballs & pasta	⅕ pkg	10.0	220	41%
veal parmigiana				
w/cheese & tomato sauce	⅙ box	8.0	210	34%
DINNER PARTNERS				
BBQ rib patties	⅙ pkg	14.0	260	48%
beef patties	¼ pkg	18.0	270	60%
gravy & meat loaf				
mashed potatoes	¼ pkg	13.0	240	49%
gravy & Salisbury steaks				
w/macaroni	¼ pkg	14.0	270	47%
gravy & sliced turkey	⅙ pkg	4.0	70	51%
macaroni & cheese	⅕ pkg	4.0	190	19%
READI-SERVE				
beef (breaded & cooked)				
chuckwagon patties	1 patty	17.0	250	61%
chicken (breaded & cooked)				
nibblers	2.85 oz	13.0	220	53%
cheddar cheese	2.85 oz	17.0	260	59%
patties	¼ pkg	14.0	210	60%
strips	⅓ pkg	18.0	260	62%
chicken (buffalo-style)				
nibblers	¼ pkg	14.0	210	60%
veal patties				
(breaded & cooked)	¼ pkg	18.0	320	51%
■ (Ore Ida)				
BAGEL BITES				
3-cheese	3.14 oz	6.0	200	27%
cheese & pepperoni	3.14 oz	7.0	210	30%

Food and Description	Amount	Fat Grams	Total Calories	% Fat Calories
cheese, sausage				
& pepperoni	3.14 oz	6.0	200	27%
extra				
meat	3.14 oz	10.0	240	38%
pepperoni	3.14 oz	10.0	240	38%
spicy nacho	3.14 oz	10.0	240	38%
BAGEL BITES/stuffed				
pepperoni & cheese	3 oz	7.0	210	30%
3-cheese	3 oz	5.0	210	21%
ultra 5-cheese	3.14 oz	7.0	220	29%
■ (Pepperidge Farm) potpie				
beef	1 pie	31.0	530	53%
chicken				
& broccoli	1 pie	30.0	490	55%
chunky Parmesan	1 pie	26.0	520	45%
creamy Alfredo w/broccoli	1 pie	40.0	600	60%
primavera	1 pie	31.0	530	53%
roasted	1 pie	32.0	410	56%
white meat	1 pie	32.0	510	56%
turkey	1 pie	26.0	420	56%
roasted	1 pie	33.0	500	59%
■ (Popper's)				
BREADED				
mushrooms	⅓ box	5.0	140	32%
zucchini	⅓ box	12.0	210	51%
CHEESE				
crisps/nacho cheddar	4 oz	28.0	460	55%
nuggets/mozzarella	⅛ box	5.0	90	50%
sticks/mozzarella				
8-oz box	⅛ box	4.5	90	45%
17-oz box	1 oz	4.5	90	45%
32-oz box	~1 oz	3.5	70	45%
MINI-TAQUITOS				
beef	3 oz	7.0	200	32%
chicken	3 oz	8.0	210	34%
POPCORN SHRIMP				
bourbon-glazed	2.8 oz	7.0	210	30%
plain	2.6 oz	10.0	210	43%
STUFFED JALAPEÑOS				
cheddar cheese				
8 oz box	2.66 oz	14.0	220	57%
32 oz box	1 oz	7.0	110	57%
cheddar cheese/big size	2.5 oz	14.0	220	57%
cheddar cheese/mild	3.5 oz	18.0	290	56%
cream cheese	2.66 oz	16.0	240	60%
cream cheese/mild	3.5 oz	20.0	310	58%
3-cheese	~1 oz	5.0	80	56%
■ (Schwan's)				
APPETIZERS & SNACKS				
American appetizer collection	3 oz	7.0	160	39%

Food and Description	Amount	Fat Grams	Total Calories	% Fat Calories
chicken				
& cheese quesadilla	1 whole	9.0	230	35%
bites	12 bites	7.0	160	39%
drummies	3 pieces	17.0	240	64%
pattie nuggets	6 pieces	15.0	230	59%
wings				
BBQ	4 pieces	11.0	170	58%
buffalo-style/boneless	4 pieces	12.0	210	51%
hot	9 pieces	10.0	170	53%
Oriental-style				
teriyaki boneless	4 pieces	14.0	250	50%
onion rings/beaded	4 medium	14.0	270	47%
potato skins				
cheddar & bacon	1 portion	5.0	80	56%
Potato Teasers/cheese Ole	4 pieces	12.0	190	57%
pretzels				
soft stuffed pretzels				
w/cheese	3 pieces	5.0	210	21%
sweet cream cheese–stuffed	1 pretzel	16.0	280	19%
twisted pizza–stuffed	1 pretzel	7.0	280	23%
COMPLETE MEALS				
beef				
& broccoli w/rice	1 cup	4.0	210	17%
casserole	1 cup	17.0	340	45%
home-style goulash	1 cup	12.0	270	40%
potpie/sirloin	1 pie	33.0	600	50%
pot roast/sliced				
w/chunky mashed potatoes	¼ tray	5.0	220	20%
w//noodles	1 cup	6.0	230	23%
w/roasted Yukon gold				
potatoes meal kit	¼ pkg	8.0	220	33%
shepherd's pie	1 cup	12.0	250	43%
cheese				
casserole	1 cup	16.0	360	40%
ravioli	5 ravioli	12.0	370	29%
w/red sauce	1 serving	15.0	350	39%
stuffed shells				
w/marinara sauce	7 oz	18.0	350	46%
tortellini	1 cup	8.0	220	33%
cheesy broccoli soup	1 bowl	27.0	360	68%
chicken				
& dumplings meal kit	1 cup	8.0	200	36%
Alfredo lasagna	1 cup	12.0	280	39%
Boston clam chowder	1 cup	8.0	190	38%
breaded cutlet	1 piece	15.0	260	52%
breast				
stir-fry w/rice	1½ cup	2.0	210	9%
tenderloin fajita	1 fajita	2.0	140	13%
cheesy chicken & broccoli				
w/rice meal kit	1 cup	8.0	260	28%

Food and Description	Amount	Fat Grams	Total Calories	% Fat Calories
casserole	1 cup	16.0	360	40%
herb-roasted breast dinner	1 meal	6.0	300	18%
Kiev	1 serving	24.0	370	58%
Marco Polo	1 serving	13.0	280	42%
potpie	1 pie	41.0	670	55%
potato, sausage				
& egg meal kit/prepared	1 cup	16.0	280	51%
ravioli	5 ravioli	11.0	310	32%
soup				
old-fashioned creamy chicken				
noodle soup	1 bowl	14.0	280	45%
wild rice soup	1 bowl	18.0	310	52%
Southwestern-style				
meal kit	¼ pkg	3.0	200	14%
sweet & sour w/rice	1 cup	1.5	260	5%
tortellini	1 cup	4.0	230	16%
English-style fish & chips	1 serving	27.0	480	51%
home-style				
beef goulash	1 cup	13.0	280	42%
pot roast dinner	1 meal	8.0	320	23%
lasagna				
family-size				
Italian-style	1 cup	16.0	340	42%
vegetable	1 cup	8.0	280	26%
w/beef sauce	1 cup	13.0	350	33%
single-serve				
traditional	1 tray	19.0	500	34%
vegetable	1 tray	18.0	420	39%
zesty	1 tray	28.0	580	60%
lemon pepper fish dinner	1 meal	7.0	340	19%
macaroni & cheese	1 cup	20.0	340	53%
mostaccioli	1 cup	18.0	350	46%
potato				
baked, topped				
w/broccoli & cheese	2 halves	14.0	370	34%
w/ham & cheese	2 halves	16.0	400	36%
sausage penne Italiano				
meal kit	¼ pkg	14.0	270	47%
shrimp meal kit				
& broccoli Alfredo	¼ pkg	13.0	270	43%
stir-fry	¼ pkg	2.0	220	8%
stuffed pasta shells	3 shells	14.0	320	39%
w/red sauce	1 serving	20.0	440	41%
INTERNATIONAL FOODS				
apple flautas	1 flauta	4.5	150	27%
Barquito				
beef taco	1 taco	17.0	350	44%
meat-trio	1	21.0	380	50%
beef				
& bean burrito	1	13.0	270	43%

Food and Description	Amount	Fat Grams	Total Calories	% Fat Calories
Oriental w/broccoli				
and rice	1 serving	6.0	290	19%
taco boat/hard shell	1 taco	16.0	270	53%
taquito	5 taquitos	12.0	340	32%
stuffed nachos	5 nachos	16.0	260	55%
chicken				
& cheese quesadilla	1 whole	9.0	230	35%
meal kits				
Alfredo rigatoni	¼ pkg	15.0	270	50%
breast fajita	2 fajitas	6.0	290	19%
breast stir-fry	¼ bag	0.5	260	2%
breast w/fried rice	¼ bag	1.0	320	3%
Szechuan shrimp	¼ pkg	14.0	270	47%
sweet & sour w/rice	⅓ pkg	1.0	240	4%
sweet & spice				
w/Japanese-				
style noodles	¼ bag	3.5	250	13%
corn dogs/mini	4 pieces	18.0	290	56%
eggrolls				
chicken	2 pieces	8.0	220	33%
pork	2 pieces	12.0	240	45%
mini	4 pieces	10.0	200	45%
Southwest chcken	2 pieces	9.0	280	29%
vegetable	2 pieces	4.5	170	24%
jalapeño peppers				
cheese-stuffed	3 pieces	15.0	230	59%
tamales	1 tamale	10.0	210	43%
won ton rolls				
pizza-flavored	5 pieces	18.0	410	40%
SANDWICHES				
bagel dogs w/cheese	1 sandwich	18.0	360	45%
cheeseburger	1 sandwich	19.0	360	48%
corn dog	1 sandwich	11.0	180	55%
grilled chicken	1 sandwich	3.5	180	18%
ranchero	1 sandwich	19.0	440	39%
■ (Stouffer's)				
BOWL CUISINE				
beef stew	1 bowl	11.0	260	38%
chunky beef & bean chili	1 bowl	12.0	330	33%
hearty chicken & vegetables	1 bowl	15.0	330	41%
home-style chicken				
& noodles	1 bowl	14.0	380	33%
steak & portabello				
mushroom	1 bowl	9.0	280	29%
ENTRÉES (Stouffer's)				
beef pie	1 pie	25.0	440	51%
broccoli au gratin	1 serving	5.0	100	45%
cheese manicotti	1 meal	16.0	360	40%
cheesy spaghetti bake				
12 oz	1 meal	21.0	430	44%

Food and Description	Amount	Fat Grams	Total Calories	% Fat Calories
chicken				
à la king	1 meal	11.0	350	28%
enchilada & Mexican rice	1 serving	11.0	220	45%
lasagna	1 serving	15.0	310	44%
potpie				
10-oz pkg	1 pie	47.0	740	57%
16-oz pkg	½ pkg	38.0	500	54%
creamed chipped beef	½ cup	9.0	150	54%
escalloped chicken				
& noodles	1 meal	23.0	370	56%
fettuccini				
Alfredo	1 meal	28.0	520	48%
primavera	1 meal	15.0	370	36%
5-cheese lasagna	1 meal	12.0	350	31%
lasagna				
bake	1 meal	15.0	410	33%
lasagna w/meat sauce				
10-oz pkg	1 meal	14.0	370	34%
21-oz pkg	⅓ pkg	8.0	250	29%
40-oz pkg	⅕ pkg	10.0	270	33%
96-oz pkg	1/12 pkg	11.0	300	33%
w/meat & sauce				
10½-oz pkg	1 meal	13.0	370	32%
21-oz pkg	⅓ pkg	8.0	250	29%
w/tomato sauce & Italian sausage	1 meal	18.0	410	40%
macaroni & beef w/tomatoes	1 meal	9.0	330	25%
macaroni & cheese				
12-oz pkg	6 oz	15.0	320	42%
20-oz pkg	8 oz	18.0	340	48%
macaroni & cheese				
& broccoli	1 meal	15.0	350	39%
(Maxaroni)				
cheese pizza minis	1 pkg	22.0	470	42%
chicken nuggets	1 pkg	22.0	430	46%
fish sticks	1 pkg	16.0	380	38%
mac & cheese				
9-oz pkg	1 meal	17.0	390	39%
19-oz pkg	9.5 oz	17.0	390	39%
ravioli				
cheese	1 pkg	12.0	390	28%
roasted chicken/Italian-style	1 meal	13.0	360	33%
rigatoni				
cheese-stuffed rigatoni				
& ravioli Italian-style	1 meal	22.0	470	42%
Italian sausage-stuffed				
/Italian-style	1 meal	16.0	380	38%
w/roasted white meat				
chicken Italian-style	x	x	x	x
spaghetti				
w/meat sauce	1 pkg	10.0	330	27%

Food and Description	Amount	Fat Grams	Total Calories	% Fat Calories
w/meatballs in sauce	1 pkg	14.0	380	33%
stuffed green pepper				
10-oz pkg	1 pkg	12.0	240	45%
stuffed peppers w/beef				
in tomato sauce	½ pkg	7.0	180	35%
Swedish meatballs	1 pkg	26.0	510	46%
tuna				
noodle casserole	1 meal	16.0	340	42%
tetrazzini	1 meal	18.0	370	44%
turkey potpie				
10 oz	1 pkg	48.0	740	58%
16 oz	½ pkg	39.0	600	59%
vegetable lasagna	1 pkg	20.0	410	44%
Welsh rarebit	~¼ pkg	8.0	120	60%
FAMILY-STYLE RECIPES				
chicken				
Alfredo	~⅐ pkg	20.0	380	47%
& broccoli bake	~⅕ pkg	17.0	340	45%
Cordon Bleu pasta	~¼ pkg	4.5	330	12%
enchiladas	⅙ pkg	7.0	310	20%
escalloped w/noodles	~⅕ pkg	23.0	370	56%
grandma's chicken &				
vegetable rice bake	~⅕ pkg	23.0	370	56%
lasagna				
39 oz	~⅕ pkg	17.0	330	46%
96 oz	~1⁄11 pkg	13.0	320	37%
parmigiana	¼ pkg	18.0	490	33%
ravioli/Italian-style	1 meal	13.0	360	33%
5-cheese lasagna	~1⁄11 pkg	11.0	280	35%
lasagna w/meat & sauce				
40 oz	~⅕ pkg	10.0	270	33%
57 oz	⅐ pkg	13.0	320	37%
96 oz	~1⁄12 pkg	14.0	320	39%
macaroni & cheese				
40 oz	~⅕ pkg	18.0	370	44%
76 oz	~⅑ pkg	18.0	380	43%
meat loaf in gravy	⅙ pkg	12.0	210	51%
stuffed green peppers	¼ pkg	7.0	180	35%
Thanksgiving Tonight	~¼ pkg	9.0	270	30%
vegetable lasagna	1⁄12 pkg	18.0	370	44%
FRENCH BREAD PIZZA				
cheese	1 pizza	16.0	380	38%
deluxe	1 pizza	21.0	430	44%
extra cheese	1 pizza	18.0	400	41%
5-cheese	1 pizza	18.0	410	40%
grilled vegetable	1 pizza	12.0	350	31%
pepperoni	1 pizza	21.0	430	44%
pepperoni & mushroom	1 pizza	19.0	410	42%
sausage	1 pizza	18.0	420	39%
sausage & pepperoni	1 pizza	24.0	470	46%

Food and Description	Amount	Fat Grams	Total Calories	% Fat Calories
3-meat	1 pizza	25.0	480	47%
white	1 pizza	23.0	470	44%
HOME-STYLE				
beef				
green pepper steak	1 meal	7.0	280	23%
meat loaf	1 meal	16.0	340	42%
pot roast	1 meal	9.0	250	32%
Stroganoff	1 meal	15.0	350	39%
chicken				
baked beast	1 meal	11.0	270	37%
breast/fried	1 meal	17.0	380	40%
breast in mushroom gravy	1 meal	17.0	370	41%
breast tenders in				
BBQ sauce	1 meal	24.0	460	47%
fettuccini	1 meal	13.0	370	32%
parmigiana	1 meal	16.0	440	33%
roasted w/stuffing	1 meal	24.0	460	47%
fish fillet w/macaroni				
& cheese	1 meal	17.0	410	37%
pork				
breaded boneless cutlet	1 meal	20.0	350	51%
roasted	1 meal	12.0	320	20%
Salisbury steak	1 meal	16.0	350	41%
turkey/roasted beast	1 meal	10.0	280	32%
veal pamigiana	1 meal	17.0	430	36%
HOME-STYLE DINNERS				
beef				
country-fried steak	1 meal	33.0	590	50%
meat loaf	1 meal	29.0	560	47%
pot roast	1 meal	14.0	380	33%
Salisbury steak	1 meal	18.0	470	34%
slow-roasted beef				
& gravy	1 meal	14.0	370	34%
Southwestern-style				
mesquite-flavored steak	1 meal	18.0	440	37%
chicken				
fettuccini	1 meal	17.0	490	31%
Southwestern-style				
grilled lime chicken	1 meal	13.0	490	24%
Monterey chicken	1 meal	18.0	440	37%
smothered chicken	1 meal	16.0	490	29%
turkey/roasted breast	1 meal	13.0	450	26%
veal parmigiana	1 meal	17.0	490	31%
LEAN CUISINE (See (LEAN CUISINE) listings within this category)				
SIDE DISHES				
cheddar potato bake	½ pkg	16.0	250	58%
corn soufflé	1 serving	8.0	180	40%
creamed spinach	½ pkg	20.0	230	78%
harvest apples	½ pkg	4.0	210	17%
potatoes au gratin	½ serving	5.0	150	30%

Food and Description	Amount	Fat Grams	Total Calories	% Fat Calories
spinach soufflé	⅓ pkg	8.0	130	55%
whipped potatoes and gravy	~½ pkg	4.5	150	26%
SKILLET SENSATIONS				
beef				
& broccoli..40 oz	~⅓ pkg	3.0	180	15%
home-style..25 oz	~⅓ pkg	6.0	170	21%
Stroganoff..40 oz	~⅕ pkg	10.0	250	36%
Yankee pot roast 24 oz	⅓ pkg	6.0	190	28%
chicken				
Alfredo..25 oz	~⅓ pkg	9.0	240	34%
& dumplings..24 oz	~⅓ pkg	7.0	200	32%
garlic..23 oz	~ ¼ pkg	4.0	190	19%
grilled w/vegetables..25 oz	~⅓ pkg	9.0	260	31%
home-style w/noodles 25 oz	~⅓ pkg	8.0	260	28%
savory w/rice..40 oz	~⅕ pkg	3.0	230	12%
teriyaki..25 oz	~⅓ pkg	2.0	160	11%
steak teriyaki..23.5 oz	⅓ pkg	3.0	190	14%
■ (Swanson)				
DINNERS				
chicken				
classic fried	1 pkg	36.0	640	51%
grilled white meat	1 pkg	11.0	310	32%
mesquite-grilled	1 pkg	9.0	380	21%
potpie	1 pkg	21.0	380	50%
Salisbury steak	1 pkg	16.0	320	45%
scalloped potatoes & ham	1 pkg	13.0	300	39%
turkey				
glazed medallions	1 pkg	11.0	380	26%
roasted/carved/breast				
w/stuffing/potatoes/peas	1 pkg	15.0	420	32%
w/dressing & potatoes	1 pkg	11.0	290	34%
w/stuffing & green beans	1 pkg	11.0	380	26%
HUNGRY MAN DINNERS				
Angus beef				
meat loaf..XXL w/mashed potatoes	1 pkg	48.0	860	50%
Salisbury steak w/onion gravy & potatoes	1 pkg	29.0	470	56%
boneless chicken Southern-fried	1 pkg	41.0	1010	37%
cheeseburger sandwiches Hearty Hero	1 sdw	43.0	730	53%
chopped beef steak	1 pkg	37.0	640	52%
fried chicken				
dark	1 pkg	45.0	860	47%
white	1 pkg	46.0	870	48%
Salisbury steak	1 pkg	41.0	680	54%

Food and Description	Amount	Fat Grams	Total Calories	% Fat Calories
sliced beef	1 pkg	12.0	450	24%
veal parmigiana	1 pkg	26.0	590	40%
■ (T.G.I. Friday's)				
chicken				
crispy baked breast strips	⅓ pkg	8.0	190	38%
popcorn				
bourbon-glazed	⅓ pkg	6.0	180	30%
quesadilla rolls	⅓ pkg	5.0	100	45%
wings				
BBQ..honey	½ pkg	10.0	180	50%
buffalo	⅓ pkg	7.0	100	63%
double-glazed	⅓ pkg	7.0	100	63%
Cheese Teasers..mozzarella	~1 oz	6.0	100	54%
dip				
black bean & cheese	2 Tbs	2.5	50	45%
spinach, cheese & artichoke	2 Tbs	3.5	45	70%
egg rolls..Southwestern	⅓ box	9.0	190	43%
pizzas..mini deep-dish				
buffalo-style chicken	⅓ pizza	4.5	140	28%
chicken				
w/honey BBQ sauce	⅓ pizza	5.5	150	27%
potato skins				
bacon & cheddar	2.2 oz	9.0	160	51%
stuffed				
broccoli & cheddar	⅓ pkg	6.0	140	39%
cheddar & bacon	⅓ pkg	9.0	170	48%
4-cheese & pepperoni	⅓ pkg	8.0	160	45%
■ (Tyson)				
FROZEN/READY-TO-EAT				
beef				
strips/seasoned	⅙ pkg	6.0	140	34%
chicken				
bites/popcorn				
diced breast fritters	⅑ pkg	9.0	210	39%
breast				
diced w/rib meat	⅐ pkg	1.0	90	10%
fillets/breast fritters	⅙ pkg	16.0	290	50%
mesquite-flavored				
w/rib meat	1/15 pkg	6.0	110	49%
patties/breaded				
28.8 oz	⅙ pkg	16.0	290	50%
32 oz	1/12 pkg	11.0	180	55%
48 oz	1/16 pkg	14.0	220	57%
strips	⅙ pkg	3.5	120	26%
Southwest seasoned	⅐ pkg	3.0	110	25%
teriyaki-flavored				
w/rib meat	⅛ pkg	7.0	170	37%
drumsticks/honey				
BBQ-style	2 pieces	7.0	160	39%
meatballs..Italian-style	⅑ pkg	11.0	180	55%

Food and Description	Amount	Fat Grams	Total Calories	% Fat Calories
nuggets..breaded				
32-oz bag	1/10 pkg	14.0	240	53%
56-oz bag	1/17 pkg	14.0	230	55%
strips				
buffalo-style				
w/seasoning	1/8 pkg	10.0	230	39%
crispy fritters				
w/rib meat	1/8 pkg	10.0	200	45%
fajita	1/7 pkg	5.0	120	38%
tenders				
breaded	3.2 oz	9.0	200	41%
breaded w/rib meat	2.5 oz	14.0	240	53%
honey-battered	3 oz	11.0	200	50%
wings				
BBQ	3 pieces	13.0	200	59%
buffalo-style hot				
32-oz bag	1/6 pkg	15.0	220	61%
64-oz bag	1/13 pkg	15.0	220	61%
honey BBQ				
32-oz bag	1/6 pkg	14.0	220	57%
64-oz bag	1/13 pkg	14.0	220	57%
■ **(Weight Watchers)**				
HIGHER-PROTEIN ENTRÉES				
beef				
sirloin & Asian-style vegetables	1 meal	9.0	230	35%
chicken				
creamy Parmesan	1 meal	8.0	230	31%
Tuscan	1 meal	9.0	210	39%
grilled in garlic herb sauce	1 meal	9.0	210	39%
marsala w/broccoli	1 meal	5.0	170	26%
turkey medallions				
w/mushroom gravy	1 meal	8.0	200	36%
MAIN STREET BISTRO SELECTIONS				
bowls				
beef & vegetable rice	1 bowl	7.0	260	24%
chicken stir-fry	1 bowl	6.0	300	18%
seafood linguini	1 bowl	4.5	290	14%
Southwestern-style chicken	1 bowl	2.5	230	10%
teriyaki chicken	1 bowl	3.0	280	10%
other bistro selections				
fire-grilled chicken				
& vegetables	1 meal	5.0	280	16%
pizza				
BBQ-style chicken	1 pizza	7.0	380	17%
4-cheese	1 pizza	7.0	400	16%
pepperoni	1 pizza	9.0	400	20%
spicy sausage	1 pizza	10.0	390	23%
veggie ultimate crust	1 pizza	5.0	400	11%
SMART ONES/ Meals				
angel-hair pasta	1 meal	4.0	240	15%

Food and Description	Amount	Fat Grams	Total Calories	% Fat Calories
baked potato, broccoli & cheese	1 meal	6.0	260	21%
beef pot roast	1 meal	9.0	220	37%
broccoli & cheddar				
& roasted potatoes	1 meal	6.0	250	22%
chicken				
chow mein	1 meal	2.0	200	9%
enchilada suiza	1 meal	10.0	340	26%
fajita supreme	1 meal	7.0	260	24%
fiesta chicken	1 meal	2.0	210	9%
fire-grilled w/vegetables	1 meal	3.5	280	11%
glazed	1 meal	2.5	260	9%
golden-baked, garlic	1 meal	5.0	270	17%
honey Dijon	1 meal	3.5	210	15%
lemon herb picatta	1 meal	5.0	250	18%
marsala	1 meal	2.0	150	12%
Mirabella	1 meal	2.0	180	10%
Oriental	1 meal	4.5	230	18%
oven-roasted	1 meal	6.0	260	21%
penne pollo	1 meal	6.0	290	19%
roasted w/sour cream				
& chive mashed potatoes	1 meal	3.5	190	17%
Santa Fe	1 meal	6.0	230	23%
tenderloins w/BBQ Sauce	1 meal	5.0	300	13%
Thai w/noodles	1 meal	4.0	290	12%
fettuccini Alfredo	1 meal	6.0	270	20%
lasagna				
Bolognese	1 meal	2.5	240	9%
Florentine	1 meal	8.0	290	25%
traditional w/meat sauce	1 meal	7.0	300	21%
macaroni & cheese				
3-cheese	1 meal	7.0	290	22%
traditional	1 meal	2.5	240	9%
meat loaf w/gravy	1 meal	8.0	260	28%
pepper steak	1 meal	5.0	230	20%
radiatore romano	1 meal	8.0	280	26%
peppercorn fillet of beef	1 meal	7.0	220	29%
ravioli Florentine	1 meal	5.0	220	20%
rigatoni..creamy				
w/broccoli & chicken	1 meal	3.5	240	13%
roast beef w/gravy	1 meal	8.0	230	31%
Salisbury steak	1 meal	6.0	260	21%
Santa Fe rice & beans	1 meal	8.0	300	24%
shrimp marinara	1 meal	2.0	180	10%
spaghetti				
Bolognese	1 meal	5.0	280	16%
marinara	1 meal	7.0	280	23%
spicy Szechuan-style				
vegetables & chicken	1 meal	5.0	220	20%
sundae w/chocolate chip				
cookie dough	½ pkg	4.5	190	21%

Food and Description	Amount	Fat Grams	Total Calories	% Fat Calories
Swedish meatballs	1 meal	7.0	280	23%
tuna noodle gratin	1 meal	7.0	270	22%
turkey				
roasted medallions	1 meal	2.0	200	9%
slow-roasted breast	1 meal	8.0	220	33%
stuffed breast	1 meal	7.0	270	23%
ziti..3-cheese marinara	1 meal	7.0	290	22%
■ (WOLFGANG PUCK) *(See also* PIZZA)				
cannelloni..ricotta	1 meal	21.0	420	45%
lasagna				
4-cheese	1 meal	22.0	480	41%
Italian vegetable	1 meal	16.0	410	35%
mushroom	1 meal	16.0	440	33%
spicy chicken	1 meal	21.0	470	40%
Parmesan..eggplant	1 plate	17.0	300	51%
pasta wrap..chicken & spinach	1 container	11.0	460	22%
ravioli				
4-cheese	1 meal	20.0	330	55%
mushroom & spinach	1 meal	18.0	260	62%
sweet potato	1 meal	21.0	360	53%
tortellini				
mushroom	1 meal	18.0	430	38%
spicy chicken	1 meal	24.0	490	44%

■ YU SING *(See* ASIAN FOOD)

FROZEN NONDAIRY DESSERT *(See* FRUIT ICES, BARS & POPS; ICE CREAM & ICE CREAM-LIKE FROZEN DESSERTS; RICE FROZEN DESSERT; SHERBET; TOFU FROZEN DESSERT)

FRUCTOSE *(See* SUGAR SUBSTITUTE)

FRUIT, MIXED *(See also* SNACKS)

CANDIED

(S&W)				
glacé fruit				
cake mix	2 Tbs	–	90	–
cherries				
green	5 pieces	–	80	–
red	5 pieces	–	80	–
citron	58 pieces	–	80	–
lemon peel	58 pieces	–	80	–
orange peel	58 pieces	–	80	–
pineapple				
green	1 piece	–	180	–
red	1 piece	–	180	–
wedges				
sliced natural	5 pieces	–	80	–
tri-color	5 pieces	–	80	–

CANNED/JARRED

(Del Monte)				
cherry mixed				
individual pull-top cans	½ cup	–	90	–
plastic cups	1 cup	–	70	–

Food and Description	Amount	Fat Grams	Total Calories	% Fat Calories
very cherry mixed	½ cup	–	90	–
chunky mixed				
in extra light syrup/light	½ cup	–	60	–
individual pull-top can	½ cup	–	60	–
in heavy syrup	½ cup	–	100	–
in 100% juice	½ cup	–	60	–
fruit cocktail	½ cup	–	100	–
in 100% juice	½ cup	–	60	–
individual pull-top cans	½ cup	–	100	
light	½ cup	–	60	–
individual pull-top cans	½ cup	–	60	
plastic cups	1 cup	–	70	–
mixed fruit				
pull-top can	½ cup	–	80	–
light	½ cup	–	50	–
in 100% juice	½ cup	–	50	–
tropical fruit				
in individual pull-top cans	4.5 oz	–	80	–
in plastic cups	1 cup	–	70	–
(Dole) tropical fruit salad				
in light syrup	½ cup	–	80	–
(S&W)				
fruit cocktail..orchard ripe				
in heavy syrup	½ cup	–	90	–
mixed fruit				
natural-style/chunky	½ cup	–	80	–
DRIED				
(Del Monte)	½ cup	–	110	–
(Mariani)				
fruit medley	¼ cup	1.0	150	5%
tropical	1 oz	1.0	90	10%
(Sun Maid)				
fruit bits	1.4 oz	–	120	–
goldens & cherries	1.5 oz	–	130	–
mixed fruit	1.4 oz	–	100	–
tropical trio				
pineapple/papaya/mango	1.4 oz	–	130	–
(Traverse Bay)				
fruit medley..apples/				
cherries/raisins	1.5 oz	–	110	–
FRESH..REFRIGERATED				
(Del Monte)				
Fruit Naturals				
tropical medley	½ cup	–	70	–
Orchard Select				
premium mixed fruit	½ cup	–	80	–
Sunfresh				
papaya/extra light syrup	½ cup	–	70	–

Food and Description	Amount	Fat Grams	Total Calories	% Fat Calories
Sunfresh				
tropical fruit salad				
in light syrup	½ cup	–	80	–
in pineapple & passion				
fruit juices	½ cup	–	80	–
(Dole)				
Fruit Bowls.. tropical	1 bowl	–	60	–

FRUIT/FRUIT JUICE DRINK (*See also* LEMONADE/LEMONADE-FLAVORED DRINK; TEA; FRUIT PUNCH; SOFT DRINK; SOFT DRINK MIX; individual *BOTTLED, BOXED, POUCH, OR CANNED*)

Food and Description	Amount	Fat Grams	Total Calories	% Fat Calories
(After the Fall) bottle				
spritzers				
banana Casablanca				
83% juice	12 oz	–	100	–
black cherry				
83% juice	12 oz	–	180	–
Key West lime cooler				
83% juice	12 oz	–	100	–
Mango Montage				
90% juice	12 oz	–	110	–
raspberry				
70% juice	12 oz	–	170	–
tangerine				
77% juice	12 oz	–	180	–
(Capri Sun) Juice Drink				
6.75-oz pouch				
grape	6.75 oz	–	100	–
Mountain Cooler	6.75 oz	–	90	–
orange	6.75 oz	–	100	–
Pacific cooler	6.75 oz	–	100	–
red berry	6.75 oz	–	100	–
strawberry	6.75 oz	–	90	–
strawberry kiwi cooler	6.75 oz	–	100	–
Surfer Cooler	6.75 oz	–	100	–
wild cherry	6.75 oz	–	110	–
11.25-oz pouch				
all flavors	11.25 oz	–	160	–
All Natural Fruit Waves				
all flavors	6.75 oz	–	100	–
Refreshers 16.5 oz				
all flavors	16.5 oz	–	110	–
Hawaiian Punch/bottles				
Berry Blue Typhoon	8 Oz	–	120	–
Bodacious Berry	8 Oz	–	110	—
Fruit Juicy Red	8 oz	–	120	–
Hawaiian punch/light	8 oz	–	45	–
Orange Ocean	8 Oz	–	120	–
Tropical Vibe	8 oz	–	110	–

Food and Description	Amount	Fat Grams	Total Calories	% Fat Calories
Wild Purple Smash	8 oz	–	110	–
(Fruitopia) Chilled				
Fruit Integration				
10% juice	8 oz	–	110	–
Grape Beyond				
5% juice	8 oz	–	120	–
Strawberry Passion				
Awareness				
5% juice	8 oz	–	110	–
Tangerine Wavelength				
5% juice	8 oz	–	110	–
10% juice	8 oz	–	120	–
(Hi-C) See (Minute Maid) below				
(Minute Maid)				
bottles				
berry kiwi	12 oz	–	160	–
Strawberry Passion	12 oz	–	170	–
tropical citrus	12 oz	–	160	–
cans				
light				
guava	12 oz	–	10	–
mango	12 oz	–	10	–
Raspberry Passion	12 oz	–	15	–
Hi-C Blast/box				
Boppin' Strawberry	6.75 Oz	–	100	–
Blue Watermelon	6.75 Oz	–	100	–
Orange Lavaburst	6.75 oz	–	90	–
Hi-C Sour Blast/pouch				
green apples	6.75 oz	–	100	–
strawberry	6.75 oz	–	100	–
wild cherry	6.75 oz	–	110	–
(Odwalla) smoothies				
blackberry fruit shake	8 oz	–	140	–
Mango Tango	8 oz	–	150	–
strawberry banana	8 oz	–	120	–
(R. W. Knudsen)				
fruit juice spritzers/can				
black cherry	12 oz	–	170	–
boysenberry	12 oz	–	160	–
cherry cola	12 oz	–	170	–
cranberry	12 oz	–	190	–
grape	12 oz	–	170	–
kiwi lime	12 oz	–	130	–
lemon lime	12 oz	–	170	–
mandarin lime	12 oz	–	170	–
Mandango Fandango	12 oz	–	190	–
orange passionfruit	12 oz	–	160	–
peach	12 oz	–	160	–
red raspberry	12 oz	–	170	–
strawberry	12 oz	–	170	–

Food and Description	Amount	Fat Grams	Total Calories	% Fat Calories
tangerine	12 oz	–	170	–
vanilla crème	12 oz	–	160	–
sparkling juice drink/bottle				
celebratory				
cherry	8 oz	–	110	–
cranberry	8 oz	–	130	–
(Snapple) bottle				
Go Bananas	8 oz	–	120	–
grapeade	8 oz	–	120	–
Kiwi Strawberry	8 oz	–	110	–
Mango Madness	8 oz	–	110	–
orangeade	8 oz	–	120	–
raspberry peach	8 oz	–	120	–
ruby red	8 oz	–	120	–
Snapple apple	8 oz	–	`120	–
Snapricot orange	8 oz	–	120	–
Summer Peach	8 oz	–	120	–
Vitamin Supreme	8 oz	–	150	–
(Sunny D) bottle				
mango	8 oz	–	130	–
orange	8 oz	–	130	–
smooth California-style	8 oz	–	130	–
w/calcium	8 oz	–	140	–
tangy original Florida-style	8 oz	–	120	–
tropical punch				
Caribbean-style	8 oz	–	140	–
(Tropicana) bottle				
smoothies				
cherry vanilla	11 oz	–	250	–
peach	11 oz	–	250	–
piña colada	11 oz	–	250	–
Pineapple Mango Medley	11 oz	–	250	–
Raspberry Chocolate Dip	11 oz	–	250	–
strawberry	11 oz	–	250	–
Tropical Orange	11 oz	–	250	–
Twister				
Apple Berry Blast	8 oz	–	130	–
	11.5 oz	–	180	–
Blue Raspberry Rush	8 oz	–	130	–
	10 oz	–	160	–
Cherry Raspberry Riptide	8 oz	–	130	——
Grape Wild Strawberry	8 oz	–	130	–
Grapefruit Tangerine Tango	8 oz	–	130	–
Kiwi Strawberry Cyclone	8 oz	–	120	–
Orange Citrus Spark	8 oz	–	130	–
Orange Cranberry Clash	8 oz	–	130	–
	10 oz	–	160	–
Tropical Fruit Fury	8 oz	–	120	–
	10 oz	–	150	–
Watermelon Strawberry Swirl	8 oz	–	130	–

Food and Description	Amount	Fat Grams	Total Calories	% Fat Calories
white grape kiwi	8 oz	–	130	–
(V8 Splash) juice drink				
diet				
berry blend	8 oz	–	10	–
strawberry kiwi	8 oz	–	10	–
tropical blend	8 zo	–	10	–
regular				
berry blend	8 oz	–	110	–
citrus blend	8 oz	–	110	–
fruit medley	8 oz	–	110	–
guava passionfruit	8 oz	–	110	–
mango peach	8 oz	–	110	–
orange pineapple	8 oz	–	110	–
peach lemonade	8 oz	–	110	–
raspberry lemonade	8 oz	–	100	–
strawberry banana	8 oz	–	110	–
strawberry kiwi	8 oz	–	110	–
tropical blend	8 oz	–	110	–
(Welch's)				
grape juice beverage	8 fl oz	–	150	–
harvest blend	8 fl oz	–	140	–
mango passion	8 fl oz	–	180	–
mountain berry blackberry	8 fl oz	–	140	–
orange pineapple apple	8 fl oz	–	140	–
sparkling cocktail				
red	8 fl oz	–	160	–
white	8 fl oz	–	160	–
white grape cranberry	8 fl oz	–	160	–
strawberry breeze	8 fl oz	–	130	–
tropical punch drink	10 fl oz	–	160	–
tropical cocktail	11.5 fl oz	–	210	–
FROZEN/PREPARED				
(Welch's) from concentrate				
cherry	8 fl oz	–	130	
strawberry breeze	8 fl oz	–	140	–
FRUIT ICES, BARS & POPS (*See also* SHERBET)				
(Blue Bunny)				
REGULAR TREATS				
banana pops	1 bar	–	35	–
Buzz mini bomb pops	1 pop	–	35	–
Chamoy & Chili	1 bar	–	70	–
Chill'n Juice pops				
fruit punch	1 pop	–	40	–
orange tangerine	1 pop	–	40	–
strawberry kiwi	1 pop	–	40	–
citrus snacks	1 bar	–	50	–
Mickey Shimmy pops	1 pop	–	50	–
Peluca's Tamarina & Chili	1 bar	–	80	–

Food and Description	Amount	Fat Grams	Total Calories	% Fat Calories
Polar pops				
12-pack				
cherry	1 pop	–	35	–
grape	1 pop	–	35	–
orange	1 pop	–	35	–
24-pack				
cherry	1 pop	–	40	–
lemon lime	1 pop	–	40	–
orange	1 pop	–	40	–
root beer pops	1 pop	–	40	–
slush pops	1 pop	–	45	–
Stitch Bomb pop	1 pop	–	50	–
twin pops				
cherry	1 pop	–	70	–
grape	1 pop	–	70	–
lemon lime	1 pop	–	70	–
orange	1 pop	–	70	–
zesty lemon lime	1 bar	–	70	–
SUGAR-FREE POPS	1 pop	–	15	–
(Dole)				
fruit juice/juice pops				
no sugar added				
grape	1 pop	–	30	–
raspberry	1 pop	–	30	–
strawberry	1 pop	–	30	–
regular				
grape	1 pop	–	45	–
raspberry	1 pop	–	45	–
strawberry	1 pop	–	50	–
Fruit 'n' Juice Bars				
lemonade	2.5 oz	–	70	–
mango guava twist	2.5 oz	–	80	–
pineapple orange twist	2.5 oz	–	90	–
raspberry	2.5 oz	–	70	–
strawberry	2.5 oz	–	70	–
(Dreyer's)				
fruit bars				
all flavors	1 bar	–	80	–
variety packs				
no sugar added..all flavors	1 bar	–	30	–
regular				
cherry	1 bar	–	70	–
grape	1 bar	–	70	–
lime	1 bar	–	60	–
strawberry	1 bar	–	60	–
tropical	1 bar	–	70	–
wild berry	1 bar	–	60	–
(Edy's)				
fruit bars				
all flavors	1 bar	–	80	–

Food and Description	Amount	Fat Grams	Total Calories	% Fat Calories
variety packs				
no sugar added..all flavors	1 bar	–	30	–
regular				
cherry	1 bar	–	70	–
grape	1 bar	–	70	–
lime	1 bar	–	60	–
strawberry	1 bar	–	60	–
tropical	1 bar	–	70	–
wild berry	1 bar	–	60	–
(Eskimo)				
Rainbow Twin Pops	1 pop		60	–
Welch's Double Dare pops				
double sours	1 pop	–	40	–
mega sours	1 pop	–	40	–
(Good Humor)				
Bubble Play Sports	1 bar	–	110	–
Cherry Torpedo	1 bar	–	35	–
Hyper Stripe	1 bar	–	80	–
Jumbo Jet Star	1 bar	–	80	–
Micro Pops	1 pop	–	80	–
Smile	1 bar	–	110	–
The Great White Bar	1 bar	–	70	–
(Häagen-Dazs) Sorbet				
bars				
chocolate	1 bar	–	80	–
pints				
mango	½ cup	–	120	–
orange	½ cup	–	120	–
orchard peach	½ cup	–	120	–
raspberry	½ cup	–	120	–
strawberry	½ cup	–	120	–
zesty lemon	½ cup	–	120	–
(Hendrie's)				
ice pops/assorted				
no sugar added..citrus & berries				
orange	1 pop	–	15	–
raspberry lime	1 pop	–	15	–
strawberry	1 pop	–	15	–
regular				
citrus stix				
lime	1 pop	–	45	–
orange	1 pop	–	45	–
raspberry	1 pop	–	45	–
(Hood)				
fruit smoothies				
lemon lime	1 bar	0.5	70	6%
orange	1 bar	0.5	70	6%
raspberry	1 bar	0.5	70	6%
Hawaiian Punch				
Arctic Surfers				
Fruit Juicy Red	1 bar	–	50	–

Food and Description	Amount	Fat Grams	Total Calories	% Fat Calories
Green Berry Rush	1 bar	–	50	–
Ocean Orange	1 bar	–	50	–
Strawberry Surfin'	1 bar	–	50	–
Hoodsie pops				
banana	1 pop	–	60	–
blue raspberry	1 pop	–	60	–
cherry	1 pop	–	60	–
grape	1 pop	–	60	–
orange	1 pop	–	60	–
root beer	1 pop	–	60	–
lemonade pop	1 bar	–	45	–
Lifesavers Pops				
no sugar added				
lime	1 pop	–	10	–
orange	1 pop	–	10	–
pineapple	1 pop	–	10	–
wild cherry	1 pop	–	10	–
regular				
lime	1 pop	–	40	–
orange	1 pop	–	40	–
pineapple	1 pop	–	40	–
wild cherry	1 pop	–	40	–
Red, White & Blue pop	1 pop	0.5	70	6%
(Kemp's)				
fruit bars..12-count box				
strawberry	1 pop	–	50	
raspberry	1 pop	–	50	–
ice pops				
All-American	1 pop	–	80	–
berries & cherries	1 pop	–	40	–
Pop Jr.'s..24-count box				
all flavors	1 pop	–	180	–
Twin pops..6-count box				
all flavors	1 pop	–	60	–
(Kool-Aid) Kool-pops/all flavors	1 bar	–	50	–
(Luigi's) Real Italian Ice cups				
Bubblegum Burst & Cherry				
Lime Chiller..swirl cups	6 oz	–	150	–
cherry	6 oz	–	110	–
chocolate fudge	6 oz	–	160	–
lemon	6 oz	–	100	–
lemon & strawberry	6 oz	–	110	–
strawberry	6 oz	–	120	–
Strawberry Blast & Blue				
Razzin' Lemonade..swirl cups	6 oz	–	150	–
(Minute Maid) Fruit Juice Bars				
all flavors	1 bar	–	60	–
(Nestlé) IceScreamers				
Bug Pops				
cherry	1 pop	–	90	–
grape w/orange	1 pop	–	90	–

Food and Description	Amount	Fat Grams	Total Calories	% Fat Calories
Itzakadoozie				
cherry	1 pop	–	90	–
lemon	1 pop	–	90	–
lime	1 pop	–	90	–
orange	1 pop	–	90	–
Tiger Ice				
orange & grape striped	1 pop	–	60	–
(Pet) Ice Pops				
assorted				
banana	1 pop	–	70	–
jr.	1 pop	–	40	–
magic wands	1 pop	–	40	–
regular	1 pop	–	70	–
sparklers	1 pop	–	40	–
(Popsicle)				
single-serve				
Bart Simpson	1 bar	–	110	–
Big Bang	1 bar	1.0	100	9%
Big Stick				
cherry/pineapple	1 bar	–	50	–
Lick-A-Color	1 bar	–	90	–
rainbow	1 bar	–	90	–
bubble gum swirl	1 bar	–	60	–
Bubble Play	1 bar	–	100	–
cotton candy swirl	1 bar	–	60	–
cups				
cherry	1 cup	–	240	–
lemon	1 cup	–	230	–
Dora the Explorer	1 bar	–	100	–
Firecracker				
fire & ice	1 bar	–	80	–
root beer float	1 bar	–	80	–
supersicle	1 bar	2.0	150	12%
supersicle red/white/blue	1 bar	–	80	–
Firecracker Jr.	1 pop	–	40	–
Incredible Hulk Bar	1 bar	–	100	–
Jimmy Neutron	1 bar	–	100	–
Mega Warheads	1 bar	–	100	–
Pop Ups				
orange burst	1 bar	1.0	80	11%
Reckless Rainbow	1 bar	1.0	90	10%
Popsicle Red Zone	1 bar	–	80	–
Power Rangers Force	1 bar	–	100	–
Rainbow	1 bar	–	90	–
Red, White & Blue				
firecracker bar	1 bar	–	80	–
Scribblers	1 bar	–	60	–
Spider-Man bar	1 bar	–	100	–
Sponge Bob	1 bar	–	100	–
Super Mario Brothers	1 bar	–	100	–

Food and Description	Amount	Fat Grams	Total Calories	% Fat Calories
Super Twin				
cello	1 bar	–	70	–
paper	1 bar	–	70	–
Supersicle				
Intense Fruit Shots	1 tube	0.5	40	11%
Neon Traffic Signal	1 bar	–	80	–
Razzle Dazzle	1 bar	–	80	–
Sour Tower	1 bar	–	80	–
Torpedo cherry pop	1 bar	–	35	–
Towering Tornado	1 pop	–	90	–
sugar-free				
cherry	1.75 oz	–	15	–
creamsicle	1.75 oz	2.0	40	45%
grape	1.75 oz	–	15	–
orange	1.75 oz	–	15	–
tropical fruits	1.75 oz	–	15	–
Tingle Twister	1.75 oz	–	45	–
(Schwan's)				
Schwan's Pops	1 pop	–	15	–
specialty items				
Garfield	1 bar	–	90	–
Screwball Cup	1 cup	1.0	100	9%
Snow Cone	1 cone	–	60	–
Super Mario	1 bar	1.0	120	8%
The Great White bar	1 bar	–	70	–
Twin Pops/assorted	1 pop	–	60	–
(Welch's) fruit juice bars				
no sugar added..1.75 oz	1 bar	–	25	–
grape	1 bar	–	25	–
raspberry	1 bar	–	25	–
strawberry	1 bar	–	25	–
regular				
1.75-oz bar				
grape	1 bar	–	45	–
raspberry	1 bar	–	45	–
strawberry	1 bar	–	45	–
3-oz bar				
grape	1 bar	–	80	–
strawberry banana	1 bar	–	80	–
tropical coolers..1.75 oz				
orange	1 bar	–	45	–
lemonade	1 bar	–	45	–
strawberry banana	1 bar	–	45	–
tropical fruit juice bars..1.75 oz				
orange pineapple banana	1 bar	–	45	–
pineapple	1 bar	–	45	–
strawberry banana	1 bar	–	45	–

FRUIT JUICE DRINK (*See* FRUIT/FRUIT JUICE DRINK; FRUIT PUNCH; individual listings)

Food and Description	Amount	Fat Grams	Total Calories	% Fat Calories
FRUIT PECTIN				
(Certo)	1 Tbs	–	2	–
(Sure-Jell)				
light	¼ tsp	–	5	–
sweetened	¼ tsp	–	5	–
FRUIT PROTECTOR (See also FRUIT PECTIN)				
(Sure-Jell) Ever-Fresh	¼ tsp	–	5	–
FRUIT PUNCH (See also FRUIT/FRUIT JUICE DRINK; SOFT DRINK; SOFT DRINK MIX; SPORTS DRINK)				
BOTTLED, BOXED, CANNED, or POUCH				
(Capri Sun)				
fruit/all-natural	6.75 fl oz	–	100	–
mountain cooler	6.75 fl oz	–	90	–
Pacific cooler	6.75 fl oz	–	100	–
super cooler	6.75 fl oz	–	100	–
tropical punch	6.75 fl oz	–	90	–
Thunder Punch/sports drink	6.75 fl oz	–	90	–
(Hawaiian Punch)				
light				
Hawaiian punch	8 oz	–	45	–
regular				
Berry Blue Typhoon	8 oz	–	120	–
Bodacious Berry	8 oz	–	110	–
Fruit Juicy Red	8 oz	–	120	–
'Mazin Melon Mix	8 oz	–	110	–
Orange Ocean	8 oz	–	120	–
Tropical Vibe	8 oz	–	110	–
Wild Purple Smash	8 oz	–	110	–
(Hi-C)				
Hi-C Blast/box				
fruit	6.75 oz	–	100	–
	8.45 fl oz	–	130	–
Hula	8 fl oz	–	110	–
	8.45 fl oz	–	120	–
(Kool Aid)				
Bursts/tropical	6.75 oz	–	100	–
Crystal Light/low-calorie	8 fl oz	–	5	–
Splash				
grape berry	8 fl oz	–	120	–
tropical	8 fl oz	–	120	–
(Libby's) 100% juice				
Juicy Juice punch	4.23 fl oz	–	60	–
	6.75 fl oz	–	100	–
	7.65 fl oz	–	120	–
(Minute Maid) can				
fruit/natural	12 oz	–	150	–
(Snapple)				
fruit	8 oz	–	110	–

Food and Description	Amount	Fat Grams	Total Calories	% Fat Calories
(Sunny D)				
tropical				
Caribbean-style	8 oz	–	140	–
(Tropicana)				
berry	8 fl oz	–	130	–
citrus	8 fl oz	–	140	–
cranberry	8 fl oz	–	140	–
	11.5 fl oz	–	200	–
fruit	8 fl oz	–	130	–
	11.5 fl oz	–	180	–
fruit punch/light	8 oz	–	60	–
pineapple	8 fl oz	–	130	–
tropical	8 fl oz	–	130	–
(Welch's)				
fruit	11.5 fl oz	–	180	–
Fruit Harvest	8.45 fl oz	–	140	–
Juice Cocktail				
fruit punch	8 fl oz	–	130	–
tropical punch	8.45 fl oz	–	160	–
strawberry	8 fl oz	–	140	–
Welchade				
Screaming Wild Berry	8 fl oz	–	130	–
strawberry punch	8 fl oz	–	140	–
FROZEN OR REFRIGERATED/prepared				
(Minute Maid)				
berry	8 fl oz	–	120	–
citrus	8 fl oz	–	120	–
fruit				
concentrate	2 oz	–	110	–
prepared	8 fl oz	–	120	–
grape	8 fl oz	–	120	–
tropical	8 fl oz	–	120	–
(Schwan's)				
tropical punch				
concentrate	1 oz	–	100	–
prepared	8 fl oz	–	100	–
MIX				
(Kool-Aid) soft drink mix/prepared				
tropical/sweetened	8 fl oz	–	60	–
FRUIT SNACK (See also individual fruit listings; CANDY)				
(Betty Crocker)				
Fruit-by-the-Foot				
all flavors	1 roll	1.5	80	17%
Fruit Roll-Ups				
all flavors	1 roll	1.0	50	18%
Fruit Snacks				
all flavors	1 pouch	–	80	–

Food and Description	Amount	Fat Grams	Total Calories	% Fat Calories
Fruit String Thing				
all flavors	1 pouch	1.0	80	11%
Gushers				
all flavors	1 pouch	1.0	90	10%
(Nabisco)				
Capri fruit rolls				
fruit punch	1 pkg	2.0	80	23%
strawberry kiwi	1 pkg	2.0	80	23%
fruit snacks				
Blue's Clues/assorted	1 pkg	–	60	–
Dora the Explorer	1 pkg	–	60	–
Fairly Odd Parents/assorted	1 pkg	–	80	–
Jimmy Neutron/assorted	1 pkg	–	80	–
Rugrats/assorted	1 pkg	–	80	–
Spongebob Squarepants /assorted	1 pkg	–	80	–
variety/value pack	1 pkg	–	80	–
rolls				
Rugrats/strawberry	1 pkg	2.0	70	26%

FRUIT SPREAD (*See* JAM/JELLY/PRESERVES)

G

Food and Description	Amount	Fat Grams	Total Calories	% Fat Calories
GARBANZO BEAN (*See* CHICKPEA/GARBANZO BEAN)				
GARLIC (*See also* SEASONINGS)				
FRESH/RAW				
(Frieda's Elephant)	1 Tbs	–	5	–
minced	1 clove	–	4	–
whole	1 clove	–	5	–
JAR				
(Christopher Ranch)				
chopped	1 tsp	1.0	10	90%
roasted	2 cloves	–	10	–
(Frieda's)				
marinated	1 oz	–	30	–
POWDERED				
(Spice Island)	1 tsp	–	5	–
GARLIC SALT (*See also* SEASONINGS)				
(Lawry's)	1 tsp	–	4	–

Food and Description	Amount	Fat Grams	Total Calories	% Fat Calories
GEFILTE FISH				
(Manischewitz)				
jelled broth				
fish only	1 piece	3.0	70	39%
w/jell	1 piece	3.0	70	39%
non-jelled				
fish only	1 piece	5.0	70	64%
sweet				
14.5 oz jar	1 piece	1.5	80	17%
24 oz jar	1 piece	2.0	90	20%
4 lb jar	1 piece	1.0	60	15%
whitefish & pike				
jelled broth				
fish only	1 piece	1.5	50	27%
w/jell	1 piece	1.5	70	19%
(Mother's)				
all whitefish				
jelled..1.5 oz	1 piece	2.0	45	40%
in liquid..1.5 oz	1 piece	1.5	40	34%
d'oeuvres..in liquid broth	5 balls	3.0	60	45%
fish d'oeuvres..liquid broth	5 balls	3.0	60	45%
old world				
regular	1 ball	1.0	70	13%
sweet	1 ball	1.0	55	16%
unsalted	1 ball	1.0	45	20%
whitefish-pike				
jelled..1.5 oz	1 piece	2.0	40	45%
in liquid..1.5 oz	1 piece	1.5	40	34%
in liquid..2 oz	1 piece	2.0	50	36%
whitefish-pike..old-fashioned				
jelled..2 oz	1 piece	2.5	50	45%
(Rokeach)				
Old Vienna	1.5 oz	1.5	40	34%
regular	1.5 oz	2.0	45	40%
GELATIN				
(Knox)				
Nutra Joint drink mix/orange	1 scoop	–	40	–
unflavored gelatin	1 pkt	–	25	–
GELATIN DESSERT MIX				
(Best Yet)				
regular				
all flavors..prepared	½ cup	–	80	–
sugar-free/prepared				
all flavors	½ cup	–	10	–
(Con-Gelli)				
Rompope	⅛ pkg	–	100	–
strawberry	⅛ pkg	–	100	–

Food and Description	Amount	Fat Grams	Total Calories	% Fat Calories
(Hain) SuperFruits dessert mix				
cherry				
prepared	½ cup	–	70	–
orange				
prepared	½ cup	–	70	–
raspberry				
prepared	½ cup	–	70	–
strawberry				
prepared	½ cup	–	90	–
(Jell-O) prepared				
Jell-O 1–2–3				
strawberry	⅔ cup	1.5	130	10%
original				
regular..all flavors	½ cup	–	80	–
sugar-free..all flavors	½ cup	–	10	–
(Jell-Well)				
regular..all flavors	½ cup	–	80	–
sugar-free..all flavors	½ cup	–	10	–
(Royal)				
apple..regular	½ cup	–	70	–
blackberry..regular	½ cup	–	70	–
cherry				
regular	½ cup	–	70	–
sugar-free	½ cup	–	10	–
Concord grape..regular	½ cup	–	80	–
Jamaica..regular	½ cup	–	70	–
lemon..regular	½ cup	–	80	–
lime				
regular	½ cup	–	70	–
sugar-free	½ cup	–	10	–
mango..regular	½ cup	–	70	–
mixed berry..regular	½ cup	–	80	–
orange				
regular	½ cup	–	70	–
sugar-free	½ cup	–	10	–
peach..regular	½ cup	–	80	–
pineapple..regular	½ cup	–	80	–
raspberry				
regular	½ cup	–	70	–
sugar-free	½ cup	–	10	–
strawberry				
regular	½ cup	–	70	–
sugar-free	½ cup	–	10	–
strawberry banana..regular	½ cup	–	80	–
tamarindo..regular	½ cup	–	70	–
GELATIN, READY TO SERVE				
(Hunt's) Snack Pack				
juicy gels/cups				
all flavors	1 cup	–	100	–

Food and Description	Amount	Fat Grams	Total Calories	% Fat Calories
(Jell-O)				
GELATIN SNACKS				
black cherry/sugar-free	1 snack	–	10	–
cherry				
regular	1 snack	–	70	–
sugar-free	1 snack	–	10	–
orange				
regular	1 snack	–	70	–
sugar-free	1 snack	–	10	–
Mystery Magical Twist	1 snack	–	80	–
raspberry				
regular	1 snack	–	70	–
sugar-free	1 snack	–	10	–
raspberry & orange				
sugar-free	1 snack	–	10	–
Spaceship Strawberry				
& tropical punch w/yogurt	1 snack	1.0	110	8%
strawberry				
fat-free	1 snack	–	80	–
regular	1 snack	–	60	–
sugar-free	1 snack	–	10	–
strawberry & orange	1 snack	–	70	–
strawberry & raspberry	1 snack	–	70	–
tropical berry/sugar-free	1 snack	–	10	–
tropical fruit punch	1 snack	–	70	–
watermelon/sugar-free	1 snack	–	10	–
Wild Watermelon	1 snack	–	70	–
X-treme				
blue raspberry/sticks	1 stick	–	60	–
cherry & blue raspberry	1 snack	–	100	–
cotton candy				
& bubble gum	1 snack	–	140	–
variety/sticks	1 snack	–	60	–
watermelon	1 snack	–	100	–
watermelon				
& cotton candy	1 snack	–	60	–
& green apple	1 snack	–	100	–
wild berry	1 snack	–	80	–
GIN (*See* LIQUOR, DISTILLED)				
GINGER ALE (*See* SOFT DRINK)				
GINGER ROOT				
candied	1 oz	–	95	–
fresh/raw/sliced	5 slices	–	8	–
	¼ cup	–	17	–
powdered-ground	1 tsp	–	6	–
GINGERBREAD (*See* BREAD; CAKE)				
GINKGO				
canned	1 oz	0.5	32	14%
dried	1 oz	0.6	99	5%
raw	1 oz	–	52	–

Food and Description	Amount	Fat Grams	Total Calories	% Fat Calories
GIZZARD (*See* CHICKEN; GOOSE; TURKEY)				
GOAT/boneless				
raw	4 oz	3.0	125	22%
roasted	3 oz	3.0	122	22%
roasted/diced	1 cup	4.0	200	18%
GOOSE (*See also* PÂTÉ)				
domesticated/roasted				
gizzard, raw	3 oz	4.5	119	34%
liver raw	3 oz	3.6	114	28%
meat & skin	~2 lb	170.0	2362	65%
meat only	4 oz	14.5	270	48%
	1¼ lbs	75.0	1406	48%
GOOSEBERRY				
canned/in light syrup	½ cup	–	93	–
raw	1 cup	0.9	67	12%
GOULASH (*See* BEEF DISH/ENTRÉE; FROZEN ENTRÉE/DINNER)				
GOURD				
dishcloth				
boiled/drained	½ cup	0.5	65	7%
boiled/drained/sliced	½ cup	0.3	50	5%
raw	~ 8.5 oz	0.5	40	11%
raw/sliced	½ cup	–	10	–
wax				
boiled/drained	½ cup	–	15	–
boiled/drained/chopped	½ cup	–	11	–
raw	~1 lb	<1.0	45	10%
raw/chopped	½ cup	–	8	–
white				
boiled/drained	½ cup	–	17	–
boiled/drained/chopped	½ cup	–	11	–
raw	~1 lb	<1.0	45	10%
raw/chopped	½ cup	–	8	–
GRAHAM CRACKER (*See* COOKIE; CRACKER)				
GRAHAM CRACKER CRUMBS (*See* CRACKER CRUMBS/MEAL)				
GRANADILLA (*See* PASSIONFRUIT/GRANADILLA)				
GRANOLA (*See* CEREAL)				
GRANOLA/GRANOLA-TYPE BAR (*See* also BREAKFAST/CEREAL BAR)				
(Atkins)				
Advantage bar				
almond brownie	1 bar	10.0	230	39%
chocolate				
coconut	1 bar	13.0	250	47%
mocha crunch	1 bar	10.0	220	41%
peanut butter	1 bar	13.0	218	54%
cookie 'n' cream	1 bar	11.0	220	45%
(Barbara's)				
Dipped Dessert bars				
chocolate				
coconut almond	1 bar	4.5	120	34%

Food and Description	Amount	Fat Grams	Total Calories	% Fat Calories
espresso bean	1 bar	3.0	120	23%
roasted peanut	1 bar	4.5	130	31%
granola bars				
carob chip	1 bar	2.0	80	23%
cinnamon & raisin	1 bar	2.0	80	23%
oats 'n' honey	1 bar	2.0	80	23%
peanut butter	1 bar	3.0	80	34%
(Carb Solutions) Taste Sensations!				
high-protein				
chocolate				
chip cookie dough	1 bar	10.0	230	39%
fudge almond	1 bar	12.0	250	43%
peanut butter	1 bar	12.0	250	43%
toffee hazelnut	1 bar	11.0	240	41%
(Carbolite)				
Nutrition Bars				
lemon crispy	1 bar	4.5	110	37%
peanut butter crispy	1 bar	5.0	120	38%
s'mores crispy	1 bar	5.0	110	41%
Snack Bars				
caramel bar	1 bar	14.0	170	74%
CarbAway caramel				
nougat	1 bar	5.0	100	45%
Carborite crisp wafer	1 bar	8.0	120	60%
chocolate				
coconut	1 bar	8.0	110	65%
coconut almond	1 bar	8.0	120	60%
crispy caramel bar	1 bar	9.0	130	55%
peanut butter cup	1 bar	5.0	100	45%
peanut caramel nougat	1 bar	14.0	170	71%
pecan cluster	1 bar	8.0	120	60%
toffee bar	1 bar	6.0	110	49%
(Doctor's)				
CarbRite Diet				
blueberry cheesecake	1 bar	3.5	199	16%
chocolate				
banana nut	1 bar	4.0	195	18%
brownie bar	1 bar	3.3	185	16%
mint	1 bar	3.3	185	16%
peanut butter	1 bar	4.0	190	19%
s'mores	1 bar	4.0	190	19%
raspberry chocolate truffle	1 bar	4.0	206	17%
diet				
cinnamon bun bar	1 bar	3.5	200	16%
diet sugar-free				
chocolate				
dark	½ piece	2.0	31	58%
dark w/almonds	½ piece	2.5	33	68%
milk	½ piece	2.25	32	63%

Food and Description	Amount	Fat Grams	Total Calories	% Fat Calories
w/soy crisps	1 square	2.0	30	60%
mint	½ piece	2.25	32	63%
white	½ piece	2.25	32	63%
(EAS) AdvantEdge Carb Control				
apple cinnamon	1 bar	5.0	210	21%
chocolate				
chip brownie	1 bar	6.0	210	26%
cream pie	1 bar	6.0	220	25%
peanut butter	1 bar	7.0	220	29%
cookies & cream	1 bar	5.0	210	21%
lemon cheesecake	1 bar	5.0	210	21%
(Full Circle) granola bars chewy				
apple cinnamon	1 bar	1.0	100	9%
peanut crunch	1 bar	3.0	110	25%
wild berry/all-natural	1 bar	1.0	100	9%
(Genisoy)				
Genisoy Xtreme..1.6-oz bars				
Carrot Cake Quake	1 bar	7.0	190	33%
crunch				
low-carb				
chocolate	1 bar	6.0	160	34%
lemon	1 bar	4.5	150	27%
peanut butter	1 bar	6.0	160	34%
raspberry	1 bar	4.5	150	27%
regular				
Island Blast	1 bar	2.0	160	11%
Lemon Shot	1 bar	3.5	170	19%
Peanut Butter Fix	1 bar	8.0	200	36%
Raspberry Rush	1 bar	7.0	190	33%
Rocky Road Trip	1 bar	7.0	190	33%
Rugged Trails	1 Bar	4.0	170	21%
Summit Smash	1 bar	3.0	160	17%
Genisoy Soy Protein..2.2-oz bars				
Arctic Frost Crispy				
chocolate mint	1 bar	4.5	240	17%
~¾ oz	1 bar	1.5	70	19%
Dutch crunch sour				
apple crisp	1 bar	4.5	230	18%
Fair Trade Arabica Café				
mocha fudge	1 bar	4.0	230	16%
New York–style blue-				
berry cheesecake	1 bar	3.5	220	14%
Obsession Fudge cookies				
& crème	1 bar	4.5	240	17%
pure golden honey creamy				
peanut yogurt	1 bar	5.0	230	20%
Southern-style chunky				
peanut butter fudge	1 bar	7.0	240	26%
Ultimate Chocolate				
fudge brownie	1 bar	4.5	230	18%

Food and Description	Amount	Fat Grams	Total Calories	% Fat Calories
(Glenny's) brown rice treat				
carob mint w/oat bran	1 bar	2.0	180	10%
cinnamon & raisin	1 bar	1.0	170	5%
peanut & raisin	1 bar	5.0	210	21%
plain & fancy	1 bar	1.0	120	8%
raisin bran	1 bar	1.0	170	5%
toasted almond w/oat bran	1 bar	5.0	200	23%
(Golden Temple)				
Wha Guru Chew snack bars				
almond ginger	1 bar	9.0	150	54%
cashew				
almond	1 bar	10.0	160	56%
vanilla	1 bar	9.0	150	54%
peanut cashew	1 bar	11.0	160	62%
sesame almond	1 bar	11.0	160	62%
(Health Valley)				
Bakes..fat-free				
apple	1 bar	–	70	–
date	1 bar	–	70	–
raisin	1 bar	–	70	–
Café creations				
chocolate				
espresso	1 bar	3.0	130	21%
raspberry	1 bar	3.0	130	21%
cinnamon Danish	1 bar	2.5	130	17%
granola bar				
fat-free				
blueberry	1 bar	–	140	–
chocolate-flavor chip	1 bar	–	140	–
Dutch apple	1 bar	1.0	100	9%
moist & chewy				
peanut crunch	1 bar	3.0	110	25%
raisin	1 bar	–	140	–
raspberry	1 bar	–	140	–
strawberry	1 bar	–	140	–
wild berry	1 bar	1.0	100	9%
peanut butter bars				
w/chocolate	1 bar	2.5	130	17%
w/grape	1 bar	2.5	130	17%
w/strawberry	1 bar	2.5	130	17%
sandwich bars				
low-fat				
Bavarian creme	1 bar	2.0	130	8%
vanilla crème	1 bar	2.0	130	8%
(Kashi) GoLean Bars				
high protein/fiber				
chocolate almond toffee	1 bar	6.0	290	19%
cookies 'n' cream	1 bar	6.0	290	19%
frosted spice cake	1 bar	5.0	290	16%
honey vanilla yogurt	1 bar	5.0	290	16%

Food and Description	Amount	Fat Grams	Total Calories	% Fat Calories
malted chocolate crisp	1 bar	6.0	290	19%
mocha java	1 bar	6.0	290	19%
oatmeal raisin cookie	1 bar	5.0	280	16%
peanut butter & chocolate	1 bar	6.0	290	19%
strawberries 'n' cream	1 bar	5.0	290	16%
(Kellogg's)				
crunchy granola bar/low-fat				
almond & brown sugar	1 bar	1.5	80	17%
apple spice	1 bar	1.5	80	17%
cinnamon raisin	1 bar	1.5	80	17%
Krave Bars				
chocolate delight	1 bar	7.0	200	32%
chocolate peanut	1 bar	7.0	200	32%
Nutri-Grain				
bars..~1 oz				
Chocolaty chips	1 bar	3.5	100	32%
honey, oat & raisin	1 bar	3.0	110	25%
chewy bites				
caramel nut crunch	1 pouch	6.0	130	42%
chocolaty chip	1 pouch	6.0	120	45%
Rice Krispies Treats Squares				
chocolaty drizzle	1 bar	3.0	100	27%
double chocolaty chunk	1 bar	4.0	100	36%
original	1 bar	2.0	90	20%
rainbow	1 bar	3.0	100	27%
(KETO) High Protein				
chocolate				
fudge	1 bar	7.0	260	24%
peanut butter	1 bar	9.0	270	30%
(Kudos) whole-grain bar				
chocolate chip	1 bar	4.5	120	34%
chocolate fudge	1 bar	4.5	120	34%
milk chocolate				
chocolate chip	1 bar	5.0	130	35%
fruit & nut	1 bar	3.0	90	30%
M&M's milk chocolate minis	1 bar	3.0	100	27%
peanut butter	1 bar	6.0	130	42%
Snickers bar	1 bar	3.5	100	32%
(Luna)				
Glow snack bar				
low-carb				
chocolate peanut crunch	1 bar	7.0	140	45%
fudge almond brownie	1 bar	7.0	140	45%
strawberry caramel sundae	1 bar	7.0	140	45%
Nutrition bar for women				
caramel apple	1 bar	2.5	180	13%
chai tea	1 bar	4.0	180	20%
cherry-covered chocolate	1 bar	4.0	180	20%
chocolate peppermint stick	1 bar	4.0	180	20%
chocolate pecan pie	1 bar	4.5	180	23%

Food and Description	Amount	Fat Grams	Total Calories	% Fat Calories
dulce de leche	1 bar	2.5	180	13%
key lime pie	1 bar	4.0	180	20%
lemon zest	1 bar	4.0	180	20%
Nutz over Chocolate	1 bar	4.5	180	23%
Orange Bliss	1 bar	4.0	180	20%
peanut butter 'n' jelly	1 bar	2.5	170	13%
s'mores	1 bar	4.5	180	23%
sesame raisin crunch	1 bar	3.0	170	16%
toasted nuts 'n cranberry	1 bar	3.0	180	15%
Sweet Dreams	1 bar	4.0	180	20%
tropical crisp	1 bar	4.5	180	23%
(Nature Valley)				
granola bar				
banana nut	2 bars	7.0	190	33%
cinnamon	2 bars	6.0	180	30%
maple brown sugar	2 bars	6.0	180	30%
oats 'n' honey	2 bars	6.0	180	30%
peanut butter	2 bars	6.0	180	30%
roasted almond	2 bars	7.0	190	33%
variety pack	2 bars	6.0	180	30%
Trail Mix Bar				
apple cinnamon	1 bar	6.0	150	36%
fruit & nut	1 bar	4.0	140	26%
Nutri-Grain (See (Kellogg's) in this section)				
(Odwalla) Odwalla Bar Caddys				
carrot	1 bar	3.0	220	12%
chocolate	1 bar	6.0	240	23%
chocolate chip peanut	1 bar	7.0	250	25%
Cranberry C Monster	1 bar	2.5	220	10%
peanut crunch	1 bar	7.0	260	24%
super protein	1 bar	5.0	240	19%
superfood	1 bar	5.0	230	20%
(PowerBar)				
PowerBar Energy bites				
chocolate crisp	1.78 oz	5.0	200	23%
oatmeal raisin crisp	1.78 oz	5.0	210	21%
peanut butter crisp	1.78 oz	5.0	210	21%
PowerBar Performance bar				
apple cinnamon	1 bar	2.5	230	10%
banana	1 bar	2.0	230	8%
cappuccino	1 bar	2.0	230	8%
chocolate	1 bar	2.0	230	8%
chocolate peanut butter	1 bar	3.0	240	11%
cookies & cream	1 bar	2.5	230	10%
malt nuts	1 bar	2.5	230	10%
oatmeal raisin	1 bar	2.5	230	10%
peanut butter	1 bar	3.5	240	13%
raspberry & cream stripes	1 bar	2.0	230	8%
vanilla crisp	1 bar	2.5	230	10%

Food and Description	Amount	Fat Grams	Total Calories	% Fat Calories
wild berry	1 bar	2.5	230	10%
(Pria)				
bars..1 oz				
chocolate				
honey graham	1 bar	3.0	110	25%
peanut crunch	1 bar	3.5	110	29%
crème caramel crisp	1 bar	3.0	110	25%
double chocolate cookie	1 bar	3.0	110	25%
French vanilla	1 bar	3.0	110	25%
strawberry shortcake	1 bar	3.0	110	25%
Carbselect triple-layer nutrition bar				
caramel nut brownie	1 bar	8.0	170	42%
cookies 'n' caramel	1 bar	7.0	170	37%
peanut butter caramel nut	1 bar	8.0	170	42%
(Quaker)				
CHEWY				
Dips				
caramel nut	1 bar	6.0	140	30%
chocolate chip	1 bar	6.0	150	36%
peanut butter	1 bar	8.0	150	48%
fruit 'n' crunch bars				
apple crisp	1 bar	3.5	160	20%
raspberry	1 bar	3.5	160	20%
strawberry	1 bar	3.5	160	20%
granola bars				
Blastin' Chocolate	1 bar	3.0	110	25%
chocolate				
chip	1 bar	4.0	120	30%
Graham Slam	1 bar	2.0	110	16%
Chunk	1 bar	2.0	110	16%
cookies 'n' cream/low-fat	1 bar	2.5	110	20%
oatmeal raisin	1 bar	2.0	220	16%
peanut butter	1 bar	3.5	110	29%
& chocolate chunk	1 bar	3.0	120	23%
Peanut Butter Graham Slam	1 bar	2.0	110	16%
s'mores/low-fat	1 bar	2.0	110	16%
WHOLESOME				
baked apple	1 bar	2.0	110	16%
cinnamon sugar	1 bar	2.0	110	16%
oatmeal raisin	1 bar	2.0	110	16%
(Slim Fast)				
CARB OPTIONS/MEAL BARS				
chocolate				
chip brownie	1 bar	8.0	200	36%
delight	1 bar	8.0	200	36%
peanut	1 bar	8.0	200	36%
cinnamon delight	1 bar	8.0	200	36%
MEAL OPTIONS/MEAL BARS				
chewy chocolate chip				
1.97-oz single	1 bar	6.0	330	16%

Food and Description	Amount	Fat Grams	Total Calories	% Fat Calories
cranberry apple				
1.97-oz single	1 bar	5.0	220	20%
mixed berry				
1.97-oz single	1 bar	5.0	220	20%
peanut butter				
1.97-oz single	1 bar	6.0	220	25%
SLIM-FAST OPTIMA SNACK BARS				
chocolate peanut nougat	1 bar	4.0	120	30%
crispy peanut caramel	1 bar	4.0	120	30%
peanut butter crunch	1 bar	4.0	120	30%
SLIM-FAST OPTIONS SNACK BARS				
chewy chocolate nougat	1 bar	3.5	120	26%
crispy peanut caramel	1 bar	4.0	120	30%
peanut butter crunch	1 bar	4.0	130	28%
peanut nougat	1 bar	4.0	120	30%
rich chewy caramel	1 bar	4.0	120	30%
SLIM-FAST SUCCEED LOW-CARD				
snack bars				
banana nut	1 bar	3.0	120	23%
chocolate peanut	1 bar	3.0	120	23%
cookies 'n' cream	1 bar	3.0	120	23%
SNACK BARS				
low-carb				
caramel nut	1 bar	5.0	120	38%
chocolate peanut				
w/chocolate coating	1 bar	3.0	120	23%
coconut almond	1 bar	5.0	120	23%
cookies 'n' cream	1 bar	3.0	120	23%
peanut butter crunch	1 bar	4.5	120	34%
rocky road	1 bar	5.0	130	35%
(Sunbelt)				
chewy granola bars				
chocolate chip				
fudge-dipped/1.5-oz bar	1 bar	13.0	270	43%
regular 1.78-oz bar	1 bar	10.0	230	39%
coconut/fudge-dipped	1 bar	16.0	300	48%
oats & honey/1.7 oz	1 bar	9.0	220	37%
GRAPE				
CANNED/PLASTIC CONTAINER				
(Oregon) fruit products				
Thompson/seedless grapes				
in light syrup	4.5 oz	–	100	–
(Welch's) single serve	¾ cup	1.0	90	10%
FRESH WITH OR WITHOUT SEEDS				
Concord	10 grapes	<1.0	15	15%
	½ cup	<1.0	30	15%
(Dole)	½ cups	1.0	90	10%

Food and Description	Amount	Fat Grams	Total Calories	% Fat Calories
muscat	10 grapes	<1.0	40	8%
	½ cup	<1.0	55	8%
Thompson	10 grapes	<1.0	40	8%
	½ cup	<1.0	55	8%
tokay	10 grapes	<1.0	40	8%
(Welch's)				
all types	1½ cups	1.0	90	10%
GRAPE JUICE/JUICE BLEND				
BOTTLED/BOXED OR CANNED				
(After the Fall)				
sparkling grape juice	8 fl oz	–	130	–
special harvest Concord				
grape	8 fl oz	–	120	–
(Apple & Eve)				
Light & Fruitful..low-carb				
cranberry grape blend	8 fl oz	–	40	–
Sesame Street, Grover's				
white grape	8 fl oz	–	130	–
white grape strawberry/pouch	6.75 oz	–	90	–
(Libby's) Juicy Juice				
100% grape juice	4.23 fl oz	–	70	–
	6.75 fl oz	–	100	–
	8 fl oz	–	130	–
	8.45 fl oz	–	160	–
(Meier's)				
sparkling				
pink Catawba	8 fl oz	–	150	–
white Catawba	8 fl oz	–	140	–
(Minute Maid) 100% juice	6.75 fl oz	–	100	–
(R. W. Knudsen)				
Concord	8 fl oz	–	160	–
(Seneca)				
purple grape	8 fl oz	–	160	–
white grape	8 fl oz	–	160	–
(Welch's)				
Concord grape				
cranberry	8 fl oz	–	140	–
mango	8 fl oz	–	140	–
strawberry	8 fl oz	–	140	–
grape	8 fl oz	–	170	–
	10 fl oz	–	210	–
	11.5 fl oz	–	240	–
grape apple	8 fl oz	–	150	–
purple grape	5.5 fl oz	–	120	–
	8 fl oz	–	170	–
Juicemakers	8 fl oz	–	170	–
red grape	8 fl oz	–	170	–
	8.45 fl oz	–	170	–
sparkling				
red grape	8 fl oz	–	160	–
white	8 fl oz	–	150	–

Food and Description	Amount	Fat Grams	Total Calories	% Fat Calories
USDA grape	8 fl oz	–	170	–
white grape				
berry	8 fl oz	–	140	–
cherry	8 fl oz	–	140	–
cranberry	8 fl oz	–	160	–
juice cocktail	8 fl oz	–	150	–
peach	8 fl oz	–	160	–
pear	8 fl oz	–	150	–
raspberry	8 fl oz	–	150	–
regular	5.5 fl oz	–	110	–
	8 fl oz	–	160	–
	8.45 fl oz	–	160	–
strawberry	8 fl oz	–	140	–
w/calcium	8 fl oz	–	170	–
FROZEN/CHILLED/REFRIGERATED				
(Old Orchard)				
grape juice concentrate	2 oz	–	160	–
prepared	8 fl oz	–	160	–
white grape juice				
concentrate	2 oz	–	160	–
prepared	8 fl oz	–	160	–
(Seneca) prepared				
blush grape	8 fl oz	–	160	–
purple grape	8 fl oz	–	160	–
white grape	8 fl oz	–	140	–
(Welch's) prepared				
100% grape	8 fl oz	–	160	–
purple grape				
regular	8 fl oz	–	170	–
sweetened	8 fl oz	–	130	–
red grape	8 fl oz	–	170	–
white grape				
regular	8 fl oz	–	170	–
sweetened	8 fl oz	–	140	–
w/all combinations	8 fl oz	–	150	–
GRAPE JUICE DRINK (See also FRUIT PUNCH; SOFT DRINK; SOFT DRINK MIX)				
BOTTLED/BOXED OR CANNED				
(Capri Sun) pouch	6.75 fl oz	–	100	–
(Hi-C)				
box	8.45 fl oz	–	130	–
can	7.7 fl oz	–	110	–
(Libby's) Juicy Juice	6 fl oz	–	90	–
	8.45 fl oz	–	130	–
(Snapple) Grapeade	8 fl oz	–	120	–
(R. W. Knudsen)				
fruit juice spritzer..grape	12 fl oz	–	170	–
(TreeTop) Juice Rivers grape punch	1 box	–	130	–
(Topicana) Chilled				
grape punch..light	8 fl oz	–	60	–
Trop 50 grape				

Food and Description	Amount	Fat Grams	Total Calories	% Fat Calories
50% juice	10 fl oz	–	65	–
Tropicana classics grape	11.5 oz	–	230	–
Twister white grape kiwi wave (Welch's)	8 fl oz	–	130	–
Concord grape juice cocktail	8 fl oz	–	130	–
grape juice cocktail	8 fl oz	–	150	–
	10 fl oz	–	170	–
grape juice drink	8 fl oz	–	130	–
	8.45 fl oz	–	150	–
	10 fl oz	–	170	–
grape apple juice cocktail	8 fl oz	–	150	–
grape apple juice drink	8.45 fl oz	–	150	–
	10 fl oz	–	160	–
grape peach juice cocktail	8 fl oz	–	130	–
	10 fl oz	–	160	–
sparkling red grape juice drink	8 fl oz	–	160	–
sparkling white grape juice drink	8 fl oz	–	160	–
sparkling white grape				
cranberry	8 fl oz	–	160	–
Welchade	8 fl oz	–	130	–
white grape				
juice cocktail	8.45 fl oz	–	160	–
FROZEN/prepared				
(Seneca) cocktail	10 fl oz	–	130	–
(Welch's)				
Concord grape	8 fl oz	–	150	–
	10 fl oz	–	170	–
grape juice cocktail..light	8 fl oz	–	50	–
passionfruit blended juice	8 fl oz	–	140	–
Welchade	8 fl oz	–	130	–
white grape				
cranberry juice cocktail	8 fl oz	–	140	–
peach juice blend	8 fl oz	–	150	–
pear	8 fl oz	–	150	–
raspberry				
juice blend	8 fl oz	–	150	–
juice cocktail..low-cal	8 fl oz	–	15	–
GRAPE LEAVES				
FRESH				
generic	1 cup	–	13	–
	1 leaf	–	5	–
CAN or JAR				
(Alma)				
California	2 leaves	–	10	–
imported	2 leaves	–	10	–
(Fancifoods)	2 leaves	–	5	–
(Krinos)	1 leaf	–	5	–
(Orlando California) drained	1 leaf	–	5	–
(Peloponnese) stuffed				
traditional Greek appetizer	3.3 oz	7.0	140	45%

Food and Description	Amount	Fat Grams	Total Calories	% Fat Calories
GRAPE SODA (See SOFT DRINK)				
GRAPEFRUIT				
*CAN, JAR, or POUCH/*sections				
(Del Monte)				
Fruit Naturals..red				
grapefruit/pouch	½ cup	–	60	–
red grapefruit..can	½ cup	–	80	–
Sunfresh..jar				
citrus salad	½ cup	–	45	–
red grapefruit	½ cup	–	80	–
in slightly sweetened				
fruit juice	½ cup	–	60	–
white in real fruit juice	½ cup	–	80	–
*FRESH/*whole				
(Dole)	½ medium	–	60	–
(Ocean Spray)				
pink	½ medium	–	50	–
white	½ medium	–	50	–
GRAPEFRUIT JUICE/JUICE BLEND				
BOTTLED, BOXED, OR CANNED				
(Dole) juice blend				
sunripe grapefruit..100%	8 fl oz	–	130	–
	10 fl oz	–	160	–
	11.5 oz	–	185	–
(Haggen) ruby-red grapefruit				
& tangerine juice	8 fl oz	–	130	–
(Minute Maid)				
grapefruit	8 fl oz	–	100	–
pink grapefruit blend	8 fl oz	–	125	–
100% grapefruit	8 fl oz	–	100	–
(Odwalla) Essentials				
grapefruit juice	8 fl oz	–	110	–
(Ocean Spray)				
Premium 100%				
pink grapefruit	8 fl oz	–	110	–
ruby red	8 fl oz	–	130	–
white grapefruit juice	8 fl oz	–	100	–
(R. W. Knudsen) 100% juice				
Rio red grapefruit	8 fl oz	–	140	–
(Tree Sweet)				
100% grapefruit				
original from concentrate	8 fl oz	–	90	–
individual cans	5.5 fl oz	–	60	–
100% pink grapefruit				
original from concentrate				
individual cans	5.5 fl oz	–	60	–
(Tropicana)				
pure premium				
golden	6 fl oz	–	80	–
	8 fl oz	–	90	–

Food and Description	Amount	Fat Grams	Total Calories	% Fat Calories
ruby red	6 fl oz	–	70	–
	8 fl oz	–	90	–
	10 fl oz	–	110	–
	14 fl oz	–	160	–
plus calcium	8 fl oz	–	90	–
plus calcium				
& vitamin D	8 fl oz	–	110	–
ruby red orange	8 fl oz	–	120	–
sweet	7 fl oz	–	130	–
Twister				
Grapefruit Tangerine Tango	8 fl oz	–	130	–
ruby red	10 fl oz	–	160	–
(V8 Splash) Juice drink				
citris blend	8 fl oz	–	110	–
(Welch's) single-serve				
100% grapefruit juice				
bottle	10 fl oz	–	130	–
can	5.5 fl oz	–	70	–
white grapefruit juice	8 fl oz	–	100	–
FROZEN				
(Cascadian Farm)				
grapefruit juice				
juice concentrate	2 oz	–	100	–
prepared	8 fl oz	–	100	–
GRAPEFRUIT JUICE DRINK (*See also* FRUIT PUNCH)				
BOTTLED, BOXED, or CANNED				
(Dole) ruby red grapefruit				
juice drink	8 fl oz	–	130	–
	10 fl oz	–	160	–
	11.5 fl oz	–	185	–
(Ocean Spray)				
juice cocktail				
ruby red grapefruit	8 fl oz	–	120	–
ruby lemonade	8 fl oz	–	120	–
ruby mango	8 fl oz	–	120	–
ruby strawberry	8 fl oz	–	130	–
ruby tangerine	8 fl oz	–	120	–
juice drink..light ruby				
red grapefruit juice	8 fl oz	–	40	–
(Snapple Farms) ruby red	8 fl oz	–	120	–
cocktail	12 fl oz	–	190	–
(Tropicana) chilled				
pink grapefruit cocktail	8 fl oz	–	130	–
(Welch's) juice cocktail				
pink grapefruit	10 fl oz	–	120	–
ruby red grapefruit	10 fl oz	–	140	–
	11.5 fl oz	–	200	–
from concentrate	8 fl oz	–	140	–
FROZEN/prepared				
(Dole) Pacific pink grapefruit				
juice drink	8 fl oz		140	–

Food and Description	Amount	Fat Grams	Total Calories	% Fat Calories
(Tropicana) Twister/light pink grapefruit				
juice drink	10 fl oz	–	40	–
GRAPEFRUIT PEEL/candied	1 oz	–	90	–
GRAVY (*See also* SAUCE; SEASONINGS)				
■ **CANNED OR JARRED** (Ready-to-serve)				
(Franco-American)				
au jus	¼ cup	–	5	–
beef				
brown w/ onions	¼ cup	1.0	25	36%
fat-free	¼ cup	–	15	–
slow-roasted	¼ cup	–	20	–
regular	¼ cup	1.0	25	36%
slow-roasted	¼ cup	0.5	25	18%
w/onions	¼ cup	1.0	25	36%
w/roasted garlic	¼ cup	0.5	25	18%
chicken				
fat-free				
slow-roasted	¼ cup	–	15	–
giblet	¼ cup	1.5	25	54%
regular	¼ cup	4.0	40	90%
slow-roasted	¼ cup	0.5	25	18%
w/roasted garlic	¼ cup	2.0	35	51%
country-style				
cream	¼ cup	2.5	35	64%
sausage	¼ cup	4.5	70	58%
mushroom				
creamy	¼ cup	0.5	20	45%
regular	¼ cup	1.0	20	45%
pork/golden	¼ cup	3.0	40	68%
turkey				
fat-free				
regular	¼ cup	–	20	–
slow-roasted	¼ cup	–	20	–
regular	¼ cup	1.0	25	36%
slow-roasted	¼ cup	0.5	25	18%
(Heinz)				
au jus/bistro-style	¼ cup	–	10	–
beef/home-style				
regular	¼ cup	1.0	25	36%
w/onions	¼ cup	1.0	25	36%
brown/savory	¼ cup	1.0	25	36%
chicken				
classic	¼ cup	1.0	30	30%
fat-free	¼ cup	–	15	–
country..home-style	¼ cup	1.0	25	36%
mushroom..home-style	¼ cup	1.0	25	36%
pork/home-style	¼ cup	1.0	25	36%
turkey				
fat-free	¼ cup	–	15	–
home-style	¼ cup	1.0	25	36%

Food and Description	Amount	Fat Grams	Total Calories	% Fat Calories
(Libby's)				
sausage/country	¼ cup	5.0	70	64%
■ **MIX** (Note: Unless stated otherwise, 1 serving of mix = the amount in ¼ cup prepared)				
(Durkee) mix/prepared				
au jus	1 serving	–	5	–
brown				
chicken	1 serving	1.0	20	45%
country	1 serving	2.0	35	51%
herb	1 serving	1.0	15	60%
home-style	1 serving	1.0	10	90%
mushroom	1 serving	–	15	–
onion	1 serving	–	10	–
original	1 serving	1.0	10	90%
pork	1 serving	–	10	–
sausage	1 serving	2.0	35	51%
Swiss steak	1 serving	–	15	–
turkey	1 serving	–	20	–
(Knorr) mix only				
au jus	⅕ pkg	–	15	–
brown/classic	⅙ pkg	0.5	20	23%
chicken/roasted	⅕ pkg	1.0	30	30%
hunter mushroom/classics	⅕ pkg	1.0	25	36%
turkey	⅕ pkg	0.5	25	18%
(Lawry's)				
au jus	⅛ pkt	–	10	–
brown	¼ pkt	–	20	–
chicken	¼ pkt	1.0	25	36%
turkey	¼ pkt	1.0	25	36%
(Loma Linda)..Quik..Mix only				
brown	1 Tbs	–	20	–
chicken	1 Tbs	–	20	–
country	1 Tbs	0.5	20	23%
mushroom	1 Tbs	–	15	–
onion	1 Tbs	–	15	–
(McCormick/Schilling) mix only				
au jus	½ tsp	–	5	–
beef & herb	¼ pkg	1.0	30	30%
brown				
herb	2 tsp	0.5	20	23%
regular	1 Tbs	0.5	20	23%
chicken & herb /roasted	¼ pkg	1.0	25	36%
country				
low-fat	⅛ pkg	2.0	40	45%
original	⅛ pkg	3.5	50	63%
sausage	⅛ pkg	3.0	45	60%
home-style	1 Tbs	1.0	20	36%
mushroom	1 Tbs	0.5	20	23%
onion	2 tsp	0.5	20	23%
pork	1 Tbs	–	20	–
turkey	⅙ pkg	–	20	–

Food and Description	Amount	Fat Grams	Total Calories	% Fat Calories
(Pillsbury) mix only				
all types	¼ pkt	–	15	–
(Pioneer Brand)				
biscuit gravy	⅛ pkt	3.0	50	54%
brown	⅛ pkt	–	20	–
Cajun brown w/Zatarain's				
seasonings	⅛ pkt	–	20	–
chicken	⅛ pkt	1.0	30	30%
country	.31 oz	3.0	50	54%
country sausage	⅛ pkt	2.5	40	56%
peppered	⅛ pkt	3.0	50	54%
turkey	⅛ pkt	1.0	25	36%
(White Lily)				
biscuit gravy	⅛ pkt	3.0	45	60%
brown	⅛ pkt	1.0	30	30%
country	⅛ pkt	3.0	45	60%
pepper	⅛ pkt	3.0	45	60%
■ FROZEN/REFRIGERATED				
(Bob Evans)				
original				
white gravy/pouch	8 oz	23.0	310	67%
white w/pork sausage	9 oz	24.0	330	65%
restaurant brown				
w/pork sausage	9 oz	24.0	330	65%
sausage, gravy & biscuits				
w/original white gravy	13.5 oz	23.0	390	53%
GREAT NORTHERN BEAN				
CANNED				
(Bush's Best)	4.5 oz	0.5	110	4%
(Eden)	½ oz	1.0	110	8%
(Haggen) recipe-ready	5 oz	–	100	–
(Joan of Arc)	½ cup	0.5	100	5%
(Luck's)				
mixed w/pinto beans	4.28 oz	2.0	130	14%
seasoned w/pork	5 oz	3.0	130	21%
(Trappey's) flavored w/sausage	4.28 oz	1.0	110	8%
DRY				
(Bean Cuisine)	½ cup	1.0	115	8%
GREEN BEAN/SNAP BEAN				
CANNED				
(Blue Boy)				
cut	½ cup	–	25	–
french sliced	½ cup	–	25	–
(Bush's Best)				
Blue Lake	½ cup	–	20	–
cut	½ cup	–	20	–
french-style	½ cup	–	20	–
whole	½ cup	–	20	–
w/shelly beans	½ cup	–	45	–

Food and Description	Amount	Fat Grams	Total Calories	% Fat Calories
(Del Monte)				
cut & potatoes w/ham	3 oz	–	30	–
Italian cut	½ cup	–	30	–
other cuts..all types	½ cup	–	20	–
(Festal)				
Blue Lake..cut	½ cup	–	20	–
cut	½ cup	–	20	–
french-style	½ cup	–	20	–
(Green Giant)				
all types	½ cup	–	20	–
(Joan of Arc)				
all types	½ cup	–	20	–
(Libby's)				
cut Blue Lake	½ cup	–	25	–
french-style	½ cup	–	25	–
whole	½ cup	–	25	–
(S&W) young & tender				
all types	½ cup	–	20	–
(Stokely)				
cut	½ cup	–	20	–
cut/no salt or sugar	½ cup	–	20	–
shellie	½ cup	–	45	–
(Stokely's Gold)				
European slender whole	½ cup	–	20	–
Italian flat-cut	½ cup	–	20	–
(The Allen's)				
cut Italian	½ cup	–	35	–
Kentucky wonder–style	½ cup	–	35	–
seasoned Southern-style..fat-free	½ cup	–	45	–
w/potatoes..Kentucky wonder-style	½ cup	–	35	–
French-style..sliced	½ cup	–	25	–
(The Allen's Sunshine)				
cut Italian				
Kentucky wonder–style	½ cup	–	35	–
seasoned Southern-style	½ cup	–	45	–
w/potatoes Kentucky wonder–style	½ cup	–	35	–
long-cut	½ cup	–	30	–
(Veg-All)				
cut	½ cup	–	20	–
French-style Ejotes al estilo frances	½ cup	–	20	–
FRESH/raw	½ cup	–	20	–
FROZEN				
(Birds Eye) green beans				
& spaetzle pasta w/bacon	9 oz	15.0	150	90%
& toasted almonds	4 oz	3.5	80	39%

Food and Description	Amount	Fat Grams	Total Calories	% Fat Calories
cut	½ cup	–	25	–
french-cut	½ cup	–	25	–
Italian	½ cup	–	30	–
whole				
deluxe	½ cup	–	45	–
(C&W)				
all styles	¾ cup	–	25	–
(Cascadian Farm)				
cut green beans	½ cup	–	30	–
french green bean casserole	½ cup	5.0	90	50%
green beans w/almonds	½ cup	3.0	70	39%
(Freshlike)				
french-style	3 oz	–	25	–
Italian-style	3 oz	–	30	–
whole	3 oz	–	25	–
(Green Giant)				
cut	½ cup	–	20	–
green bean casserole				
boil-in-bag	⅔ cup	2.5	110	20%
3-bean salad	½ cup	–	90	–
whole green beans	1 cup	–	20	–
(Veg-All)				
French	3 oz	–	30	–
Italian	3 oz	–	30	–
whole	3 oz	–	25	–

GREEN ONION (*See* SCALLION/GREEN ONION/SPRING ONION)
GRENADINE (*See* COCKTAIL MIXER)
GRITS (*See* CORN GRITS)
GROUND CHERRY

raw	½ cup	0.5	37	12%

GROUPER

cooked—dry heat	3 oz	1.0	100	9%
raw	3 oz	0.9	78	10%

GUACAMOLE (*See* DIP; SEASONINGS)
GUAVA
canned

(Herdez) guavas	7 oz	–	190	–
fresh	1 medium	0.5	45	10%

GUAVA, STRAWBERRY

raw	1 medium	<1.0	4	8%
	1 cup	1.5	169	8%

GUAVA JUICE/JUICE BLEND (*See also* FRUIT/FRUIT JUICE DRINK)

(Kern's) nectar	6 fl oz	–	110	–
(Knudsen) guava strawberry	8 fl oz	–	110	–
(Welch's) frozen, prepared	8 fl oz	–	140	–

GUAVA JUICE DRINK (*See also* FRUIT/FRUIT JUICE DRINK; FRUIT PUNCH; SOFT DRINK MIX)
   BOTTLE or CAN
     (Minute Maid)

guava citrus..light	12 fl oz	–	10	–
fridge pack	12 fl oz	–	10	–

Food and Description	Amount	Fat Grams	Total Calories	% Fat Calories
(V8 Splash)				
guava passionfruit	8 fl oz	–	110	–
GUAVA SAUCE/cooked	½ cup	–	43	–
GUINEA HEN/raw				
meat & skin	1 lb	23.0	568	36%
meat only	3.5 oz	2.5	110	20%
GUINEA PIG/raw	3 oz	1.7	82	19%
GUM				
(Altoids) sugar-free	1 piece	–	5	–
(Bazooka)				
bubble	1 piece	–	15	–
soft				
regular	1 piece	–	30	–
(Beech-Nut)..all flavors	1 piece	–	10	–
spearmint	1 piece	–	10	–
(Bubbaloo)				
burstin' liquid center	1 piece	–	20	–
(Bubble Yum) bubblegum				
mega	1 piece	–	25	–
sugar-free	1 piece	–	15	–
variety	1 piece	–	25	–
all flavors	1 piece	–	25	–
(Cadbury)				
Cinnaburst w/flavor crystals	1 piece	–	10	–
(Carefree) sugarless				
bubblegum	1 piece	–	10	–
cinnamon	1 piece	–	5	–
peppermint	1 piece	–	5	–
spearmint	1 piece	–	5	–
variety	1 piece	–	10	–
wintergreen	1 piece	–	10	–
(Chiclets)				
regular				
fruit	1 piece	–	10	–
tiny size..coated	½ pkg	–	10	–
sugarless..all types	1 piece	–	5	–
(Clorets) w/actizol	1 piece	–	10	–
(Dentyne)				
cinnamon	1 piece	–	10	–
regular	1 piece	–	10	–
sugar-free..all flavors	1 piece	–	5	–
(Dubble Bubble) bubblegum	1 piece	–	20	–
(Dentyne Fire) sugarless				
spicy cinnamon	1 piece	–	5	–
(Dentyne Ice) assorted				
sugarless	1 piece	–	5	–
(Eclipse Fresh Strips)				
thin ice	1 strip	–	–	–
winterfresh	1 strip	–	–	–
(Extra) sugar-free				
all flavors	1 piece	–	5	–

Food and Description	Amount	Fat Grams	Total Calories	% Fat Calories
original	1 piece	–	5	–
(Freedent)..all flavors				
all flavors	1 stick	–	10	–
(Fresh 'n' Up)	1 stick	–	10	–
(Fruit Stripe)				
assorted flavors	1 piece	–	10	–
(Juicy Fruit)	1 piece	–	10	–
(Orbit)	1 piece	–	5	–
(Trident)	1 piece	–	5	–
(Wrigley's)				
Big Red	1 stick	–	10	–
Doublemint	1 stick	–	10	–
Juicy Fruit	1 stick	–	10	–
spearmint	1 stick	–	10	–
Winter Fresh	1 stick	–	10	–

H

Food and Description	Amount	Fat Grams	Total Calories	% Fat Calories
HADDOCK (See also SEAFOOD ENTRÉE/DINNER)				
breaded & fried	3 oz	9.7	194	45%
cooked—dry heat	3 oz	0.8	95	8%
raw	3 oz	0.6	74	7%
smoked	3 oz	0.8	99	7%
HAKE (See WHITING)				
HALIBUT (See also SEAFOOD ENTRÉE/DINNER)				
Atlantic & Pacific				
batter-fried	3 oz	6.0	153	35%
broiled w/butter	3 oz	6.0	140	39%
cooked—dry heat	3 oz	2.5	119	19%
raw	3 oz	2.0	93	19%
smoked	3 oz	12.7	190	60%
Greenland				
raw	3 oz	12.0	160	68%
HAM (See also LUNCHEON MEAT; PORK; TURKEY)				
(Alpine Lace) cooked	2 oz	2.0	60	30%
(Boar's Head)				
Black Forest smoked	2 oz	1.0	60	15%

Food and Description	Amount	Fat Grams	Total Calories	% Fat Calories
Branded deluxe				
50% lower sodium	2 oz	1.0	60	15%
regular	2 oz	1.0	60	15%
Cappy brand	2 oz	1.5	60	23%
gourmet pepper	2 oz	1.0	60	15%
Maple-Glazed Honey Coat	2 oz	1.0	60	15%
pesto Parmesan				
oven-roasted	2 oz	4.0	90	40%
rosemary & sun-dried tomato	2 oz	2.5	70	32%
seasoned fresh ham	2 oz	3.0	80	34%
smoked Virginia ham	2 oz	1.0	60	15%
Sweet Slice boneless smoked	2 oz	3.5	100	32%
tavern	2 oz	1.0	60	15%
Virginia brand				
pineapple topped	2 oz	1.0	60	15%
(Bob Evans)				
ham steaks..sliced	2 oz			
96% fat-free		4.0	120	30%
(Briar Street Market)				
water added				
pre-sliced..3 slices				
honey	2 oz	1.5	60	23%
smoked	2 oz	1.5	60	23%
Slicemaster ham	3 oz	2.5	80	28%
(Bryan)				
bone-in				
Classic Perfection ham steak	8 oz	24.0	370	58%
	5 oz	15.0	230	59%
diced ¼" cube	3 oz	8.0	130	55%
ham & water				
Slicemaster				
chopped	2 oz	2.5	50	45%
regular	3 oz	2.5	80	28%
natural juice				
Classic Carving ham	3 oz	9.0	140	58%
cooked ham	3 oz	9.0	140	58%
pre-sliced				
hickory-smoked	2.5 oz	2.5	90	25%
shaved honey	6 slices	7.0	100	63%
sliced-to-serve	2.5 oz	2.5	90	25%
	2.28 oz	1.0	60	15%
96% fat-free	3 oz	2.5	80	28%
smoked	3 oz	7.0	130	48%
water added				
Hickory Gold Foil Wrap	3 oz	9.0	140	58%
pit ham	3 oz	9.0	140	58%
(DAK) Danish				
baked w/natural juices				
fat-free	1 oz	1.0	30	30%
canned ham	2 oz	7.0	100	63%

Food and Description	Amount	Fat Grams	Total Calories	% Fat Calories
chopped..canned	2 oz	15.0	170	79%
chunk	2 oz	6.0	100	54%
deli-sliced smoked				
97% fat-free	2 oz	2.0	60	30%
honey ham w/natural juices	1 oz	1.0	30	30%
imported slices				
98% fat-free	1.6 oz	1.0	45	20%
premium				
97% fat-free	1 oz	1.0	30	30%
98% fat-free	1.6 oz	1.0	45	20%
premium				
imported..97% fat-free	2 oz	1.5	50	27%
slices..97% fat-free	1 oz	1.0	30	30%
turkey ham..95% fat-free	1 oz	1.5	35	39%
variety pack..ham, honey ham,				
turkey breast..97% fat-free	1 oz	–	20	–
(Danola)				
baked brown sugar	2 oz	1.5	60	23%
Black Forest..smoked	1.6 oz	2.0	60	30%
hickory-smoked	2 oz	1.5	60	23%
imported				
lower sodium				
w/natural juices				
96% fat-free	1.6 oz	2.0	60	30%
regular w/natural juice	2 oz	1.0	50	18%
pepper-smoked..97% fat-free	1.8 oz	1.5	50	27%
premium sliced..98% fat-free	1.8 oz	1.0	45	20%
smoked honey	2 oz	1.5	60	23%
w/natural juices				
97% fat-free	1.6 oz	1.0	50	18%
smoked				
maple-flavored honey	2 oz	2.0	70	26%
pepper	2 oz	1.5	60	23%
Virginia Brand	2 oz	1.5	60	23%
(Dubuque)				
Royal Buffet..can				
extra-lean	3 oz	5.0	110	41%
(Eckrich)				
cooked	1 oz	1.0	30	30%
deli..thin-sliced	1.8 oz	1.5	60	23%
lean smoked..slender-sliced	3 oz	9.0	150	54%
(Farmer John)				
bone-in				
Gold Wrap				
whole	2 oz	7.0	110	57%
butt	2 oz	7.0	110	57%
ham steak	3 oz	7.0	140	45%
shank	2 oz	9.0	130	62%

Food and Description	Amount	Fat Grams	Total Calories	% Fat Calories
boneless				
Golden Tradition ham..smoked				
97% fat-free	2 oz	1.5	70	19%
half	2 oz	1.5	70	19%
honey	2 oz	1.5	70	19%
premium cut	2 oz	1.5	70	19%
sliced	2 oz	1.5	70	19%
spiral-cut	2 oz	1.5	70	19%
whole	2 oz	1.5	70	19%
(Healthy Choice) deli-thin sliced				
cooked	2 oz	1.5	60	23%
honey	2 oz	1.5	60	23%
honey				
maple	2 oz	1.5	60	23%
mustard	2 oz	1.5	60	23%
smoked	2 oz	1.5	60	23%
Virginia Brand	2 oz	1.5	60	23%
(Hillshire Farm)				
ham.. bone-in..spiral-sliced				
brown sugar-cured	3 oz	6.0	120	45%
ham...honey-cured				
spiral-sliced	3 oz	6.0	120	45%
ham—other..cured				
baked				
brown sugar..half	2 oz	2.0	70	26%
honey..half	2 oz	2.0	60	30%
ham..sliced				
cooked	1.85 oz	1.0	60	30%
lower salt	1.85 oz	1.0	60	30%
honey	1.85 oz	1.0	60	26%
honey maple	1 oz	1.0	60	15%
(Hormel) 7				
deli products				
Black Label				
canned	3 oz	4.5	100	41%
chopped				
regular	2 oz	11.0	140	71%
sweet	2 oz	11.0	140	71%
Black Forest..97% fat-free	2 oz	2.0	60	30%
chunk..lean	2 oz	6.0	90	40%
cooked..97% fat-free	2 oz	3.0	60	45%
Cure 81 ham..bone-in				
w/honey glaze				
spiral-sliced	3 oz	8.0	140	51%
Cure 81 ham..boneless				
extra lean..half	3 oz	4.5	100	41%
extra lean..whole	3 oz	4.5	100	41%
thin-sliced	3 oz	4.5	100	41%
Cure 81 w/natural juices	2 oz	4.5	100	41%
Curemaster	3 oz	2.5	80	28%

Food and Description	Amount	Fat Grams	Total Calories	% Fat Calories
deviled	2 oz	12.0	150	72%
double-smoked	2 oz	3.0	70	39%
extra-lean	2 oz	2.0	60	30%
honey ham..sliced	2 oz	3.0	70	39%
97% fat-free	2 oz	3.0	70	39%
snack size w/natural juice	2 oz	2.0	70	26%
Light & Lean..cooked				
97% fat-free	1 oz	1.0	25	36%
patties..fully cooked				
ham	1 patty	16.0	180	80%
ham & cheese	1 patty	17.0	180	85%
smoked..honey-cured	2 oz	3.0	70	39%
(Jones Dairy Farm)				
Country Carved	3 oz	4.0	100	36%
ham steak	3 oz	4.0	100	36%
(Kahn's) 97% fat-free	1 oz	1.0	30	30%
(Louis Rich and Oscar Mayer)				
turkey ham				
50% less fat	1 oz	1.5	35	39%
smoked	1 oz	1.5	35	39%
smoked..chopped	1 oz	2.0	35	51%
(Oscar Mayer)				
deli-style				
brown sugar				
shaved	1.8 oz	1.5	60	23%
thin-sliced	2 oz	1.5	70	19%
honey..shaved	1.8 oz	1.0	50	18%
smoked				
shaved	1.8 oz	1.0	45	20%
thin-sliced	2 oz	1.5	50	27%
Lunchables..boxed				
ham & American cheese	3.8 oz	19.0	450	38%
ham & cheddar	4.5 oz	23.0	420	49%
(Owens) ham steaks..fully cooked	4 oz	4.0	120	30%
(Plumrose) Danish				
baked..96% fat-free	1 oz	1.5	35	39%
baked..brown sugar				
97% fat-free	1 oz	1.0	35	26%
baked..honey brown sugar				
97% fat-free	1 oz	1.0	35	26%
chopped	1 oz	6.0	80	68%
cooked..boneless..skinless	2 oz	2.0	60	30%
ham steaks..smoked				
97% fat-free	5.3 oz	4.5	150	27%
	4 oz	3.0	120	23%
honey..96% fat-free	1 oz	1.5	35	39%
premium	2 oz	2.5	60	38%
95% fat-free	1 oz	1.5	35	39%
97% fat-free	1 oz	1.0	30	30%
baked..97% fat-free	1 oz	1.0	30	30%

Food and Description	Amount	Fat Grams	Total Calories	% Fat Calories
smoked pepper	1.7 oz	1.5	50	27%
Supreme				
Black Forest..smoked	2 oz	1.5	60	23%
brown sugar..baked				
97% fat-free	2 oz	1.5	60	23%
hickory-smoked..97% fat-free	2 oz	1.5	60	23%
imported..97% fat-free	2 oz	1.5	50	27%
smoked..97% fat-free				
honey	2 oz	1.5	60	23%
maple-flavored honey	2 oz	2.0	70	26%
pepper	2 oz	1.5	60	23%
Virginia	2 oz	1.5	60	23%
Thin & Tasty..97% fat-free	2 oz	2.0	50	36%
turkey ham	1 oz	1.5	35	39%
(West Virginia Brand)				
cooked..pre-sliced..97% fat-free	1 oz	1.0	35	26%
cooked honey..pre-sliced				
97% fat-free	1 oz	1.0	35	26%
fillets..boneless	3 oz	2.5	90	25%
golden..boneless..97% fat-free	3 oz	2.5	90	25%
lean original..semi-boneless				
50% less fat	3 oz	8.0	130	55%
regular	3 oz	8.0	130	55%

HAM SPREAD (See LUNCHEON MEAT SPREAD)
HAMBURGER (See BEEF; BEEF DISH/ENTRÉE; BUFFALO/BISON; FROZEN ENTRÉE/DINNER; TURKEY; VEGETARIAN FOODS)
HASH (See BEEF DISH/ENTRÉE; SAUSAGE DISH; TURKEY ENTRÉE/DINNER)
HAZELNUT (See also FILBERT/HAZELNUT)

Food and Description	Amount	Fat Grams	Total Calories	% Fat Calories
(Diamond of California)				
chopped	¼ cup	18.0	200	81%
shelled 1 oz	~22 nuts	18.0	200	81%
(Planters) hazelnuts..filberts	1 oz	17.0	190	81%

HAZELNUT BUTTER/SPREAD

Food and Description	Amount	Fat Grams	Total Calories	% Fat Calories
(Ferrero) Nutella chocolate	1 Tbs	5.0	85	53%
(Roaster Fresh) hazelnut butter	2 Tbs	19.0	188	91%

HERBS (See SEASONINGS; individual listings)
HERRING (See also HERRING ROE)

Food and Description	Amount	Fat Grams	Total Calories	% Fat Calories
Atlantic				
breaded & fried	3 oz	18.0	279	58%
canned/in tomato sauce	2 oz	6.0	100	54%
cooked—dry heat	3 oz	9.9	172	52%
dried	1 oz	5.0	72	63%
kippered	~ 1.5 oz	5.0	87	51%
pickled	~½ oz	2.7	39	62%
	3 oz	15.0	220	61%
raw	3 oz	7.7	134	52%
(King Oscar)				
Kipper Snacks				
fillets of herring..lightly salted	3.25 oz	13.0	190	62%
kippered				
in mustard	¼ cup	8.0	100	72%

Food and Description	Amount	Fat Grams	Total Calories	% Fat Calories
in salsa picante	¼ cup	6.0	90	60%
smoked	¼ cup	8.0	110	65%
(Lascco) chilled				
sour cream fillet	2 oz	7.0	120	53%
spice cut	2 oz	6.0	110	49%
wine snacks	2 oz	5.0	100	45%
(Nathan's) snacks in wine sauce	¼ cup	4.0	90	40%
Pacific				
cooked—dry heat	3 oz	15.0	215	63%
raw	3 oz	11.8	166	64%
(Vita Lunch)				
pickled..jarred	2 oz	8.0	130	55%
HERRING ROE/raw	3 oz	1.7	111	14%
HICKORY NUT				
dried/shelled	1 oz	18.0	187	87%
HOKI/raw	3.5 oz	0.8	74	10%
HOLLANDAISE SAUCE (*See* SAUCE)				
HOMINY (*See also* CORN GRITS)				
canned				
(Allen's)				
golden	½ cup	<1.0	120	4%
malz blanco para				
para pozole..Mexican				
white	½ cup	0.5	100	5%
white	½ cup	<1.0	100	5%
(Bush's Best)				
golden	½ cup	–	60	–
white	½ cup	1.0	70	13%
(Goya)				
golden	½ cup	–	120	–
white	½ cup	0.5	100	5%
(Springfield)				
fancy Mexican-style	½ cup	–	60	–
fancy white	½ cup	1.0	80	11%
(Van Camp's)				
golden	½ cup	1.0	80	11%
white	½ cup	1.0	80	11%
HOMINY GRITS (*See* CORN GRITS)				
HONEY				
(Aunt Sue's)				
raw-wild pure..squeeze bottle	1 Tbs	–	60	–
(Bee Maid)				
cinnamon	1 Tbs	–	70	–
natural/creamed	1 Tbs	–	60	–
regular	1 Tbs	–	60	–
(Burleson's)				
clover	1 Tbs	–	60	–
creamed	1 Tbs	–	60	–
natural	1 Tbs	–	60	–

Food and Description	Amount	Fat Grams	Total Calories	% Fat Calories
raw	1 Tbs	–	60	–
Rocky Mountain Clover	1 Tbs	–	60	–
(Golden Blossom)	1 tsp	–	20	–
	1 Tbs	–	60	–
(Knott's Berry Farm)	1 Tbs	–	60	–
pure honey	½ oz	–	45	–
(Sioux)	1 Tbs	–	60	–
(SueBee)				
honey..liquid	1 Tbs	–	60	–
(Tree of Life)				
all types	1 Tbs	–	60	–
HONEY BUTTER				
(Downey's)				
cinnamon	1 Tbs	1.0	60	15%
original	1 Tbs	1.0	60	15%
HONEYDEW MELON/fresh				
cut up	1 cup	<1.0	50	9%
(Chiquita) cubed	1 cup	–	70	–
whole	⅒ melon	<1.0	47	10%
(Dole)	⅒ melon	–	50	–
HORSE/meat only				
roasted	4 oz	7.0	200	32%
roasted/chopped	1 cup	3.0	245	11%
HORSERADISH (*See also* SAUCE)				
fresh/raw	1 oz	–	18	–
jarred				
(Boar's Head)				
horseradish	1 tsp	–	–	–
(Gold's) hot	1 tsp	–	4	–
(Hebrew National)				
red	1 Tbs	–	7	–
	½ cup	–	25	–
white	1 Tbs	–	7	–
	½ cup	–	25	–
(Koop's) squeeze				
mustard horseradish	1 tsp	–	–	–
(Kraft)				
cream-style	1 tsp	–	–	–
mustard	1 tsp	–	–	–
prepared	1 tsp	–	–	–
sauce	1 tsp	1.5	20	7%
(Marzetti) squeeze bottle				
horseradish sauce	1 Tbs	4.5	50	81%
(Plochman's) premium				
spicy mustard horseradish	1 tsp	–	–	–
(Rosoff's)				
red	1 Tbs	–	8	–
white	1 Tbs	–	7	–

HOT DOG (*See* FRANKFURTER; individual FAST FOOD listings)

Food and Description	Amount	Fat Grams	Total Calories	% Fat Calories
HUMMUS (*See also* DIP)				
READY-TO-SERVE				
(Athenos)				
14-oz tub				
black olive	2 Tbs	3.0	50	54%
cucumber dill	2 Tbs	4.0	60	60%
Greek	2 Tbs	3.0	50	54%
original	2 Tbs	3.5	60	53%
pesto	2 Tbs	3.5	50	63%
roasted eggplant	2 Tbs	2.5	45	50%
roasted garlic	2 Tbs	3.5	60	53%
roasted red pepper	2 Tbs	3.5	60	53%
scallion	2 Tbs	3.5	50	63%
spicy 3-pepper	2 Tbs	3.5	60	63%
Athenos Travelers				
1 serving = 2 Tbs hummus w/2 pitas				
original	1 serving	6.0	130	42%
roasted eggplant	1 serving	5.0	120	38%
roasted garlic	1 serving	6.0	130	42%
roasted red pepper	1 serving	6.0	140	39%
spicy 3-pepper	1 serving	6.0	130	42%
MIX				
(Casbah) prepared	¼ cup	5.0	120	38%
HUSHPUPPY (*See* BREAD)				
HYACINTH BEAN				
mature				
boiled	½ cup	0.6	114	4%
raw	½ cup	2.0	350	5%
immature	½ cup	–	20	–

Food and Description	Amount	Fat Grams	Total Calories	% Fat Calories
ICE CREAM & ICE CREAM–LIKE FROZEN DESSERTS (*See also* FRUIT ICES, BARS & POPS; ICE CREAM BARS, SANDWICHES & FROZEN NOVELTIES; RICE FROZEN DESSERT; SHERBET; TOFU FROZEN DESSERT; YOGURT, FROZEN)				
■ (Alaskan Ice Cream)				
Bear Claw	½ cup	7.0	150	42%
Caramel Caribou	½ cup	7.0	150	42%

Food and Description	Amount	Fat Grams	Total Calories	% Fat Calories
Extreme Moose Track	½ cup	11.0	170	58%
Glacier Mint	½ cup	7.0	150	42%
Moose Tracks	½ cup	10.0	170	53%
Otter Paws	½ cup	9.0	160	51%
The Mother Lode	½ cup	6.0	150	36%
vanilla bean	½ cup	9.0	150	51%
■ (Baskin-Robbins)				
BLASTS				
cappuccino				
decaf	16 oz	12.0	300	36%
	24 oz	19.0	460	37%
w/whipped cream	16 oz	14.0	320	39%
	24 oz	21.0	480	39%
chocolate	16 oz	12.0	450	24%
	24 oz	19.0	680	25%
low-fat	16 oz	2.0	220	8%
non-fat	16 oz	–	210	–
regular	16 oz	12.0	300	36%
w/whipped cream	16 oz	14.0	320	39%
	24 oz	21.0	480	39%
mintopia	16 oz	17.0	430	36%
	24 oz	25.0	630	36%
	32 oz	31.0	800	35%
mocha	16 oz	12.0	350	31%
	24 oz	18.0	540	31%
w/whipped cream	16 oz	13.0	370	32%
	24 oz	20.0	560	32%
mocha decaf	16 oz	12.0	350	31%
	24 oz	18.0	540	30%
w/whipped cream	16 oz	13.0	370	32%
	24 oz	20.0	560	32%
turtle	16 oz	17.0	540	28%
	24 oz	25.0	790	28%
	32 oz	31.0	1010	28%
CLASSIC FLAVORS				
banana nut	½ cup	16.0	260	55%
black walnut	½ cup	19.0	280	61%
chocolate almond	½ cup	18.0	310	52%
chocolate chip	½ cup	16.0	270	53%
chocolate chip cookie dough	½ cup	15.0	290	47%
chocolate fudge	½ cup	15.0	270	50%
chocolate ice cream	½ cup	14.0	260	48%
chocolate ribbon	½ cup	12.0	240	45%
French vanilla	½ cup	18.0	280	58%
fudge brownie	½ cup	19.0	300	57%
German chocolate cake	½ cup	13.0	260	45%
Gold Medal Ribbon	½ cup	8.0	150	48%
Jamoca almond fudge	½ cup	15.0	270	50%
Jamoca ice cream	½ cup	13.0	240	49%
nutty coconut ice cream	½ cup	20.0	300	60%

Food and Description	Amount	Fat Grams	Total Calories	% Fat Calories
old-fashioned butter pecan	½ cup	18.0	280	58%
Oreo Cookies 'n' Cream ice cream	½ cup	15.0	280	48%
Peanut butter'n chocolate				
ice cream	½ cup	20.0	320	56%
pistachio almond	½ cup	19.0	290	59%
pralines 'n' cream	½ cup	14.0	270	47%
Reese's peanut butter	½ cup	18.0	300	54%
rocky road	½ cup	15.0	290	47%
vanilla	½ cup	16.0	260	55%
Very Berry strawberry	½ cup	11.0	220	45%
World-Class chocolate ice cream	½ cup	15.0	270	50%
ICE CREAM CAKES				
roll				
chocolate chip ice cream				
w/chocolate cake	1 slice	14.0	290	43%
mint chocolate chip				
w/chocolate cake	1 slice	14.0	290	43%
vanilla ice cream				
w/chocolate cake	1 slice	13.0	270	43%
round				
chocolate chip ice cream				
w/devil's food 9" cake	1 slice	22.0	410	48%
Oreo Cookies 'n' Cream ice cream				
w/devil's food.. 9" cake	1 slice	22.0	430	46%
pralines 'n' cream ice cream				
w/devil's food 9" cake	1 slice	19.0	430	40%
sheet				
chocolate chip ice cream				
w/devil's food cake	1 slice	17.0	330	46%
mint chocolate chip ice cream				
w/devil's food cake	1 slice	16.0	290	50%
Oreo Cookies 'n' Cream ice cream				
w/white sponge cake	1 slice	14.0	300	42%
pralines 'n' cream ice cream				
w/white sponge cake	1 slice	13.0	300	39%
vanilla ice cream w/devil's				
food cake	1 slice	16.0	300	48%
special occasion & holiday				
chocolate chip ice cream				
w/devil's food heart cake	1 slice	17.0	320	48%
Oreo Cookies 'n' Cream heart				
ice cream cake	1 slice	16.0	300	48%
Oreo Cookies 'n' Cream ice cream				
w/devil's food heart cake	1 slice	17.0	330	46%
vanilla ice cream heart				
ice cream cake	1 slice	18.0	290	56%
vanilla ice cream				
w/devil's food heart cake	1 slice	18.0	330	49%
LOW-FAT..NO SUGAR ADDED				
berries 'n' banana	½ cup	2.0	110	16%

Food and Description	Amount	Fat Grams	Total Calories	% Fat Calories
Call Me Nuts	½ cup	2.0	110	16%
cherry cordial	½ cup	2.0	100	18%
chocolate chip	½ cup	4.5	170	24%
chocolate, chocolate chip	½ cup	4.5	150	27%
Mad About Chocolate	½ cup	3.0	170	16%
pineapple coconut	½ cup	2.0	150	12%
tin roof sundae	½ cup	3.0	190	14%
SEASONAL FLAVORS				
bananas 'n' strawberries	½ cup	9.0	220	37%
Baseball Nut	½ cup	14.0	270	47%
blueberry cheesecake	½ cup	14.0	270	47%
Bobsled Brownie	½ cup	18.0	320	51%
Candy Cookie Commotion	½ cup	16.0	300	48%
Chocoholic's Resolution	½ cup	16.0	300	48%
Chocolate Mousse Royale	½ cup	17.0	300	51%
cinnamon bun swirl	½ cup	12.0	280	39%
eggnog	½ cup	13.0	250	47%
Jamoca Roca	½ cup	14.0	280	45%
key lime pie	½ cup	14.0	270	47%
lemon custard	½ cup	13.0	260	45%
Love Gone Sour	½ cup	14.0	270	17%
Love Potion #31	½ cup	14.0	270	17%
macadamia nuts 'n' ceam	½ cup	18.0	270	60%
Mississippi mud	½ cup	13.0	270	43%
New York cheesecake	½ cup	16.0	280	51%
Nutcracker Sweet	½ cup	18.0	300	54%
oatmeal cookie	½ cup	12.0	270	40%
Oregon blackberry	½ cup	12.0	240	45%
peppermint	½ cup	14.0	270	40%
pink bubblegum	½ cup	12.0	260	42%
pumpkin pie	½ cup	12.0	230	47%
Quarterback Crunch	½ cup	16.0	290	50%
strawberry cheesecake	½ cup	14.0	270	47%
Tax Crunch	½ cup	18.0	300	54%
Trick Oreo Treat	½ cup	16.0	300	48%
Winter White Chocolate	½ cup	14.0	270	47%
SUNDAES				
2-scoop hot fudge	1 serving	29.0	430	61%
3-scoop hot fudge	1 serving	41.0	750	49%
banana royale	1 serving	27.0	630	39%
banana split	1 serving	39.0	1030	34%
Donkey sundae	1 serving	23.0	530	39%
Shrek's hot fudge sundae	1 serving	25.0	620	36%
■ (Ben & Jerry's)				
LOW-FAT				
Blondies Are a Swirl's Best Friend	½ cup	2.0	200	9%
coconut cream pie	½ cup	2.5	160	14%
mocha latte	½ cup	2.0	150	12%
s'mores	½ cup	2.0	190	9%

Food and Description	Amount	Fat Grams	Total Calories	% Fat Calories
ORGANIC				
chocolate fudge brownie	½ cup	13.0	260	45%
strawberry	½ cup	12.0	200	54%
sweet cream & cookies	½ cup	15.0	240	56%
vanilla	½ cup	14.0	220	57%
ORIGINAL				
brownie batter	½ cup	18.0	310	52%
butter pecan	½ cup	21.0	290	65%
Cherry Garcia	½ cup	15.0	250	54%
chocolate chip cookie dough	½ cup	16.0	280	51%
chocolate chocolate cookie	½ cup	14.0	280	45%
Chocolate for a Change	½ cup	17.0	270	57%
Cocolate Fudge Brownie	½ cup	14.0	280	45%
Chubby Hubby	½ cup	21.0	330	57%
Chunky Monkey	½ cup	19.0	300	57%
Coffee for a Change	½ cup	15.0	240	56%
Coffee Heath Bar Crunch	½ cup	18.0	310	52%
Everything but the...	½ cup	19.0	320	53%
Fudge Central	½ cup	18.0	300	54%
Half Baked	½ cup	14.0	280	45%
Karamel Sutra	½ cup	15.0	290	47%
Makin' Whoopie Pie	½ cup	14.0	270	47%
mint chocolate cookie	½ cup	16.0	270	53%
New York Super Fudge Chunk	½ cup	20.0	310	58%
oatmeal cookie chunk	½ cup	16.0	280	51%
One Sweet Whirled	½ cup	15.0	280	48%
peanut butter cup	½ cup	26.0	380	62%
Phish Food	½ cup	13.0	280	42%
Pistachio Pistachio	½ cup	19.0	280	61%
Uncanny Cashew	½ cup	19.0	290	59%
Vanilla for a Change	½ cup	16.0	240	60%
Vanilla Heath Bar Crunch	½ cup	19.0	300	57%
SINGLES				
Cherry Garcia	1 cont	13.0	220	53%
cookie dough	1 cont	13.0	240	49%
Chocolate Fudge Brownie	1 cont	11.0	230	43%
Vanilla for a Change	1 cont	13.0	200	59%
■ **(Blue Bunny)**				
CARB FREEDOM				
butter pecan	½ cup	8.0	110	65%
chocolate almond fudge	½ cup	8.0	120	60%
double strawberry	½ cup	6.0	100	54%
mint chip	½ cup	8.0	110	65%
vanilla bean	½ cup	6.0	100	54%
CUPS				
chocolate	1 cup	5.0	100	45%
malt	1 cup	7.0	220	29%
strawberry & chocolate sundae	1 cup	5.0	110	41%
vanilla	1 cup	6.0	100	54%
vanilla & chocolate	1 cup	6.0	100	54%

Food and Description	Amount	Fat Grams	Total Calories	% Fat Calories
DISNEY				
Mickey Chocn'illa	½ cup	3.0	110	25%
Monsters, Inc.				
Bubble Gum Scream	½ cup	2.5	110	20%
Tigger Cookie-rrific	½ cup	3.0	120	23%
FAT-FREE..NO SUGAR ADDED				
brownie sundae	½ cup	–	90	–
burgundy cherry	½ cup	–	90	–
caramel toffee crunch	½ cup	–	90	–
chocolate	½ cup	–	90	–
mint fudge swirl	½ cup	–	80	–
vanilla	½ cup	–	80	–
NO SUGAR ADDED..REDUCED-FAT				
banana split	½ cup	5.0	120	37%
Bunny Tracks	½ cup	8.0	150	48%
butter pecan	½ cup	6.0	130	42%
cherry vanilla	½ cup	4.5	120	34%
double strawberry	½ cup	4.0	110	33%
Exquisite Mint	½ cup	6.0	130	42%
Neapolitan	½ cup	4.5	110	37%
rocky road	½ cup	6.0	130	42%
tin roof sundae	½ cup	6.0	130	42%
turtle sundae	½ cup	7.0	140	45%
vanilla	½ cup	5.0	110	41%
PREMIUM				
Chocolate Amore	½ cup	8.0	170	42%
Chocolate Bunny Tracks	½ cup	11.0	200	50%
Bordeaux cherry chocolate	½ cup	8.0	160	45%
Bunny Tracks	½ cup	11.0	190	52%
butter pecan	½ cup	9.0	150	54%
chocolate chip	½ cup	8.0	150	48%
cookies & cream	½ cup	8.0	150	48%
double strawberry	½ cup	6.0	140	39%
Exquisite Mint	½ cup	8.0	170	42%
French vanilla	½ cup	8.0	150	48%
homemade chocolate	½ cup	7.0	150	42%
homemade turtle sundae	½ cup	9.0	180	45%
homemade vanilla	½ cup	7.0	150	42%
NASCAR Speedway Sundae	½ cup	10.0	190	47%
natural vanilla bean	½ cup	9.0	160	51%
Peanut Butter Panic	½ cup	12.0	200	54%
pistachio almond	½ cup	8.0	150	48%
praline pecan	½ cup	8.0	170	42%
rocky road	½ cup	7.0	150	42%
super fudge brownie	½ cup	8.0	170	42%
toasted almond fudge	½ cup	9.0	160	51%
triple raspberry temptation	½ cup	6.0	150	36%
vanilla	½ cup	8.0	140	51%
■ (Breyers)				
ALL-NATURAL				
banana fudge chunk	½ cup	8.0	160	45%

Food and Description	Amount	Fat Grams	Total Calories	% Fat Calories
butter almond	½ cup	10.0	160	56%
butter pecan	½ cup	11.0	170	58%
calcium-rich natural vanilla	½ cup	7.0	130	48%
caramel fudge	½ cup	7.0	160	39%
caramel praline crunch	½ cup	7.0	170	37%
cherry chocolate chip	½ cup	8.0	150	48%
cherry vanilla	½ cup	7.0	140	45%
chocolate	½ cup	8.0	150	48%
extra-creamy	½ cup	7.0	140	45%
chocolate chip	½ cup	9.0	160	50%
chocolate chip cookie dough	½ cup	9.0	170	48%
chocolate chocolate chip	½ cup	10.0	180	50%
coffee	½ cup	8.0	140	51%
cookies & cream	½ cup	8.0	160	45%
dulce de leche	½ cup	7.0	150	42%
French vanilla	½ cup	8.0	150	48%
fresa banana	½ cup	5.0	140	32%
fudge twirl	½ cup	7.0	140	45%
mint chocolate chip	½ cup	5.0	130	35%
mocha almond fudge	½ cup	9.0	170	48%
peach	½ cup	5.0	120	38%
peanut butter & fudge	½ cup	10.0	170	53%
rocky road	½ cup	8.0	170	42%
strawberry	½ cup	6.0	120	45%
Take Two				
vanilla & chocolate	½ cup	8.0	140	51%
vanilla & orange sherbet	½ cup	4.5	130	31%
vanilla	½ cup	8.0	140	51%
calcium-rich	½ cup	7.0	130	48%
extra-creamy	½ cup	8.0	150	48%
homemade	½ cup	7.0	140	45%
lactose-free	½ cup	7.0	130	48%
vanilla & chocolate checks	½ cup	8.0	160	45%
vanilla fudge brownie	½ cup	9.0	160	51%
vanilla fudge twirl	½ cup	8.0	150	48%
vanilla/chocolate/strawberry	½ cup	8.0	140	51%
ALL NATURAL..LIGHT				
French chocolate	½ cup	5.0	150	30%
French vanilla	½ cup	4.0	120	30%
mint chocolate chip	½ cup	5.0	140	32%
natural vanilla	½ cup	3.0	120	23%
pralines & caramel	½ cup	3.5	140	23%
rocky road	½ cup	4.5	140	29%
strawberry	½ cup	2.5	110	20%
vanilla/chocolate/strawberry	½ cup	3.0	120	23%
FAT-FREE				
vanilla	½ cup	–	90	–
HOMEMADE				
butter pecan	½ cup	11.0	170	58%
double chocolate fudge	½ cup	8.0	170	42%
fudge brownie	½ cup	9.0	180	45%

Food and Description	Amount	Fat Grams	Total Calories	% Fat Calories
Neapolitan	½ cup	8.0	150	48%
vanilla	½ cup	8.0	140	51%
ICE CREAM PARLOR				
Almond Joy	½ cup	9.0	170	48%
Banana Split	½ cup	9.0	180	45%
Chips Ahoy! chocolate chip cookie	½ cup	8.0	160	45%
Creamsicle	½ cup	5.0	130	35%
Fudgesicle chocolate fudge	½ cup	7.0	140	45%
Heath English Toffee	½ cup	9.0	180	45%
Hershey's chocolate w/almonds	½ cup	8.0	170	42%
M&M's				
mint	½ cup	9.0	170	48%
vanilla fudge	½ cup	10.0	170	53%
Mint ice cream w/Oreo	½ cup	7.0	170	37%
Oreo Cookies & Cream	½ cup	8.0	160	45%
Reese's Peanut Butter Cups	½ cup	9.0	180	45%
Snickers	½ cup	8.0	160	45%
Snickers Cruncher	½ cup	8.0	160	45%
SpongeBob cookie dough	½ cup	7.0	160	37%
strawberry shortcake	½ cup	6.0	160	34%
Twix	½ cup	7.0	160	39%
Twix..peanut butter	½ cup	10.0	170	53%
LIGHT & LOW-FAT TASTY ALTERNATIVE				
2% milk light vanilla	½ cup	4.5	130	31%
98% fat-free				
chocolate	½ cup	1.5	90	15%
vanilla-flavored	½ cup	1.5	90	15%
98% fat-free..no sugar added				
chocolate fudge brownie	½ cup	1.5	90	15%
All Natural Light				
French				
chocolate	½ cup	5.0	140	32%
vanilla	½ cup	4.0	120	30%
mint chocolate chip	½ cup	4.5	130	31%
vanilla	½ cup	3.0	110	25%
vanilla/chocolate/strawberry	½ cup	3.0	110	25%
LOW-CARB				
CarbSmart				
butter pecan	½ cup	10.0	120	75%
chocolate	½ cup	10.0	130	69%
chocolate almond	½ cup	10.0	130	69%
chocolate & vanilla	½ cup	4.5	70	58%
mint chocolate chip	½ cup	10.0	140	64%
rocky road	½ cup	11.0	140	71%
strawberry	½ cup	9.0	130	62%
vanilla				
frozen dairy dessert	½ cup	9.0	130	62%
ice cream	½ cup	9.0	130	62%
NO SUGAR ADDED				
98% fat-free				
chocolate fudge brownie	½ cup	1.5	90	15%

Food and Description	Amount	Fat Grams	Total Calories	% Fat Calories
butter pecan	½ cup	7.0	120	53%
chocolate caramel	½ cup	4.0	100	36%
French vanilla	½ cup	4.5	100	41%
vanilla	½ cup	4.5	100	41%
vanilla fudge twirl	½ cup	4.0	110	33%
vanilla/chocolate/strawberry	½ cup	4.0	90	40%
PINTS PLUS				
CarbSmart				
butter pecan	½ cup	12.0	120	90%
chocolate almond	½ cup	10.0	130	69%
vanilla	½ cup	8.0	110	65%
M&M's mint	½ cup	9.0	170	48%
natural vanilla	½ cup	8.0	140	51%
Oreo	½ cup	8.0	160	45%
Reese's Peanut Butter Cups	½ cup	9.0	180	45%
Snickers	½ cup	8.0	160	45%
strawberry shortcake	½ cup	6.0	160	34%
Twix	½ cup	7.0	160	39%
■ **(Carb Watchers)**				
PREMIUM GOURMET ICE CREAM				
butter pecan	½ cup	13.0	150	78%
chocolate fudge swirl	½ cup	13.0	145	81%
cookies 'n' cream	½ cup	10.0	160	56%
dulce de leche	½ cup	10.0	160	56%
vanilla	½ cup	10.0	140	64%
Neapolitan	½ cup	7.0	130	48%
orange float sherbet & ice cream	½ cup	4.0	120	30%
peppermint candy	½ cup	7.0	140	45%
rocky road	½ cup	8.0	160	45%
spumoni	½ cup	7.0	130	48%
summer strawberry	½ cup	6.0	120	45%
tin roof classic	½ cup	7.0	150	42%
Totally Chocolate	½ cup	7.0	140	45%
Very Vanilla	½ cup	7.0	130	48%
■ **(Dreamery)**				
Banana Boogie	½ cup	17.0	290	53%
Black Raspberry Avalanche	½ cup	14.0	250	50%
Blue Ribbon Berry Pie	½ cup	13.0	260	45%
Caramel Toffee Bar Heaven	½ cup	14.0	270	47%
Cashew Praline Parfait	½ cup	13.0	260	45%
chocolate peanut butter chunk	½ cup	18.0	310	52%
Chocolate Truffle Explosion	½ cup	15.0	280	48%
Cool Mint	½ cup	14.0	280	45%
crème caramel	½ cup	12.0	260	42%
Cuppa Joe	½ cup	13.0	230	51%
Galactic Chocolate Swirl	½ cup	12.0	280	39%
Grandma's Cookie Jar	½ cup	14.0	270	47%
Harvest Peach	½ cup	11.0	220	45%
Hot Chilly Chili	½ cup	14.0	260	48%
New York strawberry cheesecake	½ cup	13.0	250	47%

Food and Description	Amount	Fat Grams	Total Calories	% Fat Calories
Nuts About Malt	½ cup	15.0	280	48%
sticky bun	½ cup	14.0	270	47%
vanilla	½ cup	15.0	260	52%
■ (Dreyer's)				
FAT-FREE..NO SUGAR				
chocolate fudge	½ cup	–	100	–
raspberry vanilla	½ cup	–	80	–
vanilla	½ cup	–	80	–
chocolate	½ cup	–	100	–
'n' caramel	½ cup	–	80	–
GRAND				
CARB BENEFIT				
butter pecan	½ cup	12.0	170	64%
chocolate	½ cup	10.0	150	60%
chocolate chip	½ cup	11.0	160	62%
mint chocolate chip	½ cup	11.0	160	62%
vanilla bean	½ cup	9.0	140	58%
HOMEMADE				
chocolate	½ cup	7.0	150	42%
Grovestand Peach	½ cup	5.0	120	38%
mint chocolate chunk	½ cup	8.0	160	45%
old-fashioned butter pecan	½ cup	9.0	150	54%
strawberries & cream	½ cup	6.0	130	42%
vanilla	½ cup	7.0	140	45%
vanilla custard	½ cup	8.0	150	48%
LIGHT				
butter pecan	½ cup	5.0	120	38%
chocolate chip sandwich	½ cup	3.5	120	26%
chocolate fudge chunk	½ cup	4.0	120	30%
cookie dough	½ cup	4.0	130	28%
cookies 'n' cream	½ cup	4.0	120	30%
Crazy for Caramel	½ cup	3.0	110	25%
espresso fudge chip	½ cup	4.0	120	30%
French silk	½ cup	4.5	120	34%
Fudge Tracks	½ cup	4.0	120	30%
gingerbread man	½ cup	4.0	120	30%
Girl Scouts				
Tagalongs Cookie	½ cup	5.0	130	35%
Thin Mint Cookie	½ cup	3.5	120	26%
mint chocolate chip	½ cup	4.5	120	34%
mocha almond fudge	½ cup	4.5	120	34%
peppermint	½ cup	3.5	110	29%
rocky road	½ cup	4.0	120	30%
S'mores & More	½ cup	4.0	130	28%
Strawberry Cheesecake Delight	½ cup	4.0	120	30%
strawberry shortcake	½ cup	3.5	110	29%
vanilla	½ cup	3.5	100	32%
vanillaberry bar	½ cup	2.5	100	23%
Vanilla Raspberry Escape	½ cup	3.5	120	26%

Food and Description	Amount	Fat Grams	Total Calories	% Fat Calories
LIGHT..SLOW-CHURNED RICH & CREAMY				
50/50 bar	½ cup	2.5	100	23%
butter pecan	½ cup	5.0	120	38%
chocolate	½ cup	3.5	110	29%
chocolate chip	½ cup	4.5	120	34%
cookie dough	½ cup	4.5	130	31%
cookies 'n cream	½ cup	4.0	120	30%
French silk	½ cup	4.5	130	31%
French vanilla	½ cup	3.5	100	32%
Fudge Tracks	½ cup	4.0	120	30%
mint chocolate chip	½ cup	4.5	120	34%
mocha almond fudge	½ cup	3.0	100	27%
Neapolitan	½ cup	4.0	120	30%
rocky road	½ cup	4.0	120	30%
strawberry	½ cup	2.5	100	23%
vanilla	½ cup	3.5	100	32%
vanillaberry bar	½ cup	2.5	100	23%
LIMITED EDITION				
50/50 Bar..Grand Light	½ cup	2.5	100	23%
Drumstick Sundae..Nestlé	½ cup	10.0	180	50%
Grovestand Peach	½ cup	10.0	150	60%
LOW-FAT				
chocolate fudge chunk	½ cup	2.0	110	16%
cookies 'n' cream	½ cup	2.0	110	16%
espresso chip	½ cup	2.0	100	18%
Heath toffee & caramel	½ cup	2.0	120	15%
rocky road	½ cup	2.0	110	16%
vanilla	½ cup	2.0	100	18%
NO SUGAR ADDED (also see Fat-Free section)				
butter pecan	½ cup	5.0	110	41%
chips 'n' swirls	½ cup	3.0	90	30%
chocolate	½ cup	3.0	90	30%
cookie dough	½ cup	4.0	110	33%
double fudge brownie	½ cup	3.0	100	27%
mint chocolate chip	½ cup	4.5	110	37%
Neapolitan	½ cup	3.0	90	30%
strawberry	½ cup	3.0	90	30%
triple chocolate	½ cup	3.0	90	30%
vanilla	½ cup	3.0	90	30%
REGULAR				
almond praline	½ cup	8.0	170	42%
America's vanilla	½ cup	10.0	150	60%
Andes Cool Mint				
Amazing Flavor	½ cup	9.0	170	48%
apple pie	½ cup	7.0	140	45%
blue ribbon chocolate cake	½ cup	10.0	180	50%
butter pecan	½ cup	10.0	170	53%
chocolate	½ cup	8.0	150	48%
chocolate caramel swirl	½ cup	9.0	170	48%
chocolate chip	½ cup	9.0	170	48%

Food and Description	Amount	Fat Grams	Total Calories	% Fat Calories
chocolate peanut butter	½ cup	13.0	200	59%
coffee	½ cup	8.0	140	51%
cookie dough	½ cup	9.0	180	45%
cookies 'n' cream	½ cup	8.0	160	45%
double fudge brownie	½ cup	9.0	170	48%
eggnog	½ cup	7.0	140	45%
dulce de leche	½ cup	10.0	160	56%
French vanilla	½ cup	10.0	160	56%
French vanilla fudge pie	½ cup	8.0	160	45%
fudge tracks	½ cup	11.0	180	55%
Galactic Chocolate	½ cup	7.0	160	39%
Girl Scout				
Samoas Cookie	½ cup	8.0	170	40%
Thin Mint Cookie	½ cup	10.0	170	53%
ice cream sandwich	½ cup	4.0	120	30%
mint chocolate chip	½ cup	9.0	170	48%
mocha almond fudge	½ cup	9.0	160	51%
Neapolitan	½ cup	7.0	140	45%
Nestlé Toll House				
Cookie Swirl	½ cup	9.0	170	48%
Nutty Cone Crunch	½ cup	10.0	180	50%
peanut butter				
brownie	½ cup	12.0	200	54%
cup	½ cup	10.0	180	50%
peppermint	½ cup	8.0	150	48%
pumpkin	½ cup	7.0	140	45%
real strawberry	½ cup	6.0	130	42%
rocky road	½ cup	10.0	170	53%
strawberry cupcake	½ cup	6.0	140	39%
tin roof sundae	½ cup	9.0	170	48%
toasted almond	½ cup	9.0	150	54%
toffee bar	½ cup	9.0	170	48%
Triple Chocolate Thunder				
Amazing Flavor	½ cup	9.0	160	51%
turtle sundae	½ cup	9.0	160	51%
Ultimate Caramel Cup				
Amazing Flavor	½ cup	8.0	170	42%
vanilla	½ cup	10.0	150	56%
bean	½ cup	8.0	140	51%
chocolate	½ cup	8.0	150	48%
Treasure	½ cup	8.0	160	45%
vanillaberry bar	½ cup	5.0	130	35%
▣ (Edy's)				
GRAND				
CARB BENEFIT				
butter pecan	½ cup	12.0	170	64%
chocolate	½ cup	10.0	150	60%
chocolate chip	½ cup	11.0	160	62%
mint chocolate chip	½ cup	11.0	160	62%

Food and Description	Amount	Fat Grams	Total Calories	% Fat Calories
vanilla bean	½ cup	9.0	140	58%
FAT-FREE..NO SUGAR				
chocolate fudge	½ cup	–	100	–
raspberry vanilla	½ cup	–	80	–
vanilla	½ cup	–	80	–
chocolate	½ cup	–	100	–
'n' caramel	½ cup	–	80	–
HOMEMADE				
chocolate	½ cup	7.0	150	42%
Grovestand Peach	½ cup	5.0	120	38%
mint chocolate chunk	½ cup	8.0	160	45%
old-fashioned butter pecan	½ cup	9.0	150	54%
strawberries & cream	½ cup	6.0	130	42%
vanilla	½ cup	7.0	140	45%
vanilla custard	½ cup	8.0	150	48%
LIGHT				
butter pecan	½ cup	5.0	120	38%
chocolate chip sandwich	½ cup	3.5	120	26%
chocolate fudge chunk	½ cup	4.0	120	30%
cookie dough	½ cup	4.0	130	28%
cookies 'n' cream	½ cup	4.0	120	30%
Crazy for Caramel	½ cup	3.0	110	25%
espresso fudge chip	½ cup	4.0	120	30%
French silk	½ cup	4.5	120	34%
Fudge Tracks	½ cup	4.0	120	30%
gingerbread man	½ cup	4.0	120	30%
Girl Scouts				
Tagalongs Cookie	½ cup	5.0	130	35%
Thin Mint Cookie	½ cup	3.5	120	26%
mint chocolate chips	½ cup	4.5	120	34%
mocha almond fudge	½ cup	4.5	120	34%
peppermint	½ cup	3.5	110	29%
rocky road	½ cup	4.0	120	30%
S'mores & More	½ cup	4.0	130	28%
Strawberry Cheesecake				
Delight	½ cup	4.0	120	30%
strawberry shortcake	½ cup	3.5	110	29%
vanilla	½ cup	3.5	100	32%
vanillaberry bar	½ cup	2.5	100	23%
Vanilla Raspberry Escape	½ cup	3.5	120	
LIGHT..SLOW-CHURNED RICH & CREAMY				
50/50 bar	½ cup	2.5	100	23%
butter pecan	½ cup	5.0	120	38%
chocolate	½ cup	3.5	110	29%
chocolate chip	½ cup	4.5	120	34%
cookie dough	½ cup	4.5	130	31%
cookies 'n' cream	½ cup	4.0	120	30%
French silk	½ cup	4.5	130	31%
French vanilla	½ cup	3.5	100	32%
Fudge Tracks	½ cup	4.0	120	30%

Food and Description	Amount	Fat Grams	Total Calories	% Fat Calories
mint chocolate chip	½ cup	4.5	120	34%
mocha almond fudge	½ cup	3.0	100	27%
Neapolitan	½ cup	4.0	120	30%
rocky road	½ cup	4.0	120	30%
strawberry	½ cup	2.5	100	23%
vanilla	½ cup	3.5	100	32%
vanillaberry bar	½ cup	2.5	100	23%
LIMITED EDITION				
50/50 Bar..Grand Light	½ cup	2.5	100	23%
Drumstick Sundae..Nestlé	½ cup	10.0	180	50%
Grovestand Peach	½ cup	10.0	150	60%
LOW-FAT				
chocolate fudge chunk	½ cup	2.0	110	16%
cookies 'n' cream	½ cup	2.0	110	16%
espresso chip	½ cup	2.0	100	18%
Heath toffee & caramel	½ cup	2.0	120	15%
rocky road	½ cup	2.0	110	16%
vanilla	½ cup	2.0	100	18%
NO SUGAR ADDED (also see Fat-Free section)				
butter pecan	½ cup	5.0	110	41%
chips 'n' swirls	½ cup	3.0	90	30%
chocolate	½ cup	3.0	90	30%
cookie dough	½ cup	4.0	110	33%
double fudge brownie	½ cup	3.0	100	27%
mint chocolate chip	½ cup	4.5	110	37%
Neapolitan	½ cup	3.0	90	30%
strawberry	½ cup	3.0	90	30%
triple chocolate	½ cup	3.0	90	30%
vanilla	½ cup	3.0	90	30%
REGULAR				
almond praline	½ cup	8.0	170	42%
America's vanilla	½ cup	10.0	150	60%
Andes Cool Mint Amazing Flavor	½ cup	9.0	170	48%
apple pie	½ cup	7.0	140	45%
black cherry vanilla	½ cup	7.0	140	45%
Blue Ribbon chocolate cake	½ cup	10.0	180	50%
butter pecan	½ cup	10.0	170	53%
cherry chocolate chip	½ cup	8.0	160	45%
chocolate	½ cup	8.0	150	48%
chocolate caramel swirl	½ cup	9.0	170	48%
chocolate chip	½ cup	9.0	170	48%
chocolate fudge mousse	½ cup	8.0	160	45%
chocolate fudge sundae	½ cup	9.0	170	48%
chocolate peanut butter	½ cup	13.0	200	59%
coffee	½ cup	8.0	140	51%
cookie dough	½ cup	9.0	180	45%
cookies 'n' cream	½ cup	8.0	160	45%
double cookie swirl	½ cup	8.0	160	45%
double fudge brownie	½ cup	9.0	170	48%

Food and Description	Amount	Fat Grams	Total Calories	% Fat Calories
eggnog	½ cup	7.0	140	45%
espresso chip	½ cup	8.0	150	48%
dulce de leche	½ cup	10.0	160	56%
Finding Nemo				
Fish 'n' Chips	½ cup	9.0	170	48%
Mint Cookie Crush	½ cup	7.0	160	39%
French vanilla	½ cup	10.0	160	56%
French vanilla fudge pie	½ cup	8.0	160	45%
Fudge Tracks	½ cup	11.0	180	55%
Galactic Chocolate	½ cup	7.0	160	39%
Girl Scout				
Samoas Cookie	½ cup	8.0	170	40%
Thin Mint Cookie	½ cup	10.0	170	53%
ice cream sandwich	½ cup	4.0	120	30%
mint chocolate chip	½ cup	9.0	170	48%
mocha almond fudge	½ cup	9.0	160	51%
Neapolitan	½ cup	7.0	140	45%
Nestlé Toll House				
Cookie Swirl	½ cup	9.0	170	48%
Nutty Cone Crunch	½ cup	10.0	180	50%
peanut butter				
blitz	½ cup	10.0	170	53%
bones	½ cup	8.0	160	45%
butter brownie	½ cup	12.0	200	54%
cup	½ cup	10.0	180	50%
peppermint	¼ cup	8.0	150	48%
pumpkin	½ cup	7.0	140	45%
real strawberry	½ cup	6.0	130	42%
rocky road	½ cup	10.0	170	53%
spumoni	½ cup	8.0	150	48%
strawberry cupcake	½ cup	6.0	140	39%
tin roof sundae	½ cup	9.0	170	48%
toasted almond	½ cup	9.0	150	54%
toffee bar	½ cup	9.0	170	48%
Triple Chocolate Thunder				
Amazing Flavor	½ cup	9.0	160	51%
turtle sundae	½ cup	9.0	160	51%
Ultimate Caramel Cup				
Amazing Flavor	½ cup	8.0	170	42%
vanilla	½ cup	10.0	150	56%
bean	½ cup	8.0	140	51%
chocolate	½ cup	8.0	150	48%
Treasure	½ cup	8.0	160	45%
vanillaberry bar	½ cup	5.0	130	35%
■ (Godiva)				
Super-Premium Ice Cream				
Belgian dark chocolate	½ cup	17.0	280	55%
chocolate-covered cookies				
& cream	½ cup	18.0	300	54%

Food and Description	Amount	Fat Grams	Total Calories	% Fat Calories
chocolate				
cheesecake	½ cup	17.0	310	49%
raspberry truffle	½ cup	16.0	290	50%
w/chocolate hearts	½ cup	20.0	330	55%
classic milk chocolate	½ cup	18.0	290	56%
vanilla				
caramel pecan	½ cup	16.0	290	50%
chocolate				
w/chocolate caramel hearts	½ cup	18.0	310	52%
white chocolate raspberry	½ cup	16.0	290	50%
■ (Häagen-Dazs)				
ICE CREAM				
Bailey's Irish Cream	½ cup	17.0	270	57%
bananas Foster	½ cup	15.0	260	52%
black walnut	½ cup	27.0	300	81%
butter pecan	½ cup	23.0	310	67%
café mocha	½ cup	19.0	310	55%
cherry vanilla	½ cup	15.0	240	56%
chocolate	½ cup	18.0	270	60%
chocolate chip	½ cup	20.0	300	60%
mousse	½ cup	19.0	310	55%
peanut butter	½ cup	24.0	360	60%
raspberry torte	½ cup	15.0	270	50%
coffee	½ cup	18.0	270	60%
cookies & cream	½ cup	17.0	270	57%
Cookie Dough Chip	½ cup	20.0	310	58%
crème bûlée	½ cup	19.0	280	61%
dulce de leche caramel	½ cup	17.0	290	53%
French vanilla mousse	½ cup	20.0	310	58%
macadamia brittle	½ cup	20.0	360	50%
mango	½ cup	14.0	250	50%
mint chip	½ cup	19.0	300	57%
mocha almond fudge	½ cup	23.0	340	61%
peaches & cream	½ cup	12.0	240	45%
peanut butter fudge chunk	½ cup	23.0	340	61%
pineapple coconut	½ cup	13.0	230	51%
pistachio	½ cup	20.0	290	62%
rocky road	½ cup	18.0	300	54%
rum raisin	½ cup	17.0	270	57%
strawberry	½ cup	16.0	250	58%
strawberry cheesecake	½ cup	16.0	270	53%
Tres Leches	½ cup	18.0	270	60%
vanilla	½ cup	18.0	270	60%
caramel brownie	½ cup	18.0	300	54%
chocolate chip	½ cup	20.0	310	58%
fudge	½ cup	18.0	290	56%
vanilla Swiss almond	½ cup	20.0	300	60%
white chocolate				
raspberry truffle	½ cup	18.0	310	52%

Food and Description	Amount	Fat Grams	Total Calories	% Fat Calories
■ (Healthy Choice)				
ICE CREAM				
Brownie Bliss	½ cup	2.0	130	14%
butter pecan crunch	½ cup	2.0	100	18%
cappuccino chocolate chunk	½ cup	2.0	120	15%
caramel fudge brownie	½ cup	2.0	120	15%
Cherry Chocolate Mambo	½ cup	2.0	130	14%
chocolate chocolate chunk	½ cup	2.0	120	15%
cookies 'n' cream	½ cup	2.0	120	15%
Crazy Caramel	½ cup	2.0	120	15%
Double Karma	½ cup	2.0	140	13%
French Silk	½ cup	1.5	120	11%
Happy Together	½ cup	2.0	150	12%
Jumpin' Java	½ cup	2.0	130	14%
milk chocolate chip	½ cup	2.0	120	15%
peanut butter cup	½ cup	2.0	120	15%
praline & caramel	½ cup	2.0	120	15%
rocky road	½ cup	2.0	130	14%
tin roof sundae	½ cup	2.0	120	15%
turtle fudge cake	½ cup	2.0	130	14%
vanilla	½ cup	3.0	110	25%
vanilla bean	½ cup	2.0	120	15%
ICE CREAM..NO SUGAR ADDED				
chocolate fudge brownie	½ cup	2.0	120	15%
coffee almond fudge	½ cup	2.0	110	16%
mint chocolate chip	½ cup	2.0	110	16%
vanilla	½ cup	2.0	100	18%
■ (Hood's)				
ALL-NATURAL..PEAK TREASURES				
Black Raspberry Ripple	½ cup	7.0	150	42%
Caramel Cup Goldmine	½ cup	8.0	170	42%
Chocolate				
Brownie Mudslide	½ cup	8.0	170	42%
Chip Canyon	½ cup	9.0	150	54%
Peanut Butter Avalanche	½ cup	9.0	170	48%
Cookie Sandwich Snowstorm	½ cup	9.0	170	48%
French Vanilla Summit	½ cup	8.0	160	45%
Fudge River Rapids	½ cup	7.0	150	42%
Java Chip Trails	½ cup	9.0	160	51%
Mint Cookie Caverns	½ cup	9.0	170	48%
orange & vanilla swirls	½ cup	5.0	130	35%
Triple Peaks	½ cup	8.0	140	51%
Twin Peaks	½ cup	8.0	140	51%
Vanilla Snow Drift	½ cup	8.0	150	48%
FAT-FREE				
apple crisp	½ cup	–	130	–
Chocolate Passion	½ cup	–	100	–
chocolate trio	½ cup	–	100	–
double brownie sundae	½ cup	–	120	–
heavenly hash	½ cup	–	120	–

Food and Description	Amount	Fat Grams	Total Calories	% Fat Calories
Vanilla Fudge Twist	½ cup	–	120	–
Very Vanilla	½ cup	–	100	–
LIGHT				
Almond Praline Delight	½ cup	4.5	140	29%
brownie sundae	½ cup	4.0	140	29%
butter pecan	½ cup	6.0	140	39%
Caribbean Coffee Royale	½ cup	3.5	110	29%
chocolate almond chip	½ cup	5.0	140	32%
chocolate, chocolate chip cookie dough	½ cup	5.0	140	32%
Classic Trio	½ cup	3.5	110	29%
cookies 'n' cream	½ cup	4.0	130	28%
creamy vanilla	½ cup	3.5	110	29%
heavenly hash	½ cup	3.5	130	24%
Mud Pie Medley	½ cup	5.0	140	32%
raspberry swirl	½ cup	3.0	120	23%
triple-nut sundae	½ cup	5.0	140	32%
LOW-FAT..NO SUGAR ADDED				
chocolate				
chip	½ cup	2.5	120	19%
Frenzy	½ cup	2.5	120	19%
Classic Trio	½ cup	2.5	100	23%
Mocha Madness	½ cup	2.5	110	20%
Vanilla Dream	½ cup	2.5	100	23%
TRADITIONAL				
Butterscotch Blast	½ cup	7.0	160	39%
Chippedy Chocolately	½ cup	9.0	150	54%
chocolate	½ cup	7.0	140	37%
Classic Trio	½ cup	7.0	140	37%
Cookie Dough Delight	½ cup	8.0	160	45%
cookies 'n' cream	½ cup	8.0	160	45%
Creamy Coffee	½ cup	7.0	140	37%
eggnog	½ cup	8.0	150	48%
Fudge Twister	½ cup	7.0	140	37%
Golden Vanilla	½ cup	7.0	140	37%
Grasshopper Pie	½ cup	7.0	160	39%
maple walnut	½ cup	8.0	150	48%
Natural Vanilla Bean	½ cup	7.0	140	37%
Patchwork	½ cup	7.0	140	37%
peppermint stick	½ cup	5.0	140	32%
spumoni	½ cup	7.0	140	37%
strawberry	½ cup	7.0	130	48%
■ (Imagine)				
NON-DAIRY FROZEN DESSERT				
cappuccino	½ cup	6.0	150	36%
carob	½ cup	6.0	150	35%
carob almond	½ cup	8.0	170	42%
cocoa marble fudge	½ cup	6.0	150	36%
cookies 'n' dream	½ cup	7.0	170	37%

Food and Description	Amount	Fat Grams	Total Calories	% Fat Calories
mint				
carob chip	½ cup	8.0	170	42%
chocolate chip	½ cup	8.0	170	42%
Neapolitan	½ cup	6.0	150	36%
orange vanilla swirl	½ cup	6.0	150	36%
strawberry	½ cup	5.0	140	32%
vanilla	½ cup	6.0	150	36%
vanilla Swiss almond	½ cup	8.0	180	40%
RICE DREAM SUPREME				
Pralines 'n' Dream	½ cup	9.0	180	45%
■ (Kemp's)				
CARB PROMISE ICE CREAM				
butter pecan	½ cup	11.0	130	76%
Caramel Cow Tracks	½ cup	8.0	130	55%
chocolate peanut butter cup	½ cup	12.0	160	68%
toffee fudge chunk	½ cup	9.0	120	68%
vanilla	½ cup	8.0	110	65%
vanilla fudge nut	½ cup	11.0	140	71%
ROUND CONTAINER ICE CREAM				
all-natural vanilla	½ cup	8.0	150	48%
apple pie	½ cup	8.0	160	45%
Bear Tracks	½ cup	9.0	180	45%
black raspberry	½ cup	8.0	150	45%
butter pecan	½ cup	11.0	170	58%
Caramel Cow Tracks	½ cup	8.0	170	42%
Caramel Fudge Cow Tracks	½ cup	7.0	170	37%
Caramel Invasion	½ cup	8.0	170	42%
cherry fudge chunk	½ cup	8.0	160	45%
chocolate chip	½ cup	9.0	160	51%
cookies 'n' cream	½ cup	9.0	170	48%
Deep Dark Secrets	½ cup	8.0	170	42%
Double Fudge Moose Tracks	½ cup	11.0	180	55%
French vanilla	½ cup	8.0	150	45%
homemade vanilla	½ cup	8.0	160	45%
Jamaican Me Crazy	½ cup	8.0	160	45%
Las Vegas Fudge Chunk	½ cup	11.0	190	52%
maple nut	½ cup	9.0	160	51%
Mint Cow Tracks	½ cup	11.0	190	52%
Moose Tracks	½ cup	12.0	190	57%
New York strawberry cheesecake	½ cup	7.0	150	42%
New York vanilla	½ cup	8.0	150	45%
Northern Exposure	½ cup	11.0	190	52%
Peanut Butter 'n' Fudge				
Cow Tracks	½ cup	12.0	190	57%
Peanut Fudgester	½ cup	10.0	180	50%
Pearson's				
Mint Pattie	½ cup	9.0	160	51%
Nut Goodie	½ cup	9.0	170	48%
peppermint bonbon	½ cup	9.0	160	51%
Raspberry Fudge Cow Tracks	½ cup	11.0	190	52%

Food and Description	Amount	Fat Grams	Total Calories	% Fat Calories
rocky road	½ cup	9.0	170	48%
Seriously Chocolate	½ cup	10.0	190	47%
snicker doodles	½ cup	9.0	180	45%
strawberries 'n' cream	½ cup	6.0	130	42%
toasted almond fudge	½ cup	8.0	170	42%
Torch Truffle	½ cup	7.0	160	39%
Twist and Shout	½ cup	12.0	200	54%
vanilla	½ cup	8.0	150	48%
vanilla custard	½ cup	8.0	160	45%
white chocolate raspberry truffle	½ cup	7.0	160	39%
SQUARE CONTAINER ICE CREAM				
Bear Creek Caramel	½ cup	7.0	150	42%
Black Jack Cherry	½ cup	7.0	140	45%
black walnut	½ cup	8.0	140	51%
Blackberry Creek Swirl	½ cup	7.0	140	45%
butter pecan	½ cup	9.0	150	54%
candy cane	½ cup	7.0	140	45%
caramel cashew crunch	½ cup	8.0	150	48%
chocolate	½ cup	6.0	130	42%
chocolate almond cluster	½ cup	8.0	150	48%
chocolate chip	½ cup	8.0	140	51%
chocolate chip cookie dough	½ cup	7.0	150	42%
Chocolate Monster	½ cup	7.0	150	42%
cinnamon	½ cup	7.0	130	48%
cookies 'n' cream	½ cup	7.0	150	42%
Cookies 'n' Scream	½ cup	7.0	140	45%
cotton candy	½ cup	7.0	130	48%
Dreaming of Mint	½ cup	7.0	150	42%
dulce de leche	½ cup	7.0	140	45%
French Silk Pie	½ cup	6.0	150	36%
German chocolate cake	½ cup	8.0	150	48%
Gone Fishin'	½ cup	7.0	160	39%
Holiday Dazzle	½ cup	8.0	150	48%
Holiday Mint Cookie	½ cup	8.0	150	48%
Holiday Mint Fudge	½ cup	6.0	140	39%
Homemade Vanilla	½ cup	7.0	140	45%
key lime	½ cup	7.0	150	42%
mango	½ cup	5.0	120	38%
maple nut	½ cup	8.0	140	51%
mint chocolate chip	½ cup	7.0	140	45%
Moose Lake Fudge	½ cup	10.0	170	53%
Neapolitan	½ cup	8.0	130	55%
New York Vanilla	½ cup	7.0	130	48%
Nuts to You	½ cup	8.0	150	48%
Orange Cream Dream	½ cup	4.0	130	28%
peanut butter pie	½ cup	11.0	180	55%
Pecan Turtle Trail	½ cup	8.0	160	45%
pineapple coconut	½ cup	6.0	140	39%
pink peppermint	½ cup	7.0	140	45%

Food and Description	Amount	Fat Grams	Total Calories	% Fat Calories
rocky road	½ cup	7.0	150	42%
strawberry	½ cup	6.0	120	45%
Timber Lodge Mint	½ cup	10.0	170	53%
tin roof sun	½ cup	7.0	140	45%
Tres Leches	½ cup	7.0	150	42%
Turtle Tracks	½ cup	6.0	150	36%
Under the Stars	½ cup	11.0	180	55%
vanilla	½ cup	7.0	130	48%
vanilla/chocolate	½ cup	6.0	130	42%
SQUARE CONTAINER ICE CREAM..LIGHT				
After Dinner Mint	½ cup	4.5	130	31%
caramel brownie fudge	½ cup	4.0	130	28%
chocolate chip	½ cup	4.0	120	30%
cookies 'n' cream	½ cup	4.5	130	31%
French silk chocolate	½ cup	5.0	130	35%
mint chocolate chip	½ cup	4.0	120	30%
Neapolitan	½ cup	3.0	110	25%
vanilla	½ cup	3.0	100	27%
■ (Lactaid)				
Scoopfuls				
cappuccino swirl	½ cup	7.0	150	42%
classic vanilla	½ cup	8.0	150	48%
creamy butter pecan	½ cup	10.0	170	53%
double chocolate chip	½ cup	8.0	160	45%
mint chocolate chip	½ cup	8.0	160	45%
■ (LeCarb)				
cinnamon	½ cup	7.0	100	63%
chocolate	½ cup	7.0	90	70%
chocolate almond	½ cup	9.0	120	68%
Homemade Vanilla	½ cup	7.0	100	63%
lemon	½ cup	6.0	100	54%
strawberry	½ cup	6.0	100	54%
vanilla	½ cup	7.0	100	63%
■ (M&M's Brand)				
brownie chocolate	½ cup	9.0	180	45%
mint	½ cup	11.0	190	52%
vanilla	½ cup	9.0	180	45%
■ (Pet)				
CARB LIMIT				
butter pecan	½ cup	10.0	120	75%
chocolate	½ cup	8.0	110	65%
Neapolitan	½ cup	8.0	110	65%
HOMEMADE				
banana split	½ cup	14.0	160	79%
Buttery Pecan Madness	½ cup	11.0	180	55%
peach cobbler	½ cup	7.0	150	42%
vanilla	½ cup	8.0	150	48%
SIGNATURE COLLECTIONS				
hot fudge sundae	½ cup	11.0	180	55%
Moose Tracks	½ cup	12.0	190	57%

Food and Description	Amount	Fat Grams	Total Calories	% Fat Calories
Nuttin' but Turtles	½ cup	8.0	160	45%
Oozle Doozle	½ cup	7.0	150	42%
pistachio almond	½ cup	10.0	160	56%
vanilla bean	½ cup	8.0	140	51%
TRADITIONAL				
black walnut	½ cup	9.0	150	54%
butter pecan	½ cup	11.0	160	62%
vanilla	½ cup	8.0	110	65%
cherry vanilla	½ cup	7.0	140	45%
chocolate	½ cup	7.0	120	53%
cookies 'n' cream	½ cup	9.0	160	51%
French vanilla	½ cup	8.0	150	48%
heavenly hash	½ cup	7.0	130	48%
Neapolitan	½ cup	7.0	130	48%
Nutty Buddy Chocolate Nut Sunday Cone	½ cup	9.0	160	51%
strawberry	½ cup	7.0	130	48%
vanilla	½ cup	7.0	140	45%
■ **(Schwan's)**				
CARBS				
Carb Comfort				
butter pecan	½ cup	8.0	130	55%
chocolate	½ cup	6.0	110	49%
Carblicious Vanilla Vanilla	½ cup	7.0	110	57%
PREMIUM..PREMIUM PLUS				
Black Jack Cherry	½ cup	8.0	160	45%
chocolate peanut butter	½ cup	11.0	190	52%
Chunky Chocolate Peanut Butter Binge	½ cup	12.0	190	57%
Raspberry Rumble	½ cup	8.0	160	45%
strawberry cheesecake	½ cup	7.0	150	42%
SIMPLY SUPREME				
Manhattan strawberry cheesecake	½ cup	12.0	230	47%
Peanut Butter Passion	½ cup	18.0	300	54%
TRADITIONAL				
banana nut	½ cup	8.0	150	48%
black raspberry	½ cup	7.0	130	48%
butter crunch	½ cup	8.0	150	48%
butter pecan	½ cup	9.0	150	54%
cherry nut	½ cup	7.0	140	45%
cherry vanilla	½ cup	7.0	140	45%
chip & mint	½ cup	8.0	150	48%
chocolate	½ cup	7.0	140	45%
chocolate almond	½ cup	8.0	150	48%
chocolate chip	½ cup	8.0	150	48%
chocolate chip cookie dough	½ cup	8.0	150	48%
chocolate fudge ripple	½ cup	7.0	140	45%
chocolate malt twist	½ cup	7.0	160	45%
chocolate marshmallow ripple	½ cup	6.0	140	39%

Food and Description	Amount	Fat Grams	Total Calories	% Fat Calories
coffee	½ cup	7.0	140	45%
Confetti Cake	½ cup	7.0	140	45%
cookies 'n' cream	½ cup	8.0	160	45%
Dark Sweet Cherry	½ cup	6.0	140	39%
dulce de leche	½ cup	7.0	150	42%
Dutch chocolate	½ cup	8.0	150	48%
maple nut	½ cup	9.0	150	54%
Neapolitan	½ cup	8.0	140	51%
peaches & cream	½ cup	5.0	130	35%
Pecan Caramel Quake	½ cup	9.0	180	45%
pecan praline sundae	½ cup	7.0	150	42%
Race Trax	½ cup	8.0	160	45%
rocky road	½ cup	7.0	150	42%
strawberry	½ cup	6.0	130	42%
Summer's Dream	½ cup	5.0	130	35%
Sweet Impressions				
Holiday Slices	1 slice	12.0	180	60%
vanilla	½ cup	7.0	140	45%
vanilla bean	½ cup	8.0	140	51%
■ (Starbuck's)				
caramel cappuccino swirl	½ cup	12.0	240	45%
classic coffee	½ cup	18.0	270	60%
coffee almond fudge	½ cup	18.0	270	60%
Java Chip	½ cup	11.0	270	37%
latte..low-fat	½ cup	3.0	170	16%
mud pie	½ cup	11.0	240	41%
white chocolate	½ cup	15.0	280	48%
■ (Tofutti) Non-Dairy Pints				
CHEESECAKE SUPREME				
cheesecake				
blueberry	½ cup	12.0	200	54%
chocolate	½ cup	12.0	200	54%
strawberry	½ cup	12.0	200	54%
LOW-FAT SUPREME				
chocolate fudge	½ cup	4.0	145	25%
coffee marshmallow swirl	½ cup	3.0	120	23%
vanilla fudge	½ cup	4.0	130	28%
NO SUGAR ADDED				
chocolate	½ cup	5.0	115	39%
strawberry	½ cup	5.0	110	41%
PREMIUM				
better pecan	½ cup	13.0	210	56%
chocolate cookie crunch	½ cup	11.0	210	47%
chocolate supreme	½ cup	11.0	180	55%
mint chocolate chip	½ cup	13.0	210	56%
vanilla	½ cup	11.0	190	52%
vanilla almond bark	½ cup	13.0	210	56%
vanilla fudge	½ cup	9.0	190	43%
wildberry supreme	½ cup	9.0	190	43%

Food and Description	Amount	Fat Grams	Total Calories	% Fat Calories
SUPER SOY SUPREME				
Bella Vanilla	½ cup	8.0	160	45%
Cool Cappuccino	½ cup	9.0	170	48%
Plum Crazy	½ cup	8.0	160	45%
NY NY Chocolate	½ cup	9.0	170	48%
■ **(Turkey Hill)**				
CARB IQ				
butter pecan	½ cup	11.0	140	71%
LIGHT				
chocolate mint chip	½ cup	4.5	160	25%
vanilla & chocolate	½ cup	3.0	110	25%
LOW FAT..NO SUGAR				
Dutch chocolate	½ cup	2.0	80	23%
TRADITIONAL				
black cherry	½ cup	7.0	140	45%
choco malt chip..				
Creamy Commotions	½ cup	9.0	170	48%
Denali Original Moose Tracks..				
Creamy Commotions	½ cup	12.0	190	90%
Eagles Touchdown Sundae	½ cup	11.0	190	52%
Neapolitan	½ cup	8.0	150	48%
Peanut Butter Kandy Kake..				
Creamy Commotions	½ cup	14.0	230	55%
Philadelphia-style vanilla bean	½ cup	9.0	160	51%
Phillies Graham Slam	½ cup	11.0	190	52%
■ **(Weight Watchers)**				
SCROUNDS				
low-fat				
vanilla/chocolate				
giant sundae cups	1 cup	0.5	150	3%
reduced-fat..no sugar added				
butter pecan	½ cup	7.0	110	57%
crunchy peanut butter cup	½ cup	7.0	110	57%
Moose Tracks	½ cup	8.0	130	55%
Neapolitan	½ cup	4.0	90	40%
vanilla	½ cup	4.0	90	40%

ICE CREAM BARS, SANDWICHES & FROZEN NOVELTIES (See also FRUIT ICES, BARS & POPS; RICE FROZEN DESSERT; SHERBET; TOFU FROZEN DESSERT)

Food and Description	Amount	Fat Grams	Total Calories	% Fat Calories
■ **(Atkins)** *ENDULGE*				
NOVELTIES..Bars				
butter pecan	1 bar	16.0	180	80%
caramel turtle sundae	1 bar	16.0	180	80%
chocolate fudge	1 bar	11.0	130	76%
chocolate fudge swirl	1 bar	16.0	180	80%
peanut butter swirl	1 bar	16.0	180	80%
vanilla fudge swirl	1 bar	16.0	180	80%
vanilla milk chocolate	1 bar	16.0	180	80%
NOVELTIES..Sandwiches				
chocolate	1 sdw	10.0	150	60%
peanut butter	1 sdw	10.0	150	60%

Food and Description	Amount	Fat Grams	Total Calories	% Fat Calories
vanilla	1 sdw	10.0	150	60%
SINGLE-SERVE BARS				
butter pecan	1 bar	16.0	180	80%
chocolate fudge swirl	1 bar	16.0	180	80%
vanilla w/milk chocolate				
coating	1 bar	16.0	180	80%
■ **(Ben & Jerry's)**				
PEACE POPS				
Cherry Garcia	1 pop	18.0	280	58%
cookie dough	1 pop	22.0	380	52%
One Sweet Whirled	1 pop	16.0	270	53%
vanilla	1 pop	20.0	300	60%
vanilla w/Heath toffee	1 pop	21.0	320	59%
■ **(Blue Bunny)**				
BARS				
4-pack novelties..bars				
NASCAR Speedway				
Sundae	1 bar	20.0	300	60%
6-pack novelties..bars				
black raspberry	1 bar	16.0	230	63%
crunch	1 bar	13.0	190	62%
fudge	1 bar	1.5	110	12%
Goin' Bananas	1 bar	1.0	110	8%
Heath	1 bar	13.0	190	62%
root beer float	1 bar	2.5	90	25%
Star Bars..reduced fat	1 bar	8.0	130	55%
Sundae Crunch				
chocolate	1 bar	9.0	170	48%
strawberry	1 bar	9.0	170	48%
12-pack novelties..bars				
English toffee	1 bar	9.0	130	62%
Homemade Vanilla	1 bar	11.0	150	66%
Krunch	1 bar	10.0	150	60%
Star Bars..reduced-fat	1 bar	7.0	110	57%
CARB FREEDOM..Bars				
almond	1 bar	13.0	160	73%
fudge	1 bar	4.0	90	40%
vanilla	1 bar	12.0	140	77%
CONES				
6-pack novelties				
The Champ!				
caramel	1 cone	19.0	350	49%
chocolate lover's	1 cone	15.0	300	45%
vanilla	1 cone	18.0	320	51%
vanilla nutty sundae	1 cone	10.0	240	38%
8-pack novelties				
classic sundae	1 cone	14.0	270	47%
DISNEY				
Buzz Lightyear S'wiches	1 sdw	4.0	110	33%
Mickey S'wiches	1 sdw	2.5	100	23%

Food and Description	Amount	Fat Grams	Total Calories	% Fat Calories
mud 'n' fudge bars	1 bar	1.0	80	11%
Power Ranger Cool Tubes	1 tube	0.5	80	6%
Winnie the Pooh Cool Tubes	1 tube	1.0	80	11%
HEALTH SMART				
raspberry & orange crème	1 bar	–	70	–
SANDWICHES				
10-pack novelties				
Homemade Vanilla	1 Sdw	8.0	180	40%
Mississippi Mud	1 sdw	8.0	190	38%
strawberry cheesecake	1 sdw	7.0	180	35%
vanilla	1 sdw	7.0	170	37%
12-pack novelties				
Neapolitan	1 sdw	7.0	180	35%
vanilla	1 sdw	7.0	170	37%
SWEET FREEDOM..12-pack novelties				
Lites				
Krunch	1 bar	6.0	90	60%
sandwiches				
double vanilla	1 sdw	2.0	150	12%
mini	1 sdw	1.5	140	10%
vanilla..low-fat	1 sdw	1.5	140	10%
■ **(Breyers)** Ice Cream Bar				
Hershey's almond	1 bar	9.0	270	30%
■ **CARNATION** (*See* (Nestlé) in this section)				
■ **(Dove)**				
ICE CREAM BARS				
almond				
multipack	1 bar	18.0	270	60%
singles	1 bar	23.0	340	61%
milk chocolate caramel toffee crunch				
multipack	1 bar	16.0	270	53%
singles	1 bar	20.0	330	55%
Original Chocolate				
w/chocolate ice cream				
multipack	1 bar	17.0	260	59%
singles	1 bar	21.0	320	59%
vanilla				
w/dark chocolate coating				
multipack	1 bar	17.0	260	43%
singles	1 bar	21.0	320	59%
w/milk chocolate coating				
multipack	1 bar	17.0	260	43%
singles	1 bar	21.0	330	57%
LIMITED EDITION DOVE BAR				
Crunchy Cookies w/Cream	1 bar	18.0	280	58%
MINIATURES				
Flavor Collection	5 pieces	20.0	310	58%
milk chocolate				
w/French vanilla ice cream	5 pieces	20.0	320	56%
w/vanilla ice cream	5 pieces	20.0	320	56%

Food and Description	Amount	Fat Grams	Total Calories	% Fat Calories
■ **DRUMSTICK** (*See* Nestlé, within this category)				
■ **(Eskimo Pie)**				
BARS				
chocolate éclair bars	1 bar	12.0	220	49%
Frosty Snowman	1 bar	5.0	100	45%
ice cream bar				
w/dark chocolate coating	2.5 oz bar	10.0	160	56%
king-size	4 oz bar	14.0	220	57%
w/milk chocolate coating	1 bar	11.0	160	62%
Jolly Santas	1 bar	5.0	90	50%
strawberry shortcake	1 bar	12.0	220	49%
thin mint	1 bar	17.0	250	61%
toasted almond	1 bar	12.0	220	49%
vanilla w/milk chocolate coating	1 bar	15.0	220	61%
CHIPWICH				
ice cream sandwiches				
king-size..single-serve	1 sdw	13.0	310	38%
vanilla	1 sdw	11.0	250	40%
no sugar added	1 sdw	8.0	190	38%
vanilla fudge..low-fat	1 sdw	5.0	200	23%
NO SUGAR ADDED..BARS & SANDWICHES				
cookies 'n' cream	1 bar	8.0	130	55%
chocolate crisp rice	1 bar	8.0	120	60%
fudge bar	1 bar	1.0	60	15%
ice cream cone..vanilla				
reduced-fat	1 cone	12.0	200	54%
ice cream sandwich..chocolate				
slender pie clamshell	1 sdw	1.5	120	11%
ice cream sandwich..vanilla				
slender pie clamshell	1 sdw	1.5	120	11%
ice cream sandwich..vanilla fudge				
slender pie clamshell	1 sdw	1.5	120	11%
vanilla traditional ice cream				
sandwich..reduced-fat	1 sdw	4.0	160	23%
vanilla w/dark chocolate				
reduced-fat	1 bar	8.0	120	60%
SANDWICHES				
Chilly Bears cookies 'n' cream	1 sdw	9.0	180	40%
gingerbread men	1 sdw	6.0	160	34%
SINGLE-SERVE				
bars				
king-size				
candy center crunch	1 bar	16.0	230	63%
chocolate éclair	1 bar	29.0	410	64%
premium	1 bar	12.0	220	49%
ice cream bar	1 bar	17.0	250	61%
giant	1 bar	29.0	410	64%
strawberry shortcake	1 bar	13.0	250	47%
premium	1 bar	12.0	220	49%

Food and Description	Amount	Fat Grams	Total Calories	% Fat Calories
toasted almond	1 bar	16.0	230	63%
premium	1 bar	17.0	250	61%
cones				
king size..vanilla w/chocolate				
topping and peanuts	1 cone	13.0	250	47%
cups				
cookies 'n' cream	1 cup	13.0	310	38%
sandwiches				
cookies 'n' cream	1 sdw	9.0	230	35%
Giant King Size				
Neapolitan	1 sdw	10.0	250	36%
vanilla	1 sdw	10.0	250	36%
■ (Good Humor)				
ICE CREAM BARS				
multi-packs				
chocolate éclair bar	1 bar	8.0	160	45%
cookies 'n' cream bar	1 bar	12.0	190	57%
dark chocolate	1 bar	13.0	190	62%
milk chocolate	1 bar	13.0	180	65%
strawberry shortcake	1 bar	9.0	170	48%
toasted almond	1 bar	10.0	180	50%
single-serve				
candy-center crunch	1 bar	23.0	310	67%
chocolate éclair bar	1 bar	11.0	220	45%
Number 1 Bar	1 bar	11.0	200	50%
Oreo cookie	1 bar	15.0	250	54%
premium vanilla	1 bar	17.0	260	59%
Reese's Peanut Butter	1 bar	21.0	310	61%
strawberry shortcake	1 bar	12.0	230	47%
toasted almond	1 bar	12.0	230	47%
ICE CREAM CONES & CUPS..Singles				
Giant King Cone	1 cone	22.0	400	50%
King Cone	1 cone	13.0	250	47%
Premium Sundae	1 cone	15.0	270	50%
Sundae Twist Cup	1 cup	2.6	160	14%
ICE CREAM SANDWICHES..Singles				
giant				
Neapolitan	1 sdw	10.0	250	36%
vanilla	1 sdw	10.0	250	36%
premium				
cookie	1 sdw	13.0	290	40%
vanilla	1 sdw	6.0	160	34%
■ (Häagen-Dazs)				
Multipack Bars				
caramel & almond crunch	1 bar	19.0	300	57%
chocolate & dark chocolate	1 bar	20.0	290	62%
chocolate peanut butter swirl	1 bar	23.0	320	65%
chocolate sorbet	1 bar	–	80	–
coffee & almond crunch	1 bar	22.0	310	64%
cookies 'n' cream crunch	1 bar	22.0	310	64%
dulce de leche caramel	1 bar	19.0	300	57%

Food and Description	Amount	Fat Grams	Total Calories	% Fat Calories
raspberry cheesecake	1 bar	19.0	300	57%
strawberry cheesecake	1 bar	25.0	370	60%
vanilla & almonds	1 bar	23.0	320	65%
vanilla & dark chocolate	1 bar	20.0	280	64%
vanilla & milk chocolate	1 bar	20.0	280	64%
■ (Healthy Choice)				
BARS				
low-fat				
fudge				
6-pack	1 bar	1.0	80	11%
12-pack	1 bar	1.5	90	15%
mocha fudge..6-pack	1 bar	1.5	90	15%
sorbet & cream	1 bar	1.0	100	9%
strawberry & cream				
6-pack	1 bar	1.5	90	15%
12-pack	1 bar	1.5	110	12%
SANDWICHES				
caramel	1 sdw	3.0	140	19%
fudge swirl	1 sdw	3.0	140	19%
vanilla	1 sdw	3.0	130	21%
■ (Hood)				
BARS				
chocolate-covered ice cream bar				
original	1 bar	12.0	160	68%
reduced-fat	1 bar	6.0	100	54%
chocolate éclair	1 bar	10.0	150	60%
Cream Surfers..Hawaiian Punch Bars				
Fruit Juicy Red	1 bar	1.5	90	15%
Ocean Orange 98% fat-free	1 bar	1.5	90	15%
fudge bars				
dipped delights				
chocolate fudge	1 bar	0.5	95	5%
no sugar added	1 bar	1.5	50	27%
Java Smoothie	1 bar	2.5	90	25%
peanut butter chocolate	1 bar	8.0	135	53%
orange cream..regular	1 bar	1.5	90	15%
Rocket	1 bar	5.0	120	38%
Sport Sundae	1 bar	17.0	250	61%
CONES				
Nutty Royale	1 cone	12.0	220	49%
SANDWICHES				
Hoodsie				
light	1 sdw	3.5	160	20%
low-fat	1 sdw	1.5	90	15%
mint	1 sdw	4.0	100	36%
original	1 sdw	7.0	180	35%
■ (Imagine) Non-Dairy Desserts				
DREAM BARS				
chocolate	1 bar	15.0	270	50%
chocolate nutty	1 bar	18.0	270	60%

Food and Description	Amount	Fat Grams	Total Calories	% Fat Calories
vanilla	1 bar	14.0	270	47%
vanilla nutty	1 bar	18.0	260	62%
DREAM PIES				
chocolate	1 pie	18.0	320	51%
mint	1 pie	18.0	320	51%
mocha	1 pie	17.0	320	48%
vanilla	1 pie	17.0	320	48%
■ (Kemps)				
BARS	1 bar	12.0	160	68%
Cookie Crunch Jr.				
2.6 oz	1 bar	7.0	100	63%
3 oz	1 bar	8.0	120	60%
English toffee	1 bar	11.0	160	62%
float bars	2 bars	1.5	100	14%
fudge bar				
6-pack	1 bar	0.5	80	5%
JR's	2 bars	0.5	160	3%
Kemp's ice cream bar w/chocolate coating				
2.5 oz	1 bar	12.0	160	68%
King	1 bar	16.0	240	60%
Kemp's Krunch Bar				
12-pack	1 bar	9.0	140	58%
Kemp's toffee bars	1 bar	12.0	170	64%
Krunch				
JR	2 bars	14.0	210	60%
King	1 bar	15.0	230	59%
King Malt Ball crunch bar	1 bar	20.0	280	64%
Koala bar	1 bar	19.0	290	59%
Moo Jr's	2 bars	11.0	190	52%
orange crème bar				
1.78 oz	1 bar	3.0	80	34%
King	1 bar	5.0	120	38%
Scooter				
cream	2 bars	1.5	90	15%
fudge	2 bars	12.0	170	64%
Trios..vanilla	2 bars	15.0	210	64%
CARB PROMISE				
ice cream bars	1 bar	11.0	140	71%
CONES				
ice cream cones/vanilla mini	1 cone	10.0	160	56%
Kemps Sundae cone	1 cone	17.0	290	53%
caramel	1 cone	16.0	290	50%
combination	1 cone	17.0	290	53%
Nutty Royale	1 cone	12.0	220	49%
old-fashioned sundae..vanilla	1 cone	17.0	290	53%
NO SUGAR ADDED				
fudge bar..12-pack	1 bar	5.0	110	41%
ice cream bar..12-pack	1 bar	7.0	100	63%
ice cream sandwich..vanilla	1 sdw	4.0	140	26%

Food and Description	Amount	Fat Grams	Total Calories	% Fat Calories
SANDWICHES				
chocolate chip	1 sdw	7.0	140	45%
cookies 'n' cream	1 sdw	6.0	170	32%
6-pack	1 sdw	6.0	140	39%
Cow Tracks	1 sdw	9.0	190	43%
double chocolate	1 sdw	6.0	160	34%
Kemp's King..Neapolitan	1 sdw	11.0	280	35%
Kemp's mint chocolate chip	1 sdw	7.0	170	37%
Kempwich	1 sdw	18.0	340	48%
Pearson's Mint Pattie	1 sdw	7.0	180	35%
vanilla				
mini	1 sdw	3.5	100	32%
mini..reduced-fat	1 sdw	1.5	90	15%
King	1 sdw	12.0	280	39%
regular..12-pack	1 sdw	6.0	160	34%
■ (Klondike)				
BARS				
cappuccino	1 bar	19.0	280	61%
Caramel Krunch	1 bar	17.0	270	57%
chocolate éclair	1 bar	8.0	160	45%
Chocolate for Chocoholics	1 bar	19.0	280	61%
dark chocolate	1 bar	19.0	280	61%
Heath...single	1 bar	20.0	300	60%
Hershey's w/almond	1 bar	18.0	250	65%
Krunch				
multipack	1 bar	19.0	280	61%
single	1 bar	17.0	260	59%
Minis Snack-Size Vanilla	1 bar	11.0	170	58%
Movie Bites..4.48-oz pkg	1 pkg	22.0	310	64%
Neapolitan	1 bar	19.0	280	61%
original vanilla	1 bar	19.0	280	61%
Planters caramel & peanut				
multipack	1 bar	19.0	290	59%
single	1 bar	20	300	60%
Slim-a-Bear..no sugar added				
reduced-fat vanilla	1 bar	9.0	170	48%
premium fudge bar..chocolate 98% fat-free..sweetened w/Splenda	1 bar	1.5	90	15%
strawberry shortcake	1 bar	9.0	170	48%
toasted almond	1 bar	10.0	180	50%
York Peppermint Pattie	1 bar	19.0	280	61%
CARB SMART				
ice cream bar				
multipack	1 bar	16.0	210	69%
single	1 bar	15.0	170	79%
ice cream cone	1 cone	16.0	210	69%
ice cream fudge bar	1 bar	7.0	100	63%
ice cream sandwich	1 sdw	4.5	80	51%

Food and Description	Amount	Fat Grams	Total Calories	% Fat Calories
CONES				
Big Bear Sundae Kone				
vanilla	1 cone	17.0	300	51%
w/caramel center	1 cone	18.0	320	51%
chocolate	1 cone	16.0	280	51%
vanilla	1 cone	16.0	280	51%
caramel	1 cone	16.0	300	48%
fudge	1 cone	16.0	300	48%
Slim-a-Bear 96% fat-free cones				
chocolate	1 cone	3.0	180	15%
vanilla	1 cone	3.0	170	16%
CUPS				
Sundae w/chocolate coating	1 cup	17.0	280	55%
SANDWICHES				
Big Bear				
ice cream cookie	1 sdw	12.0	270	40%
Neapolitan	1 sdw	7.0	190	33%
single-serve	1 sdw	12.0	300	36%
vanilla	1 sdw	7.0	190	33%
single-serve	1 sdw	12.0	300	36%
Giant Cookie w/Hershey's				
Chips..single-serve	1 sdw	20.0	470	38%
Mini Reese's Pieces..4.2 oz	1 pkg	12.0	260	42%
Oreo Cookie	1 sdw	9.0	230	35%
Slim-a-Bear				
98% fat-free				
chocolate	1 sdw	1.5	130	10%
mint	1 sdw	1.5	130	10%
vanilla	1 sdw	1.5	130	10%
no sugar added..vanilla	1 sdw	3.0	120	23%
TACOS...singles				
Choco Taco	1 taco	16.0	290	50%
■ (M&M BRAND)				
ICE CREAM				
cone	1 cone	11.0	230	43%
sandwich				
brownie	1 sdw	10.0	220	41%
vanilla	1 sdw	11.0	220	45%
■ (Nestlé)				
Bon Bons				
dark chocolate	8 pieces	22.0	330	60%
milk chocolate	8 pieces	22.0	330	60%
Butterfinger	1 bar	15.0	210	64%
Carnation				
sandwiches				
Neapolitan..single	1 sdw	10.0	240	38%
Neapolitan..multipack	1 sdw	8.0	290	38%
vanilla..single	1 sdw	10.0	240	38%
vanilla..multipack	1 sdw	8.0	200	36%

Food and Description	Amount	Fat Grams	Total Calories	% Fat Calories
sundae cups				
w/chocolate topping	1 cup	10.0	200	45%
w/strawberry topping	1 cup	9.0	210	39%
Crunch Bar				
caramel	1 bar	14.0	210	60%
chocolate & vanilla	1 bar	16.0	230	63%
reduced-fat	1 bar	8.0	150	48%
vanilla	1 bar	15.0	220	61%
Drumstick				
caramel	1 cone	19.0	340	50%
chocolate	1 cone	19.0	340	50%
chocolate-dipped	1 cone	17.0	340	45%
classic				
fudge sundae	1 cone	19.0	340	50%
s'mores	1 cone	19.0	340	50%
strawberry cheesecake	1 cone	19.0	340	50%
cookies 'n' cream	1 cone	19.0	340	50%
fudge	1 cone	19.0	340	50%
w/chocolate layers	1 cone	16.0	280	51%
reduced-fat	1 cone	13.0	280	42%
triple chocolate	1 cone	13.0	260	45%
vanilla	1 cone	19.0	340	50%
Husky Bar	1 bar	22.0	340	58%
Toll House Cookie Sandwich				
chocolate chip cookie	1 cookie	23.0	520	40%
chocolate chocolate chip cookie	1 sdw	29.0	550	47%
■ (Pet)				
BARS				
BROWN MULE	1 bar	10.0	150	60%
vanilla ice cream				
w/orange sherbet	1 bar	2.5	90	25%
CONES				
Nutty Royale..6-count	1 cone	13.0	210	56%
SANDWICHES				
chocolate & vanilla wafers	1 sdw	6.0	160	34%
mini	1 sdw	4.5	110	37%
Neapolitan...strawberry/ vanilla/chocolate	1 sdw	7.0	170	38%
vanilla & chocolate wafers				
light	1 sdw	3.0	140	19%
original	1 sdw	6.0	150	36%
■ (Popsicle)				
Characters..singles				
Col. Crunch				
chocolate éclair	1 bar	8.0	160	45%
strawberry	1 bar	9.0	170	48%
Snoopy ice cream bar	1 bar	8.0	150	48%
WWE ice cream bar	1 bar	9.0	180	45%

Food and Description	Amount	Fat Grams	Total Calories	% Fat Calories
Creamsicle				
CarbSmart pops..1.75 oz				
all flavors	1 pop	1.0	20	45%
no sugar added..multi-packs				
all flavors	1 bar	–	25	–
original..single..orange	1 bar	3.0	110	25%
original..multi-packs..2.5 oz				
all flavors	1 bar	2.5	100	23%
pop..1.75 oz				
all flavors	1 pop	2.0	70	26%
pop..no sugar added..multi-packs	1 pop	–	25	–
sugar-free..1.65 oz each				
all flavors	2 pops	2.0	40	45%
Fudge Pop	1 pop	1.0	60	15%
Fudgsicle				
chocolate..single	1 bar	1.5	90	15%
chocolate vanilla swirl	1 bar	1.5	120	11%
fat-free	1 bar	–	60	–
mini...1.2 oz each	2 pops	1.5	80	17%
no sugar added..multi-packs				
1.65 oz	2 pops	0.5	70	6%
1.75 oz	2 pops	1.0	90	10%
original				
bar...2.5 oz	1 bar	1.5	90	15%
pop	1 pop	1.0	60	15%
vanilla	1 bar	2.0	120	15%
Heath Bar	1 bar	20.0	300	60%
ice cream bar..vanilla..single	1 bar	11.0	160	62%
ice cream pops..mini	2 pops	13.0	200	59%
ice cream sandwich..mini	2 oz	3.5	100	32%
Krunch Bar	1 bar	17.0	270	57%
Sprinklers Bar..single	1 bar	6.0	130	42%
sundae cup	1 cup	17.0	280	55%
■ (Schwan's)				
BARS				
caramel premium	1 bar	14.0	210	60%
chocolate fudge sticks	1 bar	1.5	110	12%
chocolate sundae crunch	1 bar	9.0	180	45%
double crunch	1 bar	21.0	260	73%
English toffee	1 bar	13.0	200	59%
fudge stick	1 bar	1.5	110	12%
Gold 'n' Nugit	1 bar	16.0	250	58%
Krispie Krunch	1 bar	8.0	120	60%
peanut stick	1 bar	14.0	200	62%
premium	1 bar	15.0	210	64%
rainbow stick	1 bar	1.0	90	10%
root beer float	1 bar	3.0	90	30%
Schwan's ice cream	1 bar	14.0	190	66%
Silver Mint	1 bar	10.0	150	60%
strawberry crunch	1 bar	8.0	170	42%

Food and Description	Amount	Fat Grams	Total Calories	% Fat Calories
Trim Creations				
chocolate fudge stick	1 bar	–	50	–
CONES				
banana fudge sundae	1 cone	11.0	250	40%
caramel round top	1 cone	19.0	350	49%
chip & mint sundae	1 cone	11.0	260	38%
pecan praline sundae	1 cone	12.0	260	42%
Race Trax	1 cone	14.0	270	47%
rocky road sundae	1 cone	11.0	260	38%
vanilla	1 cone	10.0	210	47%
vanilla fudge chocolate sundae	1 cone	11.0	260	38%
HEALTHY CREATIONS Fat-Free				
fudge swirl sundae cup	1 cup	–	100	–
rainbow bar	1 bar	–	60	–
raspberry and orange	1 bar	–	70	–
strawberry sundae cup	1 cup	–	70	–
ICE CREAM CUPS				
apple pie à la mode	½ cup	10.0	260	35%
brownie à la mode	½ cup	13.0	280	42%
caramel cappuccino	1 cup	15.0	300	45%
chocolate fudge sundae	1 cup	5.0	120	38%
confetti	1 cup	7.0	140	45%
frozen hot chocolate	½ cup	8.0	160	45%
root beer float	1 cup	3.5	140	23%
sundae				
chocolate	1 cup	5.0	120	38%
confetti	1 cup	7.0	140	45%
strawberry	1 cup	5.0	120	38%
vanilla	1 cup	6.0	110	49%
SANDWICH				
chocolate				
chip cookie	1 sandwich	13.0	260	45%
mini lite	1 sandwich	2.0	100	18%
Glacier Bay Lemon	1 sandwich	7.0	190	33%
Mississippi Mud	1 sandwich	8.0	200	36%
Neapolitan	1 sandwich	7.0	160	39%
Race Trax	1 sandwich	10.0	210	43%
vanilla	1 sandwich	7.0	170	34%
■ (Slim-Fast)				
chocolate fudge bar	1 bar	1.5	110	12%
ice cream sandwich				
chocolate	1 sdw	1.5	130	10%
vanilla	1 sdw	1.0	130	7%
■ (Starbucks)				
FRAPPUCCINO COFFEE BARS				
caffe vanilla	1 bar	1.5	110	12%
java fudge	1 bar	2.0	130	14%
mocha	1 bar	2.0	120	15%
■ (Tofutti))				
BARS				
Hooray Hooray	1 bar	9.0	150	54%

Food and Description	Amount	Fat Grams	Total Calories	% Fat Calories
Marry Me	1 bar	8.0	168	43%
Monkey...peanut butter	1 bar	13.0	220	53%
SANDWICHES..Cuties				
blueberry wave	1 sdw	6.0	140	39%
chocolate	1 sdw	5.0	130	35%
chocolate wave	1 sdw	6.0	140	39%
coffee break	1 sdw	5.0	130	35%
cookies 'n' cream	1 sdw	6.0	120	45%
jazzy	1 sdw	5.0	120	38%
mint chocolate chip	1 sdw	5.0	120	38%
peanut butter	1 sdw	8.0	165	44%
strawberry wave	1 sdw	6.0	140	39%
totally vanilla	1 sdw	5.0	120	38%
vanilla	1 sdw	5.0	120	38%
no sugar added	1 sdw	5.0	100	45%
wild berry	1 sdw	6.0	140	39%
SANDWICHES..Too-Too's				
vanilla chocolate chip	1 sdw	11.0	230	43%
STICKS				
Chocolate Fudge Treats	1 Stick	–	30	–
Coffee Break Treats	1 Stick	–	30	–
Totally Fudge	1 stick	1.5	95	14%
■ (Weight Watchers)				
BARS				
chocolate mousse	1 bar	–	40	–
chocolate treat	1 bar	1.5	100	14%
English toffee crunch	1 bar	6.0	110	49%
fudge treat	1 bar	0.5	100	5%
Giant...low-fat				
cookies 'n' cream	1 bar	2.0	120	15%
fudge	1 bar	–	80	–
orange vanilla treat	1 bar	0.5	40	11%
CONES				
chocolate sundae	1 cone	2.5	130	17%
peanut butter fudge	1 cone	2.5	130	17%
vanilla	1 cone	2.5	130	17%
vanilla fudge	1 cone	2.5	130	17%
CUPS...Sundae..Giant				
chocolate chocolate	1 cup	0.5	150	3%
peanut butter chocolate	1 cup	1.0	150	6%
SANDWICHES				
chocolate...round	1 sdw	1.5	130	10%
mint...round	1 sdw	1.5	130	10%
peanut butter 'n' fudge...round	1 sdw	1.5	130	10%
vanilla ice cream	1 sdw	1.5	130	10%
vanilla...round	1 sdw	1.5	130	10%
ICE CREAM CONES & CUPS				
(Baskin-Robbins) cones				
cake..plain	1 cone	–	25	–
sugar	1 cone	–	60	–

Food and Description	Amount	Fat Grams	Total Calories	% Fat Calories
waffle				
Keebler pre-made	1 cone	5.0	400	11%
large	1 cone	1.5	120	11%
(Comet)				
cones				
Oreo chocolate	1 cone	0.5	50	9%
sugar	1 cone	–	60	–
cups..plain/colors	1 cup	–	20	–
(Joy Cone)				
cones				
kid's cone	3 cups	–	15	–
sugar	1 cone	–	50	–
cups				
cake				
jumbo	1 cup	–	30	–
regular	1 cup	–	20	–
sundae	1 up	–	30	–
flavored color	1 cup	–	20	–
waffle				
bowls	1 bowl	0.5	80	6%
cones	1 cone	0.5	90	5%
(Keebler)				
fudge-dipped cup	1 cup	1.5	35	39%
ice cream cup/vanilla	1 cup	–	15	–
sugar cone	1 cone	0.5	50	9%
waffle				
bowl	1 bowl	1.0	50	18%
cone	1 cone	1.0	50	18%
(Let's Do Organic)				
waffle				
bowls	1 bowl	3.0	111	24%
cones	1 cone	3.0	120	23%
(Little Debbie) ice cream cups	1 cup	–	15	–

ICE CREAM SANDWICH (*See* ICE CREAM BARS, SANDWICHES & FROZEN NOVELTIES)
ICE CREAM TOPPING (*See also* CREAM; CUSTARD; DIP; WHIPPED TOPPING)
BOTTLED..CANNED or JARRED

Food and Description	Amount	Fat Grams	Total Calories	% Fat Calories
(Fisher)				
nut topping				
chef's natural	1 oz	14.0	170	74%
mixed nut variety	~½ oz	9.0	100	81%
(Hershey's)				
CHOCOLATE SHOPPE TOPPINGS				
double chocolate	2 Tbs	2.0	120	15%
hot fudge				
fat-free	2 Tbs	–	100	–
regular	2 Tbs	5.0	130	35%
DESSERT TOPPINGS..Sprinkles				
Reese's peanut butter				
& milk chocolate	2 Tbs	4.0	90	40%
triple chocolate	2 Tbs	3.0	90	30%

Food and Description	Amount	Fat Grams	Total Calories	% Fat Calories
SHELL TOPPINGS				
chocolate fudge cookie	2 Tbs	14.0	190	66%
Heath	2 Tbs	17.0	230	67%
Krackel	2 Tbs	14.0	190	66%
milk chocolate	2 Tbs	18.0	230	70%
Reese's	2 Tbs	17.0	220	70%
SUNDAE SYRUPS				
caramel	2 Tbs	–	100	–
double chocolate fudge	1 Tbs	4.0	50	72%
SYRUP..Hershey's				
chocolate				
light	2 Tbs	–	50	–
malt..Whoppers	2 Tbs	–	100	–
original	2 Tbs	–	100	–
strawberry	2 Tbs	–	100	–
TOPPING..HERSHEY'S CANNED				
chocolate fudge	2 Tbs	6.0	130	42%
(Kraft)				
butterscotch	2 Tbs	1.5	130	10%
caramel	2 Tbs	–	120	–
chocolate-flavored	2 Tbs	–	110	–
hot fudge	2 Tbs	4.5	140	29%
pineapple	2 Tbs	–	110	–
strawberry	2 Tbs	–	110	–
(Planters) nut topping	2 Tbs	9.0	100	81%
(Smucker's)				
PLATE SCRAPERS DESSERT TOPPINGS				
caramel	2 Tbs	–	100	–
chocolate	2 Tbs	1.0	100	9%
raspberry	2 Tbs	–	100	–
white chocolate	2 Tbs	2.5	110	20%
SPECIALTY ICE CREAM TOPPINGS				
Dove Toppings				
dark chocolate	2 Tbs	5.0	140	32%
milk chocolate	2 Tbs	4.0	130	28%
dulce de leche milk				
caramel spread	2 Tbs	1.5	110	12%
pecans in syrup	1 Tbs	10.0	170	53%
special recipe				
butterscotch caramel	2 Tbs	1.0	130	7%
hot fudge	2 Tbs	4.0	140	26%
sugar-free..spoonable	2 Tbs	–	90	–
walnuts in syrup	2 Tbs	9.0	170	48%
TOPPINGS, OTHER				
3 Musketeers..sundae syrup	2 Tbs	2.0	110	16%
butterscotch..sundae syrup	2 Tbs	–	100	–
butterscotch & caramel syrup				
regular..spoonable	2 Tbs	–	130	–

Food and Description	Amount	Fat Grams	Total Calories	% Fat Calories
sundae	2 Tbs	–	110	–
butterscotch & caramel topping				
regular..spoonable	2 Tbs	–	130	–
special recipe	2 Tbs	1.0	130	7%
caramel				
fat-free microwavable	2 Tbs	–	110	–
hot	2 Tbs	3.0	120	23%
sundae syrup	2 Tbs	–	100	–
chocolate-flavored sundae syrup	2 Tbs	–	110	–
chocolate-flavored syrup				
sugar-free	2 Tbs	–	100	–
chocolate fudge				
microwavable	2 Tbs	1.5	130	10%
regular..spoonable	2 Tbs	1.5	130	10%
sundae syrup	2 Tbs	–	110	–
dulce de leche milk caramel				
spoonable	2 Tbs	4.0	140	26%
hot caramel	2 Tbs	3.0	120	23%
hot fudge				
light/fat-free	2 Tbs	–	90	–
microwavable				
fat-free	2 Tbs	–	110	–
original	2 Tbs	2.5	130	17%
regular..spoonable	2 Tbs	4.0	140	26%
special recipe	2 Tbs	4.0	140	26%
sugar-free	2 Tbs	–	100	–
Magic Shell toppings				
caramel	2 Tbs	18.0	220	74%
chocolate	2 Tbs	18.0	220	74%
chocolate fudge	2 Tbs	18.0	220	74%
Twix	2 Tbs	15.0	210	64%
marshmallow..spoonable	2 Tbs	–	120	–
Milky Way..spoonable	2 Tbs	3.5	130	24%
pecans in syrup	2 Tbs	10.0	170	53%
pineapple..spoonable	2 Tbs	–	110	–
strawberry				
regular..spoonable	2 Tbs	–	100	–
sundae syrup	2 Tbs	–	110	–
walnuts in syrup	2 Tbs	9.0	170	48%
(Steel's) sugar-free toppings				
amaretto fudge	2 Tbs	2.5	70	32%
butterscotch	2 Tbs	–	60	–
espresso fudge	2 Tbs	2.5	70	32%
fudge	2 Tbs	2.5	65	35%
Grand Marnier fudge	2 Tbs	2.5	70	32%
praline	2 Tbs	3.0	80	34%

ICED TEA (See TEA)
ICES (See FRUIT ICES, BARS & POPS)
ICING (See CAKE FROSTING/ICING)

Food and Description	Amount	Fat Grams	Total Calories	% Fat Calories

ITALIAN SAUSAGE (*See* SAUSAGE)

J

Food and Description	Amount	Fat Grams	Total Calories	% Fat Calories
JACKFRUIT/raw	1 medium	–	107	–
JALAPEÑO (*See* MEXICAN FOOD; PEPPER)				
JAM/JELLY/PRESERVES				
(Bama)				
JAM				
grape	1 Tbs	–	50	–
red plum	1 Tbs	–	50	–
strawberry	1 Tbs	–	60	–
JELLY				
apple	1 Tbs	–	50	–
grape	1 Tbs	–	50	–
easy squeeze	1 Tbs	–	50	–
grape w/peanut butter	1 Tbs	5.0	120	38%
PRESERVES				
apricot	1 Tbs	–	50	–
blackberry	1 Tbs	–	50	–
peach	1 Tbs	–	30	–
strawberry	1 Tbs	–	50	–
SPREAD..strawberry	1 Tbs	–	50	–
(Braswell's) fig preserves	1 Tbs	–	45	–
(Cascadian Farm) organic				
FANCY FRUIT SPREADS				
all flavors	1 Tbs	–	40	–
(Crosse & Blackwell)				
lemon curd	1 tbs	–	50	–
fruit spreads..all flavors	1 Tbs	–	60	–
(Fifty/50)				
FRUIT SPREAD				
All flavors	1 Tbs	–	10	–
(Jok'n Al)				
FRUIT SPREAD..low-carb				
all flavors	1 Tbs	–	10	–

Food and Description	Amount	Fat Grams	Total Calories	% Fat Calories
(Knott's Berry Farm)				
JAM				
all flavors	½ oz	–	35	–
JELLY				
all flavors	½ oz	–	35	–
JELLY..light				
all flavors	1 tsp	–	8	–
ORANGE MARMALADE	1 oz	–	50	–
PRESERVES				
all flavors	1 oz	–	70	–
SPREAD				
all flavors	½ oz	–	35	–
(Mary Ellen)				
jam				
all flavors	1 Tbs	–	50	–
jelly				
all flavors	1 Tbs	–	50	–
(Polaner)				
JAM				
grape	1 Tbs	–	40	–
JELLY				
mint..real	1 Tbs	–	60	–
other flavors	1 Tbs	–	40	–
PRESERVES				
all flavors	1 Tbs	–	40	–
PRESERVES..60% less sugar				
strawberry	1 Tbs	–	20	–
PRESERVES..sugar-free				
all flavors	1 Tbs	–	10	–
SPREADABLES				
all flavors	1 Tbs	–	40	–
(R. W. Knudsen) all-fruit spread				
ORGANIC..all flavors	1 Tbs	–	50	–
REGULAR				
all flavors	1 Tbs	–	50	–
(Smucker's)				
FRUIT SPREADS				
home-style..all flavors	1 tbs	–	45	–
jam..all flavors	1 tbs	–	50	–
jelly..all flavors	1 Tbs	–	50	–
low-sugar..all flavors	1 Tbs	–	25	–
marmalade...orange	1 Tbs	–	50	–
preserves..all flavors	1 Tbs	–	50	–
Simply 100% Fruit Spread				
all flavors	1 Tbs	–	40	–
sugar-free..all flavors	1 Tbs	–	10	–
(Steel's)				
JAM..no sugar added				
champagne peach	1 Tbs	–	30	–
crimson strawberry	1 Tbs	–	30	–

Food and Description	Amount	Fat Grams	Total Calories	% Fat Calories
red raspberry	1 Tbs	–	30	–
sour cherry	1 Tbs	–	30	–
wild blueberry	1 Tbs	–	30	–
(Welch's)				
jam..all flavors	1 tbs	–	50	–
jelly..all flavors	1 tbs	–	50	–
preserves..all flavors	1 tbs	–	50	–
spread..strawberry	1 Tbs	–	50	–
Totally Fruit..grape	1 Tbs	–	40	–
(Wolferman's)				
FRUIT SPREADS				
all flavors	1 Tbs	–	40	–
JAPANESE FOOD (*See* ASIAN FOOD)				
JELLY (*See* JAM/JELLY/PRESERVES)				
JERKY STICKS & STRIPS (*See* MEAT SNACK)				
JERUSALEM ARTICHOKE				
raw/sliced	½ cup	–	57	–
JICAMA/YAM BEAN-TUBER				
cooked	½ cup	<1.0	46	10%
raw/sliced	1 cup	<1.0	50	9%
JUICE (*See* FRUIT/FRUIT JUICE DRINK; individual listings)				
JUJUBE				
dried	3 oz	0.9	246	3%
raw	3 oz	–	68	–

K

Food and Description	Amount	Fat Grams	Total Calories	% Fat Calories
KALE				
CANNED				
(The Allens) seasoned				
Southern-style	½ cup	0.5	35	13%
FRESH..cooked	½ cup	–	21	–
FROZEN..cooked	½ cup	–	20	–
(Best Yet) chopped	½ cup	–	30	–
RAW	½ cup	–	17	–
KANPYO/DRIED GOURD STRIP	3 strips	–	49	–
KASHA (*See* BUCKWHEAT GROATS/KASHA)				
KELP (*See* SEAWEED)				
KETCHUP (*See* CATSUP/KETCHUP)				

Food and Description	Amount	Fat Grams	Total Calories	% Fat Calories
KIDNEY BEAN				
(Bush's Best)				
dark red	½ cup	1.0	130	7%
light red	½ cup	–	110	–
(Eden) 100% Organic				
cannellini..white	½ cup	1.0	100	9%
red..no salt added	½ cup	–	100	–
refried..lightly salted	½ cup	1.0	80	11%
(Full Circle) 100% Organic				
dark	½ cup	–	110	–
(Goya) habichuelas coloradas..red	½ cup	1.0	90	10%
(Joan of Arc)..all types	½ cup	–	110	–
(Progresso)				
cannellini/white	½ cup	0.5	100	5%
red	½ cup	–	110	–
(S&W)				
dark red	½ cup	0.5	100	5%
50% less sodium	½ cup	–	100	–
(Sharianns) Organic/vegan				
cannellini	½ cup	2.0	110	16%
kidney beans				
(Stokely)..all types	½ cup	0.5	120	4%
(The Allens)..all types	½ cup	0.5	120	4%
(Trappey's)				
dark red	½ cup	0.5	130	3%
jalapeño	½ cup	0.5	120	4%
light red	½ cup	1.0	110	8%
New Orleans–style w/bacon	½ cup	0.5	110	4%
w/chili gravy	½ cup	1.0	110	8%
(Westbrae)	½ cup	–	100	–
DRY..bag				
(Best Yet)				
light red	½ cup	–	70	–
(Springfield)				
light red	1.35 oz	–	70	–
KIELBASA (*See* SAUSAGE)				
KINGFISH				
cooked—dry heat	3 oz	11.0	219	4 5%
raw	3 oz	2.6	90	26%
KIWI JUICE/JUICE BLEND (*See also* FRUIT/FRUIT JUICE DRINK; FRUIT PUNCH; SOFT DRINK MIX; individual listings)				
(Ocean Spray)..Cravin' Less Sugar				
kiwi strawberry juice drink	8 oz	–	70	–
(R. W. Knudsen)				
kiwi strawberry	8 oz	–	120	–
(Snapple) kiwi strawberry				
diet	8 fl oz	–	20	–
regular	8 fl oz	–	110	–
KIWIFRUIT				
fresh/raw	1 medium	<1.0	46	10%
	1 large	<1.0	55	8%
(Dole)	2 medium	1.0	90	10%

Food and Description	Amount	Fat Grams	Total Calories	% Fat Calories
KNOCKWURST (*See* FRANKFURTER; SAUSAGE)				
KOHLRABI				
fresh/sliced				
cooked/drained	½ cup	–	24	–
raw	½ cup	–	19	–
KOOL-AID (*See* SOFT DRINK MIX)				
KRAUT (*See* SAUERKRAUT)				
KRAUT JUICE (*See* SAUERKRAUT JUICE)				
KUMQUAT				
fresh/raw	1 medium	–	12	–

Food and Description	Amount	Fat Grams	Total Calories	% Fat Calories
LAMB				

(NOTE: All serving sizes are cooked portions, unless otherwise stated. "Lean" means lamb trimmed of all separable fat before cooking. "Lean & fat" means untrimmed and cooked or eaten as purchased. In most cases, 4 ounces of raw meat yields 3 ounces cooked.)

Food and Description	Amount	Fat Grams	Total Calories	% Fat Calories
domestic				
composite cuts/leg & shoulder				
lean				
braised/cubed	3 oz	7.5	190	36%
broiled				
cubed	3 oz	6.0	160	23%
ground	3 oz	17.0	240	64%
stewed/cubed	4 oz	10.0	255	35%
leg/foreshank				
lean				
braised	3 oz	5.0	160	28%
braised/diced	1 cup	8.5	260	29%
broiled/ground	3 oz	17.0	240	64%
stewed/diced	1 cup	8.5	265	29%
leg/shank				
lean				
roasted	3 oz	5.7	155	33%
roasted/diced	1 cup	9.0	250	32%
lean & fat				
roasted	3 oz	10.5	190	50%
roasted/diced	1 cup	17.5	315	50%

Food and Description	Amount	Fat Grams	Total Calories	% Fat Calories
leg/sirloin				
lean				
roasted	3 oz	8.0	175	41%
roasted/diced	1 cup	13.0	290	40%
lean & fat				
roasted	3 oz	17.5	250	63%
roasted/diced	1 cup	29.0	410	64%
leg/whole				
lean				
roasted	3 oz	6.5	165	35%
roasted/diced	1 cup	11.0	270	37%
lean & fat				
roasted	3 oz	14.0	220	57%
roasted/diced	1 cup	23.0	360	57%
loin				
lean				
broiled	3 oz	8.5	190	40%
roasted	3 oz	8.5	175	44%
lean & fat				
broiled	3 oz	19.5	270	65%
roasted	3 oz	20.0	265	68%
organs				
brain				
braised	3 oz	8.5	125	61%
pan-fried	3 oz	19.0	235	73%
heart				
braised	3 oz	7.0	160	39%
simmered	3 oz	7.0	160	39%
kidney				
braised	3 oz	3.0	120	23%
liver				
braised	3 oz	7.5	190	36%
pan-fried	3 oz	11.0	205	48%
lung/braised	3 oz	2.5	95	24%
pancreas/braised	3 oz	13.0	200	59%
spleen/braised	3 oz	4.0	135	27%
tongue/braised	3 oz	17.0	235	65%
rib				
lean				
broiled	3 oz	11.0	200	50%
roasted	3 oz	11.0	200	50%
lean & fat				
broiled	3 oz	25.0	305	74%
roasted	3 oz	25.5	305	75%
shoulder/arm				
lean				
braised	3 oz	12.0	235	46%
broiled	3 oz	7.5	170	40%
roasted	3 oz	8.0	165	44%

Food and Description	Amount	Fat Grams	Total Calories	% Fat Calories
shoulder/blade				
lean				
braised	3 oz	14.0	245	51%
broiled	3 oz	9.5	180	48%
roasted	3 oz	10.0	180	50%
shoulder/whole				
lean				
braised	3 oz	7.5	240	28%
braised/diced	1 cup	22.0	400	50%
broiled	3 oz	9.0	180	45%
roasted	3 oz	9.0	175	46%
roasted/diced	1 cup	10.0	320	28%
stewed	3 oz	7.5	240	28%
stewed/diced	1 cup	22.0	400	50%
New Zealand/frozen				
composite cuts				
lean/cooked	3 oz	7.5	175	39%
leg/foreshank				
lean				
braised	3 oz	5.0	160	28%
braised/diced	1 cup	8.5	260	29%
stewed	3 oz	5.0	160	28%
stewed/diced	1 cup	8.5	260	29%
leg/whole				
lean				
roasted	3 oz	6.0	155	35%
roasted/diced	1 cup	10.0	255	35%
loin				
lean				
broiled	3 oz	7.0	170	37%
roasted	3 oz	7.0	170	37%
lean & fat				
broiled	3 oz	20.5	270	68%
rib				
lean/roasted	3 oz	8.5	165	46%
lean & fat/roasted	3 oz	24.5	290	76%
shoulder/whole				
lean				
braised	3 oz	13.0	245	48%
braised/diced	1 cup	22.0	400	50%
stewed	3 oz	13.0	240	49%
stewed/diced	1 cup	22.0	400	50%
LAMB'S QUARTERS				
fresh/cooked	1 cup	0.6	29	19%
LARD (*See also* FAT; PORK)	1 Tbs	12.8	115	100%
	1 cup	205.0	1850	100%
LASAGNA (*See* BEEF DISH/ENTRÉE; FROZEN ENTRÉE/DINNER; PASTA ENTRÉE/DINNER)				
LAVER (*See* SEAWEED)				
LEEK				
freeze-dried	¼ cup	–	3	–

Food and Description	Amount	Fat Grams	Total Calories	% Fat Calories
fresh				
cooked	¼ cup	–	8	–
raw	¼ cup	–	16	–
	1 medium	–	17	–
LEMON/fresh	1 medium	–	17	–
	1 large	–	25	–
LEMON JUICE				
BOTTLED				
(Haggen)				
from concentrate, natural	2 tsp	–	–	–
(ReaLemon)	1 fl oz	–	6	–
(Seneca)	1 Tbs	–	5	–
FRESH	1 Tbs	–	4	–
	½ cup	–	20	–
FROZEN				
(Sunkist)	1 oz	–	7	–
LEMON PEEL				
candied				
(S&W)	58 pieces	–	80	–
fresh..grated	1 Tbs	–	–	–
LEMONADE/LEMONADE-FLAVORED DRINK (*See also* SOFT DRINK; SOFT DRINK MIX; TEA)				
BOTTLED, BOXED, OR CANNED				
(Capri Sun)				
lemonade..pouch	6.75 oz	–	100	–
(Crystal Light)				
all flavors	8 fl oz	–	5	–
(Minute Maid)				
Coolers				
lemonade..pouch	6.75 oz	–	100	–
pink lemonade	6.75 oz	–	90	–
	12 fl oz	–	150	–
raspberry	12 fl oz	–	160	–
regular				
all-natural	6.75 oz	–	90	–
light..fruit drink	12 fl oz	–	5	–
(Newman's Own)				
all flavors	8 fl oz	–	110	–
Lemon Aided Ice Tea	8 fl oz	–	110	–
(Odwalla) Organic				
lemonade	8 fl oz	–	90	–
strawberry	8 fl oz	–	120	–
(R. W. Knudsen)				
Recharge..lemon	8 fl oz	–	70	–
Simply Nutritious				
lemon ginger Echinacea	8 fl oz	–	110	–
spritzer..lemon lime	12 fl oz	–	170	–
(Santa Cruz Organics)				
sparkling lemonade	12 fl oz	–	100	–
(Snapple)				

Food and Description	Amount	Fat Grams	Total Calories	% Fat Calories
pink				
can	11.5 oz	–	160	–
diet	8 fl oz	–	10	–
regular	8 fl oz	–	110	–
original	8 fl oz	–	110	–
supersour	8 fl oz	–	130	–
(Tropicana)				
light	8 fl oz	–	50	–
regular	8 fl oz	–	120	–
	10 fl oz	–	140	–
	11.5 fl oz	–	160	–
(Welch's)				
lemonade juice cocktail	10 fl oz	–	160	–
	11.5 fl oz	–	190	–
single serve	8 fl oz	–	130	–
low-cal lemonade drink	8.45 fl oz	–	15	–
FROZEN..prepared				
(Minute Maid)				
country-style	8 fl oz	–	120	–
pink				
concentrate only	2 oz	–	110	–
prepared	8 fl oz	–	110	–
raspberry	8 fl oz	–	110	–
regular				
concentrate only	2 oz	–	110	–
prepared	8 fl oz	–	110	–
(Old Orchard)				
all flavors				
concentrate only	2 oz	–	110	–
prepared	8 fl oz	–	110	–
(Seneca)	8 fl oz	–	110	–
MIX...prepared...unless otherwise noted				
(Country Time)				
lemonade iced tea				
classic	8 fl oz	–	90	–
peach	8 fl oz	–	90	–
raspberry	8 fl oz	–	80	–
pink				
sugar-free	8 fl oz	–	5	–
sweetened	8 fl oz	–	70	–
regular				
sugar-free	8 fl oz	–	5	–
sweetened	8 fl oz	–	70	–
sweetened lemonade drink mix				
cranberry raspberry	8 fl oz	–	90	–
raspberry	8 fl oz	–	80	–
strawberry	8 fl oz	–	80	–
wild berry	8 fl oz	–	90	–
(Crystal Light)				
all flavors	8 fl oz	–	5	–

Food and Description	Amount	Fat Grams	Total Calories	% Fat Calories
(Kool-Aid) prepared w/sugar and water				
pink				
regular	8 fl oz	–	100	–
sugar-free	8 fl oz	–	5	–
traditional				
regular	8 fl oz	–	100	–
sugar-free	8 fl oz	–	5	–
LEMON LIME DRINK (*See* SOFT DRINK; SOFT DRINK MIX; SPORTS DRINK)				
LENTIL (*See also* SOUP; VEGETARIAN FOODS)				
CANNED				
(Eden) w/sweet onion & bay leaf	½ cup	–	90	–
(Goya)	¼ cup	–	70	–
(Health Valley) Fast Menu				
fat-free lentil				
w/couscous soup cup	⅓ cup	–	130	–
DRY				
(Arrowhead Mills)				
green or red..raw	¾ cup	–	150	–
(Springfield) dry..bag	1.14 oz	–	70	–
SPROUTED	½ cup	–	40	–
LENTIL SOUP (*See* SOUP; VEGETARIAN FOODS; FAST FOOD)				
LETTUCE				
Bibb	med head	–	21	–
butterhead	med head	–	21	–
cos/shredded	½ cup	–	2	–
iceberg	med head	–	70	–
looseleaf or Simpson/shredded	½ cup	–	5	–
romaine/shredded	½ cup	–	4	–
LICHEE NUT/LYCHEE NUT/LITCHI NUT				
dried/shelled	1 oz	<1.0	80	4%
	3 oz	1.0	235	4%
raw	~6 nuts	0.5	40	10%
shelled & seeded	½ cup	0.5	65	7%
LIMA BEAN (*See also* BUTTER BEAN)				
CANNED				
(Aunt Nellie's) Reber butter beans	½ cup	1.0	140	6%
(Bush's Best)				
green				
butter beans	½ cup	1.0	110	8%
limas..medium	½ cup	1.0	110	8%
green & white	½ cup	1.0	110	8%
speckled butter beans	½ cup	0.5	110	4%
(Del Monte) green	½ cup	–	80	–
(Eden) Baby	½ cup	1.0	100	9%
(Glory) Seasoned				
butter beans	½ cup	1.0	120	8%
limas	½ cup	–	140	–
(Joan of Arc) butter	½ cup	–	90	–
(Luck's) seasoned w/pork				
giant	½ cup	3.0	150	18%

Food and Description	Amount	Fat Grams	Total Calories	% Fat Calories
small	½ cup	2.0	140	13%
(The Allen's)				
green..medium	½ cup	–	120	–
green & white	½ cup	1.0	110	8%
(The Allens East				
Texas Fair).green limas	½ cup	–	120	–%
(Trappey's) baby green				
flavored w/slab bacon	½ cup	1.0	120	8%
baby white	½ cup	1.5	130	10%
(Veg-All)				
baby green habas verdes				
tiernas de lima	½ cup	0.5	90	5%
DRIED..bag				
(Best Yet)				
baby lima	1.33 oz	–	70	–
fordhook	3.2 oz	–	90	–
large	1.23 oz	–	70	–
tiny green	3.2 oz	0.5	110	4%
FROZEN				
(Birds Eye)				
baby	½ cup	1.0	110	8%
butter	½ cup	–	100	–
speckled butter	½ cup	–	100	–
(C&W)..all styles	½ cup	0.5	90	5%
(Green Giant) baby	½ cup	–	80	–
(McKenzie's)				
baby	½ cup	1.0	110	8%
speckled butter	½ cup	–	100	–
(Seneca)				
fordhook	⅔ cup	–	90	–
regular	⅔ cup	–	110	–
LIME	1 medium	–	20	–
LIME JUICE				
BOTTLED				
(Herdez) vegetable juice..spicy lime	11.3 oz	–	90	–
(Jero) cocktail mix..sweetened				
West India–style	1 oz	–	35	–
(Major Peters') from concentrate				
sweetened..West India–style	1 tsp	–	10	–
(T. Marzetti) Key Largo lime juice				
from concentrate	1 tsp	–	–	–
(ReaLime)	1 fl oz	–	6	–
FRESH	⅓ cup	–	22	–
LIME JUICE DRINK (See also SOFT DRINK; SOFT DRINK MIX)				
BOTTLED OR CANNED				
(Kern's) from Libby's..limeade	8 fl oz	–	120	–
(La Croix) natural lime	12 fl oz	–	–	–
(Minute Maid)				
limeade..cherry	8 fl oz	–	120	–
premium w/real limes	8 fl oz	–	120	–

Food and Description	Amount	Fat Grams	Total Calories	% Fat Calories
(Snapple a Day)				
mango lime..low-carb	11.5 fl oz	–	90	–
FROZEN				
(Minute Maid)				
premium..frozen concentrate	1.5 oz	–	100	–
prepared	8 fl oz	–	100	–
(Old Orchard)				
frozen concentrate	1.5 oz	–	115	–
prepared	8 fl oz	–	115	–
LING				
baked or broiled	3 oz	1.0	95	9%
raw	3 oz	0.5	75	6%
LING COD				
baked or boiled	3 oz	1.0	90	10%
raw	3 oz	1.0	75	12%
LINGUINE (*See* FROZEN ENTRÉE/DINNER; PASTA ENTRÉE/DINNER; VEGETARIAN FOODS)				
LIQUEUR (*See also* COCKTAIL/COCKTAIL MIXES; LIQUOR, DISTILLED)				
anisette	¾ fl oz	–	74	–
B&B	1 fl oz	–	94	–
Benedictine	¾ fl oz	–	69	–
brandy/coffee	1.5 fl oz	–	132	–
brandy/fruit-flavored	1.5 fl oz	–	129	–
Cherry Hering	1.5 fl oz	–	120	–
coffee	1.5 fl oz	–	174	–
coffee w/cream	1.5 fl oz	7.0	154	41%
crème d'amande	1.5 fl oz	–	151	–
crème de banana	1.5 fl oz	–	144	–
crème de cacao	1.5 fl 0z	–	150	–
crème de cassis	1.5 fl oz	–	122	–
crème de menthe	1.5 fl oz	–	186	–
Curaçao	¾ fl oz	–	54	–
Drambuie	1.5 fl oz	–	165	–
gin/citrus	1.5 fl oz	–	114	–
kirsch	1.5 fl oz	–	124	–
maraschino	1.5 fl oz	–	112	–
peppermint schnapps	1.5 fl oz	–	124	–
Pernod	1.5 fl oz	–	117	–
rock & rye	1.5 fl oz	–	140	–
rum..Bacardi Superior	1.5 fl oz	–	66	–
sloe gin	1.5 fl oz	–	124	–
Southern Comfort	1.5 fl oz	–	180	–
Tia Maria	1.5 fl oz	–	138	–
triple sec	1.5 fl oz	–	121	–
vodka/citrus	1.5 fl oz	–	150	–
LIQUOR, DISTILLED				
(NOTE: In all cases, the higher the proof [the % of alcohol], the higher the calories.)				
80 proof	1 fl oz	–	67	–
84 proof	1 fl oz	–	70	–
86 proof	1 fl oz	–	72	–

Food and Description	Amount	Fat Grams	Total Calories	% Fat Calories
86.8 proof	1 fl oz	–	72	–
90 proof	1 fl oz	–	75	–
90.4 proof	1 fl oz	–	75	–
94 proof	1 fl oz	–	78	–
94.6 proof	1 fl oz	–	79	–
97 proof	1 fl oz	–	81	–
100 proof	1 fl oz	–	83	–
LIVER (See BEEF; CHICKEN; GOOSE; LAMB; PÂTÉ; PORK; TURKEY)				
LIVER LOAF (See LUNCHEON MEAT)				
LIVERWURST (See LUNCHEON MEAT)				
LOBSTER (See also SEAFOOD ENTRÉE/DINNER)				
fresh				
northern				
boiled	3 oz	0.5	83	5%
	1 cup	0.9	142	6%
raw/~5-oz lobster	1 lobster	1.0	140	6%
spiny				
cooked—moist heat	3 oz	1.5	120	11%
raw	3 oz	1.0	95	10%
LOBSTER, IMITATION				
(Louis Kemp) Lobster Delights				
chunk-style	½ cup	–	80	–
flake-style	½ cup	–	80	–
salad-style	½ cup	–	80	–
LOBSTER BISQUE (See SOUP; SEAFOOD ENTRÉE/DINNER)				
LOBSTER PASTE	1 Tbs	2.0	39	46%
LOGANBERRY				
CANNED				
(Oregon) in light syrup	½ cup	0.5	100	5%
FRESH	½ lb	1.5	140	10%
FROZEN	1 cup	0.5	80	5%
LOGANBERRY JUICE	8 oz	–	100	–
LOQUAT	1 medium	–	5	–
	½ lb	–	65	–
LOTUS ROOT				
cooked	½ cup	–	75	–
raw	10 slices	–	45	–
	1 root	–	60	–
LOTUS SEED				
dried	1 oz	0.5	94	5%
	1 cup	0.6	106	5%
raw	1 oz	–	25	–
LOX (See SALMON)				
LUNCHEON LOAF (See LUNCHEON MEAT)				
LUNCHEON MEAT (See also BEEF; CHICKEN; HAM; LUNCHEON MEAT SPREAD; TURKEY; VEGETARIAN FOODS)				
■ (Alpine Lace)				
deli meats				
fat-free turkey breast	2 oz	–	50	–
97% fat-free ham..all types	2 oz	1.5	60	23%
97% fat-free roast beef	2 oz	1.5	70	19%

Food and Description	Amount	Fat Grams	Total Calories	% Fat Calories
■ (Armour)				
beef				
dried/95% fat-free	1 oz	1.5	60	27%
bologna..w/chicken & turkey	1 oz	7.0	90	70%
Lunch Makers...Cracker Crunchers				
cooked ham	2.6 oz	7.0	360	18%
ham	2.6 oz	7.0	240	26%
pepperoni pizza	3.3 oz	11.0	240	41%
fun kit	3.5 oz	13.0	440	27%
turkey	2.6 oz	14.0	360	35%
fun kit	2.6 oz	14.0	360	35%
spreads				
chicken w/white meat	7.5 oz	11.0	210	47%
ham..smoke-flavored	2.2 oz	8.0	110	65%
	3 oz	8.0	130	55%
potted meat	½ oz	9.0	130	62%
Treet luncheon loaf				
light..50% less fat	2 oz	8.0	110	65%
original	2 oz	11.0	130	76%
Vienna sausage				
barbecue	2.17 oz	13.0	150	78%
chicken	1.89 oz	9.0	110	74%
hot 'n' spicy	2.17 oz	13.0	150	78%
jalapeño	1.89 oz	16.0	170	85%
light..50% less fat	1.89 oz	7.0	90	70%
original	1.89 oz	14.0	150	84%
smoked	1.89 oz	14.0	150	84%
■ (Boar's Head)				
bologna				
28% lower sodium	2 oz	13.0	150	78%
beef	2 oz	13.0	150	78%
garlic	2 oz	13.0	150	78%
Lebanon	2 oz	5.0	100	45%
pork & beef	2 oz	13.0	150	78%
ham				
Tavern	2 oz	1.0	60	15%
Italian delicacies				
Abruzzese..hot & sweet	1 oz	8.0	100	72%
capocollo..hot & sweet	1 oz	5.0	80	56%
imported porketta	2 oz	2.0	70	26%
mortadella	2 oz	14.0	160	79%
w/pistachio nuts	2 oz	14.0	170	74%
pepperoni..sandwich-style	1 oz	12.0	130	83%
prosciutto riserva stradolce	1 oz	3.0	60	45%
sopressata..hot & sweet	1 oz	8.0	100	72%
liverwurst				
braunschweiger..lite	2 oz	8.0	120	60%
onion	2 oz	13.0	160	73%
smoked	2 oz	15.0	170	79%
Strassburger Brand	2 oz	15.0	170	79%

Food and Description	Amount	Fat Grams	Total Calories	% Fat Calories
loaves				
Dutch	2 oz	12.0	150	72%
olive	2 oz	12.0	130	83%
pickle & pepper	2 oz	13.0	150	78%
spiced ham	2 oz	10.0	120	75%
salami				
beef	2 oz	9.0	120	68%
Bianco D'Oro..Italian dry	1 oz	8.0	110	74%
cooked	2 oz	11.0	130	76%
Genoa	2 oz	14.0	180	70%
hard	1 oz	9.0	110	74%
sausages				
hot smoked	1 link	22.0	250	79%
Kielbasa	2 oz	10.0	120	75%
smoked..natural casing	1 link	31.0	360	78%
■ (Butterball)				
turkey breast				
honey-roasted & smoked				
deli-thin..fat-free	2 oz	–	50	–
hearty deli-sliced	1 oz	0.5	30	15%
oven-roasted..97% fat-free	1.6 oz	1.5	60	23%
98% fat-free	1 oz	0.5	30	15%
oven-roasted..premium carved	1.6 oz	1.5	60	23%
■ (Carl Buddig)/sliced				
1.5-oz pkgs..lean smoked				
ham	1 pkg	4.0	65	55%
ham..honey	1 pkg	4.0	70	51%
turkey	1 pkg	4.0	65	55%
turkey..honey	1 pkg	4.0	70	51%
2.5-oz pkgs..lean smoked				
beef	1 pkg	7.0	120	53%
chicken	1 pkg	7.0	110	57%
corn beef	1 pkg	7.0	120	53%
ham	1 pkg	7.0	120	53%
ham..honey	1 pkg	7.0	120	53%
pastrami	1 pkg	7.0	120	53%
turkey	1 pkg	7.0	110	57%
honey	1 pkg	7.0	120	53%
oven-roasted	1 pkg	7.0	110	57%
8-oz pkgs..lean smoked				
beef	¼ pkg	5.0	90	50%
chicken	¼ pkg	5.0	85	53%
corned beef	¼ pkg	5.0	90	50%
ham..honey	¼ pkg	5.0	90	50%
turkey..honey	¼ pkg	5.0	90	50%
PREMIUM..2.5-oz pkgs				
chicken breast				
honey-smoked	1 pkg	1.0	70	13%
oven-roasted..cured	1 pkg	1.0	60	15%
ham				
baked	1 pkg	2.0	90	20%

Food and Description	Amount	Fat Grams	Total Calories	% Fat Calories
baked..honey	1 pkg	2.0	90	20%
brown sugar..baked	1 pkg	2.0	90	20%
smoked	1 pkg	2.0	80	23%
turkey breast				
honey roasted..cured	1 pkg	1.0	60	15%
oven-roasted..cured	1 pkg	1.0	60	15%
smoked	1 pkg	1.0	60	15%
■ (Certified Angus Beef) Angus Beef				
DELI MEATS				
corned beef	2 oz	3.0	80	34%
pastrami	2 oz	3.0	80	34%
roast beef				
angus				
savory garlic	2 oz	2.5	70	32%
seasoned	2 oz	2.5	80	28%
EMMBER CLASSIC				
USDA choice..97% fat-free	2 oz	–	50	–
■ (Dak)				
beef..corned beef..can	2 oz	7.0	120	53%
ham				
chopped..can	2 oz	15.0	170	79%
deli-smoked ham..97% fat-free	2 oz	2.0	60	30%
imported..98% fat-free	1.6 oz	1.0	45	20%
premium				
97% fat-free	1 oz	1.0	30	30%
98% fat-free	1.6 oz	1.0	45	20%
honey..97% fat-free	1 oz	1.0	30	30%
imported..97% at-free	2 oz	1.5	50	27%
natural juices..97% fat-free	2 oz	1.0	30	30%
luncheon meat..can	2 oz	16.0	180	80%
turkey ham..95% fat-free	1 oz	1.5	35	39%
■ (Danola) HAM				
Black Forest..smoked				
97% fat-free	1.6 oz	2.0	60	30%
imported..lower sodium..98% fat-free	1.6 oz	1.0	40	23%
pepper smoked..97% fat-free	1.8 oz	1.5	50	27%
smoked honey..97% fat-free	1.6 oz	1.0	50	18%
Supreme				
baked brown sugar	2 oz	1.5	60	23%
Black Forest..smoked	2 oz	1.5	60	23%
hickory-smoked	2 oz	1.5	60	23%
imported w/natural juices	2 oz	1.0	50	18%
smoked honey	2 oz	1.5	60	23%
smoked maple-flavored honey	2 oz	2.0	70	26%
smoked Virginia Brand	2 oz	1.5	60	23%
■ (Dubuque) HAM				
ham & water...lean	3 oz	4.0	100	36%
cooked..96% fat-free	2 oz	2.5	60	38%
Royal Buffet..extra lean	3 oz	5.0	110	41%

Food and Description	Amount	Fat Grams	Total Calories	% Fat Calories
■ (Eckrich)				
bologna				
German	1 oz	7.0	80	90%
regular	1 oz	8.0	90	80%
ham				
cooked	1 oz	1.0	30	30%
deli-thin	1.8 oz	1.5	60	23%
honey & clove	1 slice	1.0	30	30%
honey-smoked	1 slice	1.0	30	30%
smoked..lean..slender-sliced	3 oz	9.0	150	54%
Virginia baked	1 slice	1.0	30	30%
honey loaf	1 oz	3.0	50	54%
pickle loaf	1 oz	5.0	70	64%
salami..cotto	1 oz	6.0	70	77%
Smok-Y-links	1.66 oz	13.0	150	78%
turkey breast..oven-roasted				
deli-thin	1 oz	1.5	60	23%
■ (Farmer John)				
bologna..beef..sliced	2 slices	13.0	150	78%
bologna..roll..sliced	2 slices	17.0	190	81%
cotto salami	2 slices	12.0	150	72%
ham				
cooked..sliced	2 slices	1.5	60	23%
extra-lean	1 slice	1.0	40	23%
roll..sliced	2 slices	2.0	60	30%
steak	2 oz	1.5	70	19%
head cheese..sliced	1 slice	9.0	110	74%
liverwurst..w/bacon	2 oz	17.0	190	81%
mission loaf..sliced	2 slices	4.5	80	51%
■ (Galileo)				
coppacola..hot	2 oz	11.0	140	71%
cotto salami	2 oz	14.0	170	74%
Genoa salami	2 oz	15.0	180	75%
hard salami	1 oz	11.0	120	83%
mortadella	2 oz	14.0	160	79%
salami..Italian dry				
light	5 slices	4.0	60	60%
no burn	8 slices	11.0	120	83%
thin-sliced	5 slices	8.0	110	65%
whole	1 oz	10.0	120	75%
■ (Healthy Choice)				
COLD CUTS..Deli-thin-sliced				
chicken breast..honey-roasted	4 slices	1.5	60	23%
chicken breast..honey-roasted				
& smoked	4 slices	1.5	70	19%
chicken breast..oven-roasted	4 slices	1.5	60	23%
chicken..smoked	4 slices	1.5	60	23%
ham				
cooked..baked	4 slices	1.5	60	23%
cooked..water added	4 slices	1.5	60	23%
honey ham	4 slices	1.5	60	23%

Food and Description	Amount	Fat Grams	Total Calories	% Fat Calories
honey maple	4 slices	1.5	60	23%
honey mustard	4 slices	1.5	60	23%
Virginia Brand..smoked	4 slices	1.5	60	23%
pastrami	4 slices	1.5	60	23%
turkey breast				
mesquite flavor..smoked	4 slices	1.5	60	23%
oven-roasted	4 slices	1.5	60	23%
rotisserie-seasoned	4 slices	1.5	60	23%
turkey breast & white meat				
honey-roasted & smoked	4 slices	1.5	60	23%
smoked	4 slices	1.5	60	23%
COLD CUTS..Regular				
bologna	2 slices	3.0	80	34%
chicken breast				
oven-roasted	1 oz slice	1.0	30	30%
smoked	1 oz slice	1.0	35	26%
ham				
baked cooked	1 oz slice	1.0	30	30%
cooked	1 oz slice	1.0	30	30%
honey..square	1 oz slice	1.0	30	30%
smoked	1 oz slice	1.0	30	30%
turkey breast				
honey-roasted & smoked	1 oz slice	1.0	35	26%
oven-roasted	1 oz slice	1.0	30	30%
smoked	1 oz slice	1.0	30	30%
COLD CUTS...resealable				
chicken breast..oven-roasted	1 slice	1.0	35	26%
ham				
cooked	1 slice	1.0	30	30%
honey	1 slice	1.0	30	30%
honey maple	1 slice	1.0	30	30%
virginia brand..smoked	1 slice	1.0	30	30%
turkey breast				
honey-roasted	1 slice	1.0	35	26%
oven-roasted	1 slice	1.0	30	30%
■ (Hebrew National)				
bologna				
beef				
lean	1 oz	5.0	90	50%
regular..sliced	1 oz	8.0	80	90%
corned beef				
Deli Express	2 oz	3.0	90	30%
knockwurst..beef	1 link	25.0	260	86%
pastrami..deli slices	2 oz	3.0	70	38%
salami				
beef..chub	2 oz	14.0	170	74%
beef..lean	1 oz	2.5	45	50%
beef..slices	1 oz	7.0	80	79%
turkey breast				
oven-roasted	5 slices	0.5	50	9%

Food and Description	Amount	Fat Grams	Total Calories	% Fat Calories
smoked	2 oz	0.5	50	9%
■ (Hillshire Farm)				
beef..Deli Select				
oven-roasted/cured	2 oz	1.0	60	15%
roast	2 oz	1.0	60	15%
smoked/97% fat-free	2 oz	1.0	60	15%
bologna..deluxe club				
pre-sliced	1 slice	8.0	90	80%
bratwurst	2.5 oz link	20.0	250	72%
bratwurst..beer	2.5 oz link	20.0	250	72%
chicken breast..Deli Select				
oven-roasted	2 oz	–	50	–
corned beef/Deli Select	2 oz	1.0	50	18%
ham				
baked..97% fat-free	2 oz	1.5	60	23%
brown sugar.. baked	2 oz	2.0	70	26%
brown sugar cured..bone in	3 oz	6.0	120	45%
honey-cured..baked	2 oz	2.0	70	26%
regular	2 oz	2.0	60	30%
spiral-sliced	3 oz	6.0	120	45%
spiral-sliced brown sugar cured half	3 oz	6.0	120	45%
Italian sausage	2.5 oz	20.0	250	72%
pepperoni	1 oz	14.0	150	84%
pickle loaf	1 oz	6.0	70	77%
Polska kielbasa..turkey	2 oz link	5.0	90	50%
Smokeys..Big Red				
8-count..smoked..skinless	2 oz link	16.0	180	80%
Smokeys...Lit'l	2 oz	15.0	170	79%
summer sausage				
9-oz stick	2 oz	16.0	190	76%
beef..Old World	2 oz	15.0	180	75%
Yard-O-Beef	2 oz	17.0	190	81%
■ (Hormel)				
BEEF				
chuck roast	2 oz	2.0	60	30%
dried	10 slices	1.5	50	27%
seasoned	2 oz	3.0	70	39%
seasoned..prime rib..boneless				
ready-to-eat	2 oz	12.0	140	77%
top round roast	2 oz	1.0	50	18%
CHICKEN..Chunk meat				
chicken	2 oz	3.0	70	39%
chicken breast				
no salt	2 oz	1.5	60	23%
regular	2 oz	1.5	60	23%
CORNED BEEF	2 oz	7.0	120	53%
HAM				
Black Label				
canned	3 oz	4.5	100	41%

Food and Description	Amount	Fat Grams	Total Calories	% Fat Calories
chopped				
regular	2 oz	11.0	140	71%
sweet	2 oz	11.0	140	71%
Black Forest..97% fat-free	2 oz	2.0	60	30%
chunk..lean	2 oz	6.0	90	40%
cooked..97% fat-free	2 oz	3.0	60	45%
Cure 81 ham..bone in				
w/honey glaze...spiral-sliced	3 oz	8.0	140	51%
Cure 81 ham..boneless				
extra-lean..half	3 oz	4.5	100	41%
extra-lean..whole	3 oz	4.5	100	41%
thin-sliced	3 oz	4.5	100	41%
Cure 81 w/natural juices	2 oz	4.5	100	41%
Curemaster	3 oz	2.5	80	28%
deviled	2 oz	12.0	150	72%
double-smoked	2 oz	3.0	70	39%
extra-lean	2 oz	2.0	60	30%
honey ham..sliced	2 oz	3.0	70	39%
97% fat-free	2 oz	3.0	70	39%
snack-size w/natural juice	2 oz	2.0	70	26%
Light & Lean..cooked				
97% fat-free	1 oz	1.0	25	36%
smoked..honey-cured	2 oz	3.0	70	39%
CHICKEN..chunk				
breast	2 oz	1.0	50	18%
no salt	2 oz	1.0	50	18%
chunk chicken	2 oz	2.5	60	38%
lemon	2 oz	1.0	50	18%
tomato basil..w/garlic	2 oz	1.0	50	18%
Southwest	2 oz	1.0	50	18%
CHICKEN SALAD				
lunch kit	1 kit	9.0	220	37%
PASTRAMI..cooked	2 oz	3.0	70	39%
PEPPERONI				
chunk	1 oz slice	13.0	140	84%
sliced	1 oz slice	13.0	140	84%
SPAM...luncheon meat				
BBQ	2 oz	13.0	160	73%
Camouflage	2 oz	16.0	180	80%
garlic	2 oz	14.0	160	79%
hot & spicy	2 oz	16.0	180	80%
less salt	2 oz	16.0	180	80%
light	2 oz	8.0	110	65%
oven-roasted turkey	2 oz	4.0	80	45%
regular	2 oz	16.0	180	80%
smoked	2 oz	16.0	180	80%
Spam				
w/cheese	2 oz	15.0	170	79%
TURKEY				
breast				
honey-smoked	2 oz	1.0	70	13%

Food and Description	Amount	Fat Grams	Total Calories	% Fat Calories
roasted	2 oz	1.0	50	18%
smoked turkey	2 oz	1.0	60	15%
chunk	2 oz	3.0	60	45%
white	2 oz	1.5	50	27%
■ (Jenny-O/Turkey Store)				
oven-roasted chicken breast	2 oz	1.5	50	27%
oven-roasted turkey breasts				
browned	2 oz	0.5	50	9%
oven-roasted	2 oz	0.5	50	9%
premium turkey hams				
Black Forest	2 oz	3.0	70	39%
regular	2 oz	3.0	70	39%
premium seasoned turkey breasts				
all flavors	2 oz	–	50	–
rotisserie-ready turkey breasts	4 oz	3.0	140	19%
smoked turkey breasts/natural smoked				
all flavors	2 oz	1.0	60	15%
turkey...*pre-sliced*				
Blue Ribbon breast..deli-shaved	2 oz	1.0	50	18%
Grand Champion..w/caramel	2 oz	2.0	70	26%
Jennie-O	2 oz	1.0	50	18%
breast..w/caramel	2 oz	2.0	70	26%
smoked..deli-shaved	2 oz	–	50	–
X-tra Lean turkey				
bologna	2 oz	9.0	110	74%
breast..99% fat-free	4 oz	8.0	180	40%
hickory-smoked..97% fat-free	2 oz	3.0	60	45%
honey-cured..96% fat-free	2 oz	3.0	60	45%
oven-roasted breast	1.5 oz	–	45	–
pastrami	2 oz	3.0	60	45%
salami	2 oz	2.0	70	26%
smoked turkey breast	1.5 oz	–	40	–
turkey ham	2 oz	3.0	70	38%
■ (Kahn's)				
bologna				
beef				
family pack	1 oz slice	6.0	70	77%
fat-free	1 oz slice	–	30	–
Pounder	1 oz slice	8.0	90	80%
regular sliced	1 oz slice	8.0	90	80%
beef 'n' cheddar..8-oz pkg	1 oz slice	8.0	90	80%
pickle loaf	1 oz slice	6.0	70	77%
salami				
beef				
8-oz pkg	1 oz slice	6.0	70	77%
family pack	1 oz slice	5.0	60	75%
cooked..8-oz pkg	1 oz slice	4.0	60	60%
cotto salami/regular sliced	1 oz slice	4.5	60	68%
souse loaf..8-oz pkg	1 oz slice	7.0	90	70%

Food and Description	Amount	Fat Grams	Total Calories	% Fat Calories
spice loaf				
beef/family pack	1 oz slice	5.0	60	75%
regular				
8-oz pkg	1 oz slice	7.0	80	79%
family pack	1 oz slice	6.0	70	77%
■ (Land O' Frost)				
DELI-SHAVED..12-oz pkg				
chicken	2 oz	6.0	100	54%
honey	2 oz	5.0	110	41%
ham	2 oz	5.0	70	64%
honey	2 oz	5.0	80	56%
turkey	2 oz	6.0	90	60%
honey	2 oz	5.0	100	45%
DELI STYLE..thin-sliced..2.5-oz pkg				
beef	1 pkg	7.0	120	53%
chicken	1 pkg	7.0	120	53%
honey	1 pkg	7.0	140	45%
corned beef	1 pkg	7.0	120	53%
ham	1 pkg	7.0	120	53%
honey	1 pkg	7.0	100	63%
pastrami	1 pkg	7.0	120	53%
turkey	1 pkg	7.0	110	57%
honey	1 pkg	7.0	120	53%
roasted pepper	1 pkg	7.0	120	53%
PREMIUM..1-lb pkg				
chicken breast..oven-roasted	2 oz	5.0	80	56%
ham				
honey	2 oz	3.0	80	34%
smoked	2 oz	3.0	70	39%
turkey breast				
honey-smoked	2 oz	4.0	90	40%
oven-roasted	2 oz	4.0	80	45%
smoked	2 oz	4.0	90	40%
■ (Libby's)				
corned beef..canned	2 oz	7.0	120	53%
■ (Louis Rich)				
bologna..turkey variety pack	3 oz	4.0	100	36%
lower-fat	1 oz	4.0	50	72%
Carving Board				
ham..honey..thin-carved	2.5 oz	1.5	70	19%
turkey breast				
oven-roasted..98% fat-free	2.75 oz	1.5	70	19%
smoked..98% fat-free	2.75 oz	1.5	70	19%
chicken breast				
breast cuts				
honey-roasted	3 oz	2.5	130	17%
oven-roasted	3 oz	2.5	130	17%
deli-thin variety pack	2 oz	–	40	–
cotto salami..turkey variety pack	3 oz	4.0	100	36%
50% less fat	1 oz	2.5	40	56%

Food and Description	Amount	Fat Grams	Total Calories	% Fat Calories
ham				
baked	2 slices	1.5	50	27%
honey-glazed				
thin-carved	6 slices	1.5	70	19%
traditional	2 slices	1.5	50	27%
smoked	2 slices	1.5	45	30%
turkey variety pack	3 oz	4.0	100	36%
turkey ham				
chopped..50% less fat	1 oz	2.0	35	51%
smoked..50% less fat	1 oz	1.5	35	39%
smoked..chopped..50% less fat	1 oz	2.0	35	51%
turkey breast				
deli-thin..variety pack	2 oz	–	40	–
hickory-smoked				
98% fat-free	1 oz	0.5	30	15%
fat-free	2 oz	–	50	–
honey-roasted..fat-free	2 oz	–	60	–
oven-roasted..fat-free	2 oz	–	50	–
smoked..white..95% fat-free	1 oz	1.5	35	39%
smoked..white..variety pack	3 oz	4.0	100	36%
Turkey Polska Kielbasa	2 oz	5.0	90	50%
■ **(Old Wisconsin Sausage)**				
beef sausage				
snack bites	1 oz	10.0	110	82%
snack sticks	½ oz	5.0	60	75%
beef snack sticks				
4-count pkg	1 stick	9.0	100	81%
7-count pkg	1 stick	8.0	90	80%
Bologna..ring	2 oz	15.0	170	79%
pepperoni snack				
bites	1 oz	10.0	110	82%
slices	1 oz	16.0	170	85%
sticks	½ oz	6.0	60	90%
summer sausage				
beef snack slices	2 oz	19.0	210	81%
party chub	2 oz	20.0	220	81%
premium..original	2 oz	20.0	220	81%
garlic	2 oz	20.0	220	81%
premium beef stick..chub	2 oz	19.0	220	78%
■ **(Oscar Mayer)**				
BOLOGNA..sliced				
beef	1 oz	8.0	90	80%
cheese	1 oz	8.0	90	80%
light	1 oz	4.0	60	60%
turkey	1 oz	4.0	50	72%
CHICKEN BREAST				
oven-roasted	2.5 oz	2.0	70	26%
oven-roasted..deli-stye				
thin-sliced	2 oz	1.5	60	23%

Food and Description	Amount	Fat Grams	Total Calories	% Fat Calories
HAM				
96% fat-free				
baked..cooked	1 oz	3.5	60	53%
boiled	3 oz	2.0	60	30%
chopped	1 oz	3.0	50	54%
cooked	1 oz	1.0	30	30%
honey	3 oz	2.0	70	26%
	2.28 oz	2.0	70	26%
	2.5 oz	1.5	60	23%
honey..chopped	1 oz	3.5	60	53%
smoked	2.5 oz	1.5	60	23%
deli-style				
brown sugar				
shaved	1.8 oz	1.5	60	23%
thin-sliced	1.8 oz	1.5	60	23%
honey..shaved	1.8 oz	1.5	50	27%
smoked				
shaved	1.8 oz	1.0	45	20%
thin-sliced	1.8 oz	1.0	45	20%
LOAVES & SAUSAGES				
braunschweiger..liver sausage	2 oz	17.0	290	53%
ham & cheese loaf	1 oz	4.5	60	68%
liver cheese	1.3 oz	10.0	120	75%
luncheon loaf..spiced	1 oz	4.5	60	68%
olive	1 oz	6.0	70	77%
pickle & pimiento	1 oz	6.0	80	68%
SALAMI				
beef cotto	1 oz	4.5	60	68%
cotto	1 oz	6.0	70	77%
cotto..beef	1 oz	4.5	60	68%
hard	1 oz	8.0	100	72%
TURKEY BREAST				
mesquite-smoked..thin-sliced	2 oz	1.0	60	15%
oven-roasted..thin-sliced	2 oz	1.0	60	15%
oven-roasted ..98% fat-free	1 oz	–	25	–
smoked..white..95% fat-free	1 oz	1.0	30	30%
smoked..white..honey..lean	1 oz	1.5	35	39%
white..oven-roasted..95% fat-free	1 oz	1.0	30	30%
■ **(Plumrose)**				
HAM				
baked..96% fat-free	3 oz	1.5	35	39%
brown sugar..baked..97% fat-free	1 oz	1.0	30	30%
honey..96% fat-free	1 oz	1.5	35	39%
honey-baked..97% fat-free	1 oz	1.0	35	26%
HAM..PREMUIM				
95% fat-free	1 oz	1.5	35	39%
97% fat-free	1 oz	1.0	30	30%
THIN & TASTY...97% fat-free				
ham..all types	2 oz	2.0	50	36%

Food and Description	Amount	Fat Grams	Total Calories	% Fat Calories
turkey breast				
fat-free	2 oz	–	35	–
honey	2 oz	1.0	45	20%
TURKEY BREAST				
98% fat-free	1 oz	0.5	25	18%
hickory-smoked..97% fat free	1 oz	1.0	30	30%
honey..97% fat-free	1 oz	1.0	30	30%
TURKEY HAM..95% fat-free	1 oz	1.5	35	39%
■ (Sara Lee) Deli Meats				
BEEF				
corned beef..USDA choice	2 oz	2.5	70	32%
corned beef..pre-sliced	2 slices	2.0	50	36%
pastrami..USDA choice	2 oz	2.5	70	32%
pastrami..pre-sliced	2 slices	2.5	60	38%
roast beef				
medium	2 oz	2.0	60	30%
peppered	2 oz	2.0	70	26%
rare	2 oz	2.0	60	30%
rare..pre-sliced	2 slices	2.5	60	38%
CHICKEN				
oven-roasted breast	2 oz	–	45	–
oven-roasted breast..pre-sliced	2 slices	0.5	45	10%
oven-roasted rotisserie-flavored	2 oz	–	50	–
HAM				
Bavarian Brand..oven- roasted honey ham	2 oz	3.5	70	45%
Black Forest	2 oz	1.0	60	15%
brown sugar	2 oz	1.5	70	19%
brown sugar..pre-sliced	2 slices	1.5	60	23%
cooked..pre-sliced	2 slices	0.5	40	11%
homestyle-baked	2 oz	2.0	60	30%
honey-cured	2 oz	1.5	60	23%
honey-cured..pre-sliced	2 slices	1.0	45	20%
maple honey	2 oz	1.5	70	19%
old-fashioned cooked	2 oz	1.0	50	18%
peppered	2 oz	1.0	60	15%
smokehouse	2 oz	1.5	60	23%
tavern honey	2 oz	1.0	60	15%
Virginia-baked..pre-sliced	2 slices	1.5	50	27%
SAUSAGE...salami				
Genoa salami	1 oz	10.0	110	82%
Genoa salami..pre-sliced	4 slices	10.0	110	82%
hard salami	1 oz	11.0	120	83%
hard salami..pre-sliced	4 slices	11.0	120	83%
sandwich-style pepperoni pre-sliced	7 slices	13.0	140	84%
TURKEY BREAST				
cracked pepper..pre-sliced	2 slices	–	45	–
golden-roasted	2 oz	0.5	50	9%

Food and Description	Amount	Fat Grams	Total Calories	% Fat Calories
hardwood-smoked	2 oz	0.5	60	8%
hardwood-smoked..pre-sliced	2 slices	0.5	45	10%
honey-roasted	2 oz	0.5	60	8%
honey-roasted..pre-sliced	2 slices	0.5	50	9%
honey-roasted turkey ham	2 oz	3.0	70	39%
mesquite-smoked	2 oz	0.5	60	8%
oven-roasted	2 oz	1.5	60	23%
oven-roasted	2 slices	0.5	45	10%
oven-roasted rotisserie-flavored	2 oz	2.0	70	26%
peppered	2 oz	–	50	–
■ SPAM (See also (Hormel) in this section)				
■ (Tyson)				
DELI MEATS..self-serve				
beef Bologna	1 slice	7.0	80	79%
chicken breast				
golden-roasted..smoked	3 sices	1.0	60	15%
corned beef	2 slices	2.0	70	26%
ham				
Black Forest	1 slice	1.0	30	30%
brown sugar	1 slice	1.0	35	26%
honey-cured	1 slice	1.0	35	26%
Virginia Brand	1 slice	1.0	30	30%
olive loaf	1 slice	5.0	70	64%
pastrami	2 slices	2.0	70	26%
pepperoni..sandwich	5 slices	12.0	130	83%
pickle loaf	1 slice	5.0	70	64%
roast beef	2 slices	2.0	90	20%
salami				
Genoa	4 slices	9.0	110	74%
hard	4 slices	3.0	110	25%
turkey breast				
golden-roasted	2 slices	–	70	–
hickory-smoked	2 slices	–	70	–
honey-flavored	2 slices	–	70	–
oven-roasted	2 slices	–	35	–
LUNCHEON MEAT SPREAD (See also PÂTÉ)				
(Armour)				
chicken..w/white meat	2.2 oz	6.0	110	49%
deviled ham..smoke flavor	2.2 oz	8.0	110	65%
	3 oz	8.0	130	55%
potted meat/all flavors	2.2 oz	5.0	80	56%
	3 oz	9.0	130	62%
(Hormel)				
braunschweiger	2 oz	17.0	190	81%
Cure 81 deviled ham	4 Tbs	12.0	150	72%
Hormel				
liverwurst	4 Tbs	10.0	130	69%
potted meat	4 Tbs	8.0	100	72%
Spam..meat spread	1.5 oz	12.0	140	77%

Food and Description	Amount	Fat Grams	Total Calories	% Fat Calories
(Libby's) Spreadables				
deviled meats	¼ cup	8.0	120	60%
potted meats	3 oz	13.0	160	73%
(Old Wisconsin Sausage) Spreadables..Pate				
braunschweiger				
black pepper	2 oz	18.0	210	77%
onion & parsley	2 oz	18.0	210	77%
original	2 oz	18.0	210	77%
(Oscar Mayer)				
braunschweiger liver sausage	2 oz	17.0	190	80%
sandwich spread	2 oz	10.0	130	69%
(Underwood)				
chicken..white meat	¼ cup	7.0	110	57%
ham				
deviled	¼ cup	14.0	160	79%
honey	2 oz	10.0	130	69%
liverwurst..pork..ground	¼ cup	14.0	170	74%
regular	2 oz	11.0	140	71%
liverwurst	2 oz	14.0	170	74%
roast beef	/4 cup	7.0	100	63%
LUPIN				
boiled	½ cup	2.0	98	18%
raw	½ cup	8.0	330	22%
LYCHEE				
dried	1 oz	–	80	–
fresh	1 fruit	–	5	–

M

Food and Description	Amount	Fat Grams	Total Calories	% Fat Calories
MACADAMIA NUT				
(Diamond of California) chopped	¼ cup	24.0	240	90%
(Fisher) Snack 'n' Serve Nut Bowl				
chocolate-covered	1 oz	15.0	200	68%
dry-roasted	1 oz	21.0	200	95%
halves & pieces	1 oz	21.0	210	90%
(Mauna Loa)				
candied honey-roasted	¼ cup	21.0	210	90%
butter candy-glazed	¼ cup	15.0	190	24%
chocolate-covered	1 oz	13.0	170	69%

Food and Description	Amount	Fat Grams	Total Calories	% Fat Calories
dry-roasted..unsalted	¼ cup	21.0	200	95%
honey-roasted	1 oz	17.0	200	77%
Kona coffee–glazed	¼ cup	21.0	210	90%
Maui onion & garlic	¼ cup	21.0	210	90%
(Planters)				
chopped..single package	2 oz	42.0	400	95%
jar	1 oz	21.0	200	95%

MACARONI (*See* PASTA)
MACARONI & CHEESE (*See* FROZEN ENTRÉE/DINNER; PASTA ENTRÉE/DINNER; VEGETARIAN FOODS)

MACE/ground	1 tsp	0.6	8	68%

MACKEREL (*See also* SEAFOOD ENTRÉE/DINNER)

(3 Diamonds) mackerel fillets..box				
in soybean oil	~3 oz	12.0	160	68%
water & salt added	~3 oz	3.0	70	39%
Atlantic				
cooked—dry heat	3 oz	15.0	223	61%
raw	3 oz	11.8	174	61%
Jack..canned..drained				
(Empress)	4 oz	8.0	140	51%
(Geisha) water & salt added	2.5 oz	3.5	80	39%
King				
cooked—dry heat	3 oz	5.5	135	37%
raw	3 oz	1.7	89	17%
Pacific..mixed species				
cooked—dry heat	3 oz	8.5	170	45%
raw	3 oz	6.5	135	43%
smoked				
fillets	2 oz	14.0	150	84%
Spanish				
cooked—dry heat	3 oz	5.0	134	34%
raw	3 oz	5.0	118	38%

MAHIMAHI

cooked—dry heat	3 oz	1.0	95	9%
Hawaiian-style..frozen				
skinless, boneless	4 oz	1.0	100	9%

MALT (*See* BARLEY MALT; MILK MIX)
MALT LIQUOR (*See* BEER, ALE & MALT LIQUOR)
MAMEY APPLE/MAMMEY APPLE/MAMMEE APPLE

raw				
peeled/no seeds	3 oz	<1.0	42	6%
whole	1 medium	4.4	445	9%

MANDARIN ORANGE (*See also* TANGERINE)
CANNED

(Del Monte) in light syrup				
individual pull-top can	4 oz	–	70	–
SunFresh..chilled jar	½ cup	–	80	–
(Dole) in light syrup	½ cup	–	70	–
(Empress)	½ cup	–	80	–

Food and Description	Amount	Fat Grams	Total Calories	% Fat Calories
FRESH				
(Dole)	½ cup	–	80	–
whole	1 medium	–	35	–
MANGO				
FRESH				
diced or sliced	1 cup	0.5	110	4%
(Del Monte) Sunfresh..chilled jar				
in extra-light syrup	½ cup	0.5	100	5%
whole	1 medium	0.5	135	3%
(Dole)	½ med	0.5	70	6%
FROZEN				
(C&W) chunks	1 cup	–	90	–
MANGO JUICE/JUICE BLEND/JUICE DRINK (*See also* FRUIT PUNCH)				
BOTTLED				
(Kern's from Libby's) nectar	5.5 fl oz	–	100	–
	6.59 fl oz	–	120	–
	8 fl oz	–	150	–
	12 fl oz	–	210	–
(Jumex) juice drink				
Bida from concentrate	8 fl oz	–	120	–
(Knudsen)				
Mango Montage	8 fl oz	–	110	–
mango peach	8 fl oz	–	120	–
(Libby's) nectar	8 fl oz	–	100	–
(Minute Maid) fruit drink				
mango tropical..light	12 oz	–	10	–
(Snapple) juice drink				
Mango Madness				
regular	8 fl oz	–	110	–
diet	8 fl oz	–	15	–
(Welch's single serve) juice drink				
mango passionfruit	7.5 oz	–	120	–
mango passionfruit	10 oz	–	160	–
mango passionfruit	11.5 oz	–	180	–
MIX..prepared				
(Kool Aid) soft drink mix				
Aguas Frescas Mango				
unsweetened	8 fl oz	–	–	–
MANICOTTI (*See* FROZEN ENTRÉE/DINNER; PASTA ENTRÉE/DINNER)				
MAPLE SYRUP (*See* PANCAKE & WAFFLE SYRUP)				
MARGARINE, MARGARINE SPREAD & SPRAY				
(Benecol)				
light	1 tbs	5.0	45	100%
regular	1 Tbs	9.0	80	100%
(Blue Bonnet)				
East Coast packaging..stick	1 Tbs	9.0	80	100%
light	1 Tbs	5.0	50	100%
light				
soft	1 Tbs	4.5	40	100%
sticks	1 Tbs	5.0	50	100%

Food and Description	Amount	Fat Grams	Total Calories	% Fat Calories
home-style soft	1 Tbs	7.0	60	100%
regular...stick	1 Tbs	9.0	80	100%
West Coast packaging..stick	1 Tbs	9.0	80	100%
light	1 Tbs	5.0	50	100%
(Breakstone)				
original..unsalted	1 Tbs	11.0	100	100%
whipped				
salted	1 Tbs	7.0	60	100%
unsalted	1 tbs	7.0	60	100%
(Brummel & Brown) made w/yogurt				
tub	1 tbs	5.0	50	100%
stick	1 Tbs	10.0	90	100%
(Country Morning Blend) ...See Land O'Lakes within this category				
(Fleischmann's)				
olive oil spread				
original..soft	1 tbs	9.0	80	100%
light	1 tbs	4.5	40	100%
unsalted	1 tbs	9.0	80	100%
premium blend..squeeze	1 Tbs	8.0	70	100%
(Gold-n-Sweet) w/canola oil	1 Tbs	11.0	100	100%
(Gregg's) Gold-n-Soft				
40% vegetable oil..tub	1 Tbs	6.0	50	100%
70% vegetable oil..tub	1 Tbs	10.0	90	100%
80% vegetable oil	1 Tbs	11.0	100	100%
Light	1 Tbs	6.0	50	100%
Original..tub	1 Tbs	11.0	100	100%
(Hain) safflower				
regular	1 tbs	11.0	100	100%
unsalted	1 Tbs	11.0	100	100%
(Heartlight) canola	1 Tbs	11.0	100	100%
(Hollywood) safflower				
regular	1 tbs	11.0	100	100%
unsalted sweet	1 Tbs	11.0	100	100%
(I Can't Believe It's Not Butter)				
fat-free	1 tbs	–	5	–
light spread				
stick..East Coast	1 Tbs	6.0	50	100%
tub	1 Tbs	5.0	50	100%
regular	1 tbs	10.0	90	100%
soft	1 tbs	10.0	90	100%
spray	5 sprays	–	–	–
squeeze	1 tbs	8.0	80	100%
sweet cream & calcium	1 tbs	6.0	50	100%
sweet cream buttermilk	1 tbs	10.0	90	100%
unsalted..sweet	1 tbs	10.0	90	100%
whipped..squeeze	1 Tbs	7.0	60	100%
(Imperial)				
⅓ less fat..stick	1 Tbs	7.0	70	100%
light	1 Tbs	6.0	60	100%
Savory Squeeze..all flavors	1 Tbs	10.0	90	100%

Food and Description	Amount	Fat Grams	Total Calories	% Fat Calories
soft	1 tbs	11.0	100	100%
soft..diet	1 Tbs	6.0	50	100%
(Kraft) Touch of Butter	1 Tbs	7.0	60	100%
(Keller's)				
48% vegetable oil..tub	1 Tbs	7.0	60	100%
70% vegetable oil..box	1 Tbs	10.0	90	100%
(Land O'Lakes)				
Country Morning Blend				
stick	1 Tbs	11.0	100	100%
light	1 Tbs	6.0	50	100%
tub	1 Tbs	11.0	50	100%
light	1 Tbs	6.0	50	100%
Fresh Buttery Taste				
soft	1 Tbs	8.0	80	100%
stick	1 Tbs	10.0	90	100%
tub	1 Tbs	8.0	80	100%
soybean oil..all types	1 Tbs	11.0	100	100%
(Move Over Butter)				
65% vegetable oil..whipped				
w/sweet cream..tub	1 Tbs	6.0	60	100%
regular..all types	1 Tbs	10.0	90	100%
(Mrs. Filbert's)				
corn oil family spread	1 Tbs	7.0	60	100%
Golden Quarters	1 Tbs	8.0	70	100%
soft corn	1 tbs	11.0	100	100%
vegetable oil	1 Tbs	7.0	65	100%
(Nucanola)	1 Tbs	10.0	90	100%
(Nucoa)				
Heart Beat..corn oil	1 Tbs	3.0	25	100%
Smartbeat				
light/unsalted	1 Tbs	3.0	25	100%
squeeze/fat-free	1 Tbs	–	5	–
super light/trans fat–free	1 Tbs	2.0	20	100%
tub/salted and unsalted	1 Tbs	3.0	25	100%
soft	1 Tbs	10.0	90	100%
stick	1 Tbs	11.0	100	100%
(Parkay)				
light..all types	1 Tbs	5.0	50	100%
original..60% vegetable oil				
stick	1 Tbs	10.0	90	100%
tub	1 Tbs	8.0	80	100%
spray				
for cooking	1 spray	–	–	–
for topping	5 sprays	–	–	–
Squeeze	1 Tbs	8.0	70	100%
(Promise)				
extra light	1 tbs	6.0	50	100%
fat-free	1 tbs	–	5	–
regular..stick	1 tbs	10.0	90	100%
sunflower oil	1 Tbs	10.0	90	100%

Food and Description	Amount	Fat Grams	Total Calories	% Fat Calories
Twin Tubs	1 Tbs	8.0	80	100%
Ultra..tub	1 Tbs	4.0	35	100%
(Shedd's Spread)				
canola oil blend	1 Tbs	7.0	60	100%
churn-style..East Coast				
stick	1 Tbs	9.0	80	100%
tub	1 Tbs	7.0	60	100%
Cinnamon	1 Tbs	6.0	70	100%
cooking & topping spray	5 short sprays	–	–	–
Country Crock	1 Tbs	7.0	70	100%
honey	1 tbs	6.0	70	100%
light	1 tbs	5.0	50	100%
original	1 Tbs	9.0	80	100%
Quarters Spread	1 Tbs	9.0	80	100%
Shedd's Willow..stick	1 Tbs	11.0	100	100%
soybean..stick	1 tbs	11.0	100	100%
squeeze	1 tbs	9.0	80	100%
whipped honey spread	I Tbs	9.0	90	90%
(Smart Balance)				
buttery..67% vegetable oil	1 tbs	9.0	80	100%
light..37% vegetable oil	1 tbs	5.0	45	100%
squeeze	1 Tbs	–	5	–
(Weight Watchers)				
all types	1 Tbs	4.0	45	100%
MARINADE (See also SEASONINGS)				
BAG, BOTTLE, OR JAR				
(A.1.) marinade				
Chicago	1 tbs	1.0	20	45%
steak house..New Orleans				
Cajun	1 tbs	–	25	–
steak house teriyaki	1 Tbs	–	25	–
(Andre Prost) hot adobo	1 Tbs	–	10	–
(Annie's Naturals)				
Spicy Ginger	2 Tbs	2.0	35	51%
Smokey Campfire	2 Tbs	6.0	60	90%
Paradise	2 Tbs	3.5	50	63%
(Carb Options) See (Lawry's) within this category.				
(Cardini)				
chipotle pepper	1 Tbs	–	10	–
fajita mesquite	1 Tbs	–	10	–
honey Dijon	1 Tbs	–	20	–
roasted garlic & herb	1 Tbs	–	10	–
spicy Cajun	1 Tbs	–	10	–
tangy teriyaki	1 Tbs	–	20	–
zesty lemon pepper	1 Tbs	–	15	–
(Chef Paul)				
Magic Sauce & Marinade				
California sun-dried tomato	1 Tbs	–	17	–
Louisiana red pepper	1 Tbs	–	16	–
San Francisco teriyaki	1 Tbs	–	16	–

Food and Description	Amount	Fat Grams	Total Calories	% Fat Calories
Southwest chipotle	1 Tbs	–	8	–
(Emeril's)				
marinade				
Asian	½ oz	7.0	70	90%
lemon rosemary & garlic	½ oz	7.0	70	90%
orange herb..w/poppy seed	½ oz	8.0	80	90%
roasted vegetable	½ oz	7.0	70	90%
Marinade & Grill				
ginger teriyaki	½ oz	0.5	25	18%
(Gourmet) Marinades				
bold & spice steakhouse grill	1 Tbs	–	15	–
cilantro & lime Caribbean grill	1 Tbs	–	10	–
jalapeño & lime..Southwest grill	1 Tbs	–	10	–
lemon & pepper citrus grill	1 Tbs	1.0	25	36%
roasted garlic, fine wine & herbs Mediterranean	1 Tbs	–	10	–
(KC Masterpiece)				
garlic & herb	1 Tbs	1.0	30	30%
ginger & garlic	1 Tbs	–	30	–
golden honey Dijon	1 Tbs	0.5	40	11%
honey teriyaki	1 Tbs	0.5	40	11%
mesquite	1 Tbs	1.0	40	23%
original BBQ	1 Tbs	1.5	40	34%
spiced Caribbean Jerk	1 Tbs	–	25	–
zesty lemon pepper	1 Tbs	1.0	25	36%
(Kikkoman)				
marinade & sauce				
honey & mustard teriyaki	1 Tbs	–	35	–
roasted garlic teriyaki	1 Tbs	–	25	–
teriyaki	1 Tbs	–	15	–
teriyaki light	1 Tbs	–	15	–
Quick & Easy marinade				
gourmet teriyaki	1 Tbs	–	30	–
honey mustard	1 Tbs	–	30	–
roasted garlic & herb	1 Tbs	–	20	–
toasted sesame teriyaki	1 Tbs	0.5	40	11%
Stir-Fry & Marinade				
black bean sauce..w/garlic	2 Tbs	1.0	50	18%
hoisin Sauce	2 Tbs	1.5	80	17%
Thai-style chili sauce	2 Tbs	1.0	70	13%
(Lawry's)				
Carb Options				
Asian teriyaki	1 Tbs	0.5	5	90%
Italian garlic	1 Tbs	–	–	–
regular marinades				
Caribbean Jerk	1 Tbs	–	25	–
citrus grill	1 Tbs	–	15	–
Dijon & honey	1 Tbs	–	20	–
Havana garlic & lime	1 Tbs	–	10	–

Food and Description	Amount	Fat Grams	Total Calories	% Fat Calories
Hawaiian	1 Tbs	–	20	–
herb & garlic	1 Tbs	–	10	–
lemon pepper	1 Tbs	0.5	10	45%
Mediterranean..w/lime juice	1 Tbs	–	10	–
mesquite	1 Tbs	–	5	–
red wine	1 Tbs	–	5	–
sesame ginger				
w/mandarin orange	1 Tbs	–	30	–
tequila lime	1 Tbs	–	15	–
teriyaki..w/pineapple juice	1 Tbs	–	35	–
Thai ginger	1 Tbs	–	10	–
(Litehouse)				
Simple Sensations				
Cajun garlic herb	2 Tbs	–	45	–
fajitas	2 Tbs	–	15	–
honey Dijon	2 Tbs	7.0	80	79%
Jamaican Jerk	2 Tbs	4.5	60	68%
mesquite grill	2 Tbs	0.5	35	13%
teriyaki	2 Tbs	0.5	35	13%
(Maple Grove Farms)				
Marinade & Basting Sauce				
low-carb..sugar-free				
Dijon	1 Tbs	5.0	50	90%
hickory	1 Tbs	–	20	–
lemon rosemary	1 Tbs	3.5	35	90%
sweet 'n' sour	1 Tbs	4.0	40	90%
teriyaki	1 Tbs	–	–	–
(McCormick Golden Dipt)				
seafood marinade				
Cajun-style	1 Tbs	4.5	60	68%
garlic herb	1 Tbs	6.0	60	90%
ginger teriyaki	1 Tbs	3.0	60	45%
honey mustard	1 Tbs	–	25	–
honey soy	1 Tbs	–	30	–
lemon herb	1 Tbs	8.0	80	90%
lemon pepper	1 Tbs	2.0	25	72%
mesquite	1 Tbs	0.5	10	45%
white wine	1 Tbs	1.5	20	68%
(Patak's) Original				
marinade				
golden mango..mild	1 Tbs	1.0	30	30%
honey & ginger..mild	1 Tbs	1.5	35	39%
sweet & smokey..medium	1 Tbs	1.5	35	39%
marinade & grilling sauce				
spicy ginger & garlic..mild	1 Tbs	1.0	35	36%
(S&W)				
mesquite	1 Tbs	–	10	–
Southwestern fajitas				
restaurant recipe	1 Tbs	–	10	–

Food and Description	Amount	Fat Grams	Total Calories	% Fat Calories
teriyaki				
light	1 Tbs	–	25	–
regular	1 Tbs	–	25	–
(Seapak Shrimp Co.) liquid marinade..bag				
Caesar Parmesan	3.3 oz	4.5	110	37%
garlic herb	3.3 oz	3.0	90	30%
spicy Szechuan	3.3 oz	4.5	110	37%
(UP Country Organics)				
Dijon	1 Tbs	3.0	80	34%
garlic & herb	1 Tbs	–	20	–
ginger teriyaki	1 Tbs	–	35	–
MIX..mix only				
(Adolph's)				
For the Grill				
cracked pepper..w/lemon	½ tsp	–	10	–
fajita	½ tsp	–	10	–
hickory barbecue	½ tsp	–	15	–
mesquite	½ tsp	–	10	–
teriyaki	½ tsp	–	10	–
Marinade in Minutes..tenderizing				
all flavors	½ tsp	–	5	–
tenderizers				
all flavors	½ tsp	–	–	–
(Kikkoman)	1 oz	–	60	–
(Lawry's)				
beef..tenderizing	¼ tsp	–	–	–
teriyaki	1 Tbs	–	25	–
Weekday Gourmet				
liquid mix marinade				
beef				
London broil	1 Tbs	–	10	–
teriyaki steak	1 Tbs	1.0	25	36%
(McCormick Golden Dip)				
mesquite	2 tsp	–	15	–
Montreal steak	1 tsp	–	–	–
Oriental	2 tsp	–	15	–
Southwest	2 tsp	–	15	–
spicy Caribbean	2 tsp	–	10	–
zesty herb	2 tsp	–	10	–
MARINARA SAUCE (*See* SAUCE)				
MARJORAM/dried	1 tsp	–	2	–
MARMALADE (*See* JAM/JELLY/PRESERVES)				
MARSHMALLOW				
(Kraft)				
Funmallows				
large	1.1 oz	–	100	–
miniature	~1 oz	–	100	–
	½ cup	–	100	–
Jet-Puffed	1 oz	–	90	–
miniatures	1 oz	–	100	–

Food and Description	Amount	Fat Grams	Total Calories	% Fat Calories
toasted coconut	1 oz	2.5	100	23%
(La Nouba) Zero Carb marshmallows				
regular	1 piece	–	15	–
MARSHMALLOW CRÈME				
(Kraft) Jet-Puffed	2 Tbs	–	40	–
MATZO (*See* CRACKER; MATZO MEAL & MIX)				
MATZO MEAL & MIX (*See also* SOUP)				
Meal				
(Goodman's)				
matzo ball mix				
50% less salt	2 Tbs	–	50	–
regular	2 Tbs	–	50	–
Passover	1 cup	1.0	514	2%
(Manischewitz)	1 cup	<1	243	2%
"Daily"	1 cup	1.0	514	2%
Farfel	1 cup	1.0	280	3%
Mix				
(Manischewitz) matzo ball..mix only	2 Tbs	–	50	–
MAYONNAISE/MAYONNAISE-TYPE DRESSING (*See also* SALAD DRESSING)				
(Bennett's) real	1 Tbs	12.0	110	98%
(Best Foods)				
Dijonnaise creamy Dijon	1 tsp	–	5	–
Just 2 Good..reduced-fat	1 Tbs	2.0	25	72%
light	1 Tbs	5.0	50	90%
low-fat..cholesterol-free	1 Tbs	1.0	25	36%
real	1 Tbs	11.0	100	99%
reduced-fat	1 Tbs	3.0	40	68%
squeeze..light				
all flavors	1 Tbs	5.0	50	90%
squeeze..low-fat				
cholesterol-free	1 Tbs	1.0	25	36%
(Estee)	1 Tbs	5.0	50	90%
(Featherweight) soyamaise				
mayo dressing	1 Tbs	11.0	100	99%
(Hain)				
canola				
light..reduced-calorie	1 Tbs	5.0	60	75%
regular	1 Tbs	11.0	100	100%
cold-processed	1 Tbs	12.0	110	98%
eggless	1 Tbs	12.0	110	98%
light	1 Tbs	6.0	60	90%
real	1 Tbs	12.0	110	98%
safflower	1 Tbs	12.0	110	98%
(Hellman's)				
Dijonaise	1 tsp	–	5	–
bacon & tomato twist..light	1 Tbs	5.0	50	90%
garlic paradise	1 Tbs	5.0	50	90%
herb sensation..light	1 Tbs	5.0	50	90%
Just 2 Good..reduced-fat	1 Tbs	2.0	25	72%

Food and Description	Amount	Fat Grams	Total Calories	% Fat Calories
light	1 Tbs	5.0	50	90%
real	1 Tbs	11.0	100	100%
reduced-fat	1 Tbs	3.0	40	68%
(Hollywood)...all types	1 Tbs	11.0	100	100%
(Kraft)				
mayonnaise				
hot 'n' spicy	1 Tbs	11.0	100	99%
Kraft Free..non-fat	1 Tbs	–	10	–
light	1 Tbs	5.0	50	90%
real	1 Tbs	11.0	100	99%
squeeze..easy	1 Tbs	11.0	100	99%
super-easy squeeze	1 Tbs	4.0	45	80%
Miracle Whip				
hot 'n' spicy	1 Tbs	6.0	60	90%
light	1 Tbs	3.0	35	77%
non-fat	1 Tbs	–	15	–
original	1 Tbs	7.0	70	90%
squeeze..super-easy	1 Tbs	6.0	60	90%
squeeze..super-easy..light	1 Tbs	2.5	35	64%
(La Costena) w/lime juice	1 Tbs	12.0	100	90%
(Life All Natural) egg-free	1 Tbs	8.0	70	100%
(Nasoya) tofu Nayonaise	1 Tbs	4.0	40	90%
(Nucoa) Heart Beat corn oil	1 Tbs	4.0	40	90%
(Smart Beat)				
canola oil	1 Tbs	4.0	40	90%
corn oil	1 Tbs	4.0	40	90%
fat-free	1 Tbs	–	10	–
(Spectrum) canola				
eggless..lite	1 Tbs	3.0	30	90%
real	1 Tbs	12.0	100	100%
(Weight Watchers)				
fat-free	1 Tbs	–	10	–
light..all types	1 Tbs	2.0	25	72%
whipped	1 Tbs	–	15	–

MEAL REPLACEMENT (*See* NUTRITIONAL LIQUID SUPPLEMENT)
MEAT LOAF (*See* FROZEN ENTRÉE/DINNER)
MEAT SEASONING (*See* MARINADE; SEASONINGS)
MEAT SNACK

Food and Description	Amount	Fat Grams	Total Calories	% Fat Calories
(Armour) dried, sliced				
beef..jar	~1 oz	1.5	60	23%
(Jimmy Dean)				
Beef Jerky..1-oz pkg				
original	1 pkg	0.5	70	6%
teriyaki	1 pkg	0.5	80	6%
Beef Jerky				
original	1 oz	0.5	70	6%
peppered	1 oz	0.5	70	6%
teriyaki	1 oz	0.5	80	6%
Giant Sticks..beef..1.5 oz	1 pkg	12.0	150	72%
Kippered Steak..1-oz pkg				

Food and Description	Amount	Fat Grams	Total Calories	% Fat Calories
original	1 pkg	3.0	70	39%
peppered	1 pkg	2.5	70	32%
teriyaki	1 pkg	2.5	70	32%
sausage..pickled..1 oz	1 pkg	9.0	240	34%
(Outpost)				
beef jerky	1 oz	0.5	70	6%
beef 'n' cheese	1.5 oz	13.0	150	78%
beef sticks	.25 oz	3.0	35	77%
hot sausage	.875 oz	4.5	60	68%
Kippered Beef Steak	.875 0z	2.0	60	30%
Kippered Beef Steak Nuggets	1 oz	1.0	80	11%
(Pemmican)				
Kippered Beef Steak				
BBQ	1 oz	1.0	60	15%
original	1 oz	1.0	60	15%
peppered	1 oz	1.0	60	15%
sweet & hot	1 oz	1.0	70	13%
teriyaki	1 oz	1.0	60	15 %
(Penrose) pouch items				
Big Mama	2.4 oz	16.0	190	76%
Firecracker	0.875 oz	0.5	70	6%
	1.2 oz	7.0	100	63%
giant	1.7 oz	10.0	140	64%
smoked sausage..Big Mama	2 oz	15.0	200	68%
Tijuana Mama	2.4 oz	16.0	190	76%
(Rustler's)				
beef jerky	1 stick	2.5	40	56%
spicy stick	1 stick	8.0	100	72%
(Slim Jim)				
Beef Jerky..Super Jerk	0.31 0z	2.0	35	51%
Deli Sticks..All Flavors	1.8 oz	20.0	240	75%
trial-size	0.6 oz	7.0	80	79%
Kippered Beef Steak				
original	1.4 oz	5.0	110	41%
peppered	1.4 oz	5.0	110	41%
teriyaki	1.4 oz	5.0	110	41%
meat & cheese items				
beef 'n' cheese	1.5 oz	11.0	150	66%
chili beef 'n' cheese	1.5 0z	11.0	150	66%
pepperoni	1.5 oz	12.0	150	72%
Slim Jim items				
big..spicy	0.44 oz	6.0	70	77%
giant				
chili	0.97 oz	13.0	150	78%
mild	0.97 oz	13.0	150	78%
spicy	0.97 oz	13.0	150	78%
mild..super	0.64 oz	9.0	100	81%
nacho				
giant	0.97 oz	13.0	150	78%
super	0.64 oz	9.0	100	81%

Food and Description	Amount	Fat Grams	Total Calories	% Fat Calories
sweet & spicy				
giant	0.97 oz	12.0	140	77%
super	0.64 oz	9.0	100	81%
Tabasco				
giant	0.97 oz	13.0	150	78%
super	0.64 oz	9.0	100	81%
twin..vending pkg				
spicy	0.56 oz	8.0	90	80%
(Tombstone)				
beef jerky	1 stick	–	35	–
beef sticks	1 stick	8.0	90	80%
Snappy Sticks	1 stick	8.0	90	80%
(Trail's Best)				
beef jerky				
1-oz pkg				
original	1 oz	1.0	70	13%
peppered	1 oz	1.0	70	13%
teriyaki	1 oz	1.0	80	11%
2-oz pkg				
hot teriyaki	2 oz	1.5	150	9%
original	2 oz	1.5	140	10%
peppered	2 oz	1.5	140	10%
teriyaki	2 oz	1.5	150	9%
giant sticks..1.5-oz pkg				
beef..smoked	1 pkg	12.0	150	72%
meat				
hot & spicy	1 pkg	11.0	140	71%
pepperoni	1 pkg	11.0	150	66%
teriyaki	1 pkg	10.0	140	64%
Happy Trails..meat sticks				
.35-oz pkg	1 pkg	3.0	40	68%
1.1-oz pkg	1 pkg	9.0	120	68%
Kippered..Big Steak				
1.6-oz pkg				
hot	1 pkg	3.0	120	23%
original	1 pkg	4.5	110	37%
peppered	1 pkg	4.0	110	33%
sweet & hot	1 pkg	3.5	120	26%
teriyaki	1 pkg	3.5	110	29%
Kippered..Jumbo Steak				
original	1.2 oz	3.5	80	39%
peppered	1.2 oz	3.0	80	34%
teriyaki	1.2 oz	3.0	90	30%
Kippered...King Steak				
1.1-oz pkg				
original	1 pkg	2.5	80	28%
peppered	1 pkg	2.5	80	28%
teriyaki	1 pkg	2.5	170	13%
sweet & hot	1 pkg	2.5	80	28%

Food and Description	Amount	Fat Grams	Total Calories	% Fat Calories
meat & cheese snack				
2-oz pkg				
beef	1 pkg	17.0	210	73%
ham & cheddar	1 pkg	16.0	200	72%
pepperoni & mozzarella	1 pkg	15.0	200	68%
spicy beef & jalapeño				
cheese	1 pkg	17.0	200	77%

MEAT SPREAD (*See* LUNCHEON MEAT SPREAD)
MEAT SUBSTITUTE (*See* VEGETARIAN FOODS; individual listings)
MEAT TENDERIZER (*See* MARINADE; SEASONINGS)
MELBA TOAST (*See* CRACKER)
MELON (*See* individual listings)
MEXICAN FOOD (*See also* BEEF DISH/ENTRÉE; BREAKFAST SANDWICH; DIP; FROZEN ENTRÉE/DINNER; PASTA ENTRÉE/DINNER; RICE DISH; SAUCE; SEASONINGS; TOMATO; TOMATO SAUCE; TORTILLA CHIPS/CORN CHIPS; VEGETARIAN FOODS)
■ **BEANS** (*See* Refried Beans in this section)
■ **BURRITO** (*See* MEXICAN DINNERS/ENTRÉES within this section)
■ **CHILI** (*See* BEEF DISH/ENTRÉE; CHILI/CHILI BEANS; SEASONINGS)
■ **CHILI SAUCE** (*See* SAUCE)
■ **CHILIES** (*See* PEPPERS within this section)
■ **CHURRO**

frozen				
(Tio Pepe's) cinnamon..6-oz pkg	1 piece	5.0	110	41%

■ **DIP** (*See also* DIP)

(Garden of Eatin')..dips..all flavors	2 Tbs	–	25	–

■ **ENCHILADA** (*See* MEXICAN DINNERS/ENTRÉES within this section)
■ **FLAUTA**

frozen				
(Schwan's) apple	1 flauta	4.5	150	27%

■ **GAZPACHO** (*See* SOUP)
■ **GUACAMOLE** (*See* DIP)
■ **MENUDO**

(Juanita's) hot & spicy	1 cup	7.0	170	37%
(La Costena) beef tripe & hominy stew	1 cup	8.0	180	40%
(Pico Pica)	1 cup	9.0	200	41%

■ **MEXICAN DINNERS/ENTRÉES**

FROZEN/MICROWAVABLE/REFRIGERATED				
(Delimex)				
QUESADILLAS				
chicken & cheese	⅛ box	10.0	230	39%
RICE				
gourmet bowls				
grilled chicken teriyaki	1 bowl	4.5	450	9%
kung pao–style chicken	1 bowl	10.0	510	18%
regular				
chicken–fried	6.9 oz	4.5	290	14%
TAQUITOS				
beef	5 pieces	13.0	370	32%
chicken	5 pieces	14.0	370	34%

Food and Description	Amount	Fat Grams	Total Calories	% Fat Calories
seasoned beef & cheddar				
rolled	⅓ box	20.0	410	44%
3-cheese	5 pieces	20.0	400	45%
(Don Miguel)				
burritos				
bean & cheese	1 burrito	12.0	460	23%
bean & rice	1 burrito	3.5	360	9%
chicken	1 burrito	8.0	390	18%
lean steak & rice	1 burrito	3.5	360	9%
steak burrito	1 burrito	8.0	400	18%
(El Monterey)				
APPETIZERS				
Fiesta				
family pack/classics	⅓ box	21.0	370	58%
taquitos	3 pieces	15.0	330	41%
minis				
tacos	4 pieces	12.0	260	42%
variety	4.5 oz	24.0	370	58%
BREAKFAST TAQUITOS				
egg, bacon & cheese	⅙ box	12.0	300	36%
CARB-FRIENDLY				
chicken & cheese quesadilla	1	9.0	210	39%
chipotle chicken & cheese	1	12.0	310	35%
shredded beef steak burrito	1	15.0	320	42%
shredded steak quesadilla	1	15.0	260	52%
CRUNCHEROS				
quesadilla				
3-cheese & grilled chicken	4 pieces	26.0	460	52%
taquitos				
chicken & cheese	4 pieces	16.0	410	35%
shredded steak & cheese	⅓ box	20.0	390	46%
Southwest chicken	½ box	17.0	400	37%
taco beef & cheese	4 pieces	24.0	420	51%
ENCHILADAS				
beef w/sauce				
1.5-lb tray	1	7.0	150	42%
2.5-lb tray	1	9.0	180	43%
cheese w/sauce & garnish				
1.5-lb tray	1	10.0	170	53%
2.5-lb tray	1	13.0	220	53%
chicken w/suiza sauce	1	11.0	210	47%
MEXICAN GRILL				
charbroiled				
chicken & cheese quesadilla	1	10.0	230	39%
chicken breast taquitos	3	19.0	380	45%
steak burrito	1	9.0	290	28%
MINI FRIED BURRITOS				
cream cheese & jalapeños	3 pieces	24.0	370	58%
nacho cheese & beef	3 pieces	16.0	330	44%
QUESADILLA				
grilled chicken & cheese	1	14.0	260	48%

Food and Description	Amount	Fat Grams	Total Calories	% Fat Calories
SOFT TACOS				
beef & cheese	1	22.0	440	45%
sausage, egg & cheese	1	23.0	370	56%
spicy				
beef & cheese	1	22.0	420	47%
chicken & cheese	1	11.0	340	29%
TAMALES/SHREDDED BEEF	1	9.0	200	41%
(Patio)				
BURRITOS				
bean & cheese burrito	1 burrito	9.0	300	27%
beef & bean				
green chili	1 burrito	12.0	330	33%
medium	1 burrito	10.0	310	29%
mild	1 burrito	12.0	330	33%
red-hot	1 burrito	12.0	320	34%
chicken	1 burrito	8.0	290	25%
DINNERS				
beef enchilada	1 meal	12.0	370	29%
beef tamale & enchilada	1 meal	24.0	480	45%
cheese enchilada	1 meal	10.0	350	26%
chicken enchilada	1 meal	12.0	350	31%
con queso burrito	1 meal	14.0	450	28%
enchilada combo	1 meal	12.0	370	29%
spicy hot	1 meal	13.0	390	30%
PLATTERS				
enchiladas..w/sauce	2 pieces	7.0	190	33%
cheese..w/sauce	2 pieces	7.0	190	33%
(Rosarita)				
REFRIGERATED MEALS				
enchilada				
shredded chicken	1 meal	13.0	280	42%
fajita..grilled chicken breast	1 meal	4.0	160	23%
quesadilla..grilled chicken	1 meal	13.0	250	47%
MIXES AND REFRIGERATED DINNER KITS				
(Chi-Chi's)				
Fiesta tortilla soup..mix only	⅓ pkg	1.5	80	17%
shells & seasonings				
fajita	2 shells	7.0	300	21%
soft taco	2 shells	7.0	300	21%
white corn	2 shells	7.0	200	32%
sweet corn cake..mix only	½ cup	0.5	100	5%
(Kraft) refrigerated				
dinner kits				
3-cheese chicken enchilada	⅕ kit	15.0	300	45%
fiesta taco dinner bake	⅕ kit	21.0	340	56%
Mexican-style lasagna	⅕ kit	16.0	310	46%
(Old El Paso)				
kit				
mix & 1 tortilla	1 piece	3.5	190	16%
prepared	1 piece	7.0	280	23%

Food and Description	Amount	Fat Grams	Total Calories	% Fat Calories
(Ortega)				
dinner kit				
taco..w/shells & seasoning	⅙ box	5.0	150	30%
taco kit..soft tortilla w/seasonings	⅕ box	5.0	240	19%
(Oscar Mayer)				
Lunchables..refrigerated				
nachos				
cheese dip & salsa				
1 box..4.4 oz	1 box	21.0	380	50%
1 box..4.75 oz	1 box	29.0	570	46%
Ultimate Nachos	1 box	32.0	790	36%
(Taco Bell) dinner kits				
Home Originals				
fajita dinner..15.5-oz box	⅕ box	5.0	230	20%
soft taco..16.35-oz box	⅕ box	5.0	230	20%
soft taco..12.5-oz box	⅕ box	5.0	200	23%
taco dinner..14.25-oz box	⅙ box	10.0	230	39%
taco dinner..10.75-oz box	⅙ box	4.5	130	31%
taco dinner..10.2-oz box	⅙ box	10.0	180	50%
Ultimate Nacho's	¼ box	15.0	280	48%
■ **MEXICAN FOOD SEASONINGS (*See also* SEASONINGS)**				
(Chi-Chi's)				
mix..dry				
fajita seasoning	¼ pkg	1.0	35	26%
fiesta burrito seasoning	¼ pkg	1.0	35	26%
restaurant seasoning	1 Tbs	–	10	–
taco	⅕ pkg	–	25	–
(Old El Paso) mix..dry				
burrito	2 tsp	–	15	–
chili	1 Tbs	0.5	15	30%
enchilada	2 tsp	–	10	–
fajita	1 tsp	–	10	–
taco	2 tsp	–	15	–
less sodium	2 tsp	–	15	–
mild	2 tsp	–	15	–
(Durkee) mix..dry				
family	1 serving	–	10	–
mild	1 serving	–	15	–
regular	1 serving	–	15	–
salad	1 serving	–	20	–
(Rosarita) mix..dry				
burrito	⅛ pkg	–	20	–
fajita	⅛ pkg	–	15	–
taco	⅙ pkg	–	20	–
(Taco Bell) mix only	2 Tbs	–	20	–
■ **NACHOS (See MEXICAN DINNERS/ENTRÉES within this section)**				
■ **PEPPERS**				
(Chi-Chi's)				
diced tomatoes & green chilies	¼ cup	–	20	–

Food and Description	Amount	Fat Grams	Total Calories	% Fat Calories
green chili				
diced	2 Tbs	–	10	–
whole	¾ pepper	–	10	–
jalapeño				
wheels	19 pieces	–	10	–
whole	2-½ peppers	–	10	–
(Del Monte)				
chipotle..in spice sauce	2 Tbs	–	20	–
hot yellow chili	4 peppers	–	10	–
jalapeño				
nachos	2 Tbs	–	5	–
pickled..all types	2 Tbs	–	5	–
(Embasa)				
green chilis..mild..whole	~1 oz	–	15	–
Guerito peppers	~1 oz	0.5	10	45%
jalapeño..all types	1 oz	–	5	–
nopalitos..sliced	~1 oz	–	5	–
(Clemente Jacques)				
chipotle..in adobe sauce	1 oz	1.0	25	36%
jalapeño..pickled..all types	1 oz	–	5	–
(La Victoria)				
green				
diced	2 Tbs	–	–	–
whole	1 pepper	–	5	–
jalapeño				
diced	2 Tbs	–	–	–
marinated	1½ Tbs	–	10	–
sliced	14 pieces	–	<1	–
(Old El Paso)				
green chili				
chopped	2 Tbs	–	5	–
whole	1 medium	–	10	–
jalapeño				
sliced	2 Tbs	–	15	–
whole				
peeled	3 medium	–	10	–
pickled	2 medium	–	5	–
(Ortega)..all types	1 oz	–	10	–
(Ro*tel)				
green chiles..blended In spicy tomato sauce				
chunky	½ cup	–	20	–
diced in sauce	½ cup	–	40	–
extra-hot	½ cup	–	20	–
Mexican festival	½ cup	–	30	–
milder	½ cup	–	20	–
original	½ cup	–	20	–
(Rosarita)..all types	2 Tbs	–	10	–
(Vlasic)				
jalapeño..Mexican hot	1 oz	–	8	–

Food and Description	Amount	Fat Grams	Total Calories	% Fat Calories
Mexican..tiny hot	1 oz	–	6	–
pepperoncini..mild	1 oz	–	5	–
■ REFRIED BEANS				
(Amy's) Organic				
traditional	½ cup	3.0	140	19%
vegetarian black beans	½ cup	3.0	140	19%
w/green chiles	½ cup	3.0	130	21%
(Bush's Best)				
authentic recipe..traditional	½ cup	3.0	150	18%
fat-free	½ cup	–	130	–
traditional	½ cup	3.0	150	18%
(Chi-Chi's)				
vegetable	½ cup	1.0	100	9%
(Comida Sabrosa)	½ cup	2.0	140	13%
(Eden) Refried				
black beans	½ cup	1.5	110	12%
black beans..spicy	½ cup	1.5	110	12%
black soy & black beans	½ cup	1.0	90	10%
kidney beans	½ cup	1.0	80	11%
pinto beans	½ cup	1.0	90	10%
pinto beans..spicy	½ cup	1.0	90	10%
(Full Circle) Organic				
salsa				
hot	1 oz	–	10	–
medium	1 oz	–	10	–
mild	1 oz	–	10	–
(Gebhardt)				
Mexican-style..w/jalapeño	½ cup	3.0	110	25%
traditional	½ cup	3.0	110	25%
(La Costena)				
black beans				
refried	½ cup	11.0	180	55%
whole	½ cup	1.0	70	13%
pinto..refried	½ cup	9.0	160	51%
(Kuner's Southwestern) w/lime	½ cup	3.0	170	16%
(La Sierra) w/chipotle	½ cup	6.0	150	34%
(Old El Paso)				
beans & cheese	½ cup	3.5	120	26%
beans & green chillies	½ cup	0.5	100	5%
beans & sausage	½ cup	13.0	200	59%
fat-free	½ cup	–	100	–
spicy..fat-free	½ cup	–	100	–
traditional	½ cup	0.5	100	5%
vegetarian	½ cup	1.0	100	9%
(Rosarita)				
authentic home-style	½ cup	8.0	140	51%
traditional..98% fat-free	½ cup	2.0	110	16%
traditional..no fat	½ cup	–	100	–
(Taco Bell)				
Home Originals				
original	½ cup	3.0	140	19%

Food and Description	Amount	Fat Grams	Total Calories	% Fat Calories
vegetarian blend	½ cup	3.0	140	19%
■ SALSA/SAUCE (See also SAUCE)				
(Chi-Chi's)				
enchilada	¼ cup	1.5	30	45%
picante..all types	2 Tbs	–	10	–
salsa				
con queso	2 Tbs	3.0	45	60%
fiesta..hot	2 Tbs	–	10	–
garden	2 Tbs	–	15	–
hot..medium..mild	2 Tbs	–	10	–
original				
medium..mild	2 Tbs	–	10	–
roasted tomato	2 Tbs	–	10	–
taco..thick & chunky	1 Tbs	–	10	–
(Del Monte)				
picante..all types	2 Tbs	–	10	–
salsa				
fire-roasted..medium	2 Tbs	–	10	–
garlic	2 Tbs	–	10	–
Mexicana	2 Tbs	–	5	–
taquera	2 Tbs	–	5	–
thick & chunky..all types	2 Tbs	–	10	–
(Doritos) salsa..all types	2 Tbs	–	15	–
(Embasa).salsa..all types	2 Tbs	–	5	–
salsa				
(Enrico's)				
picante sauce...all types	2 Tbs	–	10	–
salsa..all types	2 Tbs	–	10	–
(Hain) salsa/green chili				
hot	¼ cup	–	20	–
mild	¼ cup	–	20	–
(Heluva Good Cheese) salsa				
cheese	2 Tbs	6.0	80	68%
thick & chunky..all types	2 Tbs	–	10	–
(Herdez)				
Salsa Casera..all types	1 oz	–	10	–
Salsa Ranchera	1 oz	–	15	–
Salsa Taquera				
medium	1 oz	–	10	–
Mexicana picante	1 oz	–	26	–
(La Victoria)				
chile sauce..red	2 oz	0.5	15	30%
enchilada				
mild green chile	2 oz	–	15	–
red	2 oz	1.5	20	45%
salsa				
brava	1 tbs	–	0	–
other types	2 tbs	–	10	–
taco				
green..all types	1 tbs	–	0	–
red..all types	1 Tbs	–	5	–

Food and Description	Amount	Fat Grams	Total Calories	% Fat Calories
(Muir Glen) organic fat-free				
black bean & corn	2 tbs	–	15	–
hot.. habanero	2 tbs	–	10	–
medium..all types	2 tbs	–	10	–
mild	2 Tbs	–	10	
(Newman's Own) Bandito salsa				
medium & mild heat	2 Tbs	–	10	–
peach	2 Tbs	–	25	–
pineapple	2 Tbs	–	15	–
(Old El Paso)				
enchilada				
green chili	¼ cup	1.5	30	45%
hot	¼ cup	1.0	20	45%
mild	¼ cup	1.0	20	45%
picante..all types	2 tbs	–	10	–
salsa..all types	2 tbs	–	10	–
taco				
hot	1 Tbs	–	5	–
medium	1 Tbs	–	5	–
mild	1 Tbs	–	5	–
(Ortega) salsa				
garden-style..all types	2 tbs	–	10	–
home-style..all types	2 Tbs	–	10	–
Mexican-style..medium	2 Tbs	–	15	–
(Pace)				
enchilada sauce	¼ cup	–	25	–
Mexican Creations Sauce				
cilantro & lime	1cup	–	25	–
roasted ranchero	1 cup	1.0	35	26%
sweet roasted onion				
& garlic	¼ cup	–	30	–
taco				
classic	2 Tbs	–	20	–
mild	2 Tbs	–	15	–
picante sauce	2 tbs	–	10	–
salsa..all types	2 tbs	–	10	–
salsa.. con queso	2 Tbs	3.0	45	60%
verde..w/tomatillos & jalapeños	1 cup	–	20	–
(Rosarita) chunky				
picante..all types	3 tbs	–	25	–
salsa/taco..all types	3 Tbs	–	25	–
(Ro*Tel)				
salsa..diced tomatoes &				
green chilies..all types				
extra-hot	½ cup	–	20	–
regular	½ cup	–	20	–
(Taco Bell) Home Originals				
hot sauce	1 tsp	–	–	–
picante..Smooth 'n' Zesty				
mild	2 Tbs	–	15	–

Food and Description	Amount	Fat Grams	Total Calories	% Fat Calories
salsa				
con queso..all types	2 Tbs	3.0	40	68%
thick & chunky..all types	2 Tbs	–	15	–
taco sauce				
medium	2 Tbs	–	10	–
mild	2 Tbs	–	15	–
(Tostitos)				
picante..all types	2 tbs	–	15	–
salsa				
con queso..all types	2 Tbs	3.0	80	34%
other salsa..all types	2 Tbs	–	30	–
■ SHELLS				
TACO				
(Azteca) super	1 shell	12.0	200	54%
(Chi-Chi's)				
white	2 shells	8.0	170	40%
yellow	2 shells	8.0	170	40%
(Mission) 12-count	1 shell	5.0	100	45%
(Old El Paso)				
mini..fun-size	7 shells	7.0	150	42%
regular	3 shells	7.0	150	42%
salad	1 shell	6.0	110	49%
super stuffer	2 shells	8.0	180	40%
white corn	3 shells	7.0	150	42%
(Ortega)				
taco				
white corn	2 shells	4.5	120	34%
yellow corn	2 shells	5.0	120	38%
tostada	2 shells	5.0	130	35%
(Rosarita)	3 shells	8.5	155	32%
(Taco Bell) Home Originals	3 shells	6.0	150	36%
TOASTADA..corn				
(Guerrero) Nortenas				
chili chipotle	2 shells	7.0	130	48%
(Mission)				
caseras..24-count	1 shell	5.0	100	45%
nortenas amarilla..32-count	2 shells	5.0	110	41%
(Old Dutch) restaurant-style				
yellow	2 shells	6.0	140	39%
(Old El Paso)	3 shells	7.0	150	42%
(Ortega)	2 shells	5.0	130	35%

■ **TACO** (*See* BREAKFAST SANDWICH; MEXICAN FOOD SEASONINGS within this section; MEXICAN DINNER/ENTRÉES within this section; SHELLS within this section)
■ **TACO SHELL** (*See* SHELLS within this section)
■ **TAMALE** (See also MEXICAN DINNERS/ENTRÉES within this section)

CANNED				
(Derby)	2 tamales	7.0	160	39%
(Gebhardt)				
jumbo	2 tamales	30.0	400	68%
original	2 tamales	22.0	290	68%

Food and Description	Amount	Fat Grams	Total Calories	% Fat Calories
(Hormel)				
beef				
hot-spicy	2 tamales	7.0	140	45%
jumbo	2 tamales	10.0	190	47%
regular	2 tamales	7.0	140	45%
chicken	2 tamales	7.0	130	48%
(Old El Paso)	3 tamales	19.0	330	52%
(Wolf)	2 tamales	12.0	210	51%
■ TOMATILLO				
CANNED				
(La Costena)	4 medium	2.5	40	56%
■ TORTILLA				
(Abuelita)				
tortilla..6"				
yellow corn	4 tortillas	–	160	–
white corn/table	2 tortillas	1.5	150	9%
tortilla..8" lower carbs	1 tortilla	4.0	80	45%
tortilla..9"..whole wheat	1 tortilla	2.5	110	20%
tortilla..12"				
cheese	1 tortilla	9.0	217	37%
chili	1 tortilla	9.5	238	36%
pesto	1 tortilla	8.5	216	35%
plain	1 tortilla	9.0	217	37%
tomato	1 tortilla	9.0	237	34%
whole wheat	1 tortilla	7.0	179	35%
tortilla..12"..hand-stretched				
original	1 tortilla	2.5	110	20%
tortilla..12"..pressed	1 tortilla	7.0	270	23%
tortilla chips..uncooked..yellow				
triangle..w/lime	9 chips	1.0	80	11%
(Adios Carbs)				
tortillas..10-count				
garlic & herb	1 tortilla	3.2	87	33%
green onion	1 tortilla	3.2	87	33%
jalapeño pepper	1 tortilla	3.2	87	33%
regular	1 tortilla	3.2	87	33%
tortillas..burrito-size..8-count	1 tortilla	3.9	108	33%
tortillas..chocolate dessert..8-count	1 tortilla	3.2.	87	33%
tortillas..red chili pepper..10-count	1 tortilla	3.2	87	33%
(Cruz)				
tortillas				
corn..stone-ground	2 tortillas	1.0	110	8%
flour				
13.5-oz bag..8-count	1 tortilla	3.5	130	24%
97% fat-free	1 tortilla	0.5	120	4%
burrito-size	1 tortilla	1.0	130	7%
chimichanga	1 tortilla	3.0	130	21%
restaurant-style	1 tortilla	6.0	300	18%

Food and Description	Amount	Fat Grams	Total Calories	% Fat Calories
(Don Pancho)				
tortilla..flour				
gorditas				
burrito-style	1 tortilla	7.0	210	30%
fajita-style	1 tortilla	5.0	160	28%
family pack..30-count	1 tortilla	4.0	130	28%
(Guerrero)				
tortilla..corn				
50-count	2 tortillas	1.5	120	11%
90-count	2 tortillas	2.0	110	16%
Estilo ranchero				
50-count	2 tortillas	1.5	120	11%
90-count	2 tortillas	1.5	110	12%
tortilla..flour				
fajita..20-count	1 tortilla	4.0	110	33%
Fresqui Ricas..10-count	1 tortilla	6.0	140	26%
Riquisimas..12-count	1 tortilla	12.0	320	34%
Riquisimas..30-count	1 tortila	5.0	140	32%
Triguenas..whole wheat	1 tortilla	5.0	140	32%
(La Suprema)				
corn..all types	2 tortillas	1.5	100	14%
flour				
angel flour extra-soft				
burrito-size	1 tortilla	5.0	200	23%
taco-size	1 tortilla	4.0	150	24%
(Labrada)				
Tortilla Wraps				
chipotle	1 wrap	3.5	60	53%
flavors...all other	1 wrap	3.0	60	54%
(Mission)				
corn				
como hechas en casa	1 tortilla	1.0	70	13%
Estilo Casero				
regular-size	1 tortilla	1.0	70	13%
super-size	1 tortilla	5.0	100	45%
regular-size	2 tortillas	1.5	100	14%
super-size	1 tortilla	1.0	80	11%
white corn..12-count	2 tortillas	1.0	80	11%
flour				
burrito-size				
98% fat-free	1 tortilla	0.5	160	3%
regular-size	1 tortilla	5.0	220	20%
tortillas Caseras	1 tortilla	5.0	185	24%
Estilo Casero				
corditas/burrito-size	1 tortilla	9.0	260	31%
sabrositas				
burrito-size	1 tortilla	7.0	220	29%
burrito-size..98% fat-free	1 tortilla	0.5	160	3%
regular-size	1 tortilla	5.0	140	32%
super-size	1 tortilla	7.0	190	33%

Food and Description	Amount	Fat Grams	Total Calories	% Fat Calories
fajita-size	1 tortilla	3.0	120	23%
98% fat-free wheat	1 tortilla	2.5	140	16%
grande	1 tortilla	4.0	130	28%
restaurant-size	1 tortilla	3.0	120	23%
low-carb				
fajita-size	1 tortilla	2.0	80	23%
soft taco–size	1 tortilla	2.5	110	20%
whole wheat..burrito	1 tortilla	4.5	200	20%
whole wheat..fajita	1 tortilla	2.0	80	23%
soft taco–size				
fluffy home-style	1 tortilla	5.0	180	25%
98% fat-free	1 tortilla	0.5	120	4%
regular-size..20-count	1 tortilla	4.0	150	24%
restaurant-style	1 tortilla	3.0	140	19%
wraps				
garden spinach herb	1 tortilla	6.0	240	23%
Southwestern chili	1 tortilla	6.0	240	23%
zesty garlic herb	1 tortilla	6.0	240	23%
(Reser's) Baja Café				
flour tortillas				
burrito-size..10-count	1 tortilla	5.0	180	25%
home-style..10-count	1 tortilla	3.5	130	24%
soft taco size..12-count	1 tortilla	4.0	130	27%
(Thomas) Sahara wraps..6-count				
100% whole wheat	1 wrap	4.5	170	24%
Carb Counting..home-style	1 wrap	5.0	110	41%
white	1 wrap	4.5	170	24%
■ TORTILLA MIX				
(Quaker) mix only				
harina, preparada para tortillas	⅓ cup	4.5	160	25%
masa harina	¼ cup	1.5	110	12%
(White Wings) tortilla mix flour	¼ cup	7.0	220	29%
■ TOSTADA				
■ TOSTADA SHELL (*See* SHELLS within this section)				
MEXICAN POTATO (*See* JICAMA/YAM BEAN TUBER)				
MILK (*See also* MILK SUBSTITUTE; RICE; SOY MILK)				
BUFFALO	1 cup	17.0	236	65%
CAROB	1 cup	3.0	160	17%
COW..CANNED				
condensed..sweetened				
(Borden) Eagle Brand				
creamy chocolate	1.4 oz	2.5	120	19%
fat-free	1.4 oz	–	110	–
low-fat	1.4 oz	1.5	120	11%
original	1.4 oz	3.0	130	21%
(Carnation)	2 Tbs	3.0	130	21%
(Dairy Sweet)	⅓ cup	9.0	320	25%
COW..EVAPORATED				
(Carnation)				
fat-free	2 Tbs	–	25	–
	½ cup	–	100	–

Food and Description	Amount	Fat Grams	Total Calories	% Fat Calories
low-fat	2 Tbs	0.5	25	18%
whole..regular	2 Tbs	2.0	40	45%
(Milnot)				
skim	2 Tbs	–	25	–
	½ cup	–	100	–
whole	2 Tbs	2.0	40	45%
	½ cup	8.0	150	48%
(Pet)				
regular	2 Tbs	2.0	40	45%
	½ cup	10.0	170	53%
skim	2 Tbs	–	25	–
	½ cup	–	100	–
COW..FRESH				
(Blue Bunny)				
1% low-fat	1 cup	2.5	100	23%
2% reduced-fat				
chocolate milk	1 cup	5.0	180	25%
regular milk	1 cup	5.0	120	38%
sweet acidophilus	1 cup	5.0	120	38%
fat-free	1 cup	–	90	–
vitamin D	1 cup	8.0	150	48%
(Borden)				
2% reduced-fat	1 cup	5.0	120	38%
buttermilk				
Golden Churn 1.5% fat	1 cup	1.0	120	30%
chocolate-flavored				
Dutch..2% reduced-fat	1 cup	5.0	170	26%
skim	1 cup	–	80	–
whole	1 cup	8.0	150	48%
(Darigold)				
1% fat..light	1 cup	2.5	110	20%
2% fat..reduced-fat	1 cup	5.0	130	35%
acidophilus bifidus..fat-free	1 cup	–	100	–
acidophilus..low-fat	1 cup	2.5	110	20%
buttermilk..low-fat	1 cup	2.5	110	20%
calcium extra	1 cup	2.5	110	20%
fat-free	1 cup	–	90	–
fat-free..Trim Deluxe	1 cup	–	100	–
flavored milk				
chocolate..reduced-fat	1 cup	5.0	210	21%
extra chocolate	1 cup	9.0	240	34%
strawberry..reduced-fat	1 cup	5.0	210	21%
vanilla	1 cup	5.0	210	21%
homogenized	1 cup	8.0	150	48%
(Full Circle) Organic				
fat-free	8 oz	–	90	–
whole	8 oz	8.0	150	48%
(Hershey's)				
chocolate				
fat-free	1 cup	–	160	–

Food and Description	Amount	Fat Grams	Total Calories	% Fat Calories
reduced-fat	1 cup	5.0	200	23%
shake				
cookies 'n' cream	7 fl oz	5.0	200	23%
creamy chocolate	7 fl oz	5.0	200	23%
mint chocolate	7 fl oz	7.0	300	21%
strawberry	7 fl oz	7.0	280	23%
vanilla cream	7 fl oz	7.0	320	20%
2% reduced-fat	1 cup	5.0	200	23%
whole milk	1 cup	9.0	210	39%
(Hood)				
Carb Countdown..dairy beverage				
2% reduced-fat	1 cup	4.5	100	41%
chocolate	1 cup	4.5	100	41%
fat-free	1 cup	–	70	–
homogenized	1 cup	8.0	130	55%
regular milk products				
buttermilk	1 cup	–	90	–
chocolate				
1%	1 cup	3.0	170	16%
whole	1 cup	8.0	230	31%
coffee..1%	1 cup	2.5	170	13%
LightBlock				
1%	1 cup	2.5	110	20%
2%	1 cup	5.0	130	35%
fat-free	1 cup	–	80	–
whole	1 cup	8.0	150	48%
Simply Smart				
1%	1 cup	2.5	120	19%
fat-free	1 cup	–	90	–
low-fat	1 cup	2.5	120	19%
whole..w/vitamin D	1 cup	8.0	150	48%
(Horizon) Organic				
1%..low-fat	8 oz	2.5	100	23%
2%..reduced-fat	8 oz	5.0	120	38%
vitamins A & D added	8 oz	5.0	120	38%
chocolate..reduced-fat	8 oz	5.0	190	24%
fat-free	8 oz	–	90	–
vitamins A & D added	8 oz	–	90	–
vanilla..reduced-fat	8 oz	4.5	190	21%
(Kemp's)				
1% low-fat	1 cup	2.5	110	20%
2% reduced-fat	1 cup	5.0	130	35%
flavored				
café mocha..reduced-fat	12 oz	5.0	200	23%
chocolate	1 cup	8.0	220	33%
French vanilla	12 oz	8.0	210	34%
vitamin D	1 cup	8.0	150	48%
(Nestlé USA) Nesquik..ready-to-drink				
Buncha Banana	1 cup	5.0	200	23%

Food and Description	Amount	Fat Grams	Total Calories	% Fat Calories
chocolate				
fat-free	1 cup	–	160	–
whole	1 cup	8.0	230	31%
double chocolate	1 cup	9.0	230	35%
very vanilla	1 cup	8.0	220	33%
(Oberweis Dairy) bottles..flavored				
chocolate..reduced-fat	12 oz	8.0	270	26%
strawberry	12 oz	8.0	30	21%
(Pet)				
chocolate	1 cup	7.0	200	32%
whole..vitamin D	1 cup	8.0	150	48%
(Smith's) Moovers..flavored				
8-oz bottle				
chocolate..1% low-fat	8 oz	2.5	150	15%
14-oz bottle				
chocolate	7 oz	7.0	180	35%
chocolate malt shake	7 oz	4.0	240	15%
strawberry..reduced-fat	7 oz	4.5	160	25%
(The Organic Cow of Vermont)				
chocolate..low-fat	1 cup	2.5	160	14%
low-fat	1 cup	2.5	100	23%
reduced-fat	1 cup	4.5	120	34%
skim..fat-free	1 cup	–	80	–
whole				
homogenized	1 cup	8.0	150	48%
not homogenized	1 cup	8.0	150	48%
(Umpqua)				
1% low-fat	8 oz	2.5	100	23%
2% reduced-fat	8 oz	5.0	120	38%
buttermilk..low-fat	8 oz	2.5	110	20%
chocolate..Dutch-style	8 oz	7.0	190	33%
fat-free white milk	8 oz	–	80	–
homogenized..w/vitamin D	8 oz	8.0	150	48%
COW/LACTOSE-REDUCED (See MILK SUBSTITUTE)				
DRY..POWDERED				
(Alba) non-fat..prepared	1 cup	–	80	–
(Carnation) mix only				
non-fat	⅓ cup	–	80	–
(Nestlé) Nido..dry mix				
whole milk	⅓ cup	9.0	150	54%
(Saco)				
buttermilk				
mix only	4 Tbs	<1	80	5%
prepared	1 cup	<1	80	5%
non-fat milk				
mix only	⅓ cup	–	80	–
prepared	1 cup	–	80	–
GOAT				
canned..evaporated				
(Meyenberg)	8 oz	8.0	145	50%

Food and Description	Amount	Fat Grams	Total Calories	% Fat Calories
carton				
powder mixed w/water	1 cup	8.0	145	50%
refrigerated				
1% low-fat	1 cup	2.5	90	25%
whole	1 cup	7.0	145	43%
fresh	1 cup	10.0	168	54%
HUMAN	1 cup	11.0	170	58%
REINDEER	8 fl oz	48.6	580	75%
SHEEP	8 fl oz	17.0	264	58%
MILK MIX (*See also* BREAKFAST DRINK; COCOA; MILK SHAKE)				
(Carnation)..mix only..malted milk				
chocolate	2 Tbs	1.0	90	10%
original	2 Tbs	2.0	90	20%
(Country Choice Naturals)..mix only				
royal chocolate cocoa	2 Tbs	–	100	–
royal chocolate cocoa..soy	2 Tbs	1.0	100	9%
Irish chocolate mint	2 Tbs	–	100	–
(Ghirardelli)				
mix only				
cocoa..unsweetened	1 Tbs	1.5	20	68%
double chocolate hot chocolate	3 Tbs	1.5	100	14%
hazelnut	3 Tbs	1.5	100	14%
mocha	3 Tbs	1.5	100	14%
prepared..w/2% milk				
chocolate hazelnut	1 cup	6.0	210	26%
milk double chocolate	1 cup	5.0	210	21%
mocha	1 cup	6.0	210	26%
white mocha	1 cup	5.0	210	21%
(Hershey's)				
Hot Cocoa Collection				
Dutch chocolate	1 envelope	2.0	140	13%
French vanilla	1 envelope	1.5	140	10%
syrups				
(Land O'Lakes)				
Cappuccino Classics				
Amaretto Italia	1 pkt	3.0	130	21%
French vanilla	1 pkt	3.0	130	21%
mocha	1 pkt	3.0	130	21%
Suisse mocha	1 pkt	3.5	140	23%
Suprema	1 pkt	3.0	130	21%
Cocoa Classics..chocolate &				
all flavors	1 pkt	5.0	160	28%
(Nestlé)				
hot cocoa..mix only				
Butterfinger	1 pkt	3.0	120	23%
Double Chocolate Meltdown	1 pkt	3.0	150	18%
chocolate w/marshmallows	1 pkt	–	30	–
French vanilla	1 pkt	3.0	120	23%
milk chocolate..envelope	1 pkt	2.5	80	28%
Nesquik..w/bunny-shaped				
marshmallows	1 pkt	3.0	130	21%

Food and Description	Amount	Fat Grams	Total Calories	% Fat Calories
rich chocolate..envelope	1 pkt	3.0	80	34%
rich chocolate..fat-free				
envelope	1 pkt	–	25	–
rich chocolate..no sugar added				
canister	3 Tbs	–	50	–
envelopes	1 pkt	–	80	–
rich chocolate..w/mini				
marshmallows..envelope	1 pkt	3.0	80	34%
s'mores..w/marshmallows	1 pkt	3.5	130	24%
Nesquik..mix only				
chocolate	2 Tbs	0.5	90	5%
no sugar	2 Tbs	1.0	40	23%
double chocolate	2 Tbs	0.5	90	5%
strawberry	2 Tbs	–	90	–
very vanilla	2 Tbs	–	90	–
Nesquik..flavored syrup				
chocolate	2 Tbs	–	100	–
strawberry	2 Tbs	–	110	–
Quik				
chocolate				
no sugar added	2 Tbs	1.0	40	23%
regular	2 Tbs	0.5	90	5%
strawberry	2 Tbs	–	90	–
(Swiss Miss) mix only				
chocolate sensation	1 pkt	4.0	150	24%
cocoa				
diet	1 pkt	–	25	–
fat-free				
regular	1 pkt	–	50	–
French vanilla	1 pkt	2.5	120	19%
light	1 pkt	<1.0	70	6%
no sugar added..regular	1 pkt	1.0	50	18%
double rich	1 pkt	1.0	110	8%
French vanilla..fat-free	1 pkt	2.5	120	19%
marshmallow lovers				
fat-free	1 pkt	–	60	–
regular	1 pkt	3.0	140	19%
milk chocolate				
regular				
26-oz canister	¼ cup	3.0	140	19%
39-oz canister	¼ cup	3.5	140	23%
	1 pkt	2.5	120	19%
sugar-free	1 pkt	–	50	–
w/ marshmallows	1 pkt	2.5	120	19%
MILK SHAKE (See MILK; individual FAST FOOD listings)				
MILK SUBSTITUTE (See also RICE; SOY MILK; YOGURT DRINK)				
(Better Than Milk)				
carob	1 cup	5.0	130	35%
chocolate	1 cup	5.0	125	36%

Food and Description	Amount	Fat Grams	Total Calories	% Fat Calories
light	1 cup	–	80	–
natural	1 cup	5.0	90	50%
(Dairy Ease) 100% lactose-free				
fat-free	1 cup	–	80	–
reduced-fat	1 cup	5.0	130	35%
whole	1 cup	9.0	160	51%
(EdenSoy) light				
original	8 oz	2.0	93	19%
vanilla	8 oz	2.0	120	15%
(Full Circle) organic..enriched				
lactose-free				
chocolate				
bottle	8 oz	3.5	140	23%
carton	8 oz	3.5	100	32%
original	8 oz	3.5	90	35%
vanilla	8 oz	3.5	110	29%
(Lactaid) 100% lactose-free				
chocolate..2% reduced-fat	1 cup	2.5	150	15%
regular				
fat-free	1 cup	–	90	–
low-fat	1 cup	2.5	110	20%
calcium-fortified	1 cup	2.5	110	20%
reduced-fat	1 cup	5.0	130	35%
whole	1 cup	8.0	150	48%
fat-free	1 cup	–	80	–
(Le Carb) less lactose..fewer carbs				
chocolate	1 cup	8.0	130	55%
white				
2% low-fat	1 cup	4.5	110	37%
homogenized	1 cup	9.0	140	58%
(Vance's DariFree) non-dairy..powder				
chocolate..2 Tbs	8 fl oz	–	110	–
white..2 Tbs	8 fl oz	–	70	–
(VitaSoy) soy milk				
classic original	8 oz	4.5	120	34%
rich chocolate	8 oz	4.0	100	36%
smooth vanilla	8 oz	4.0	110	33%
unsweetened original	8 oz	4.0	80	45%
vanilla delight	8 oz	4.0	120	30%
MILKFISH/raw	3 oz	6.0	125	43%
MILLET (See also CEREAL; FLOUR)				
(Arrowhead Mills)/hulled	¼ cup	1.5	150	9%
MINCEMEAT (See PIE FILLING)				
MINERAL WATER (See WATER)				
MINESTRONE (See SOUP)				
MISO (See also SOUP)				
(Eden)				
genmai..brown rice	1 Tbs	1.0	25	72%
hacho..soybean	1 Tbs	1.5	35	39%

Food and Description	Amount	Fat Grams	Total Calories	% Fat Calories
mugi..soybean & barley	1 Tbs	1.0	25	36%
shiro..soybean..sweet	1 Tbs	1.0	35	26%
(Westbrae) pasteurized				
miso bags				
barley	1 tsp	–	10	–
brown rice	1 tsp	–	10	–
soybean	1 tsp	0.5	10	45%
miso soups..instant				
red	1 pkt	–	35	–
white	1 pkt	1.5	35	39%
miso tubs..mellow				
all types	1 tsp	–	10	–
MOLASSES				
(Brer Rabbit)				
blackstrap	1 Tbs	–	60	–
dark	1 Tbs	–	60	–
full flavor	1 Tbs	–	60	–
light	1 Tbs	–	60	–
(Mott's) Grandma's				
gold label	1 Tbs	–	70	–
green label	1 Tbs	–	70	–
(Up Country Organics)				
unsulphured	1 Tbs	–	60	–
MONKFISH				
cooked—dry heat	3 oz	2.0	85	21%
raw	3 oz	1.0	64	14%
MOOSE/boneless				
raw	3 oz	4.8	152	28%
roasted	3 oz	1.0	115	8%
roasted/diced	1 cup	1.5	190	7%
MORTADELLA (*See* SAUSAGE)				
MOTH BEAN				
boiled	½ cup	0.5	105	4%
raw	½ cup	1.5	335	4%
MOUNTAIN YAM				
Hawaiian/cooked	1 cup	–	119	–
MOUSSE (*See* PUDDING & MOUSSE)				
MUFFIN (*See also* BREAKFAST SANDWICH; PASTRY, TOASTER)				
■ **FROZEN**				
(Sara Lee) Thaw & Serve				
FOOD SERVICE				
large..4.25 oz				
apple cranberry nut	1 muffin	23.0	440	47%
banana nut	1 mufin	13.0	440	27%
blueberry	1 muffin	16.0	430	33%
reduced-fat	1 muffin	9.0	270	30%
bran	1 mufin	22.0	440	45%
carrot nut	1 muffin	19.0	440	39%
cheese streusel	1 muffin	22.0	440	45%
cinnamon pecan cheesecake	1 muffin	26.0	490	48%

Food and Description	Amount	Fat Grams	Total Calories	% Fat Calories
corn	1 muffin	26.0	490	48%
double chocolate chunk	1 muffin	18.0	440	37%
lemon poppyseed	1 muffin	22.0	460	43%
orange streusel	1 muffin	19.0	450	38%
triple berry	1 muffin	13.0	370	32%
small..2.125 oz				
apple cranberry nut	1 muffin	12.0	220	49%
blueberry	1 muffin	8.0	210	34%
bran	1 muffin	8.0	200	36%
cheese streusel	1 muffin	11.0	220	45%
corn	1 muffin	12.0	250	43%
double chocolate chunk	1 muffin	11.0	230	43%
(Weight Watchers)				
chocolate chocolate chip	1 muffin	2.0	290	9%
■ MIX				
(Betty Crocker)				
original..box mix..prepared				
apple streusel	1 muffin	8.0	210	34%
banana nut	1 muffin	6.0	170	32%
cranberry orange	1 muffin	5.0	150	30%
double chocolate	1 muffin	8.0	200	36%
lemon poppyseed	1 muffin	7.0	190	33%
Twice the Blueberry	1 muffin	4.0	140	26%
wild blueberry	1 muffin	5.0	170	26%
pouch..made w/water..prepared				
apple cinnamon	1 muffin	4.0	130	28%
banana nut	1 muffin	5.0	130	35%
chocolate chip	1 muffin	5.0	130	35%
lemon poppyseed	1 muffin	3.5	130	24%
triple berry	1 muffin	3.0	120	23%
(Carb Fit)				
banana nut				
mix only	3 Tbs	2.5	100	23%
prepared	1 muffin	2.5	100	23%
blueberry				
mix only	3 Tbs	1.5	100	14%
prepared	1 muffin	1.5	100	14%
(Duncan Hines)				
bakery-style..prepared				
blueberry streusel	1 muffin	4.5	170	24%
wild Maine blueberry	1 muffin	4.0	140	26%
box mix..prepared				
blueberry	1 muffin	4.5	150	27%
chocolate chip	1 muffin	7.0	190	33%
cranberry orange	1 muffin	5.0	150	30%
(Golden Dipt)..prepared				
basic	1 muffin	3.0	120	23%
blueberry	1 muffin	3.0	120	23%
corn	1 muffin	2.0	99	18%

Food and Description	Amount	Fat Grams	Total Calories	% Fat Calories
(Jiffy)..dry mix only				
apple cinnamon	¼ cup	5.0	170	26%
banana nut	¼ cup	5.0	160	28%
blueberry	¼ cup	5.0	160	28%
bran..w/dates	¼ cup	4.0	150	24%
corn	¼ cup	4.0	160	23%
raspberry	¼ cup	6.0	170	32%
(Krusteaz)				
CarbSimple				
banana nut	1 muffin	7.0	170	37%
chocolate chip	1 muffin	7.0	170	37%
cranberry orange	1 muffin	6.0	170	32%
wild blueberry	1 muffin	6.0	170	32%
Fat-free				
banana	1 muffin	–	140	–
blueberry	1 muffin	–	130	–
cinnamon apple	1 muffin	–	130	–
corn..honey cornbread & muffin	1 muffin	–	120	–
cranberry orange	1 muffin	–	140	–
Low-fat				
apple oat bran	1 muffin	2.0	170	11%
Original				
almond poppyseed	1 muffin	5.0	180	25%
apple cinnamon	1 muffin	4.5	170	24%
blueberry	1 muffin	6.0	180	30%
honey bran	1 muffin	5.0	180	25%
lemon poppyseed	1 muffin	4.5	170	24%
oat bran	1 muffin	4.0	180	20%
wild blueberry	1 muffin	4.5	150	27%
(Martha White)..prepared				
apple cinnamon	1 muffin	4.5	160	25%
banana nut	1 muffin	5.0	150	30%
blackberry	1 muffin	4.5	160	25%
blueberry	1 muffin	4.5	160	25%
blueberry cheese	1 muffin	7.0	170	37%
carrot cake	1 muffin	4.0	160	23%
chocolate chip	1 muffin	4.5	160	25%
cinnamon	1 muffin	4.5	180	23%
lemon poppyseed	1 muffin	4.5	150	27%
strawberry banana	1 muffin	4.5	160	25%
(Pillsbury)..mix only				
Quick Bread & Muffin Mix				
apple cinnamon	⅟₁₄ pkg	2.5	130	17%
banana	⅟₁₂ pkg	1.5	130	10%
blueberry	⅟₁₂ pkg	1.5	140	10%
cranberry	⅟₁₄ pkg	1.5	110	12%
lemon poppyseed	⅟₁₂ pkg	3.0	150	18%
pumpkin	⅟₁₂ pkg	1.5	130	10%

Food and Description	Amount	Fat Grams	Total Calories	% Fat Calories
muffin mix				
blueberry	⅙ pkg	5.0	170	26%
chocolate chip	⅙ pkg	6.0	180	30%
(Shawnee Mills)..prepared				
corn muffin				
Mexican	1 piece	3.0	130	21%
yellow	1 piece	2.5	120	19%
yellow buttermilk	1 piece	3.0	130	21%
(White Lily)..mix only				
apple cinnamon	⅕ pkg	6.0	190	28%
banana nut	⅕ pkg	6.0	180	30%
blackberry	⅕ pkg	6.0	190	28%
blueberry	⅕ pkg	6.0	190	28%
chocolate chip..real milk chocolate	⅕ pkg	6.0	180	30%
cinnamon raisin	⅕ pkg	6.0	180	30%
corn	⅕ pkg	5.0	190	27%
strawberry	⅕ pkg	6.0	190	28%
wild berry	⅕ pkg	7.0	200	32%
■ READY-TO-SERVE				
(Arnold) English muffins				
Bran'nola	1 muffin	1.5	130	10%
extra-crisp	1 muffin	1.0	130	7%
raisin	1 muffin	1.0	130	7%
sourdough	1 muffin	1.0	120	8%
(Awrey's)				
muffins..1½-oz				
apple	1 muffin	7.0	140	45%
banana nut	1 muffin	9.0	170	48%
blueberry	1 muffin	7.0	140	45%
raisin bran	1 muffin	8.0	160	45%
muffins..grande..4-oz				
banana nut	1 muffin	23.0	410	50%
blueberry	1 muffin	19.0	360	48%
cheese streusel	1 muffin	20.0	400	45%
chocolate chip	1 muffin	21.0	370	51%
(Bay's) English muffins				
original	1 muffin	1.5	140	10%
sourdough	1 muffin	1.0	130	7%
(Earth Grains) English muffins				
cinnamon raisin	1 muffin	1.0	150	6%
plain	1 muffin	1.0	150	6%
sourdough..premium	1 muffin	0.5	130	3%
wheatberry	1 muffin	1.0	150	6%
whole wheat	1 muffin	2.0	170	11%
(Entenmann's)				
Carb Counting				
blueberry..breakfast	1 muffin	9.0	170	48%
Little Bites..pouches				
blueberry	1 pouch	9.0	190	43%

Food and Description	Amount	Fat Grams	Total Calories	% Fat Calories
chocolate chip	1 pouch	10.0	210	43%
(Friehofer's)..corn muffin	1 muffin	9.0	250	32%
(Hostess)				
hearty muffins				
banana nut	1 muffin	31.0	620	45%
blueberry	1 muffin	28.0	590	43%
chocolate chip	1 muffin	29.0	620	42%
cranberry orange	1 muffin	28.0	590	43%
mini muffin				
banana walnut	3 muffins	9.0	160	51%
blueberry	3 muffins	8.0	150	48%
chocolate chip	3 muffins	8.0	160	45%
cinnamon apple	3 muffins	9.0	160	45%
muffin loaf				
apple spice	1 loaf	18.0	430	38%
banana nut	1 loaf	20.0	460	39%
blueberry	1 loaf	19.0	440	39%
chocolate chip	1 loaf	17.0	400	38%
raspberry	1 loaf	19.0	440	39%
oat bran..large muffin	1 muffin	8.0	160	45%
(Oroweat) Master's Best English				
blueberry	1 muffin	1.0	170	5%
cinnamon raisin	1 muffin	1.0	170	5%
extra-crisp	1 muffin	1.0	140	6%
health nut raisin	1 muffin	3.0	170	16%
oat bran	1 muffin	1.0	150	6%
oat nut raisin	1 muffin	2.0	160	11%
raisins, dates & pecans	1 muffin	3.0	200	14%
sourdough	1 muffin	1.0	140	6%
winter wheat	1 muffin	8.0	220	33%
(Otis Spunkmeyer)				
LOW-FAT.. 4-oz muffins				
apple cinnamon	½ muffin	3.0	190	14%
banana nut	½ muffin	3.0	180	15%
chocolate chocolate chip	½ muffin	3.0	190	14%
wild blueberry	½ muffin	3.0	180	15%
LOW-FAT..2.25-oz muffins				
apple cinnamon	1 muffin	3.5	210	15%
banana nut	1 muffin	3.5	200	16%
chocolate chocolate chip	1 muffin	3.5	210	15%
wild blueberry	1 muffin	3.5	200	16%
REGULAR..2-oz muffins				
banana	1 muffin	11.0	220	45%
orange	1 muffin	11.0	220	45%
REGULAR..2.25-oz muffins				
apple cinnamon	1 muffin	13.0	240	49%
banana nut	1 muffin	14.0	270	47%
chocolate chocolate chip	1 muffin	13.0	260	45%
corn	1 muffin	14.0	250	50%
harvest bran	1 muffin	10.0	230	39%

Food and Description	Amount	Fat Grams	Total Calories	% Fat Calories
wild blueberry	1 muffin	13.0	230	51%
REGULAR..4-oz muffins				
almond poppyseed	½ muffin	12.0	210	51%
apple cinnamon	½ muffin	11.0	220	45%
banana nut	½ muffin	12.0	240	45%
blueberry	½ muffin	11.0	210	47%
cheese streusel	½ muffin	10.0	220	41%
chocolate chip	½ muffin	13.0	240	49%
chocolate chocolate chip	½ muffin	12.0	230	47%
corn	½ muffin	13.0	230	51%
cranberry orange	½ muffin	12.0	210	51%
harvest bran	½ muffin	9.0	200	9%
lemon	½ muffin	13.0	230	51%
orange	½ muffin	13.0	230	51%
pumpkin walnut	½ muffin	13.0	220	53%
raspberry cheese streusel	½ muffin	8.0	190	38%
triple berry	½ muffin	11.0	210	47%
SPECIAL CAFÉ COLLECTION..6.5 oz				
banana walnut	½ muffin	20.0	380	47%
chocolate chocolate chip	½ muffin	19.0	360	48%
wild blueberry	½ muffin	17.0	330	46%
(Pepperidge Farm) English				
cinnamon raisin	1 muffin	1.0	140	6%
plain	1 muffin	1.0	140	6%
sourdough	1 muffin	1.0	130	7%
(Perkins restaurant)				
apple	1 muffin	23.0	550	38%
banana nut	1 muffin	32.5	650	45%
blueberry	1 muffin	16.0	550	26%
carrot	1 muffin	26.0	455	51%
chocolate chip	1 muffin	26.0	620	38%
cranberry nut	1 muffin	29.0	585	45%
oat bran	1 muffin	15.0	455	30%
lemon poppyseed	1 muffin	33.0	685	43%
peaches & cream	1 muffin	23.0	520	40%
pumpkin	1 muffin	26.0	550	43%
raspberry & cream	1 muffin	26.0	585	40%
(Sara Lee)				
INDIVIDUALLY WRAPPED..2.0 oz				
banana nut	1 muffin	7.0	190	33%
blueberry	1 muffin	6.0	170	32%
bran	1 muffin	9.0	190	43%
cheese streusel	1 muffin	11.0	220	45%
INDIVIDUALLY WRAPPED..4.75 oz				
banana nut	1 muffin	17.0	480	32%
blueberry	1 muffin	14.0	440	29%
bran	1 muffin	21.0	470	40%
carrot nut	1 muffin	21.0	480	39%
cheese streusel	1 muffin	25.0	500	45%
chocolate chip cookie	1 muffin	25.0	550	41%

Food and Description	Amount	Fat Grams	Total Calories	% Fat Calories
chocolate chunk	1 muffin	18.0	470	34%
cinnamon pecan coffeecake	1 muffin	27.0	560	43%
corn	1 muffin	24.0	510	42%
(Thomas') English muffins				
CARB CONSIDER				
original	1 muffin	1.5	100	14%
REGULAR				
cinnamon raisin	1 muffin	1.0	140	6%
hearty grains				
honey wheat	1 muffin	0.5	130	3%
oat bran	1 muffin	1.0	130	7%
whole wheat..100%	1 muffin	1.0	120	8%
honey wheat	1 muffin	0.5	130	3%
multigrain				
light	1 muffin	2.0	200	9%
regular-size	1 muffin	1.5	140	10%
super-size	1 muffin	2.0	230	8%
oat bran	1 muffin	1.0	130	7%
original				
regular-size	1 muffin	1.0	120	8%
super-size	1 muffin	2.0	190	9%
sourdough	1 muffin	1.0	120	8%
toasting bread..original muffin	1 slice	1.0	90	10%
Toast R cakes..corn muffins	1 muffin	3.5	110	29%
(Wenchell's)				
banana nut	1 muffin	28.0	535	47%
blueberry	1 muffin	25.0	442	51%
low-fat	1 muffin	3.0	410	7%
bran	1 muffin	20.0	425	42%
low-fat	1 muffin	3.0	405	7%
cheese	1 muffin	25.0	520	43%
chocolate chip	1 muffin	22.0	480	41%
(Wolferman's)				
CAKE MUFFINS..5-oz				
almond poppyseed	1 muffin	33.0	590	50%
apple cinnamon	1 muffin	30.0	570	47%
cherry cream cheese	1 muffin	30.0	570	47%
chocolate caramel pecan	1 muffin	31.0	570	49%
ENGLISH MUFFINS..miniature				
1910 original recipe	2 muffins	0.5	130	3%
cinnamon raisin	2 muffins	0.5	125	4%
cranberry citrus	2 muffins	0.5	140	3%
San Francisco sourdough	2 muffins	–	110	–
SIGNATURE..English muffins				
1910 original recipe	1 muffin	0.5	230	2%
apple orchard	1 muffin	3.5	260	12%
cinnamon & raisin	1 muffin	1.0	260	3%
cranberry citrus	1 muffin	0.5	250	2%
honey & oats	1 muffin	1.5	260	5%
mixed berry	1 muffin	0.5	250	2%

Food and Description	Amount	Fat Grams	Total Calories	% Fat Calories
multigrain & honey	1 muffin	1.0	240	4%
natural cheese	1 muffin	2.5	250	9%
pumpkin spice	1 muffin	1.0	250	4%
San Francisco sourdough	1 muffin	0.5	230	2%
smoked onion & garlic	1 muffin	0.5	220	2%
wild Maine blueberry	1 muffin	1.0	250	4%
MULBERRY/fresh	1 cup	0.6	61	8%
MULLET/striped				
cooked—dry heat	3 oz	4.0	127	28%
raw	3 oz	3.0	99	27%
MUNG BEAN				
dried/generic				
boiled	6 oz	–	107	–
raw	½ cup	1.0	361	3%
sprouted				
canned	½ cup	–	8	–
cooked	½ cup	–	13	–
raw	½ cup	–	16	–
MUNGO BEAN				
boiled	½ cup	–	95	–
raw	½ cup	2.0	365	5%
MUSHROOM				
CANNED OR JARRED				
(3 Diamonds)				
stems & pieces...4 oz	1 can	–	28	–
(BinB) broiled in butter				
pieces & stems	1 can	–	30	–
sliced	1 can	1.5	40	34%
sliced w/garlic	1 can	1.5	40	34%
whole	1 can	1.5	40	34%
(Cara Mia)				
marinated	1 oz	1.0	15	60%
seasoned/whole	1 oz	–	10	–
(Empress)				
button				
all types	2 oz	–	14	–
straw/broken	2 oz	–	10	–
(Geisha)..pieces & stems..4 oz	1 can	–	30	–
(Green Giant)..white				
mushrooms & garlic	½ cup	–	25	–
pieces & stems	½ cup	–	30	–
sliced	1 can	1.5	40	34%
whole	1 can	1.5	40	34%
(Libby's)..all types	? cup	–	25	–
(Seneca)				
shiitake	½ cup	–	25	–
white				
marinated				
food service	1 oz	0.5	15	30%
retail	1 oz	9.0	90	90%
pickled	1 oz	–	5	–

Food and Description	Amount	Fat Grams	Total Calories	% Fat Calories
DRIED				
(Frieda's)				
chanterelle	2 pieces	–	15	–
morel	3 pieces	–	15	–
oyster	3 pieces	–	15	–
padi straw	6 pieces	–	15	–
porcini	5 pieces	–	15	–
portabello	7 pieces	–	–	–
shiitake	¼ cup	–	10	–
FRESH				
enoki..raw	~1 oz	–	10	–
oyster..raw	2 oz	–	14	–
shiitake..cooked	4 oz	–	40	
white				
boiled	½ cup	–	21	–
fried or sautéed in butter	10 small	10.0	100	90%
raw				
pieces	½ cup	–	10	–
whole	1 medium	–	5	–
FROZEN				
(Nancy's) mushroom turnovers	12 pieces	31.0	490	57%

MUSHROOM DISH (*See* FROZEN ENTRÉE/DINNER; VEGETABLES, MIXED; individual FAST FOOD listings)
MUSHROOM SOUP (*See* SOUP)
MUSKELLUNGE/NORTH AMERICAN PIKE

Food and Description	Amount	Fat Grams	Total Calories	% Fat Calories
raw	3 oz	2.0	93	19%

MUSKMELON (*See* CANTALOUPE/MUSKMELON)
MUSKRAT

Food and Description	Amount	Fat Grams	Total Calories	% Fat Calories
roasted	3 oz	10.0	200	45%
roasted/diced	1 cup	13.0	260	45%

MUSSEL
CANNED

Food and Description	Amount	Fat Grams	Total Calories	% Fat Calories
(Reese)..in red sauce..drained	4 oz	5.0	120	38%
FRESH..blue				
cooked—moist heat	3 oz	3.8	147	23%
raw	3 oz	1.9	73	23%
	1 cup	3.0	129	21%

MUSTARD
DRY

Food and Description	Amount	Fat Grams	Total Calories	% Fat Calories
	1 tsp	<1.0	12	38%
PREPARED				
(Best Foods)				
Dijonnaise	1 tsp	–	5	–
honey	1 tsp	–	10	–
(Crystal)				
spicy brown	1 tsp	–	–	–
squeeze bottle	1 tsp	–	–	–
(Grey Poupon)..all types	1 tsp	–	6	–
(Gulden's)..all types	1 tsp	–	5	–
(Hain)..stone-ground..all types	1 Tbs	1.0	14	64%

Food and Description	Amount	Fat Grams	Total Calories	% Fat Calories
(Hebrew National)..deli mustard				
original	1 Tbs	–	4	–
w/horseradish	1 Tbs	–	4	–
(Heinz)				
mild yellow	1 Tbs	–	8	–
spicy brown	1 Tbs	1.0	14	64%
(Hellmann's)				
deli mustard	1 tsp	–	–	–
Dijonnaise	1 tsp	–	5	–
honey mustard	1 tsp	–	10	–
yellow mustard	1 tsp	–	–	–
(Jack Daniel's)..all types	1 tsp	–	5	–
(Koop's)				
Arizona heat	1 tsp	–	10	–
deli spicy brown	1 tsp	–	–	–
Dijon	1 tsp	–	–	–
honey	1 tsp	–	–	–
horseradish	1 tsp	–	–	–
(Kraft)..mustard				
horseradish	1 tsp	–	–	–
prepared	1 tsp	–	–	–
(Luzianne)..Creole mustard	1 Tbs	–	10	–
other mustards				
Chicago fire..spiked				
w/Tabasco	1 tsp	–	5	–
chili dog..squeeze	1 tsp	–	5	–
Dijon				
w/California chardonnay	1 tsp	–	5	–
honey Dijon..w/SueBee				
honey...squeeze	1 tsp	–	10	–
mild yellow..squeeze	1 tsp	–	–	–
natural stone-ground	1 tsp	–	5	–
spicy horseradish	1 tsp	–	–	–
spicy peppa..w/Louisiana				
pepper sauce..squeeze	1 tsp	–	5	–
(Plochman's)				
Celebrations..all types	1 tsp	–	5	–
(Westbrae)				
Asian-style	1 tsp	–	5	–
Dijon-style	1 tsp	–	–	–
organic..all types	1 tsp	–	5	–
(Zatarain's)..Creole	1 tsp	–	–	–
MUSTARD GREENS				
CANNED				
(Glory Foods)				
seasoned	½ cup	0.5	50	9%
(The Allens)				
seasoned Southern-style	½ cup	0.5	45	10%
w/turnips..Southern-style	½ cup	0.5	45	10%

Food and Description	Amount	Fat Grams	Total Calories	% Fat Calories
FRESH				
boiled..drained	½ cup	–	15	–
(Glory)..raw..bag	2 cups	–	20	–
FROZEN...(Birds Eye)	1 cup	–	30	–
MUSTARD SAUCE (*See* SAUCE)				
MUSTARD SEED				
yellow..whole	1 tsp	1.0	15	60%
MUSTARD SPINACH				
fresh..boiled/drained	½ cup	–	14	–
raw..chopped	½ cup	–	17	–

N

Food and Description	Amount	Fat Grams	Total Calories	% Fat Calories
NACHOS (*See* MEXICAN FOOD)				
NAPOLEON (*See* PASTRY)				
NATAL PLUM (*See* CARISSA/NATAL PLUM)				
NATTO	½ cup	9.7	187	47%
NAVY BEAN				
CANNED				
(Bush's Best)	½ cup	–	110	–
(Eden Foods)..organic	½ cup	0.5	110	4%
(Luck's)..seasoned w/pork	½ cup	4.0	140	26%
(Trappey's)..seasoned				
w/slab bacon	½ cup	1.5	110	12%
w/slab bacon & jalapeño	½ cup	1.5	110	12%
DRIED				
(Haagen)	½ cup	–	80	–
SPROUTED..raw	½ cup	–	35	–
NAVY BEAN SOUP (*See* SOUP)				
NECTARINE/fresh				
sliced	1 cup	1.0	70	13%
whole	1 medium	1.0	70	13%
NEUFCHÂTEL CHEESE (*See* CHEESE; CHEESE SPREAD)				
NONDAIRY FROZEN DESSERT (*See* ICE CREAM & ICE CREAM–LIKE FROZEN DESSERTS; ICE CREAM BARS, SANDWICHES & FROZEN NOVELTIES; RICE FROZEN DESSERT; SHERBET; TOFU FROZEN DESSERT)				
NOODLE (*See* ASIAN FOOD; PASTA)				
NORI (*See* SEAWEED)				

Food and Description	Amount	Fat Grams	Total Calories	% Fat Calories
NUTMEG/ground	1 tsp	0.8	11	66%
NUTRITION BAR (*See* GRANOLA/GRANOLA-TYPE BAR)				
NUTRITIONAL LIQUID SUPPLEMENT (*See also* BREAKFAST DRINK; SPORTS DRINK)				
(Atkins)..Advantage shakes				
café au lait	11 oz	9.0	170	48%
Chocolate Delight	11 0z	9.0	170	48%
Chocolate Royale	11 0z	9.0	170	48%
Creamy Vanilla	11 0z	9.0	170	48%
Strawberry Supreme	11 oz	9.0	170	48%
(Boost)				
Boost Plus				
chocolate	8 fl oz	14.0	360	35%
strawberry	8 fl oz	14.0	360	35%
vanilla	8 fl oz	14.0	360	35%
Boost..w/fiber				
chocolate	8 fl oz	4.0	240	15%
vanilla	8 fl oz	4.0	240	15%
Breeze				
mixed berry	8 fl oz	–	160	–
tropical fruit	8 fl oz	–	160	–
Drink..high-protein..all flavors	8 fl oz	4.0	240	15%
Drink..protein..all flavors	8 fl oz	4.0	240	15%
(Carb Solutions)				
high-protein drink				
creamy vanilla	11 oz	5.0	100	45%
rich chocolate	11 oz	5.0	110	41%
(Ensure)				
Enlive!..Clear Liquid Nutrition				
apple	8 oz	–	300	–
peach	8 oz	–	300	–
Ensure..balanced nutrition..lactose-free				
all flavors	8 oz	6.0	250	22%
Ensure..fiber w/FOS				
all flavors	8 oz	6.0	250	22%
Ensure..high-calcium				
all flavors	8 oz	6.0	225	24%
Ensure..high-protein				
all flavors	8 oz	6.0	230	23%
Ensure..light				
all flavors	8 oz	3.0	200	14%
Ensure..plus				
all flavors	8 oz	11.0	360	32%
(Odwalla)				
Future Shakes				
Dutch chocolate	8 oz	3.0	160	17%
vanilla al'mondo	8 oz	6.0	190	28%
Nutritionals..juices				
C Monster	8 oz	1.0	150	6%

Food and Description	Amount	Fat Grams	Total Calories	% Fat Calories
Mo'Beta	8 oz	–	140	–
Strawberry C Monster	8 oz	0.5	150	3%
Super Protein 2001/02	8 oz	1.0	170	5%
Superfood	8 oz	1.0	140	6%
Wellness	8 oz	1.0	150	3%
(Powerade)..energy drink				
Liquid Hydration+				
Arctic Shatter	8 oz	–	70	–
black cherry lime	8 oz	–	60	–
fruit punch	8 oz	–	60	–
Green Squall	8 Oz	–	70	–
Jagged Ice	8 oz	–	60	–
lemon lime	8 oz	–	60	–
Mountain Blast	8 oz	–	60	–
orange	8 oz	–	70	–
(Resource)				
health shake..frozen..ready-to-serve				
chocolate	4 oz	4.0	200	18%
	6 oz	6.0	300	18%
strawberry	4 oz	4.0	200	18%
	6 oz	6.0	300	18%
vanilla	4 oz	4.0	200	18%
	6 oz	6.0	300	18%
health shake..no sugar added				
chocolate	4 oz	9.0	200	41%
	6 oz	13.0	300	39%
strawberry	4 oz	9.0	200	41%
	6 oz	13.0	300	39%
vanilla	4 oz	9.0	200	41%
	6 oz	13.0	300	39%
juice drink..nutritious				
all flavors	6 oz	–	210	–
Resource Shake..lactose-free				
strawberry	6 oz	6.0	270	20%
vanilla	6 oz	6.0	270	20%
Resource Shake..frozen				
ready-to-serve..nutrient-dense				
all flavors	8 oz	16.0	480	30%
Wound-Healing Promotion				
Resource..all flavors	8 fl oz	21.0	475	40%
(Ross) (See (Ensure) within this section)				
(Slim-Fast)				
HEALTHY..ready-to-drink meal				
apple cranberry raspberry	11 oz	1.0	220	4%
banana cream	11 oz	2.5	220	10%
Cappuccino Delight	11 oz	1.0	220	4%
chocolate royale..rich	11 oz	3.0	220	12%
chocolate soy..lactose-free	11 oz	3.0	220	12%
creamy chocolate	11 oz	3.0	220	12%
dark chocolate fudge	11 oz	3.0	220	12%

Food and Description	Amount	Fat Grams	Total Calories	% Fat Calories
French vanilla	11 oz	2.5	220	10%
golden apple	11 oz	1.5	220	6%
milk chocolate	11 oz	3.0	220	12%
orange cream	11 oz	3.0	220	12%
orange pineapple..w/soy protein	11 oz	1.0	220	4%
orange strawberry banana w/soy protein	11 oz	1.0	220	4%
strawberries 'n' cream	11 oz	2.5	220	10%
vanilla..w/soy..lactose-free	11 oz	3.0	220	12%
LOW-CARB..Ready-to-drink meal				
all flavors	11 oz	9.0	190	43%
SLIM-FAST OPTIMA..Ready-to-drink meal				
all flavors	11 oz	5.0	180	25%
NUTS (*See* NUTS, FORMULATED; NUTS, MIXED; individual listings)				
NUTS, FORMULATED/wheat-based				
macadamia-flavored	1 oz	16.0	176	82%
other flavors	1 oz	18.0	184	88%
unflavored	1 oz	16.0	177	81%
NUTS, MIXED (*See also* individual nut listings)				
(Ann's House of Nuts)				
mixed nuts deluxe, no peanuts				
salted	1 oz	16.0	170	85%
unsalted	1 oz	16.0	170	85%
(Fisher)				
Fisher Chef's Naturals..nut topping	1 oz	14.0	170	74%
Fisher Deluxe..mixed..no peanuts	1 oz	17.0	170	90%
glazed nut mix & cashews				
praline	1 oz	12.0	170	64%
toffee	1 oz	11.0	160	62%
Gourmet Select..imperial				
mixed nuts	1 oz	16.0	180	80%
Holiday Selections..deluxe mixed				
premium whole cashews	1 oz	16.0	170	85%
Holiday Selections..mixed w/cashews	1 oz	16.0	170	85%
Nature's nut mix	1 oz	12.0	160	68%
Nuts & Crunches				
Bayou Blend..spicy sweet	1 oz	10.0	150	60%
Fiesta	1 oz	7.0	140	45%
golden crisp	1 oz	7.0	140	45%
honey crunch	1 oz	6.0	140	39%
Nuts & Fruits snack mix				
California-style	1 oz	8.0	140	51%
Pineapple..banana	1 oz	8.0	140	51%
raisin..cranberry	1 oz	9.0	150	54%
trail-style	1 oz	11.0	150	66%
Nuts & Seeds				
less than 50% peanuts	1 oz	15.0	170	90%
Snack 'n' Serve nut bowl				
mixed deluxe..w/no peanuts	1 oz	16.0	180	80%

Food and Description	Amount	Fat Grams	Total Calories	% Fat Calories
nuts & seeds..less than 50%				
peanuts	1 oz	16.0	180	80%
(Kettle) Roaster Fresh mixed nuts				
camping mix	1 oz	10.0	140	64%
Chocolate Lover's				
natural	1 oz	6.0	120	45%
regular	1 oz	7.0	130	48%
deluxe nut				
no salt	1 oz	16.0	170	85%
w/salt	1 oz	16.0	170	85%
honey cranberry	1 oz	6.0	120	45%
honey roast				
Harvest	1 oz	7.0	130	48%
nuts & fruit	1 oz	6.0	120	45%
plain	1 oz	13.0	160	73%
organic sunrise..soy & mango	1 oz	6.0	120	45%
Raw Hikers	1 oz	6.0	120	45%
Southwest BBQ	1 oz	10.0	150	60%
Sporting	1 Oz	11.0	150	66%
Truffle Trail	1 oz	6.0	120	45%
X-Treme Trail	1 oz	12.0	150	72%
(Planters)..mixed				
deluxe	1 oz	16.0	170	85%
lightly salted	1 oz	16.0	170	85%
Holiday Collection..mixed				
w/fancy cashews	1 oz	14.0	170	74%
honey-roasted	1 oz	13.0	160	73%
lightly salted..mixed	1 oz	15.0	170	79%
macadamia..cashew mix				
w/almonds	23 pieces	17.0	180	85%
nuts in milk chocolate..mixed	1.4 oz	15.0	220	61%
unsalted..mixed	1 oz	15.0	170	79%

O

Food and Description	Amount	Fat Grams	Total Calories	% Fat Calories
OAT BRAN (See BRAN; CEREAL)				
OATS (See also CEREAL; FLOUR)				
(Arrowhead Mills)				
groats	¼ cup	3.0	160	17%
rolled flakes	⅓ cup	2.5	130	17%

Food and Description	Amount	Fat Grams	Total Calories	% Fat Calories
steel-cut	¼ cup	3.0	170	16%
whole-grain	1 oz	2.0	110	16%
	1 cup	10.8	607	16%
OCEAN PERCH (*See also* FROZEN ENTRÉE/DINNER; SEAFOOD ENTRÉE/DINNER)				
Atlantic				
breaded & fried	3 oz	11.0	185	54%
cooked—dry heat	3 oz	1.8	103	16%
raw	3 oz	1.0	80	11%
OCTOPUS				
CANNED				
(Goya)..spiced	¼ cup	9.0	140	58%
(Reese)	¼ cup	8.0	120	60%
cooked—moist heat	3 oz	2.0	140	13%
raw	3 oz	0.9	70	11%
OIL (*See also* ASIAN FOOD; COOKING SPRAY)				
FLAVORED				
(House of Tsang)				
hot chili sesame	1 tsp	5.0	45	100%
Mongolian Fire Oil	1 tsp	5.0	45	100%
pure sesame	1 tsp	5.0	45	100%
Singapore Curry	1 tsp	5.0	45	100%
Wok	1 Tbs	14.0	130	100%
PLAIN				
all 100% vegetable & fish oils	1 tsp	5.0	45	100%
	1 Tbs	14.0	120	100%
	1 cup	218.0	1927	100%
(Smucker's)				
Baking Healthy Oil & Shortening				
oil-replacement for baking	1 Tbs	–	30	–

(NOTE: We all need to watch even our use of "healthier" (less saturated) oils in order to keep our total fat intake within acceptable boundaries. Because it is so important to select the least saturated oil that fits your needs, I have listed the most commonly used oils below, showing the percentages of saturated fat, polyunsaturated fat, and monounsaturated fat in each. Those that contain less saturated fat are listed first. Data are based on information from *USDA Nutritive Value of American Foods in Common Units, 1988.* REMEMBER—NO VEGETABLE OIL CONTAINS CHOLESTEROL!)

Vegetable Oils	% Saturated	% Unsaturated	
		% Poly	% Mono
canola	7%	35%	58%
almond	8%	19%	73%
safflower	9%	78%	13%
sunflower	11%	69%	20%
corn	13%	62%	25%
olive	14%	12%	74%
sesame	15%	43%	42%
soybean	15%	43%	42%
peanut	18%	33%	49%
soybean/cottonseed blend	19%	50%	31%

Vegetable Oils	% Saturated	% Unsaturated	
		% Poly	% Mono
wheat germ	20%	50%	31%
shortening (vegetable)	27%	26%	47%
cottonseed	27%	55%	18%
palm	52%	10%	38%
cocoa butter	62%	3%	35%
palm kernel	87%	2%	11%
coconut	92%	2%	6%

Food and Description	Amount	Fat Grams	Total Calories	% Fat Calories
OKRA (*See also* VEGETABLES, MIXED)				
CANNED..JARRED				
(Best Maid)				
pickled				
hot	1 oz	–	10	–
mild	1 oz	–	10	–
(Mt. Olive)				
pickled..all types, hot	1.5 oz	–	15	–
(Trappey's)				
Creole gumbo	½ cup	–	35	–
cut	½ cup	–	25	–
w/tomatoes	½ cup	–	30	–
w/tomatoes & corn	½ cup	–	30	–
FRESH				
boiled	½ cup	–	25	–
raw	½ cup	–	19	–
FROZEN				
(McKenzie's)				
breaded	2.66 oz	0.5	90	5%
cut	3.2 oz	–	25	–
(Veg-All)				
cut	½ cup	–	25	–
whole	½ cup	–	30	–
OLIVE				
(Alma) black/Greek	2 large	3.0	30	90%
(Angonoa)				
green	2 Tbs	2.5	30	75%
sliced ripe	2 Tbs	2.5	30	75%
(Black Pearls)..ripe				
chopped	½ oz	2.0	25	72%
colossal..pitted	½ oz	1.5	20	68%
extra-large..pitted	½ oz	2.0	25	72%
large..pitted	½ oz	2.0	25	72%
medium..pitted	½ oz	–	15	–
jalapeño slice	½ oz	2.0	25	72%
jumbo..pitted	½ oz	1.5	20	68%
jumbo..whole	½ oz	2.0	25	72%
sliced	½ oz	2.0	25	72%
small..pitted	½ oz	2.0	25	72%
Spanish salad olives	½ oz	2.5	25	90%

Food and Description	Amount	Fat Grams	Total Calories	% Fat Calories
(Burgundy Pearls)..pitted				
classic Italian	½ oz	–	25	–
roasted pepper	½ oz	–	25	–
(Early California)..pitted..ripe				
most all types	½ oz	2.5	25	90%
other types				
colossal	½ oz	2.0	20	90%
Spanish..queen	½ oz	1.5	20	68%
(Green Pearls)				
jumbo whole Sicilian-style	½ oz	1.5	20	68%
Manzanilla pimiento..sliced	½ oz	2.0	25	72%
Manzanilla pimiento..stuffed	½ oz	2.0	25	72%
queen pimiento..stuffed	½ oz	1.5	20	68%
queen..whole	½ oz	1.5	20	68%
super colossal..Sicilian-style				
whole	½ oz	1.5	20	68%
zesty sliced..Sicilian-style	½ oz	1.5	20	68%
(Krinos)				
Greek..black	2 olives	3.0	35	77%
kalamata	3 olives	4.0	45	80%
(Lindsay)..ripe				
chopped	½ oz	2.5	25	90%
extra-large..pitted	½ oz	2.5	25	90%
jumbo..pitted	½ oz	2.0	25	72%
large..pitted	½ oz	2.5	25	90%
manzanilla..pimiento-stuffed	½ oz	2.5	25	90%
queen..pimiento-stuffed	½ oz	1.5	15	90%
select..green medium..pitted	½ oz	2.5	25	90%
sliced	½ oz	2.5	25	90%
sliced..pimiento	½ oz	2.5	25	90%
small..pitted	½ oz	2.5	25	90%
spread..Olivada				
Taste of Greece	1 oz	6.0	60	90%
Taste of Sicily	1 oz	5.0	60	75%
Taste of Tuscany	1 oz	4.0	45	80%
(Peloponnese)..naturally brine-cured				
Amfissa	½ oz	4.0	40	90%
cracked	½ oz	2.0	20	90%
gourmet black olives	½ oz	4.0	40	90%
Ionian	½ oz	2.5	25	90%
kalamata	½ oz	4.0	40	90%
mixed	½ oz	4.0	40	90%
(Santa Barbara Olive Co.)				
Cajun	0.5 oz	1.5	15	90%
California black	0.5 oz	1.5	15	90%
country	0.5 oz	2.0	25	72%
garlic	0.5 oz	1.5	15	90%
pitted	0.5 oz	2.0	25	72%
stuffed	0.5 oz	1.5	15	90%
Italian/pitted	0.5 oz	1.5	15	90%
jalapeño	0.5 oz	1.5	15	90%

Food and Description	Amount	Fat Grams	Total Calories	% Fat Calories
pimiento-stuffed martini	0.5 oz	1.5	15	90%
(Star) Spanish olives				
Manzanillas	½ oz	1.0	15	60%
queens	½ oz	1.0	15	60%

OLIVE LOAF (See LUNCHEON MEAT)
OLIVE OIL (See OIL)
OMELET (See EGG DISH/MEAL)
ONION (See also SCALLION/GREEN ONION/SPRING ONION; VEGETABLES, MIXED)
CANNED or JARRED

(Aunt Nellie's)..whole Holland-style	~ 4 oz	–	40	–
(B&G)..pearl cocktail	1 Tbs	–	<5	–
(Crosse & Blackwell) cocktail	1 Tbs	–	5	–
(Durkee) French-fried	1 oz	15.0	175	77%
(Heinz) sweet	1 oz	–	40	–
(S&W)				
small..whole	½ cup	–	40	–
tiny..whole	½ cup	–	40	–
(Vlasic) cocktail				
lightly spiced	1 oz	–	4	–
plain	1 oz	–	4	–

DRIED

flakes	1 Tbs	–	16	–
powder/ground	1 tsp	–	7	–
	1 Tbs	–	23	–

FRESH..all types..mature

cooked	1 cup	–	60	–
raw				
chopped	1 Tbs	–	4	–
	½ cup	–	20	–
(Frieda's)..baby Hawaiian whole	⅓ cup	–	10	–
(Bland Farms)				
Peruvian sweet	1 medium	–	60	–
Texas 1015	1 medium	–	60	–
Vidalia sweet	1 medium	–	60	–

FROZEN

(Birds Eye)				
small..whole	½ cup	–	30	–
Southern vegetables..diced onions	⅔ cup	–	30	–
(C&W) petite..whole	⅔ cup	–	30	–

ONION, GREEN OR SPRING (See SCALLION/GREEN ONION/SPRING ONION)
ONION DISH (See also FROZEN ENTRÉE/DINNER; VEGETABLES, MIXED; VEGETARIAN FOODS)
FROZEN

(Birds Eye)				
vegetables w/sauce..pearl onions in real cream sauce	½ cup	2.0	60	30%
(Bland Farms) Vidalia O's	6 rings	7.0	180	35%
(Mrs. Paul's) onion rings	7 rings	10.0	200	45%
(Ore-Ida)				
chopped onions..fresh/frozen	2.66 oz	–	20	–

Food and Description	Amount	Fat Grams	Total Calories	% Fat Calories
gourmet onion rings	4 pieces	10.0	210	43%
Onion Ringers	6 rings	12.0	220	49%
ONION POWDER	1 tsp	–	7	–

ONION RINGS (See ONION DISH; individual FAST FOOD listings)
ONION SOUP (See SOUP)
OPOSSUM

braised or roasted	3 oz	8	190	38%
roasted/diced	1 cup	14.5	310	42%

ORANGE (See also MANDARIN ORANGE)
FRESH

California				
navel				
peeled sections	1 cup	–	75	–
whole	1 medium	–	65	–
Valencia				
peeled sections	1 cup	0.5	90	5%
whole	1 medium	–	60	–
(Dole)	1 medium	–	70	–
(SunKist)				
navel	1 medium	–	80	–
Valencia	1 medium	–	80	–
Moro (blood)	1 medium	–	80	–

ORANGE JUICE/JUICE BLEND/JUICE DRINK (See also FRUIT PUNCH; SOFT DRINK; SOFT DRINK MIX; TEA)
BOTTLED..BOXED..OR CANNED

(Dole)				
orange juice				
double vitamin C	8 fl oz	–	120	–
home-style	8 fl oz	–	120	–
original	6 fl oz	–	80	–
	8 fl oz	–	120	–
plus calcium	8 fl oz	–	120	–
orange juice blend..all types	8 fl oz	–	`120	–
(Minute Maid)				
Premium OJ..all types	8 fl oz	–	110	–
(Ocean Spray)				
orange juice	8 fl oz	–	120	–
orange citrus spritzer	11.75 fl oz	–	160	–
(Odwalla)..Essentials				
juice	8 fl oz	–	110	–
juice..organic	8 fl oz	–	110	–
(R. W. Knudsen) orange juice blend				
orange mango	8 fl oz	–	120	–
(Snapple)..juice drinks				
orange..carrot..diet	8 fl oz	–	10	–
orangeade	8 fl oz	–	120	–
(SSIPS)..juice drinks				
orange-tangerine	6.75 fl oz	–	120	–
Sabor Latino orange mango	8 fl oz	–	130	–
(Sunny D)..fruit juice drink				
orange	8 fl oz	–	130	–

Food and Description	Amount	Fat Grams	Total Calories	% Fat Calories
smooth California-style	8 fl oz	–	130	–
w/calcium	8 fl oz	–	140	–
tangy original Florida-style	8 fl oz	–	120	–
(Tree Ripe)..100% pure orange juice				
Florida Premium Extra	8 fl oz	–	120	–
Premium natural..no pulp	8 fl oz	–	90	–
Premium organic..no pulp	8 fl oz	–	120	–
(Tropicana)				
orange juice..				
Essentials..Light'n Healthy	10 fl oz	–	140	–
no calcium	8 fl oz	–	70	–
Grovestand	8 fl oz	–	110	–
Healthy Heart	8 fl oz	–	110	–
home-style	14 fl oz	–	190	–
Immunity Defense				
orange plus	8 fl oz	–	110	–
low-acid	14 fl oz	–	190	–
orange..plus calcium	6 fl oz	–	80	–
	8 fl oz	–	110	–
plus calcium	14 fl oz	–	190	–
Pure Premium				
orange	6 fl oz	–	80	–
	8 fl oz	–	110	–
Sweet Valencia..no pulp	8 fl oz	–	110	–
Sweet Valencia..w/pulp	8 fl oz	–	110	—
Orange Twisters				
orange..cranberry clash	10 fl oz	–	160	–
	8 fl oz	–	130	–
orange..strawberry..				
banana burst	10 fl oz	–	160	–
	8 fl oz	–	130	–
(V8 Splash)				
juice drink..orange pineapple	8 fl oz	–	110	–
smoothie..orange crème	8 fl oz	–	130	–
(Welch's)				
orange pineapple				
juice cocktail	8 fl oz	–	180	–
orange..Welchade	8 fl oz	–	140	–
FROZEN				
(Old Orchard)..prepared..unless noted otherwise				
all types	8 fl oz	–	120	–
(Seneca)..juice concentrate..undiluted				
Awake	2 oz	–	120	–0
orange	2 oz	–	110	–
Orange Juice Plus	2 oz	–	130	–
Valencia orange	2 oz	–	110	–
(Welch's)..prepared				
orange pineapple apple				
juice cocktail	8 fl oz	–	150	–

Food and Description	Amount	Fat Grams	Total Calories	% Fat Calories
MIX				
(Tang)..breakfast drink..prepared				
orange	8 fl oz	–	90	–
orange pineapple	8 fl oz	–	100	–
ORANGE PEEL				
CANDIED				
(S&W)	58 pieces	–	80	–
FRESH	1 Tbs	–	–	–
ORANGE ROUGHY (See also SEAFOOD ENTRÉE/DINNER)				
cooked—dry heat	3 oz	1.0	80	11%
raw	3 oz	6.0	110	50%
OREGANO/ground	1 tsp	–	5	–
ORIENTAL FOOD (See ASIAN FOOD; FROZEN ENTRÉE/DINNER; PASTA ENTRÉE/DINNER; RICE DISH; VEGETARIAN FOODS; individual listings)				
OSTRICH				
(New West)..ostrich steak	4 oz	2.5	130	10%
OYSTER (See also SEAFOOD ENTRÉE/DINNER; SOUP)				
CANNED				
(3 Diamonds)				
whole..in salted water	2 oz	2.0	60	30%
(Bumble Bee)..fancy				
Orleans..smoked	2 oz	7.0	120	53%
smoked	2 oz	7.0	120	53%
whole	2 oz	3.0	70	39%
(Chicken of the Sea)				
smoked	2.3 oz	8.0	140	51%
smoked..in oil	3.75 oz	8.0	140	51%
smoked..in water	3.75 oz	3.0	120	23%
smoked..teriyaki	3.75 oz	3.0	120	23%
whole	2 oz	3.0	80	34%
(Crown Prince)..smoked in oil	¼ cup	–	60	–
(Empress)..whole	½ cup	4.0	100	36%
(Geisha)				
smoked..in cottonseed oil..fancy	~2 oz	7.0	120	53%
whole..in water	½ cup	2.5	60	38%
(Reese)..smoked	2 oz	1.0	45	50%
(S&W)				
smoked	2 oz	6.0	100	54%
whole	2 oz	3.0	70	39%
(Shurfine)..whole cove	2 oz	3.0	80	34%
FRESH				
Eastern				
battered & fried	3 oz	10.0	180	50%
	6 medium	11.0	175	57%
breaded & fried	3 oz	11.0	170	58%
	6 medium	11.0	175	57%
meat only	1 cup	4.0	160	23%
raw	6 medium	2.0	50	30%
steamed	3 oz	4.5	120	34%
	6 medium			
	~1.5 oz	2.0	60	30%

Food and Description	Amount	Fat Grams	Total Calories	% Fat Calories
Pacific/Western				
raw	3 oz	2.0	70	26%
steamed	1 medium	1.0	40	23%
	3 oz	4.0	140	26%

P

Food and Description	Amount	Fat Grams	Total Calories	% Fat Calories
PANCAKE				
FROZEN or REFRIGERATED				
(Aunt Jemima)				
blueberry	3 pancakes	3.5	210	15%
buttermilk	3 pancakes	3.5	200	16%
home-style	3 pancakes	3.5	200	16%
low-fat	3 pancakes	2.5	190	12%
mini	13 pancakes	4.0	240	15%
original	3 pancakes	3.5	210	15%
other pancakes				
Great Starts				
pancakes & sausage	1 box	21.0	380	50%
Syrup Dunk'ers	~½ box	4.0	520	7%
(Pillsbury)				
blueberry	3 pancakes	4.0	260	14%
buttermilk	3 pancakes	4.5	260	15%
mini	11 pancakes	7.0	260	24%
original				
mini	11 pancakes	4.0	230	14%
regular	3 pancakes	4.0	260	14%
(Van's) multigrain..non-dairy	2 pancakes	1.5	180	8%
MIX (Note: Unless otherwise stated, data are for dry mix only.)				
(Arrowhead Mills)				
blue corn	⅓ cup	2.0	150	12%
buckwheat	⅓ cup	1.5	140	10%
buttermilk	¼ cup	0.5	120	4%
gluten-free	¼ cup	2.0	130	14%
griddle lite	¼ cup	3.0	260	10%
kamut	¼ cup	1.0	130	7%
multigrain	¼ cup	0.5	120	4%
oat bran	¼ cup	1.5	140	10%
whole-grain	¼ cup	0.5	120	4%

Food and Description	Amount	Fat Grams	Total Calories	% Fat Calories
wild rice	¼ cup	1.0	140	6%
(Aunt Jemima)..pancake & waffle..mix only				
buckwheat	¼ cup	1.0	100	9%
buttermilk	¼ cup	0.5	110	4%
buttermilk..complete	⅓ cup	2.5	160	14%
complete	⅓ cup	2.0	160	11%
low-carbohydrate				
buttermilk complete	⅓ cup	1.0	130	7%
original	⅓ cup	0.5	150	3%
whole wheat	¼ cup	0.5	120	4%
(Betty Crocker)..prepared				
box..mixed w/water				
buttermilk	3 pancakes	2.5	200	11%
original	3 pancakes	3.0	200	14%
pouch				
complete..mixed w/water				
buttermilk	3 pancakes	4.0	210	17%
original	3 pancakes	7.0	250	25%
(Bisquick) Shake 'n' Pour pancake & waffle mix				
prepared				
blueberry	3 pancakes	3.5	210	15%
buttermilk	3 pancakes	3.0	200	14%
original	3 pancakes	4.0	210	17%
(Hungry Jack)..mix only				
pancake & waffle				
blueberry				
4-count	⅛ pkg	2.5	200	11%
buttermilk	⅓ cup	1.5	150	9%
buttermilk				
4-count	⅛ pkg	2.0	200	9%
(Hodgson Mill)..dry mix only				
buckwheat	⅓ cup	1.0	190	5%
multigrain buttermilk				
w/milled flaxseed & soy	⅓ cup	2.0	150	12%
whole wheat buttermilk	⅓ cup	1.0	120	8%
(Jiffy) buttermilk complete				
pancake & waffle mix				
prepared	2 pancakes	2.5	160	14%
(Krusteaz)..prepared				
apple spice	2 pancakes	3.5	210	15%
blueberry	3 pancakes	3.0	240	11%
buttermilk				
fat-free	3 pancakes	–	200	–
original	3 pancakes	2.5	210	54%
CARB SIMPLE..prepared				
chocolate chip	3 pancakes	4.0	220	16%
home-style	3 pancakes	4.0	230	16%
oat bran				
light	3 pancakes	1.0	140	6%
low-fat	3 pancakes	3.0	230	12%
wheat & honey	3 pancakes	1.5	220	6%

Food and Description	Amount	Fat Grams	Total Calories	% Fat Calories
(Maple Grove Farms)				
pancake & waffle..mix only				
buckwheat				
24-oz box	⅟₁₇ box	1.0	130	7%
buttermilk..w/honey				
24-oz box	⅟₁₇ box	0.5	130	3%
(Mrs. Butterworth's)..prepared				
buttermilk complete	3-4 pancakes	2.0	160	11%
(Pillsbury)				
pancake..mix only				
buttermilk	2 oz	2.5	210	11%
buttermilk..Old West	1.9 oz	3.5	200	16%
buttermilk..Select	1.9 oz	3.0	200	14%
pancake..waffle..complete				
mix only	2 oz	4.5	220	18%
(Shawnee Mills)				
pancake..mix only				
buttermilk..complete..low-fat	1.5 oz	2.5	150	15%
pancake-waffle..mix only				
buttermilk	¼ pkg	4.0	180	20%
buttermilk..low-fat	1.5 oz	3.0	160	17%
whole wheat	⅓ pkg	5.0	170	26%
(Snoqualmie Falls Lodge)				
pancake & waffle..mix only				
nutra-rich	⅟₁₅ pkg	2.0	170	11%
old-fashioned	⅟₁₅ pkg	2.0	170	11%
(White Lily)..pancake..mix only				
blueberry..w/imitation nuggets	¼ pkg	2.0	160	11%
buttermilk	¼ pkg	–	140	–
PANCAKE & WAFFLE MIX (*See also* PANCAKE under Mix)				
PANCAKE & WAFFLE SYRUP (*See also* ICE CREAM TOPPING: SYRUP)				
(Aunt Jemima)				
butter light	¼ cup	–	100	–
butter rich	¼ cup	–	210	–
country rich				
light	¼ cup	–	100	–
regular	¼ cup	–	210	–
light	¼ cup	–	100	–
low-carbohydrate	¼ cup	–	25	–
original	¼ cup	–	210	–
(Cary's)				
pure maple	2 Tbs	–	100	–
sugar-free	¼ cup	–	35	–
(Golden Griddle)				
cinnamon	¼ cup	–	240	–
light	¼ cup	–	90	–
original	¼ cup	–	220	–
(Hungry Jack)	¼ cup	–	210	–
(Karo)				
golden	2 Tbs	–	125	–
pancake	¼ cup	–	240	–

Food and Description	Amount	Fat Grams	Total Calories	% Fat Calories
(Log Cabin)				
Country Kitchen				
light	¼ cup	–	100	–
original	¼ cup	–	200	–
original				
light	¼ cup	–	100	–
regular	¼ cup	–	210	–
(Roddenbery's) NorthWoods				
butter-maple	¼ cup	–	230	–
light	¼ cup	–	100	–
original	¼ cup	–	230	–
sugar-free	¼ cup	–	100	–
(Smucker's)				
breakfast..sugar-free				
low-calorie..squeeze	¼ cup	–	30	–
PAPAW/fresh	½ lb	2.0	194	9%
PAPAYA				
CANNED or JARRED				
(Del Monte) Sun Fresh..refrigerated				
in extra-light syrup	½ cup	–	70	–
DRIED				
(Sun-Maid)..tropical trio				
pineapple..papaya..mango	1.4 oz	–	130	–
FRESH				
cubed/peeled	1 cup	–	60	–
(Dole)	½ medium	–	70	–
PAPAYA JUICE/NECTAR (*See also* FRUIT PUNCH)				
BOTTLED, BOXED, OR CANNED				
(After the Fall)				
Pele papaya..98% juice	8 fl oz	–	120	–
(Goya)	6 fl oz	–	110	–
(Kern's)	6 fl oz	–	110	–
(Knudsen)				
nectar	8 fl oz	–	140	–
(Libby's)	6 fl oz	–	110	–
	11.5 fl oz	–	210	–
(Tree Top) Island Blends				
tangerine..papaya	10 fl oz	–	140	–
PAPRIKA/ground	1 tsp	–	6	–
PARFAIT (*See* CANDY; ICE CREAM BARS, SANDWICHES & FROZEN NOVELTIES; PUDDING & MOUSSE)				
PARSLEY				
dried	1 tsp	–	1	–
freeze-dried	any amount	–	–	–
fresh	10 sprigs	–	3	–
	½ cup	–	10	–
PARSNIP/fresh				
cooked	½ cup	–	66	–
raw/sliced	½ cup	–	50	–

Food and Description	Amount	Fat Grams	Total Calories	% Fat Calories
PASSION FRUIT/GRANADILLA				
fresh	1 medium	–	18	–
	½ lb	–	106	–
(Frieda's)	5 oz	–	140	–
PASSIONFRUIT JUICE/JUICE BLEND (*See also* FRUIT PUNCH)				
FRESH				
purple	1 cup	–	126	–
yellow	1 cup	–	149	–
FROZEN				
(Welch's) passionfruit	8 fl oz	–	140	–
PASTA (*See also* COUSCOUS)				
(Adrienne's) gourmet/wheat-free & gluten-free				
Papadini Hi-Protein pure lentil bean pasta				
cavatappi	2 oz	1.0	190	5%
conchigliette	2 oz	1.0	190	5%
orzo	2 oz	1.0	190	5%
penne	2 oz	1.0	190	5%
rotini	2 oz	1.0	190	5%
shipper	2 oz	1.0	190	5%
(American Beauty) dry				
angel hair	2 oz	1.0	210	4%
capellini	2 oz	1.0	210	4%
curly roni	2 oz	1.0	210	4%
egg noodles..all shapes	2 oz	2.5	210	11%
elbow roni	2 oz	1.0	210	4%
fettuccini..egg	2 oz	1.0	210	11%
fettuccini..Florentine	2 oz	1.0	210	11%
lasagna	2 oz	1.0	210	4%
enriched	2 oz	1.0	210	4%
oven-ready	2 oz	1.0	200	5%
manicotti	2 oz	1.0	210	4%
mostaccioli	2 oz	1.0	210	4%
penne rigate	2 oz	1.0	210	4%
rainbow shells...twirls	2 oz	1.0	210	4%
rigatoni..enriched	2 oz	1.0	210	4%
roni mac	2 oz	1.0	210	4%
rotelle	2 oz	1.0	210	4%
rotini..enriched	2 oz	1.0	210	4%
sea shells	2 oz	1.0	210	4%
shells..medium	2 oz	1.0	210	4%
shell roni..all shapes	2 oz	1.0	210	4%
Soups 'n' Sides				
Acini de pepe	2 oz	1.0	210	4%
orzo	2 oz	1.0	210	4%
spaghetti..all types	2 oz	1.0	210	4%
trio Italiano..rotini mostaccioli	2 oz	1.0	210	4%
vermicelli	2 oz	1.0	210	4%
vermicelli fideo..enriched	2 oz	0.5	200	2%

Food and Description	Amount	Fat Grams	Total Calories	% Fat Calories
(Amish Kitchens)..egg noodles	2 oz	4.0	220	16%
(Azumaya)..cooked				
pasta ..soy				
large square wrappers	8 wraps	0.5	160	3%
round	10 wraps	0.5	160	3%
spinach pasta	1 cup	0.5	210	2%
thin-cut noodles	1 cup	0.5	210	2%
(Barilla)				
angel hair	2 oz	1.0	200	5%
egg	2 oz	2.0	210	9%
campanelle	2 oz	1.0	200	5%
castellane	2 oz	1.0	200	5%
cellentani	2 oz	1.0	200	5%
ditalini	2 oz	1.0	200	5%
egg noodles				
extra-wide	2 oz	2.0	210	9%
wide	2 oz	2.0	210	9%
elbows	2 oz	1.0	200	5%
farfalle	2 oz	1.0	200	5%
fettuccini	2 oz	1.0	200	5%
gemelli	2 oz	1.0	200	5%
lasagna..oven-ready	~2 oz	2.0	190	10%
linguine..all types	2 oz	1.0	200	5%
manicotti	~2 oz	1.0	180	5%
mostaccioli	2 oz	1.0	200	5%
orzo	2 oz	1.0	200	5%
penne	2 oz	1.0	200	5%
rigatoni	2 oz	1.0	200	5%
rotini..all types	2 oz	1.0	200	5%
shells..all shapes	2 oz	1.0	180	5%
spaghetti..all types	2 oz	1.0	200	5%
tortelloni..ricotta & spinach	2 oz	8.0	220	33%
tortelloni..3-cheese	2 oz	8.0	240	30%
ziti	2 oz	1.0	200	5%
(Buitoni)..refrigerated cut pasta				
REGULAR-SIZE PASTA				
angel hair	1¼ cups	2.5	230	10%
beef ravioletti	1 cup	7.0	300	21%
cheese & roasted				
garlic tortelloni	1 cup	8.0	270	27%
chicken				
herb tortellini	1 cup	9.0	340	24%
Parmesan ravioli	1¼ cups	8.0	310	23%
& prosciutto tortelloni	1 cup	9.0	330	25%
roasted..w/garlic ravioli	1-¼ cups	11.0	340	29%
classic beef ravioli	1-¼ cup	10.0	340	27%
fettuccini	1-¼ cup	2.5	240	9%
4-cheese ravioli	1-¼ cup	14.0	330	38%
garden vegetable ravioli	1 cup	5.0	250	18%
light..4-cheese ravioli	1¼ cups	4.0	230	16%

Food and Description	Amount	Fat Grams	Total Calories	% Fat Calories
linguine	1¼ cups	2.5	240	9%
mozzarella				
& herb tortelloni	1 cup	10.0	330	27%
& pepperoni tortelloni	1 cup	10.0	330	27%
portobello mushroom				
& cheese tortelloni	1 cup	6.0	270	20%
spinach				
cheese tortelloni	1 cup	8.0	330	22%
fettuccini	1¼ cups	3.0	220	12%
sun-dried tomato tortelloni	1 cup	9.0	310	26%
sweet Italian sausage tortelloni	1 cup	9.0	330	25%
3-cheese				
ravioletti	1 cup	6.0	270	20%
tortellini	1 cup	7.0	320	20%
(Creamette) dry				
egg noodles				
enriched..wide	2 oz	3.0	220	12%
no egg yolk..all types	2 oz	2.5	210	11%
regular				
dumpling	2 oz	2.5	210	11%
extra-wide	2 oz	2.5	210	11%
fine	2 oz	2.5	210	11%
kluski	2 oz	2.0	210	9%
medium	2 oz	2.5	210	9%
wide	2 oz	1.5	210	11%
enriched pasta..all types	2 oz	1.0	210	4%
Healthy Harvest..all types	2 oz	1.5	210	6%
Kid's Club..all shapes	2 oz	1.0	210	4%
lasagna	2 oz	1.0	210	4%
linguini	2 oz	1.0	210	4%
manicotti	~2 oz	1.0	210	4%
mostaccioli..all types	2 oz	1.0	210	4%
penne rigate	2 oz	1.0	210	4%
rainbow rotini	2 oz	1.0	210	4%
ribbons..no egg yolk	2 oz	1.0	210	4%
rigatoni	2 oz	1.0	210	4%
rotelle	2 oz	1.0	210	4%
rotini..all types	2 oz	1.0	210	4%
shells..all shapes	2 oz	1.0	210	4%
spaghetti..all types				
spinach				
egg	2 oz	3.0	220	12%
no egg	2 oz	1.0	210	4%
tricolor	2 oz	1.0	210	4%
vermicelli	2 oz	1.0	210	4%
(De Boles) organic..dry..uncooked				
angel hair..Jerusalem artichoke				
garlic & parsley	2 oz	1.0	210	4%
plain	2 oz	1.0	210	4%
tomato..all types	2 oz	0.5	210	2%

Food and Description	Amount	Fat Grams	Total Calories	% Fat Calories
whole wheat	2 oz	1.5	210	6%
elbow-style..plain	2 oz	0.5	210	2%
fettuccini..all types	2 oz	0.5	210	2%
lasagna..organic	2 oz	0.5	210	2%
linguine..Jerusalem artichoke	2 oz	1.0	210	4%
penne				
garlic & parsley	2 oz	0.5	210	2%
plain	2 oz	1.0	210	4%
tomato & basil	2 oz	0.5	210	2%
whole wheat	2 oz	1.5	210	6%
ribbon				
eggless	2 oz	0.5	210	2%
garlic & parsley	2 oz	1.0	210	4%
whole wheat	2 oz	1.5	210	6%
rigatoni				
garlic & parsley	2 oz	0.5	210	2%
Jerusalem artichoke	2 oz	1.0	210	4%
tomato & basil	2 oz	0.5	210	2%
whole wheat	2 oz	1.5	210	6%
rotini..all types	2 oz	1.0	210	4%
shells/organic	2 oz	0.5	210	2%
spaghetti-style				
garlic & parsley	2 oz	0.5	210	2%
Jerusalem artichoke	2 oz	1.0	210	4%
plain	2 oz	1.0	210	4%
tomato & basil	2 oz	0.5	210	2%
w/spinach	2 oz	0.5	210	2%
whole wheat	2 oz	1.5	210	6%
ziti				
Jerusalem artichoke	2 oz	1.0	210	4%
(Di Giorno)..Refrigerated				
low-fat..cholesterol-free				
angel's hair	2 oz	1.5	160	8%
fettuccini..all types	3 oz	1.5	200	7%
linguine..all types	2.5 oz	1.5	200	7%
tortelloni				
3-cheese	3 oz	7.0	250	25%
chicken & herbs	1 cup	5.0	270	17%
mozzarella-garlic	1 cup	8.0	300	24%
pesto	1 cup	8.0	320	23%
portabello mushroom	1 cup	7.0	310	20%
(Eden)..dry				
artichoke ribbons	2 oz	1.5	210	6%
creste dei gallo..parsley garlic	2 oz	1.0	210	9%
elbows..organic..all types	2 oz	2.0	210	9%
extra-fine pasta	2 oz	1.5	210	6%
kuzu				
& sweet potato pasta	2 oz	–	200	–
kiri pasta	2 oz	–	200	–
mung bean..Harusame	2 oz	–	190	–

Food and Description	Amount	Fat Grams	Total Calories	% Fat Calories
pesto gemelli	2 oz	1.0	210	9%
quinoa..organic	~1.5 oz	3.5	180	18%
ribbons, durum..golden amber..organic				
wheat	2 oz	1.0	220	4%
wheat curry	2 oz	1.0	220	4%
wheat paella	2 oz	1.0	220	4%
wheat parsley garlic	2 oz	1.5	210	6%
wheat pesto	2 oz	1.5	210	6%
saffron	2 oz	1.5	210	6%
spelt				
100% whole-grain	2 oz	2.0	210	9%
80% whole-grain	2 oz	1.5	200	7%
whole wheat spinach	2 oz	2.0	200	9%
rice pasta..bifun	2 oz	0.5	200	2%
rigatoni..endless tubes	2 oz	1.0	210	4%
shells, durum-wheat				
vegetable..organic	2 oz	1.0	210	4%
soba				
100% buckwheat	2 oz	1.0	200	5%
40% buckwheat	2 oz	1.0	190	5%
Japanese	2 oz	1.0	190	5%
lotus-root	2 oz	1.0	190	5%
mugwort	2 oz	0.5	190	2%
wild yam jinenjo	2 oz	0.5	190	2%
somen	2 oz	2.0	200	9%
spaghetti..organic				
durum-wheat	2 oz	1.0	210	4%
kamut	2 oz	1.5	190	7%
parsley-garlic	2 oz	1.0	210	4%
whole wheat	2 oz	2.0	210	9%
spirals..organic				
durum-wheat vegetable	2 oz	1.0	210	4%
flax rice..60% whole-grain	2 oz	2.0	200	9%
kamut	2 oz	1.5	190	7%
mixed-grain	2 oz	2.0	210	9%
rye	2 oz	–	200	–
sesame rice	2 oz	2.0	200	9%
whole wheat vegetable	2 oz	2.0	210	9%
udon				
brown rice..organic	2 oz	2.0	200	9%
Japanese	2 oz	1.5	190	8%
vegetable shells..small	2 oz	2.0	210	9%
ziti rigati..parsley-garlic	2 oz	1.0	210	4%
(Foulds) no yolks..dry				
egg noodle				
broad	2 oz	0.5	210	2%
substitute	2 oz	2.0	210	9%
(Goodman's)..dry				
alphabets	2 oz	1.0	210	4%
bows..large	2 oz	3.0	220	12%

Food and Description	Amount	Fat Grams	Total Calories	% Fat Calories
egg flakes	2 oz	3.0	220	12%
egg noodles				
fine	2 oz	2.5	210	11%
medium	2 oz	2.5	210	11%
wide	2 oz	2.5	210	11%
yolk-free ribbons	2 oz	1.0	210	4%
(Hodgson Mill)..dry				
organic whole wheat..w/milled				
flaxseed & soy...all types	2 oz	2.0	200	9%
veggie..all shapes	2 oz	1.0	200	5%
whole wheat				
angel hair	2 oz	1.0	190	5%
bow ties	2 oz	1.0	190	5%
couscous	⅓ cup	1.0	210	4%
couscous..garlic & basil				
w/milled flaxseed & soy	⅓ cup	2.0	235	8%
couscous..Parmesan cheese				
w/milled flaxseed & soy	⅓ cup	2.5	240	9%
couscous..w/milled flaxseed				
& soy	⅓ cup	2.0	230	8%
egg noodles..alll types	2 oz	1.0	190	5%
elbows	2 oz	1.0	190	5%
fettuccini	2 oz	1.0	190	5%
lasagna	2 oz	1.0	190	5%
penne	2 oz	1.0	190	5%
radiatores	2 oz	1.0	190	5%
shells..medium	2 oz	1.0	190	5%
spaghetti..all types	2 oz	1.0	190	5%
yolkless pasta ribbons	2 oz	1.0	190	5%
(Lundberg Family Farms)..brown rice pasta				
organic				
penne	2 oz	2.0	210	11%
rotini	2 oz	2.0	210	11%
spaghetti	2 oz	2.0	210	11%
(Monterey)..refrigerated pasta..cooked				
Carb-Smart				
fettuccini..classic egg	3 oz	5.0	200	23%
linguine..classic egg	3 oz	5.0	200	23%
ravioli				
4-cheese & chives	3.6 oz	13.0	260	45%
seafood..w/lobster..crab	3.6 oz	9.0	220	37%
spinach ricotta	3.6 oz	11.0	240	41%
tortelloni..spinach & cheese	3.6 oz	9.0	230	35%
other pasta				
borsellini	3 oz	8.0	270	27%
fettuccini	3 oz	1.5	240	6%
grandi				
ravioli..low-fat	3 oz	4.5	230	18%
ravioli..snow crab	3 oz	5.0	240	19%
spinach ricotta	3 oz	6.0	240	23%

Food and Description	Amount	Fat Grams	Total Calories	% Fat Calories
tortelloni	3 oz	8.0	300	24%
tortellini				
classic Italian cheese	3 oz	12.0	340	32%
rainbow..5-cheese	3 oz	3.0	280	10%
tricolor..roasted chicken	3 oz	4.5	250	16%
(Mrs. Weiss')..dry				
egg bows				
small	2 oz	2.5	210	11%
egg noodles				
egg farfel	2 oz	2.0	210	9%
egg flakes	2 oz	2.0	210	9%
extra-fine	2 oz	2.0	210	9%
halushka	2 oz	2.5	210	11%
kluski	2 oz	2.0	210	11%
kluski..enriched	2 oz	2.0	210	11%
medium	2 oz	2.5	210	11%
wide	2 oz	2.5	210	11%
(Nasoya)..cooked				
pasta wrappers..for eggrolls	2.28 oz	0.5	170	3%
(Quinoa)..wheat-free..all types	2 oz	7.0	180	10%
(Reames)..frozen				
egg noodles				
golden ribbons	½ cup	2.5	210	11%
home-style	½ cup	2.0	170	11%
pre-cooked	½ cup	2.5	240	9%
hearty home-style				
chicken noodle	3 oz	2.0	130	14%
home-style				
free..no yolk	½ cup	–	160	–
quick-cook egg noodle	1 cup	2.5	230	10%
(Ronzoni)..dry				
acini pepe-44	2 oz	1.0	210	9%
angel hair..lemon pepper	2 oz	1.0	210	9%
cavatappi..elbow twists	2 oz	1.0	210	9%
egg fettuccini	2 oz	2.5	210	11%
egg noodles				
regular	2 oz	2.0	210	9%
spinach	2 oz	3.0	220	12%
egg pastina	2 oz	2.5	210	11%
fettuccini..all types	2 oz	1.0	210	4%
fusilli	2 oz	1.0	210	4%
Healthy Harvest				
noodle-style..all types	2 oz	1.5	210	6%
lasagna	2 oz	1.0	210	4%
macaroni..all types	2 oz	1.0	210	4%
macarrones	2 oz	1.0	210	4%
mostaccioli	2 oz	1.0	210	4%
rigatoni	2 oz	1.0	210	4%
rotelle	2 oz	1.0	210	4%
rotini..tricolor	2 oz	1.0	210	4%

Food and Description	Amount	Fat Grams	Total Calories	% Fat Calories
shells..all shapes	2 oz	1.0	210	4%
spinach pastina	2 oz	1.0	210	4%
Tradizione D'Italia..all types	2 oz	1.0	210	4%
(San Giorgio)..dry				
light & fluffy				
dumplings	1 oz	1.0	210	4%
egg noodles..all types				
regular				
acine di pepe	2 oz	1.0	210	4%
alphabets	2 oz	1.0	210	4%
bow ties..egg	2 oz	3.0	210	13%
capellini	2 oz	1.0	210	4%
ditalini	2 oz	1.0	210	4%
elbow macaroni	2 oz	1.0	210	4%
flakes	2 oz	1.0	210	4%
Healthy Harvest..all shapes	2 oz	1.5	210	6%
kluske	2 oz	3.0	220	12%
lasagna..rippled	2 oz	1.0	210	4%
linguine	2 oz	1.0	210	4%
mafalda..mini lasagne	2 oz	1.0	210	4%
manicotti	2 oz	1.0	210	4%
mostaccioli rigati	2 oz	1.0	210	4%
penne rigate	2 oz	1.0	210	4%
perciatelli-6	2 oz	1.0	210	4%
shells..rainbow	2 oz	1.0	210	4%
rigatoni	2 oz	1.0	210	4%
rotelle	2 oz	1.0	210	4%
rotini	2 oz	1.0	210	4%
shells..all sizes	2 oz	1.0	210	4%
jumbo	2 oz	1.0	210	4%
spaghetti	2 oz	1.0	210	4%
spaghettini	2 oz	1.0	210	4%
twists..rainbow	1 oz	1.0	210	4%
ziti..cut	1 oz	1.0	210	4%
vermicelli	2 oz	1.0	210	4%
(VitaSpelt)..whole grain pasta..dry				
angel hair	2 oz	1.5	190	7%
egg noodles	2 oz	1.5	190	7%
lasagna	2 oz	1.5	190	7%
spaghetti	2 oz	1.5	190	7%
buckwheat	2 oz	1.5	190	7%
white spelt pasta...all types	2 oz	0.5	210	2%
(Westbrae Natural)..dry				
whole wheat				
angel hair..corn	2 oz	1.5	210	6%
lasagna/whole wheat..no egg				
plain	2 oz	2.0	210	9%
spinach	2 oz	2.0	180	10%
spaghetti				
whole wheat..no egg				
plain	2 oz	1.5	200	7%
spinach	2 oz	2.0	180	10%

Food and Description	Amount	Fat Grams	Total Calories	% Fat Calories

PASTA ENTRÉE/DINNER (*See also* ASIAN FOOD; FROZEN ENTRÉE/DINNER; VEGETARIAN FOODS; individual listings)
■ **CANNED**...unless otherwise noted

Food and Description	Amount	Fat Grams	Total Calories	% Fat Calories
(Annie's)..homegrown organic				
All Stars	1 cup	1.0	150	6%
Arthur Loops	1 cup	1.0	150	6%
BernieOs	1 cup	1.0	150	6%
cheesy ravioli	1 cup	3.5	180	18%
P'Sghetti loops..w/soy meatballs	1 cup	4.0	190	19%
(Chef Boyardee)				
Beefaroni				
big..w/beef in tomato sauce	1 cup	9.0	270	30%
macaroni..w/beef in sauce	1 cup	7.0	260	24%
Chili Mac	1 cup	13.0	270	43%
lasagna..beef				
& tomato sauce..cup	10.5 oz	10.0	300	30%
macaroni..cheesy burger	1 cup	6.0	220	25%
pasta shells & meatballs..mini bites	1 cup	12.0	270	40%
Pepperoni Pizzazaroli	1 cup	11.0	320	31%
ravioli				
beef in tomato & meat sauce	1 cup	7.0	230	27%
cup	7.5 oz	5.0	190	24%
cheesy burger	1 cup	7.0	300	21%
mini beef in tomato				
& meat sauce	1 cup	7.0	240	26%
mini bites..beef & meatballs	1 cup	13.0	300	39%
overstuffed..w/sausage				
& meat sauce	1 cup	4.0	290	12%
overstuffed..w/tomato				
& meat sauce	1 cup	4.5	280	14%
rotini..in creamy tomato sauce	1 cup	7.0	260	24%
spaghetti & meatballs	1 cup	11.0	270	37%
cup	7.5 oz	9.0	210	39%
jumbo	1 cup	13.0	280	42%
mini bites..w/meatballs	1 cup	13.0	280	42%
spaghetti rings & meatballs..cup	7.5 oz	9.0	240	34%
X-Men				
in tomato & cheese sauce	1 cup	0.5	200	2%
w/meatballs	1 cup	11.0	290	34%
(Franco American)..SpaghettiOs				
beef ravioli..in meat sauce	1 cup	7.0	260	24%
beef raviolios..in meat sauce	1 cup	10.0	290	31%
Fun Shapes SpaghettiOs				
Smilers	1 Cup	1.0	180	5%
w/Meatball Smilers	1 cup	9.0	260	31%
Garfield pasta	1 cup	1.5	190	7%
Knights & Castles SpaghettioOs	1 cup	1.5	190	7%
Knights & Castles SpaghettiOs				
w/meatballs	1 cup	10.0	260	35%

Food and Description	Amount	Fat Grams	Total Calories	% Fat Calories
spaghetti..in tomato & cheese sauce	1 cup	2.0	210	9%
SpaghettiOs				
A to Z's	1 cup	1.0	180	5%
A to Z's..w/meatballs	1 cup	9.0	260	31%
A to Z's..w/sliced franks	1 cup	7.0	230	27%
in meat sauce	1 cup	2.0	170	11%
plus calcium	1 cup	1.0	180	5%
w/meatballs	1 cup	8.0	240	30%
w/sliced franks	1 cup	10.0	230	39%
Superior Beef Ravioli..meat sauce	1 cup	6.0	270	20%
(Hormel)				
chili mac	1 can	9.0	200	41%
lasagna	1 can	14.0	260	48%
spaghetti & meatballs	1 can	7.0	220	29%
■ FRESH				
(Reser's)				
pasta salads..prepared				
elbo-mac	¾ cup	22.0	320	62%
California pasta	¾ cup	4.0	160	23%
gourmet mac & cheese	¾ cup	17.0	280	55%
Italian	½ cup	9.0	160	51%
Thai noodle	⅔ cup	12.0	230	47%
traditional macaroni	¾ cup	22.0	320	62%
■ FROZEN				
(Birds Eye)				
Easy Recipe Creations				
basil herb primavera	1 cup	11.0	260	38%
roasted garlic Parmesan	1 cup	10.0	240	38%
tortellini parmigiana	1 cup	12.0	240	45%
Pasta Secrets..prepared				
Italian pesto	1 cup	9.0	240	34%
primavera	1 cup	10.0	230	39%
radiatore pasta & vegetables	1 cup	8.0	200	36%
ranch	1 cup	15.0	300	45%
3-cheese	1 cup	8.0	230	31%
white cheddar	1 cup	10.0	240	38%
zesty garlic	1 cup	10.0	240	38%
(Cascadian Farm)				
bowls..veggie				
Japanese noodles & vegetables	1 bowl	2.5	180	13%
pasta marinara	1 bowl	3.0	180	15%
pasta primavera	1 bowl	8.0	270	27%
(Freshlike)..entrées				
Pasta Combos				
garlic herb	6.5 oz	11.0	260	38%
Italian herb	6.5 oz	9.0	240	34%
pasta..vegetables..w/sauce	5.3 oz	9.0	200	41%
(Green Giant)				
Boil-in-Bag pasta				
Alfredo	1 pkg	8.0	300	24%

Food and Description	Amount	Fat Grams	Total Calories	% Fat Calories
primavera	1 pkg	10.0	300	30%
roasted garlic	1 pkg	6.0	250	22%
3-cheese	1 pkg	8.0	270	27%
Complete Skillet Meal..as packaged				
chicken Alfredo	¼ pkg	6.0	270	20%
chicken cheesy pasta	¼ pkg	6.0	270	20%
creamy chix noodle	¼ pkg	5.0	290	16%
garlic chicken pasta	¼ pkg	7.0	260	24%
Create a Meal..as packaged				
beefy noodle	1¾ cups	1.5	170	8%
cheesy pasta & vegetable	1¾ cups	8.0	210	34%
chicken Alfredo	2 cups	6.0	230	23%
garlic herb chicken	1⅓ cups	9.0	230	35%
Parmesan herb chix	1¾ cups	2.5	160	14%
skillet lasagna	1¾ cups	0.5	150	3%
Pasta Accents..as packaged				
Alfredo	2 cups	7.0	200	32%
creamy cheddar	2⅓ cups	8.0	250	29%
garden herb seasoning	2 cups	7.0	230	27%
garlic seasoning	2 cups	10.0	260	35%
3-cheese	2 cups	14.0	350	36%
white cheddar sauce	1¾ cups	11.0	290	34%
(Mrs. T's)..Pasta Pockets				
potato				
& cheddar	3 pieces	2.5	180	13%
& onion	3 pieces	2.5	210	11%
(Uncle Ben's)..Noodle & Pasta Bowls				
3-cheese ravioli	1 bowl	7.0	380	17%
cheese lasagna..w/meat sauce	1 bowl	7.0	220	19%
chicken fettuccini Alfredo	1 bowl	7.0	350	18%
garlic & herb chicken	1 bowl	7.0	380	17%
honey ginger chicken	1 bowl	5.0	430	10%
orange glaze	1 bowl	8.0	440	16%
Parmesan shrimp penne	1 bowl	7.0	380	17%
spicy peanut chicken	1 bowl	8.5	420	18%
Thai-style chicken	1 bowl	8.0	400	18%
tomato sausage rotini	1 bowl	8.0	420	17%
■ MICROWAVE CONTAINER				
(Annie's)..totally natural				
mac & cheese meals	¾ cup	4.5	230	18%
real aged Wisconsin cheddar	¾ cup	4.5	230	18%
(Betty Crocker)				
Bowl Appetit				
home-style chicken pasta	1 bowl	6.0	260	21%
macaroni & cheese	1 bowl	12.0	370	28%
pasta Alfredo	1 bowl	12.0	360	30%
3-cheese rotini	1 bowl	10.0	360	25%
tomato Parmesan penne	1 bowl	8.0	350	21%
(Dinty Moore)				
American Classics				
beef ravioli	1 bowl	9.0	300	27%

Food and Description	Amount	Fat Grams	Total Calories	% Fat Calories
chicken & noodles	1 bowl	8.0	260	28%
lasagna	1 bowl	16.0	340	42%
macaroni & cheese				
w/Cure 81 ham	1 bowl	16.0	330	44%
spaghetti..w/meatballs	1 bowl	7.0	290	22%
microwave cups				
noodles & beef	1 cup	14.0	240	53%
noodles & chicken	1 cup	9.0	190	43%
(Hormel)..shelf stable entrées				
Kid's Kitchen				
beefy macaroni	1 cup	5.0	180	25%
cheezy mac & beef	1 cup	7.0	260	24%
macaroni & cheese	1 cup	11.0	270	37%
mini ravioli	1 cup	7.0	240	26%
noodle rings & chicken	1 cup	4.0	140	26%
spaghetti & meatballs	1 cup	9.0	230	35%
spaghetti rings	1 cup	2.0	190	9%
spaghetti rings & franks	1 cup	9.0	240	34%
spaghetti rings & meatballs	1 cup	7.0	230	27%
(Kraft)..It's Pasta Anytime				
fettuccini..w/classic				
Alfredo sauce	1 meal	22.0	580	34%
spaghetti..w/tomato sauce	1 meal	8.0	550	13%
(Spice Hunter)..Pasta Cups				
creamy Alfredo fusilli	1 cup	5.0	210	21%
creamy butter fusilli	1 cup	4.5	210	19%
curly macaroni & cheese	1 cup	4.5	200	20%
(Uncle Ben's)..Pasta Bowls				
3-cheese rotini	1 bowl	7.0	380	17%
chicken fettuccini Alfredo	1 bowl	7.0	350	18%
4-cheese lasagna	1 bowl	7.0	330	19%
garlic herb chicken	1 bowl	7.0	380	17%
Parmesan shrimp penne	1 bowl	7.0	380	17%
tomato sausage rotini	1 bowl	8.0	420	17%
■ MIX				
(Annie's)..certified organic..prepared, as directed				
Deluxe Mac & Cheese				
elbows & 4-cheese sauce	1 cup	11.0	320	31%
rotini..w/white cheddar	1 cup	9.0	300	27%
shells & real aged				
Wisconsin cheddar	1 cup	11.0	320	31%
macaroni & cheese				
Alfredo shells & cheddar	1 cup	16.0	370	39%
family-size shells				
& white cheddar	1 cup	15.0	370	36%
mild Mexican shells & cheddar	1 cup	4.0	280	13%
peace & pasta Parmesan	1 cup	4.0	280	13%
shells & real aged				
Wisconsin cheddar	1 cup	15.0	370	36%
shells & white cheddar	1 cup	15.0	370	36%

Food and Description	Amount	Fat Grams	Total Calories	% Fat Calories
whole wheat shells & cheddar	1 cup	15.0	360	38%
Totally Natural Pasta Meals				
made w/organic pasta				
curly fettuccini..w/white cheddar & broccoli sauce	1 cup	12.0	350	31%
gemelli pasta..roasted garlic Parmesan	1 cup	13.0	360	33%
penne pasta..w/Alfredo cheese sauce	1 cup	13.0	360	33%
radiatore pasta..w/sun-dried tomato & basil sauce	1 cup	11.0	350	28%
rotini pasta..w/4-cheese sauce	1 cup	12.0	350	31%
(Bean Cuisine)..mix only				
country French beans..w/gemelli	¼ pkg	1.0	210	4%
Florentine beans..w/bow ties	¼ pkg	2.0	160	11%
Mediterranean black beans & fusilli	¼ pkg	1.0	210	4%
pasta & beans..w/radiatore	¼ pkg	1.0	210	4%
(Betty Crocker)				
Complete Meals..mix only				
fettuccini Alfredo	⅕ pkg	13.0	320	37%
lasagna pasta bake	⅕ pkg	9.0	250	32%
Suddenly Salad..prepared				
Caesar	1 cup	10.0	240	38%
classic	1 cup	7.0	240	26%
creamy Parmesan	1 cup	24.0	360	60%
ranch & bacon	¾ cup	23.0	330	63%
roasted garlic..Parmesan	¾ cup	22.0	340	58%
(Carapelli)..box mix				
pasta & sauce				
4-cheese..w/cavatappi pasta	½ box	1.0	240	4%
creamy Alfredo..w/penne pasta	½ box	1.0	240	4%
creamy tomato..w/spirals	½ box	0.5	240	2%
roasted garlic & Parmesan	½ box	1.0	240	4%
(DiGiorno)..mix only				
fettuccini	2.5 oz	1.5	200	7%
3-cheese..tortellini	3 oz	7.0	250	25%
(Fantastic Foods)				
Carb'tastic..Fast Naturals..ready meals				
penne..w/meat sauce	1 pkg	14.0	240	53%
penne Alfredo	1 pkg	15.0	280	48%
vegetarian pesto primavera	1 pkg	13.0	270	43%
couscous..dry mix only				
basil pesto	⅓ cup	2.5	220	10%
organic	¼ cup	1.0	190	5%
organic..whole wheat	¼ cup	1.0	210	4%
roasted garlic & red pepper couscous	⅓ cup	0.5	220	2%
ramen noodle cups				
big cup..vegetable curry	½ pkg	1.0	110	8%

Food and Description	Amount	Fat Grams	Total Calories	% Fat Calories
small cup				
vegetable miso	1 cup	1.0	130	7%
vegetarian..chicken-free	1 cup	0.5	140	3%
vegetarian..chicken free	½ pkg	0.5	100	5%
vegetable miso	½ pkg	0.5	100	5%
(Golden Grain)..Pasta Roni..prepared, as directed				
angel hair				
w/herbs	1 cup	13.0	320	37%
w/lemon & butter	1 cup	15.0	360	38%
w/Parmesan cheese	1 cup	14.0	320	39%
broccoli				
au gratin	1 cup	10.0	280	32%
regular	1 cup	15.0	340	40%
chicken				
& garlic..low-fat	1 cup	3.0	210	13%
regular	1 cup	13.0	310	38%
corkscrew pasta				
w/creamy garlic sauce	1 cup	25.0	420	54%
w/4-cheese sauce	1 cup	19.0	410	42%
fettuccini				
w/Alfredo sauce				
original	1 cup	25.0	460	49%
reduced-fat	1 cup	8.0	310	23%
w/broccoli au gratin	1 cup	10.0	290	31%
w/chicken sauce	1 cup	13.5	320	38%
w/mild cheddar sauce	1 cup	10.5	300	32%
w/Romanoff sauce	1 cup	19.0	410	42%
w/Stroganoff sauce	1 cup	14.0	370	34%
garlic Alfredo	1 cup	13.0	360	33%
herb w/butter	1 cup	19.0	380	45%
home-style chicken	1 cup	6.0	230	23%
linguine				
w/chicken & broccoli	1 cup	16.0	370	39%
w/creamy chicken Parmesan	1 cup	18.0	410	40%
mild cheddar	1 cup	10.0	290	31%
Parmesan	1 cup	17.0	390	39%
rigatoni w/white cheddar	1 cup	19.0	400	43%
& broccoli sauce				
romanoff	1 cup	19.0	400	43%
shells w/white cheddar sauce	1 cup	13.0	310	38%
Stroganoff	1 cup	14.0	370	34%
vermicelli w/roasted garlic & olive oil	1 cup	16.0	360	40%
(Knorr)				
bow tie & beans	½ pkg	2.0	260	7%
fettuccine..w/classic				
Alfredo sauce	½ pkg	7.0	280	23%
penne..w/sun-dried tomato				
Parmesan sauce	½ pkg	3.5	270	12%
rotini..w/delicate				
mushroom sauce	½ pkg	1.5	260	5%

Food and Description	Amount	Fat Grams	Total Calories	% Fat Calories
(Kraft)				
macaroni & cheese..mix only, unless noted otherwise				
Blue's Clues	2.75 oz	2.5	260	10%
Crazy Noodles..Green Wigglers	2.75 oz	3.0	260	10%
Deluxe				
4-cheese blend	3.5 oz	10.0	320	28%
half the fat	3.5 oz	4.5	290	14%
original	3.5 oz	10.0	320	29%
sharp cheddar	2.8 oz	9.0	270	30%
Nickelodeon..the				
Fairly Odd Parents	2.75 oz	2.5	260	9%
Pokémon	2.75 oz	2.5	260	9%
Rugrats	2.75 oz	2.5	260	9%
Scooby Doo!	2.75 oz	2.5	260	9%
Spirals	2.75 oz	2.5	260	9%
SpongeBob SquarePants	2.75 oz	2.5	260	9%
The cheesiest	2.4 oz	2.5	260	9%
pasta salads				
classic ranch..w/bacon	¼ pkg	0.5	130	3%
creamy Caesar	¼ pkg	2.0	190	9%
garlic Parmesan	¼ pkg	1.5	180	8%
Italian	¼ pkg	2.0	160	11%
ranch..w/tuna..prepared	¼ pkg	18.0	300	54%
Side Dishes				
deluxe rotini & white				
cheddar sauce..w/broccoli	½ box	15.0	400	34%
Spaghetti Classics				
Tangy Italian	2 oz	1.5	200	7%
spaghetti dinner..w/meat				
sauce..prepared	5.5 oz	11.0	330	30%
Velveeta..prepared				
radiatore & cheese				
herb & garlic	1 cup	13.0	360	33%
rotini & cheese..w/broccoli	1 cup	16.0	400	36%
shells & cheese				
bacon	1 cup	16.0	400	36%
light	1 cup	6.0	320	17%
original	1 cup	13.0	360	33%
salsa	1 cup	14.0	380	33%
(Lipton)				
Asian Side Dish				
beef	½ pkg	2.5	230	10%
sweet & sour	½ pkg	2.0	260	7%
teriyaki	½ pkg	3.0	250	11%
Thai sesame	½ pkg	3.5	230	14%
Fiesta Sides				
jalapeño jack	½ pkg	2.5	230	10%
nacho	½ pkg	2.5	230	10%
Noodles & Sauce..mix only				
beef	½ pkg	3.0	220	12%

Food and Description	Amount	Fat Grams	Total Calories	% Fat Calories
Pasta & Sauce..mix only				
Alfredo	½ pkg	6.0	240	23%
Alfredo broccoli	½ pkg	6.0	250	22%
butter	½ pkg	4.0	240	15%
butter & herb	½ pkg	4.5	240	17%
cheddar broccoli	½ pkg	2.0	250	7%
cheesy cheddar	½ pkg	2.0	220	8%
chicken	½ pkg	2.0	220	8%
chicken broccoli	½ pkg	2.5	220	10%
creamy chicken flavor	½ pkg	4.0	230	16%
Parmesan	½ pkg	4.5	230	18%
Stroganoff	½ pkg	2.0	210	9%
Pasta & Sauce.. Italian sides				
creamy garlic	½ pkg	5.0	270	17%
4-cheese bow tie	½ pkg	4.0	220	16%
tomato Parmesan	½ pkg	4.5	240	17%
Pasta Sides..pouch..prepared				
Alfredo	½ pkg	7.0	250	25%
butter	½ pkg	8.0	260	28%
chicken	½ pkg	4.0	230	15%
Stroganoff	½ pkg	3.5	210	15%
(Near East)..prepared, as directed				
couscous				
broccoli	1 cup	2.5	210	11%
herbed chicken	1 cup	3.5	220	14%
Mediterranean curry	1 cup	3.5	220	14%
Moroccan pasta	1¼ cups	6.0	260	21%
Parmesan	1 cup	3.0	220	12%
roasted garlic & olive oil	1 cup	4.5	230	18%
toasted pine nuts	1 cup	6.0	230	23%
tomato lentil	1 cup	3.5	220	14%
wild mushroom..herb	1 cup	4.0	230	16%
Creative Grains				
chicken & herbs	1 cup	6.0	270	20%
creamy Parmesan	1 cup	7.0	280	23%
roasted garlic	1 cup	5.0	220	20%
roasted pecan & garlic	1 cup	9.0	240	34%
pastas				
basil & herbs..w/radiatore	1 cup	6.0	240	23%
roasted garlic & olive oil w/vermicelli	1 cup	9.0	310	26%
roasted tomato..w/angel hair	1 cup	6.0	240	23%
pastas..w/delicate sauce				
angel hair..spicy tomato	1 cup	6.0	240	23%
fusilli..Parmesan & Romano	1 cup	7.0	300	21%
gemelli..tomato Parmesan	1 cup	10.0	330	27%
radiatore..basil & herb	1 cup	8.0	260	28%
vermicelli..garlic & olive oil	1 cup	8.0	260	28%

Food and Description	Amount	Fat Grams	Total Calories	% Fat Calories
(Pasta Roni)..prepared, as directed				
angel hair				
garlic & butter	1 cup	8.0	260	28%
primavera	1 cup	16.0	330	44%
tomato Parmesan	1 cup	9.0	280	29%
w/herbs	1 cup	13.0	320	37%
w/lemon & butter	1 cup	15.0	360	38%
w/Parmesan cheese	1 cup	14.0	320	39%
broccoli	1 cup	14.0	330	38%
au gratin	1 cup	10.0	280	32%
chicken	1 cup	13.0	310	38%
& garlic..low-fat	1 cup	11.0	300	33%
home-style	1 cup	6.0	230	23%
creamy garlic sauce				
w/corkscrew pasta	1 cup	17.0	350	44%
fettuccini				
Alfredo	1 cup	25.0	460	50%
Alfredo..reduced-fat	1 cup	8.0	310	23%
4-cheese sauce				
w/corkscrew pasta	1 cup	17.0	390	39%
garlic Alfredo	1 cup	14.0	360	35%
herb & butter rigatoni	1 cup	16.0	350	41%
linguine				
w/chicken & broccoli	1 cup	15.0	380	36%
w/creamy chicken Parmesan	1 cup	18.0	410	40%
Parmesano	1 cup	17.0	390	39%
Romanoff	1 cup	19.0	400	43%
shells & white cheddar	1 cup	13.0	310	38%
sour cream & chives	1 cup	15.0	320	42%
Stroganoff	1 cup	14.0	370	34%
vermicelli..w/roasted garlic				
& olive oil	1 cup	15.0	360	38%
white cheddar & broccoli				
sauce..w/rigatoni	1 cup	14.0	320	11%
(Ragu)..Ragu Express				
pasta dinners				
classic meat flavor	⅙ box	3.0	200	14%
sweet tomato & garlic	⅙ box	2.5	500	5%
traditional tomato	⅙ box	2.5	190	12%
(Ramen) noodles (See SOUP)				
(Velveeta)..See (Kraft) within this section				
(Zatarain's)				
New Orleans–style scampi	⅓ box	1.0	100	9%
PASTA SAUCE (See SAUCE)				
PASTRAMI (See LUNCHEON MEAT)				
PASTRY (See also CAKE; DONUT; PASTRY, TOASTER; PASTRY DOUGH; PIE CRUST)				
■ **FROZEN OR REFRIGERATED**				
(Allouette)..pastry kit				
baked Brie in pastry				
w/raspberries & almonds	⅓ kit	14.0	220	57%

Food and Description	Amount	Fat Grams	Total Calories	% Fat Calories
(Athens)				
baklava pastry..bite-size	2 pieces	12.0	230	47%
(Pepperidge Farm)				
dumplings				
apple	1 dumpling	11.0	250	40%
peach	1 dumpling	11.0	320	31%
turnovers				
apple	1	15.0	290	47%
blueberry	1	15.0	280	48%
peach	1	15.0	290	47%
raspberry	1	15.0	290	47%
(Nancy's)..pecan tartlets	6 tartlets	27.0	470	52%
(Pillsbury)				
sweet roll..Home-Baked Classics				
cinnamon roll..w/icing	1 roll	10.0	330	27%
sweet rolls..dulce de leche				
caramel	1 roll	7.0	160	39%
turnover				
apple	1 turnover	8.0	170	42%
cherry	1 turnover	8.0	170	42%
(Rhodes)				
Bake-N-Serv Rolls..prepared				
orange rolls..w/cream				
cheese frosting	1 roll	9.5	285	30%
raspberry..w/rich vanilla icing	1 roll	5.0	180	25%
strawberry..w/rich vanilla icing	1 roll	5.0	180	25%
Rolls Anytime!				
cinnamon..w/cream				
cheese frosting	1 roll	7.0	240	26%
orange..w/cream				
cheese frosting	1 roll	8.5	300	26%
(Rich's)..Temptations Éclairs				
Bavarian crème	1 éclair	12.0	220	49%
Bavarian crème..mini	4 eclairs	13.0	250	47%
cappuccino	1 éclair	12.0	220	49%
(Sara Lee)				
cinnamon roll..deluxe..w/icing	1 roll	15.0	320	42%
coffee cakes				
butter streusel	⅛ cake	9.0	190	43%
crumb	⅛ cake	8.0	190	38%
pecan	⅛ cake	13.0	140	84%
éclair	1 eclair	9.0	190	43%
(Schwan's)				
Freezer-to-Oven				
caramel..w/caramel icing	1 roll	11.0	310	32%
cinnamon..w/icing	1 roll	8.0	290	25%
■ READY-TO-SERVE				
(Athens)..Fillo pastries				
spanakopita..spinach & cheese				
0.5 oz	10 pieces	23.0	390	53%

Food and Description	Amount	Fat Grams	Total Calories	% Fat Calories
1.0 oz	5 pieces	23.0	390	53%
2.0 oz	2½ pieces	23.0	390	53%
Tiropita..3-cheese				
0.5 oz	10 pieces	31.0	450	62%
1.0 oz	5 pieces	31.0	450	62%
2.0 oz	2½ pieces	23.0	390	53%
(Awrey's)				
almond tea bites	1	24.0	430	19%
apple-filled pastry..petite	1	9.0	180	45%
bear claws..gourmet	1	24.0	430	19%
cinnamon rolls..w/cream				
cheese icing	1	27.0	650	37%
cinnamon swirl pastries	1	21.0	430	44%
Danish cinnamon swirl..6-pack	1	15.0	320	42%
long John coffee cake	1 slice	10.0	200	45%
raspberry cheese swirl pastries	1	19.0	400	43%
sweet roll..8-pack Danish	1	15.0	300	45%
(Dunkin' Donuts) (See DONUT and DUNKIN' DONUTS in FAST FOOD section)				
(Entenmann's)				
cinnamon buns..light	1 bun	3.0	170	16%
cinnamon raisin swirl buns	1 bun	13.0	310	38%
cinnamon swirl buns	1 roll	13.0	310	38%
coffee cake..crumb	¹⁄₁₀ cake	12.0	250	43%
crumb cake				
Crumb Delight..light	⅛ cake	6.0	210	26%
Little Bites..crumb cakes	1 pouch	14.0	280	45%
Ultimate for Crumb Lovers	¹⁄₁₀ cake	13.0	250	47%
lemon twist..fat-free	⅛ twist	–	130	–
pecan Danish ring	2-oz piece	15.0	250	54%
Raspberry Twist				
fat-free	⅛ twist	–	140	–
original	⅛ twist	11.0	220	45%
walnut danish ring	2-oz slice	15.0	240	56%
(Hostess)..snack				
cherry sweet rolls	1 roll	6.0	220	25%
cinnamon sweet rolls	1 roll	7.0	210	30%
glazed honey bun	1 bun	19.0	320	53%
iced..frosted honey bun	1 bun	24.0	410	53%
(Lance)..snack				
cinnamon roll	4-oz roll	7.0	370	17%
dunking sticks	1 piece	9.0	180	45%
honey bun	3-oz bun	13.0	320	37%
(Little Debbie)..snack				
boxed				
honey bun..1.78 oz	1 pkg	13.0	230	51%
iced..2 oz	1 pkg	13.0	250	47%
Pecan Spinwheel	1 pkg	4.0	100	36%
individual packages				
honey bun				
3-oz bun	1 bun	23.0	380	54%

Food and Description	Amount	Fat Grams	Total Calories	% Fat Calories
3.98-oz bun	1 bun	28.0	460	55%
Pecan Spinwheel	1 pkg	11.0	220	45%
2 oz	1 pkg	8.0	210	34%
(Otis Spunkmeyer)				
Café Collection				
cinnamon rolls..4 oz	½ roll	5.0	190	24%
Café Collection Crumb Cakes				
apple	1 cake	18.0	370	44%
cheese	1 cake	16.0	340	42%
Danish				
bear claw	2 oz	14.0	250	50%
breakfast claw	2 oz	12.0	240	45%
buttercrumb	2 oz	13.0	250	47%
cinnamon				
Danish	2 oz	13.0	250	47%
roll	1.3 oz	8.0	150	48%
roll	1.1 oz	7.0	140	45%
roll	2.75 oz	17.0	340	45%
roll..giant..4 oz	½ roll	13.0	250	47%
twist	1.8 oz	14.0	230	55%
fruit	2 oz	12.0	240	45%
raisin	2 oz	12.0	240	45%
(Sara Lee)				
breakfast cakes..home-style				
blueberry yogurt	1 slice	11.0	300	33%
lemon poppyseed	1 slice	10.0	300	30%
cinnamon rolls				
Cinnamon Supreme..2.25 oz	1 roll	10.0	240	38%
Cinnamon Supreme..4.25 oz	1 roll	20.0	470	38%
Nutti-Sticky bun..4.0 oz	1 bun	27.0	480	51%
original Cinnaswirl..5.75 oz	1 roll	22.0	600	33%
Danish				
Small				
Demi-Danish..1.25 oz				
apple	1	4.5	120	34%
cheese	1	6.0	130	42%
cinnamon raisin	1	6.0	140	39%
pecan	1	9.0	150	54%
raspberry	1	6.0	130	42%
individually wrapped				
cinnamon rolls				
Ultimate Cinnamon				
roll..4.25 oz	1 roll	25.0	570	39%
single-serve..microwave				
cinnamon roll..4.75 oz	1 roll	26.0	540	43%
Danish..3.25 oz				
apple orchard	1 roll	15.0	340	40%
cinnamon raisin	1 roll	18.0	370	44%
creamy cheese	1 roll	12.0	230	47%
red raspberry	1 roll	15.0	250	39%

Food and Description	Amount	Fat Grams	Total Calories	% Fat Calories
sweet cheese	1 roll	17.0	330	46%
(TastyKake)..snack				
apple fritter..Oxford	1 fritter	9.0	170	48%
honey bun				
glazed	1 bun	22.0	390	51%
iced	1 bun	22.0	400	50%
maple..iced	1 bun	21.0	390	48%
(Wolferman's)				
baklava	1 piece	19.0	337	51%
coffee cake				
blueberry	1 slice	13.0	230	51%
chocolate orange	1 slice	12.0	220	49%
cinnamon almond	1 slice	13.0	250	47%
Povitica				
cream cheese	1 slice	8.0	150	48%
English walnut	1 slice	10.0	180	50%
rugulach	1 slice	8.0	150	48%
PASTRY, TOASTER				
(Kellogg's)..Pop-Tarts				
low-fat..frosted..all flavors	1 pastry	3.0	190	14%
Pastry Swirls				
apple cinnamon	1 pastry	11.0	250	40%
cheese	1 pastry	11.0	260	38%
cheese & cherry	1 pastry	11.0	250	40%
Pop-Tarts..regular..frosted				
blueberry	2 pastries	10.0	400	23%
cinnamon	1 pastry	7.0	210	30%
s'mores	1 pastry	6.0	200	27%
Wild Magicburst	1 pastry	6.0	200	27%
Pop-Tarts..regular...frosted				
all other flavors	1 pastry	5.0	200	23%
Pop-Tarts..regular..unfrosted				
apple cinnamon	1 pastry	6.0	210	26%
blueberry	1 pastry	6.0	210	26%
brown sugar cinnamon	1 pastry	6.0	210	26%
chocolate chip	1 pastry	7.0	220	29%
French toast	1 pastry	8.0	220	33%
Snack-Stix..frosted				
caramel chocolate	1 pastry	6.0	200	26%
cookies & crème	1 pastry	5.0	200	26%
double chocolate	1 pastry	5.0	200	26%
Yogurt Blasts				
blueberry	1 pastry	6.0	210	26%
strawberry	1 pastry	6.0	210	26%
(Pillsbury) Toaster Strudel				
apple	1 pastry	8.0	190	38%
blueberry	1 pastry	8.0	190	38%
brown sugar cinnamon	1 pastry	8.0	190	38%
caramel apple	1 pastry	9.0	200	41%
cherry	1 pastry	8.0	190	38%

Food and Description	Amount	Fat Grams	Total Calories	% Fat Calories
chocolate	1 pastry	9.0	190	43%
cinnamon	1 pastry	8.0	190	38%
cream cheese	1 pastry	11.0	200	50%
cream cheese & cherry	1 pastry	10.0	200	45%
cream cheese & raspberry	1 pastry	10.0	200	45%
cream cheese & strawberry	1 pastry	10.0	200	45%
Danish-style cream cheese	1 pastry	11.0	200	50%
raspberry	1 pastry	8.0	190	38%
strawberry	1 pastry	8.0	190	38%
wild berry	1 pastry	9.0	190	43%
(Quaker)..Breakfast Squares..Toastable				
apple cinnamon brown sugar				
iced	1 pastry	4.5	190	21%
un-iced	1 pastry	5.0	190	24%
blueberry				
iced	1 pastry	4.5	190	21%
un-iced	1 pastry	5.0	190	24%
strawberry				
iced	1 pastry	4.5	190	21%
un-iced	1 pastry	5.0	190	24%
PASTRY DOUGH (*See also* PIE CRUST)				
(Apollo)..fillo dough	3 sheets	1.0	180	5%
(Athens/Apollo Foods)..ready-to-go				
baklava dough				
rectangles	2 pieces	16.0	310	46%
triangles	2 pieces	26.0	540	43%
chocolate				
almond blossoms	2 pieces	37.0	590	56%
almond rolls	4 pieces	34.0	580	53%
swirls	1 swirl	10.0	230	39%
triangles	2 pieces	29.0	550	47%
large shells				
traditional	1 shell	10.0	160	56%
mini shells				
chocolate	2 shells	1.0	35	51%
fillo..traditional	2 shells	2.0	35	51%
graham	2 shells	2.5	35	64%
pastry sheets..fillo				
14"x18"	2½ sheets	1.5	180	7%
12"x17"	3 sheets	1.5	160	8%
pecan				
blossoms	2 pieces	35.0	590	53%
tarts	9 pieces	39.0	600	59%
shredded dough..Kataifi	⅓ pkg	2.0	180	10%
(Pepperidge Farm)				
pastry shell	1 shell	13.0	190	62%
puff pastry dough sheet	⅙ sheet	11.0	170	58%
PÂTÉ (*See also* LUNCHEON MEAT; LUNCHEON MEAT SPREAD; VEGETARIAN FOODS)				
(Boar's Head)				
liverwurst	2 oz	12.0	150	72%

Food and Description	Amount	Fat Grams	Total Calories	% Fat Calories
(Bonavita)				
Swiss..vegetarian	1 oz	4.0	60	60%
(Old Wisconsin Sausage)				
black pepper	2 oz	18.0	210	77%
braunschweiger				
original	2 oz	18.0	210	77%
w/onion & parsley	2 oz	18.0	210	77%
(Sell's)				
liver	¼ cup	14.0	160	79%

PEA (*See also* BLACK-EYED PEA; PEA DISH; PIGEON PEA; PURPLE HULL PEA; SNOW PEA; VEGETABLES, MIXED)

CANNED

Food and Description	Amount	Fat Grams	Total Calories	% Fat Calories
(Blue Boy)				
sweet peas	½ cup	–	70	–
(Bush's Best)..purple hull peas	½ cup	1.0	110	8%
(Del Monte) sweet..all styles	½ cup	–	60	–
(Freshlike)				
Tender Garden	½ cup	0.5	60	8%
no salt	½ cup	0.5	60	8%
(Green Giant)...all styles	½ cup	–	60	–
(LeSueur)				
Early June				
low-salt	½ cup	–	60	–
regular	½ cup	–	60	–
(Libby's)..all styles	½ cup	–	70	–
(Luck's) seasoned w/pork	½ cup	3.0	120	23%
(S&W)				
petit pois..early June	½ cup	–	70	–
sweet..young & tender..medium	½ cup	–	70	–
w/tiny pearl onions	½ cup	–	40	–
(The Allens..East Texas Fair)				
Lady Cream Peas	½ cup	1.0	100	9%
White Acre	½ cup	1.0	100	9%
(Trappey's)..field peas				
w/bacon	½ cup	1.0	90	10%
w/snaps & bacon	½ cup	1.0	110	8%

DRIED

Food and Description	Amount	Fat Grams	Total Calories	% Fat Calories
(Arrowhead Mills)				
green split	¼ cup	0.5	170	3%
(Freida's)	⅓ cup	–	130	–

FRESH

Food and Description	Amount	Fat Grams	Total Calories	% Fat Calories
green..cooked	½ cup	–	67	–
snow..raw				
(Freida's)	1 cup	–	35	–
split..field				
boiled	½ cup	–	115	–
raw	½ cup	1.0	348	3%
sugar snap				
(Dole)	½ cup	–	40	–
(Freida's)	⅔ cup	–	35	–

Food and Description	Amount	Fat Grams	Total Calories	% Fat Calories
FROZEN				
(Birds Eye)				
Baby Pea Gourmet Blend	¾ cup	–	40	–
baby sweet	⅔ cup	0.5	70	6%
butter peas	½ cup	0.5	110	4%
crowder	½ cup	1.0	120	8%
field peas w/snaps	½ cup	0.5	110	4%
green	⅔ cup	0.5	70	6%
purple hull	½ cup	0.5	110	4%
sugar snap..deluxe	½ cup	–	45	–
sweet peas..w/pearl onions	⅔ cup	0.5	60	8%
(C&W)				
petite	⅔ cup	0.5	70	6%
sugar snap	⅔ cup	–	35	–
(Cascadian Farm)				
peas & pearl onions	¾ cup	–	60	–
sugar snap peas	¾ cup	–	35	–
(Green Giant)				
Boil-in-Bag				
baby sweet peas	⅔ cup	–	80	–
baby sweet peas & butter	¾ cup	1.5	90	15%
sugar snap peas	⅔ cup	–	50	–
sweet peas & pearl onions	½ cup	–	50	–
sugar snap peas	¾ cup	–	35	–
sweet peas				
plain	½ cup	0.5	70	6%
select	⅔ cup	0.5	60	8%
PEA, BLACK-EYED (*See* BLACK-EYED PEA)				
PEA, PIGEON (*See* PIGEON PEA)				
PEA, PURPLE HULL (*See* PURPLE HULL PEA)				
PEA, SNOW (*See* SNOW PEA)				
PEACH				
CAN OR CUP				
(Del Monte)				
cups..plastic				
diced	1 bowl	–	70	–
strawberry banana..flavored	1 bowl	–	70	–
freestone				
halves..heavy syrup	½ cup	–	100	–
individual pull-top can				
slices..heavy syrup	1 can	–	100	–
slices..heavy syrup	½ cup	–	100	–
light	½ cup	–	60	–
halves				
heavy syrup	½ cup	–	100	–
light	½ cup	–	60	–
Harvest Spice..sliced	½ cup	–	80	–
pull-top cans..4 oz				
diced..light syrup	1 can	–	80	–
in 100% juice	1 can	–	60	–

Food and Description	Amount	Fat Grams	Total Calories	% Fat Calories
light	1 can	–	50	–
sliced..light	1 can	–	60	–
pull-top cans..4.5 oz				
raspberry-flavored				
chunks..light syrup	1 can	–	80	–
slices..heavy syrup	1 can	–	100	–
sliced peaches				
100% juice	½ cup	–	60	–
heavy syrup	½ cup	–	100	–
raspberry-flavored	½ cup	–	80	–
spiced..whole	½ cup	–	100	–
yellow cling				
fruit naturals..chunks	½ cup	–	70	–
orchard select..jar				
sliced	½ cup	–	80	–
(Dole)				
Fruit Bowls				
diced	4 oz cup	–	70	–
in strawberry gel	4.3 oz cup	–	80	–
yellow cling..sliced				
in light syrup	3.5 oz	–	80	–
(Libby's)..light..in juice				
halves	½ cup	–	50	–
sliced	½ cup	–	50	–
(S&W)				
halves..light syrup	½ cup	–	70	–
slices				
heavy syrup	½ cup	–	100	–
light syrup	½ cup	-	70	–
natural-style	½ cup	–	80	–
snow peaches...light syrup	½ cup	–	80	–
sun peaches	½ cup	–	80	–
Sweet Memory..w/cinnamon	½ cup	–	80	–
Tropical Sun	½ cup	–	80	–
whole/spiced/in heavy syrup	1 peach	–	100	–
DRIED				
(Del Monte) sun-dried	⅓ cup	–	90	–
(Mariani)	¼ cup	–	140	–
(Sun Maid)	¼ cup	–	100	–
(SunSweet)	¼ cup	–	140	–
FRESH				
peeled..sliced	½ cup	–	37	–
whole	1 medium	–	37	–
(Dole)	1 medium	–	40	–
FROZEN				
(Big Valley) freestone	⅔ cup	–	50	–
(C&W) sliced	⅔ cup	–	50	–
PEACH BUTTER				
(Smucker's)	1 Tbs	–	50	–

Food and Description	Amount	Fat Grams	Total Calories	% Fat Calories

PEACH JUICE/JUICE BLEND/JUICE DRINK (*See also* FRUIT PUNCH; SOFT DRINK; SOFT DRINK MIX)
BOTTLED, BOXED, OR CANNED

Food and Description	Amount	Fat Grams	Total Calories	% Fat Calories
(Dole)				
peach mango				
100% juice blend	8 fl oz	–	140	–
	10 fl oz	–	170	–
(Goya) nectar	6 fl oz	–	110	–
(Kern's)				
nectar	11.5 oz	–	200	
	8 fl oz	–	150	–
	6.59 oz	–	110	–
from concentrate	8 fl oz	–	130	–
(Libby's) Juicy Juice	8 fl oz	–	130	–
(R. W. Knudsen)				
After the Fall..Georgia peach	8 fl oz	–	100	–
nectar	8 fl oz	–	120	-
peach spritzer	12 fl oz	–	160	–
(Snapple)..juice drinks				
peach tea..diet	8 fl oz	–	<1	–
(V8 Splash)				
juice drink..peach lemonade	8 fl oz	–	110	–
smoothie..peach mango	8 fl oz	–	120	-
FROZEN..prepared, unless otherwise noted				
(Dole)..Orchard Peach 100% juice blend	8 fl oz		140	–
PEANUT				
(Ballpark)	1 oz	15.0	180	75%
(Barcelona)..Virginia blanched				
salted peanuts	¼ cup	17.0	200	77%
unsalted peanuts	¼ cup	17.0	200	77%
(Eagle)				
lightly salted	1 oz	15.0	180	75%
oil honey-roasted	1 oz	13.0	170	69%
roasted	1 oz	15.0	180	75%
(Fisher)				
dry..honey-roasted	1 oz	13.0	170	69%
dry..roasted	1 oz	14.0	170	74%
golden..dry-roasted	1 oz	14.0	170	74%
honey-roasted	1 oz	13.0	170	68%
oil-roasted	1 oz	15.0	170	79%
party	1 oz	14.0	160	79%
raw..Chef's Naturals	1 oz	11.0	160	62%
salted in shell..dry-roasted	1 oz	14.0	160	78%
Spanish..redskin..12-oz can	1 oz	16.0	180	80%
(Guy's)				
dry-roasted	1 oz	14.0	170	74%
Spanish/salted	1 oz	14.0	170	74%
(kettle)..hand-crafted nuts				
honey-roast peanuts	1 oz	12.0	160	68%

Food and Description	Amount	Fat Grams	Total Calories	% Fat Calories
Spanish..jumbo..salted	1 oz	14.0	160	79%
Spanish..raw	1 oz	14.0	160	79%
(Lance)				
honey-roasted				
1.75-oz pkg	1 pkg	15.0	220	61%
hot 'n' spicy..1.75-oz pkg	1 pkg	21.0	290	65%
salted..original..1.75-oz pkg	1 pkg	15.0	200	68%
(Mojave)				
peanuts				
w/mild chile	1 oz	14.0	160	79%
w/spicy chile	1 oz	14.0	160	79%
(Planters)				
cocktail				
family pack	1 oz	14.0	170	74%
honey-roasted..Sweet 'n' Crunchy	1 oz	14.0	170	74%
lightly salted	1 oz	15.0	170	79%
party pack..unsalted	1 oz	14.0	170	74%
dry-roasted	1 oz	13.0	160	73%
lightly salted	1 oz	14.0	170	74%
unsalted	1 oz	14.0	160	79%
honey..dry-roasted	1 oz	13.0	160	73%
honey-roasted				
original	1 oz	13.0	160	73%
oil-roasted				
cocktail	1 oz	14.0	170	74%
lightly salted	1 oz	15.0	170	79%
unsalted	1 oz	14.0	170	74%
red-skin	1 oz	14.0	180	70%
Spanish				
oil roasted	1 oz	14.0	170	74%
raw	1 oz	13.0	150	78%
Sweet 'n' Crunchy	1 oz	7.0	140	45%
PEANUT BUTTER				
(Arrowhead Mills)				
100% Valencia/sodium-free				
creamy	2 Tbs	15.0	200	68%
crunchy	2 Tbs	15.0	200	68%
(Bama)				
creamy	2 Tbs	17.0	200	77%
crunchy	2 Tbs	17.0	200	77%
swirl				
grape..w/peanut butter	2 Tbs	5.0	120	38%
strawberry..w/peanut butter	2 Tbs	5.0	120	38%
(Erewhon)				
chunky				
regular	2 Tbs	14.0	190	66%
unsalted	2 Tbs	14.0	190	66%
creamy				
regular	2 Tbs	14.0	190	66%
unsalted	2 Tbs	14.0	190	66%

Food and Description	Amount	Fat Grams	Total Calories	% Fat Calories
(Estee)				
creamy	2 Tbs	15.0	190	71%
crunchy	2 Tbs	15.0	190	71%
(Fisher)				
creamy	2 Tbs	16.0	200	72%
crunchy	2 Tbs	16.0	200	72%
(Jif)				
original				
creamy	2 Tbs	16.0	190	76%
extra-crunchy	2 Tbs	16.0	190	76%
reduced-fat				
creamy	2 Tbs	12.0	190	57%
crunchy	2 Tbs	12.0	190	57%
Simply Jif				
creamy	2 Tbs	16.0	190	76%
crunchy	2 Tbs	16.0	190	76%
(Laura Scudder's)				
old-fashioned				
creamy				
regular	2 Tbs	16.0	200	72%
unsalted	2 Tbs	16.0	200	72%
nutty				
regular	2 Tbs	16.0	200	72%
unsalted	2 Tbs	16.0	200	72%
reduced-fat..creamy	2 Tbs	12.0	220	49%
(Peter Pan)				
creamy				
regular	2 Tbs	16.0	190	75%
very low sodium	2 Tbs	17.0	200	77%
crunchy				
regular	2 Tbs	16.0	190	75%
very low sodium	2 Tbs	17.0	200	77%
Smart Choice spread				
creamy	2 Tbs	11.0	180	55%
crunchy	2 Tbs	12.0	190	57%
whipped				
creamy	2 Tbs	13.0	150	78%
crunchy	2 Tbs	13.0	150	78%
(Roaster Fresh) gourmet..unsalted	2 Tbs	14.0	170	74%
(Skippy)				
Doubly Delicious				
w/Nestlé Crunch pieces	2 Tbs	15.0	210	64%
w/Nestlé Toll House pieces	2 Tbs	15.0	210	64%
reduced-fat				
creamy	2 Tbs	12.0	190	57%
super-chunk	2 Tbs	12.0	180	60%
roasted honey nut..creamy	2 Tbs	17.0	190	81%
super-chunk	2 Tbs	17.0	190	81%
Squeez'it..tube..creamy	2 Tbs	17.0	190	81%

Food and Description	Amount	Fat Grams	Total Calories	% Fat Calories
(Smucker's)				
Chocolate Silk Smooth Sensation	2 Tbs	12.0	190	57%
Goober PB&J				
grape	3 Tbs	13.0	230	51%
strawberry	3 Tbs	13.0	230	51%
old-fashioned natural				
all types..regular	2 Tbs	16.0	200	72%
all types..reduced-fat	2 Tbs	12.0	190	57%
PEAR				
Candied	1 oz	–	86	–
CANNED OR JARRED				
(Del Monte)				
halves				
in extra-light syrup..light	½ cup	–	60	–
in heavy syrup	½ cup	–	100	–
in light syrup				
cinnamon-flavored	½ cup	–	80	–
in pear juice..Fruit Naturals	½ cup	–	60	–
Orchard Select..sliced Bartlett	½ cup	–	80	–
Individual pull-top cans..4 oz				
diced				
in heavy syrup	1 can	–	80	–
lite	1 can	–	50	–
sliced				
in extra-light syrup..light	½ cup	–	60	–
in heavy syrup	½ cup	–	100	–
(Libby's) light				
halves	½ cup	–	60	–
sliced	½ cup	–	60	–
(S&W)				
Bartlett halves				
in heavy syrup	½ cup	–	90	–
California Sun..light syrup	½ cup	–	80	–
natural-style..Bartlett				
halved	½ cup	–	80	–
sliced	½ cup	–	80	–
quartered..in heavy syrup	½ cup	–	90	–
sliced..in pear juice	½ cup	–	80	–
FRESH				
Bartlett	1 medium	1.0	100	9%
California Sun..ready-cut	½ cup	–	80	–
D'Anjou				
sliced	1 cup	0.7	97	6%
whole	1 medium	1.0	120	8%
(Dole)	1 medium	1.0	100	9%
PEAR JUICE/NECTAR				
CANNED..Jarred				
(Goya) nectar	6 fl oz	–	120	–
(Kern's) nectar	12 fl oz	–	220	–
(Libby's) nectar	6 fl oz	–	110	–

Food and Description	Amount	Fat Grams	Total Calories	% Fat Calories
PECAN				
(Azar)..all types	1 oz	21.0	210	90%
(Diamond of California)				
all types	¼ cup	21.0	220	86%
(Fisher)..all types	1 oz	20.0	200	90%
(Planters)				
chips	2 oz	40.0	390	92%
halves				
Gold Measure	2 oz	40.0	390	92%
regular	1 oz	20.0	190	95%
honey-roasted	1 oz	16.0	180	80%
pieces	1 oz	20.0	190	95%
	2 oz	40.0	390	92%
PEPPER (*See also* MEXICAN FOOD; PEPPER, GROUND; SEASONINGS)				
CANNED or JARRED				
(Arnold's) Chilito's Encurtidos	1 oz	–	10	–
(B&G)				
hot jalapeños..slices	1 oz	–	–	–
roasted	1 oz	–	–	–
w/garlic	1 oz	0.5	15	30%
w/imported balsamic vinegar	1 oz	–	10	–
Sandwich Toppers				
peppers				
hot..chopped	1 oz	–	–	–
sweet bell	1 oz	–	20	–
sweet	1 oz	–	10	–
sweet red	2 oz	–	20	–
(Hebrew National)				
fillet peppers	1 oz	–	9	–
hot cherry	1 oz	–	11	–
red fillet peppers	1 oz	–	9	–
(Heinz)				
banana..hot	1 pepper	–	6	–
hot rings..slices	1 pepper	–	4	–
mild sweet	1 pepper	–	8	–
Sweet Pepper Momentos	1 pepper	–	6	–
(Mt. Olive)				
banana peppers..hot	1 oz	–	10	–
cherry rings	1 oz	–	10	–
chow-chow				
hot	1 oz	–	15	–
mild	1 oz	–	15	–
jalapeño slices	2 oz	–	5	–
pepper rings				
banana..hot	1 oz	–	10	–
banana..mild	1 oz	–	10	–
pepperoncini				
imported	1 oz	–	10	–
sweet 'n' hot peppers..salad	1 oz	–	40	–

Food and Description	Amount	Fat Grams	Total Calories	% Fat Calories
(Progresso) drained				
cherry	2 Tbs	2.0	30	60%
fried..sweet..w/onions	2 Tbs	1.5	20	68%
hot cherry				
sliced	2 Tbs	2.0	25	72%
whole	1 pepper	–	10	–
pepper salad	2 Tbs	1.0	15	60%
roasted	2 peppers	–	10	–
Tuscan	3 peppers	–	10	–
(Trappey's)				
banana				
slices	21 slices	–	6	–
whole	3 peppers	–	6	–
cherry				
hot	1 oz	–	10	–
mild	1 oz	–	10	–
hot..in vinegar	1 oz	–	10	–
jalapeño..hot				
sliced	1 oz	–	5	–
whole	1 oz	–	10	–
serrano..hot	1 oz	–	10	–
Tempero..Greek				
pepperoncini mild	1 pepper	–	10	–
Torrido..Santa Fe				
grande..hot	1 pepper	–	10	–
(Vlasic)				
banana..hot	1 oz	–	4	–
cherry				
hot	1 oz	–	10	–
mild	1 oz	–	8	–
Greek pepperoncini salad				
hot	1 oz	–	10	–
mild	1 oz	–	5	–
Mexican..hot	1 oz	–	8	–
Mexican..tiny hot	1 oz	–	6	–
DRIED				
green	1 Tbs	–	1	–
red	1 Tbs	–	1	–
FRESH..whole				
green chili..hot	1 medium	–	15	–
jalapeño	2 medium	–	14	–
red chili..hot	1 medium	–	18	–
red or green..sweet	1 medium	–	18	–
yellow..sweet	1 medium	–	50	–
FROZEN				
(Birds Eye) green & red..stir-fry	3 oz	–	25	–
(C&W) green & red/strips	3 oz	–	25	–
PEPPER, GROUND (See also SEASONINGS)				
(Durkee)				
black	1 tsp	–	8	–

Food and Description	Amount	Fat Grams	Total Calories	% Fat Calories
red/cayenne	1 tsp	–	8	–
white	1 tsp	–	9	–
(Lawry's) lemon	1 tsp	–	6	–
PEPPER POT SOUP (See SOUP)				
PEPPERONI (See SAUSAGE)				
PERCH (See OCEAN PERCH; SEAFOOD ENTRÉE/DINNER; WHITE PERCH)				
PERSIMMON				
Japanese/kaki				
dried	1 medium	<1.0	93	5%
fresh	1 medium	<1.0	118	4%
native/fresh	1 medium	–	32	–
PHEASANT/raw				
breast meat	~6 oz	5.9	243	22%
giblets	3 oz	4.0	119	30%
leg meat	~4 oz	4.6	143	29%
meat & skin	~1 lb	42.0	825	46%
meat only	~¾ lb	12.8	470	25%
PHYLLO DOUGH (See PASTRY DOUGH)				
PICANTE SAUCE (See MEXICAN FOOD; SAUCE)				
PICCALILLI (See PICKLE RELISH)				
PICKLE (See also PICKLE RELISH)				
(Arnold's)				
dill..all types	1 oz	–	–	–
Garden Mix..So Hot	1 oz	–	–	–
(Cascadian Farm)				
baby dills	1 oz	–	5	–
Baby Sweets	1 oz	–	30	–
bread & butter chips	1 oz	–	30	–
kosher dill..all types	1 oz	–	5	–
sweet relish	1 Tbs	–	20	–
(Claussen)				
bread 'n' butter				
chips	4 slices	–	20	–
sandwich slices	2 slices	0.5	20	23%
half-sours..New York deli-style	½ pickle	–	5	–
hamburger dills				
chips	10 chips	–	5	–
slices chips	10 slices	–	5	–
hearty garlic..deli-style				
sandwich slices	1 oz	–	5	–
wholes	1 oz	–	5	–
kosher dills..all types	1 oz	–	5	–
sweet gherkins	1 oz	–	30	–
sweet pickle relish	1 Tbs	–	15	–
(Del Monte)				
pickle relish				
hamburger-style	1 Tbs	–	20	–
hot dog–style	1 Tbs	–	15	–
sweet..all sizes	2 oz	–	40	–

Food and Description	Amount	Fat Grams	Total Calories	% Fat Calories
pickles				
Dill..all types	1 oz	–	5	–
dill chips	1 oz	–	40	–
gherkins	1 oz	–	40	–
midget	1 oz	–	40	–
sweet				
chips	1 oz	–	5	–
whole..all types	1 oz	–	40	–
(Hebrew National)				
half-sour	1 oz	–	4	–
kosher				
barrel-cured dill				
hot	1 pouch	–	23	–
regular	1 pouch	–	23	–
other..all types	1 oz	–	4	–
(Heifetz)				
kosher dill..all types	1 oz	–	–	–
Picklevator				
bread & butter chips	1 oz	–	30	–
hamburger chips	1 oz	–	–	–
sweet midgets	1 oz	–	35	–
(Heinz)				
hot garlic	1 oz	–	6	–
kosher				
dill..all types	1 oz	–	–	–
old-fashioned..all types	1 oz	–	–	–
pickled cucumbers	2 spears	–	13	–
Polish-style				
dill..all types	1 oz	–	4	–
Polskie ogorki	1 oz	–	6	–
processed dill	1 oz	–	2	–
sour	1 oz	–	3	–
sweet				
gherkins..midget or regular	1 oz	–	35	–
mixed	1 oz	–	40	–
pickles	1 oz	–	35	–
salad cubes	1 oz	–	30	–
slices	1 oz	–	35	–
sweet cucumber				
slices	1 oz	–	20	–
stix	1 oz	–	25	–
(Mrs. Klein's) fancy imported				
pepperoncini	1 oz	–	5	–
Southern hot mix	1 oz	–	–	–
(Mt. Olive)				
bread & butter	1 oz	–	25	–
no sugar added	1 oz	–	–	–
old-fashioned sweet	1 oz	–	25	–
old-fashioned sweet..strips	1 oz	–	20	–
zesty..chips	1 oz	–	25	–

Food and Description	Amount	Fat Grams	Total Calories	% Fat Calories
dill..all types	1 oz	–	–	–
hot..mixed	1 oz	–	–	–
jalapeño dill strips	1 oz	–	–	–
salad cubes				
dill	1 Tbs	–	–	–
sweet cubes	1 Tbs	–	15	–
green	1 Tbs	–	20	–
red	1 Tbs	–	20	–
sweet	1 oz	–	35	–
cucumber strips	1 oz	–	20	–
gherkins..no sugar added	1 oz	–	–	–
midgets	1 oz	–	35	–
super-sweet dill strips	1 oz	–	40	–
(Peter Piper's)				
bread & butter..all types	1 oz	–	30	–
(Rosoff's)..all types	1 oz	–	4	–
(Schorr's)				
bread & butter	1 oz	–	12	–
kosher..all types	1 oz	–	4	–
sour				
garlic whole	1 oz	–	3	–
half spears	1 oz	–	4	–
halves	1 oz	–	4	–
(Steinfeld's)				
crunchy..all types	1 oz	–	5	–
garlic dills	1 oz	–	5	–
Greek pepperoncini	1 oz	–	5	–
home-style dills	1 oz	–	5	–
kosher..all types	1 oz	–	5	–
Polish dills	1 oz	–	5	–
sandwich builders				
bread & butter	1 oz	–	35	–
kosher dill..all types	1 oz	–	5	–
Polish dill	1 oz	–	–	–
zesty dill	1 oz	–	7	–
sweet	1 oz	–	30	–
midget	1 oz	–	30	–
cucumber chips	1 oz	–	30	–
(Vlasic)				
Half-the-Salt				
hamburger dill chips	1 oz	–	2	–
kosher crunchy dills	1 oz	–	4	–
kosher dill spears	1 oz	–	4	–
sweet butter chips	1 oz	–	30	–
kosher..all types	1 oz	–	4	–
no garlic..all types	1 oz	–	4	–
refrigerated				
deli bread & butter	1 oz	–	25	–
deli dill halves	1 oz	–	4	–

Food and Description	Amount	Fat Grams	Total Calories	% Fat Calories
regular				
bread & butter chunks	1 oz	–	25	–
original dills				
original dills	1 oz	–	2	–
Polish snack chunks	1 oz	–	4	–
sweet butter chips	1 oz	–	30	–
sweet butter stix	1 oz	–	18	–
sweet gherkins	1 oz	–	35	–
zesty..all types	1 oz	–	4	–
PICKLE RELISH (See also PICKLE)				
(Arnold's) sweet	1 Tbs	–	15	–
(Cascadian Farm)				
dill	1 Tbs	–	5	–
sweet	1 Tbs	–	20	–
(Claussen)..sweet	1 Tbs	–	15	–
(Hebrew National)..sweet..green	1 Tbs	–	18	–
(Heinz)				
piccalilli	1 oz	–	30	–
relish				
dill	1 Tbs	–	–	–
hamburger	1 Tbs	–	15	–
hot dog	1 Tbs	–	15	–
sweet	1 Tbs	–	30	–
(Mt. Olive)..all types	1 Tbs	–	20	–
(Steinfeld's)..sweet relish	1 Tbs	–	20	–
(Vlasic)				
piccalilli				
green tomato	1 oz	–	35	–
hot	1 oz	–	35	–
relish				
dill	1 oz	–	2	–
hamburger	1 oz	–	40	–
hot dog	1 oz	<1.0	40	11%
India	1 oz	–	30	–
PIE & COBBLER (See also PIE CRUST; PIE FILLING)				
■ **FROZEN OR REFRIGERATED**				
(Chef Pierre)				
CREAM PIES...10"				
apples..cinnamon..cream				
Fruit de la Cream	⅛ pie	26.0	430	54%
banana..Crème de la Cream	⅒ pie	25.0	360	63%
chocolate cream layer	⅛ pie	37.0	520	64%
chocolate Crème de la Cream	⅛ pie	32.0	470	61%
coconut..Crème de la Cream	⅛ pie	20.0	350	51%
cookies & cream				
Crème de la Cream	⅛ pie	28.0	410	61%
Crème de la Cream..variety pack	⅒ pie	17.0	300	51%
double chocolate				
Crème de la Cream	⅒ pie	19.0	360	48%

Food and Description	Amount	Fat Grams	Total Calories	% Fat Calories
gourmet				
chocolate peanut butter silk	⅛ pie	35.0	500	63%
French silk	⅛ pie	40.0	570	63%
	1/10 pie	37.0	520	64%
peanut butter crème	⅛ pie	30.0	460	59%
pumpkin cream layer	⅛ pie	23.0	380	54%
strawberries & cream				
Fruit de la Cream	⅛ pie	24.0	400	54%
toffee crunch				
Crème de la Cream	1/9 pie	29.0	430	61%
MERINGUE PIES				
gourmet				
chocolate	1/10 pie	12.0	320	34%
coconut	1/10 pie	14.0	340	37%
lemon	1/10 pie	8.0	290	25%
lemon layer	1/10 pie	13.0	310	38%
traditonal				
chocolate..traditional	⅛ pie	16.0	370	39%
chocolate icebox..condensed	1/9 pie	15.0	340	40%
coconut..traditional	⅛ pie	14.0	340	37%
coconut icebox..condensed	1/9 pie	12.0	330	33%
key lime	⅛ pie	15.0	440	31%
Key West lime icebox				
condensed	⅛ pie	16.0	460	31%
lemon..traditional	⅛ pie	9.0	290	28%
lemon icebox..condensed	⅛ pie	10.0	380	24%
lime icebox..condensed	⅛ pie	9.0	360	23%
*OPEN-FACED..SPECIALTY..*10" pies				
French coconut	⅛ pie	22.0	490	40%
pumpkin	1/10 pie	11.0	320	31%
Southern pecan	1/10 pie	27.0	570	43%
sweet potato	1/9 pie	19.0	400	43%
*TRADITIONAL..*10" pies				
apple..full-crust topping	⅛ pie	15.0	350	39%
banana cream	⅛ pie	22.0	400	50%
Boston cream	3 oz slice	7.0	220	29%
chocolate cream	⅙ pie	23.0	410	50%
coconut cream	⅛ pie	25.0	430	52%
lemon cream	⅙ pie	23.0	420	49%
strawberry cream	⅙ pie	23.0	420	49%
(Edward's)				
chocolate butter pecan..limited	⅛ pie	32.0	560	51%
Family Recipe				
Georgia pecan				
22 oz	⅕ pie	23.0	450	46%
lemon meringue				
22 oz	⅕ pie	8.0	350	21%
34 oz.ready-to-serve	⅛ pie	8.0	350	21%
Gourmet				
key lime				
36 oz.ready-to-serve	⅛ pie	22.0	440	45%

Food and Description	Amount	Fat Grams	Total Calories	% Fat Calories
Mocha Mudslide				
36-oz ready-to-serve	⅛ pie	21.0	410	46%
pecan cheesecake				
36-oz ready-to-serve	⅛ pie	27.0	530	46%
turtle				
36-oz ready-to-serve	⅛ pie	21.0	390	48%
Sundae Creations..ready-to-serve				
25.5-oz ready-to-serve				
caramel	⅙ pie	25.0	440	51%
chocolate	⅙ pie	32.0	480	60%
cookie dough..ready-to-serve	⅙ pie	25.0	450	50%
strawberry	⅙ pie	22.0	410	48%
(Marie Callender's)..cobblers				
apple	¼ cobbler	20.0	370	49%
berry				
10 oz	½ cobbler	18.0	380	43%
16 oz	¼ cobbler	21.0	370	51%
cherry	¼ cobbler	19.0	380	45%
peach	¼ cobbler	18.0	400	41%
(Mrs. Smith's)				
COBBLERS				
apple	⅛ pie	10.0	270	33%
w/toasted oatmeal topping	⅛ pie	11.0	280	35%
blackberry	⅛ pie	10.0	260	35%
cherry	⅛ pie	10.0	280	32%
w/almond crumb topping	⅛ pie	11.0	290	34%
peach.. 2 # cobbler	⅛ pie	10.0	230	39%
strawberry..w/toasted oatmeal				
crumb top	⅛ pie	12.0	330	33%
PIES..CREAM				
Boston cream	⅒ pie	9.0	210	34%
Caramel Caribou..2-count	1 pie	20.0	350	51%
chocolate..Restaurant Classics				
French silk	⅛ pie	32.0	490	59%
chocolate..Soda Shoppe	⅛ pie	18.0	340	48%
coconut custard	⅛ pie	12.0	250	43%
Moose Tracks..2-count	1 pie	22.0	370	54%
Soda Shoppe..coconut cream	⅛ pie	20.0	360	50%
PIES..FRUIT				
apple				
caramel..flip-it cakes	½ pkg	13.0	480	24%
crumb..deep-dish	⅒ pie	13.0	320	37%
deep-dish	¹⁄₁₂ pie	16.0	330	44%
Dutch apple crumb	⅛ pie	16.0	360	40%
no sugar added	⅛ pie	20.0	350	51%
old-fashioned	⅛ pie	17.0	350	44%
berries..deep-dish..Festival of..	⅒ pie	13.0	300	39%
blueberry	⅛ pie	17.0	330	46%
cherry	⅛ pie	17.0	340	45%
deep-dish crumb	⅒ pie	12.0	300	36%

Food and Description	Amount	Fat Grams	Total Calories	% Fat Calories
peach				
deep-dish	1/10 pie	12.0	270	40%
traditional	1/8 pie	17.0	320	48%
strawberry..w/toasted oatmeal				
crumb-top	1/6 pie	12.0	330	33%
strawberry delight..flip-it cakes	1/2 pkg	9.0	380	21%
PIES..OTHER				
key lime..authentic				
2-count box	1/2 pkg	17.0	410	37%
restaurant classics	1/8 pie	17.0	410	37%
lemon meringue	1/8 pie	11.0	290	34%
mince	1/8 pie	17.0	380	40%
pecan				
5-lb's	1/18 pie	12.0	270	40%
Southern..Special Recipe	1/8 pie	26.0	550	43%
pumpkin				
custard	1/8 pie	9.0	240	34%
hearty	1/8 pie	10.0	260	35%
Special Recipe..homemade	1/10 pie	11.0	280	35%
red raspberry	1/8 pie	17.0	340	45%
sweet potato	1/8 pie	15.0	330	41%
(Pet-Ritz)				
COBBLERS..home-style				
apple cinnamon	1/6 pie	12.0	280	39%
blackberry	1/6 pie	12.0	260	42%
cherry	1/6 pie	11.0	300	33%
peach	1/6 pie	10.0	240	38%
PIES..home-style				
apple	1/4 pie	18.0	380	43%
berry banana cream	1/4 pie	18.0	320	51%
cherry	1/4 pie	18.0	400	41%
chocolate drizzle cream	1/4 pie	18.0	330	49%
coconut cream..toasted	1/4 pie	19.0	330	52%
lemon razz	1/4 pie	18.0	320	51%
(Sara Lee's)				
COBBLER ANYTIME..2-count box				
apple	1	17.0	350	44%
blackberry	1	17.0	350	44%
peach	1	17.0	340	45%
DESSERT CUPS				
Boston cream	1 cup	11.0	310	32%
PIES				
French silk..24 oz	1/5 pie	21.0	340	56%
lemon meringue..tangy..30 oz	1/6 pie	5.0	220	20%
tropical coconut cream..24 oz	1/5 pie	11.0	330	30%
PIES..OVEN-FRESH..37 oz				
apple	1/8 pie	16.0	340	42%
blueberry	1/8 pie	15.0	360	38%
cherry	1/8 pie	14.0	320	39%
Dutch apple	1/8 pie	15.0	350	39%

Food and Description	Amount	Fat Grams	Total Calories	% Fat Calories
mince	⅛ pie	15.0	370	36%
peach	⅛ pie	13.0	330	35%
pumpkin	⅛ pie	11.0	260	38%
raspberry	⅛ pie	16.0	360	40%
Southern sweet potato	⅛ pie	10.0	280	50%
SIGNATURE SELECTIONS				
apple..orchard deep-dish	1/10 pie	24.0	400	54%
caramel apple nut	1/9 pie	18.0	370	43%
cherry..deep-dish gourmet	1/10 pie	18.0	380	43%
cinnamon French apple	1/10 pie	15.0	360	38%
dulce de leche				
caramel swirl	⅛ pie	26.0	400	59%
Fruits of the Forest	1/9 pie	17.0	340	45%
golden peach..deep-dish	1/10 pie	16.0	340	42%
Key West lime	⅛ pie	25.0	400	56%
pumpkin..traditional	1/10 pie	9.0	250	32%
Southern pecan	⅛ pie	24.0	520	42%
strawberries & crème	⅛ pie	27.0	400	61%
(Schwan's)				
Andes mint cream pie	1 piece	28.0	500	50%
apple...old-fashioned	1/12 pie	15.0	320	42%
peach	1/10 pie	16.0	330	44%
pecan caramel cream slices	1 slice	15.0	280	48%
(Weight Watchers)..Smart Ones				
key lime pie	1 piece	6.0	200	27%
peanut butter pie	1 piece	6.0	210	26%
■ **READY TO SERVE**				
(Break Cake) snack..fried pie				
apple	1 pie	14.0	255	49%
cherry	1 pie	14.0	250	50%
(Entenmann's) pie				
original				
apple..home-style	1 serving	16.0	370	39%
coconut custard	1 serving	8.0	140	51%
(Hostess) snack				
apple	1 pie	22.0	480	45%
blackberry	1 pie	21.0	520	36%
blueberry	1 pie	21.0	480	39%
cherry	1 pie	22.0	470	42%
French apple	1 pie	22.0	480	41%
lemon	1 pie	24.0	500	43%
peach	1 pie	21.0	480	39%
pineapple	1 pie	21.0	460	41%
strawberry fruit	1 pie	23.0	510	41%
(Lance)..snack..pecan	3 oz	17.0	350	44%
(Tastykake) snack				
apple	1 pie	11.0	260	38%
banana	1 pie	15.0	370	36%
blueberry	1 pie	10.0	290	31%
cherry	1 pie	10.0	290	31%

Food and Description	Amount	Fat Grams	Total Calories	% Fat Calories
coconut crème	1 pie	20.0	370	49%
French apple	1 pie	12.0	330	33%
lemon	1 pie	13.0	300	39%
peach	1 pie	10.0	270	33%
pineapple	1 pie	12.0	290	37%
pineapple cheese	1 pie	11.0	290	34%
pumpkin	1 pie	12.0	320	34%
strawberry	1 pie	12.0	330	33%
Tastyklair	1 pie	20.0	390	46%
PIE CRUST (See also PASTRY)				
■ **FROZEN**				
(Chef Pierre)..food service..unbaked				
deep-dish..9" deep-dish crust	⅛ crust	8.0	130	55%
regular/10" crust	⅛ crust	7.0	110	57%
vegetable shortening				
9" deep-dish crust	⅛ crust	8.0	130	55%
10" crust	⅛ crust	8.0	120	60%
(Mrs. Smith's)				
flaky home-style..9" deep-dish	⅒ crust	7.0	120	53%
home-style shortbread pastry				
9" deep-dish	⅟₁₆ crust	8.0	130	55%
regular..9"	⅛ crust	7.0	100	63%
(Oronoque)				
6" crust	¼ crust	7.0	110	57%
9" deep-dish crust	⅛ crust	7.0	100	63%
9" regular	⅛ crust	6.0	80	68%
(Pepperidge Farm)..patty shells	1 shell	13.0	190	62%
(Pet-Ritz)..Ready-to-Bake				
deep-dish				
all-vegetable	⅛ crust	4.5	80	51%
9"	⅛ crust	5.0	90	50%
regular				
all-vegetable	⅛ crust	4.5	80	51%
9" crust	⅛ crust	4.0	80	45%
■ **MIX**				
(Betty Crocker) 9" crust..prepared	⅛ crust	8.0	110	65%
(Flako)..mix only	¼ cup	8.0	130	55%
(Jiffy)..mix only	¼ cup	4.0	160	23%
(Krusteaz)				
9" crust..baked	⅛ crust	5.0	90	50%
(Nabisco)..prepared				
Honey Maid..graham..9"	⅛ crust	7.0	140	45%
Nilla/cookie crumb..9"	⅛ crust	7.0	140	45%
Oreo/cookie crumb..9"	⅛ crust	7.0	140	45%
(Pillsbury)..mix only	2 Tbs	6.0	100	54%
■ **READY TO USE**				
(Keebler) Ready Crust				
chocolate				
9" pie	⅛ crust	4.5	90	45%
single-serve	1 tart	5.0	110	41%

Food and Description	Amount	Fat Grams	Total Calories	% Fat Calories
graham cracker				
9" pie	.75 oz	5.0	110	41%
	.92 oz	6.0	130	42%
reduced-fat	⅛ crust	3.5	90	35%
single-serve tarts	1 tart	6.0	120	45%
shortbread	⅛ crust	5.0	110	41%
(Pillsbury) refrigerated	⅛ crust	7.0	120	53%
PIE FILLING (*See also* PUDDING & MOUSSE)				
■ **CANNED OR JARRED**				
(Borden)..None Such mincemeat				
original..classic..condensed	½ cup	0.5	150	3%
ready-to-use				
original..classic	½ cup	0.5	190	2%
w/brandy & rum	½ cup	1.0	200	5%
(Comstock)				
apple				
banana cream	⅓ cup	1.5	130	10%
blackberry	⅓ cup	–	110	–
blueberry..More Fruit	⅓ cup	–	80	–
cherry				
dark sweet	⅓ cup	–	100	–
More Fruit				
light	⅓ cup	–	60	–
regular	⅓ cup	–	90	–
original				
light	⅓ cup	–	60	–
red ruby	⅓ cup	–	90	–
chocolate cream	⅓ cup	5.0	120	38%
cinnamon 'n' spice	⅓ cup	–	100	–
coconut cream	⅓ cup	3.0	110	25%
French	⅓ cup	–	100	–
lemon	⅓ cup	1.5	130	10%
mincemeat	⅓ cup	–	170	–
More Fruit	⅓ cup	–	80	–
original				
country	⅓ cup	–	90	–
sliced apples	⅓ cup	–	30	–
peach..More Fruit	⅓ cup	–	80	–
pineapple	⅓ cup	–	110	–
pumpkin				
pie mix	⅓ cup	–	90	–
pure pumpkin	⅓ cup	–	50	–
raisin..California	⅓ cup	–	120	–
raspberry	⅓ cup	–	100	–
reduced-calorie	⅓ cup	–	50	–
strawberry	⅓ cup	–	100	–
(Libby's)..pumpkin pie mix	⅓ cup	0.5	90	5%
(Lucky Leaf)				
apple	⅓ cup	–	90	–
premium	⅓ cup	–	90	–

Food and Description	Amount	Fat Grams	Total Calories	% Fat Calories
apricot	⅓ cup	–	90	–
blackberry..premium	⅓ cup	–	90	–
blueberry	⅓ cup	–	90	–
premium	⅓ cup	–	100	–
cherry	⅓ cup	–	100	–
lite..no sugar added	⅓ cup	–	35	–
premium	⅓ cup	–	100	–
cherries jubilee	⅓ cup	–	80	–
lemon	⅓ cup	0.5	120	4%
peach	⅓ cup	–	80	–
red raspberry..premium	⅓ cup	–	80	–
strawberry	⅓ cup	–	80	–
(S&W) mincemeat	¼ cup	2.5	180	13%
(Thank You)				
apple				
cinnamon 'n' spice	⅓ cup	–	100	–
French	⅓ cup	–	100	–
MoreFruit	⅓ cup	–	80	–
original				
country	⅓ cup	–	90	–
sliced apples	⅓ cup	–	30	–
reduced-calorie	⅓ cup	–	50	–
banana cream	⅓ cup	1.5	130	10%
blackberry	⅓ cup	–	110	–
blueberry..MoreFruit	⅓ cup	–	80	–
cherry..dark sweet	⅓ cup	–	100	–
chocolate cream	⅓ cup	5.0	120	38%
coconut cream	⅓ cup	3.0	110	25%
lemon	⅓ cup	1.5	130	10%
mincemeat	⅓ cup	–	170	–
peach/MoreFruit	⅓ cup	–	80	–
pineapple	⅓ cup	–	110	–
pumpkin				
pie mix	⅓ cup	–	90	–
pure pumpkin	⅓ cup	–	50	–
raisin..California	⅓ cup	–	120	–
raspberry	⅓ cup	–	100	–
strawberry	⅓ cup	–	100	–
(Wilderness)				
banana cream	½ cup	1.5	100	14%
cherry..light	⅓ cup	–	60	–
cherry..original red ruby	⅓ cup	–	90	–
chocolate cream	½ cup	1.5	120	11%
coconut cream	½ cup	3.0	110	25%
lemon..quick & easy	⅓ cup	–	130	–
MoreFruit				
apple	⅓ cup	–	80	–
blueberry	⅓ cup	–	80	–
cherry	⅓ cup	–	90	–
pumpkin	½ cup	–	90	–

Food and Description	Amount	Fat Grams	Total Calories	% Fat Calories

■ MIX (Note: Unless stated otherwise, 1 serving of mix = the amount in ½ cup prepared.)

(Banquet Dessert Bakes)

Food and Description	Amount	Fat Grams	Total Calories	% Fat Calories
apple crisp..w/cinnamon topping	⅙ box	3.5	210	15%
cherry cobbler	⅙ box	4.0	250	14%
peach cobbler	⅙ box	4.0	220	16%
(Calhoun Bend Mill)..mix only				
apple-cinnamon crisp topping	3 Tbs	–	140	–
cherry-oatmeal crunch topping	3 Tbs	–	120	–
chocolate-fudge/mix only	3 Tbs	5.0	140	32%
cinnamon crisp topping	¼ cup	–	140	–
fruit cobbler	¼ cup	0.5	140	3%
oatmeal crunch topping	¼ cup	0.5	140	3%
peach cobbler	3 Tbs	–	95	–
pecan pie	⅛ cup	–	110	–
(Jell-O) pudding & pie filling				
Americana pudding & custard				
custard..prepared w/2% milk	½ cup	2.5	140	16%
rice pudding..prepared w/skim milk	½ cup	–	140	–
tapioca pudding..prepared w/skim milk	½ cup	–	130	–
cook & serve				
fat-free..prepared w/skim milk				
all flavors	½ cup	–	130	–
original..prepared w/2% milk				
banana cream	½ cup	2.5	140	16%
butterscotch	½ cup	2.5	160	14%
chocolate	½ cup	2.5	150	15%
chocolate fudge	½ cup	2.5	150	15%
coconut cream	½ cup	5.0	150	30%
flan	½ cup	2.5	140	16%
lemon..prepared as directed	½ cup	2.0	140	13%
milk chocolate	½ cup	3.0	150	18%
vanilla	½ cup	2.5	140	16%
sugar-free..reduced calorie..prepared..w/2% milk				
chocolate	½ cup	2.5	90	25%
vanilla	½ cup	2.5	80	28%
instant				
fat-free..prepared w/skim milk				
all flavors	½ cup	–	140	–
fat-free..sugar-free..prepared w/skim milk				
banana	½ cup	–	70	–
butterscotch	½ cup	–	70	–
chocolate	½ cup	–	80	–
chocolate fudge	½ cup	–	80	–
vanilla	½ cup	–	70	–

Food and Description	Amount	Fat Grams	Total Calories	% Fat Calories
vanilla chocolate	½ cup	–	70	–
(Royal) mix only				
cook & serve				
banana cream	1 serving	–	80	–
butterscotch	1 serving	–	90	–
chocolate	1 serving	–	90	–
dark 'n' sweet chocolate	1 serving	–	90	–
vanilla	1 serving	–	80	–
instant				
regular				
banana cream	1 serving	–	90	–
butterscotch	1 serving	–	90	–
cherry vanilla	1 serving	–	90	–
chocolate	1 serving	–	100	–
chocolate almond	1 serving	1.0	120	8%
chocolate chocolate chip	1 serving	1.0	110	8%
chocolate peanut butter	1 serving	1.0	110	8%
dark 'n' sweet	1 serving	–	110	–
lemon	1 serving	–	90	–
pistachio	1 serving	1.0	90	10%
strawberry	1 serving	–	100	–
toasted coconut	1 serving	2.0	100	18%
vanilla	1 serving	–	90	–
vanilla chocolate chip	1 serving	1.0	90	10%

PIEROGI/POTATO DUMPLING (See POTATO DISH/ENTRÉE)
PIGEON (See SQUAB/PIGEON)
PIGEON PEA
DRIED..shelled

boiled	½ cup	–	100	–
raw	½ cup	1.5	350	4%
FRESH				
cooked	½ cup	1.0	90	10%
raw	½ cup	1.5	350	4%
shelled				
boiled-drained	½ cup	1.5	120	11%
raw	½ cup	2.0	155	12%
SEEDS..immature				
boiled—drained	½ cup	1.0	85	11%
raw	20 seeds	<1.0	10	18%

PIGNOLIA (See PINE NUT)
PIG'S FEET (See PORK; PORK ENTRÉE)
PIKE (See also PIKE ROE)
Northern

cooked—dry heat	3 oz	1.0	95	9%
raw	3 oz	1.0	75	12%
walleye				
cooked—dry heat	3 oz	1.0	100	9%
raw	3 oz	1.0	79	11%

PIKE ROE

Northern..raw	3 oz	1.7	110	14%

Food and Description	Amount	Fat Grams	Total Calories	% Fat Calories
PILAF (See RICE DISH)				
PIMIENTO/canned				
(Dromedary)	1 oz	–	10	–
(Dunbar's)	½ oz	–	4	–
(Goya)..fancy	½ oz	–	–	–
(S&W) whole	2¼ oz	–	20	–
PIÑA COLADA (See COCKTAIL/COCKTAIL MIXERS)				
PINE NUT				
CANNED				
(Diamond of California)	1 oz	17.0	180	85%
DRIED				
pignolia	1 oz	14.0	146	86%
(Frieda's)	¼ cup	15.0	150	90%
(Krino's)	½ oz	7.5	90	75%
pinyon	1 oz	17.0	161	95%
JARRED				
(Progresso)..pignolia nuts	1 oz	13.0	170	69%
PINEAPPLE				
BOWL..CAN..CUP..JAR				
(Del Monte)				
chunks				
in heavy syrup	½ cup	–	90	–
in juice	½ cup	–	70	–
crushed				
in heavy syrup	½ cup	–	90	–
in juice	½ cup	–	70	–
Fruit Naturals	½ cup	–	70	–
individual 4.3-oz pull-top cans				
tidbits..100% juice	1 can	–	50	–
wedges..100% juice	1 can	–	70	–
sliced				
in heavy syrup	2 slices	–	90	–
in juice	2 slices	–	60	–
spears or wedges/in juice	½ cup	–	70	–
SunFresh..slightly sweetened	½ cup	–	70	–
tidbits/in juice				
bowl..100% juice	1 bowl	–	70	–
canned	½ cup	–	70	–
wedges in juice	½ cup	–	70	–
(Dole)				
chunks				
in clarified juice	½ cup	–	60	–
in heavy syrup	½ cup	–	90	–
coarse-cut crushed				
in juice	½ cup	–	70	–
crushed				
in extra-heavy syrup	½ cup	–	110	–
in heavy syrup	½ cup	–	90	–
in juice	½ cup	–	70	–

Food and Description	Amount	Fat Grams	Total Calories	% Fat Calories
cubes				
in extra-heavy syrup	½ cup	–	200	–
in light syrup	½ cup	–	80	–
Dole fruit bowls	1 bowl	–	60	–
pieces				
in light syrup	½ cup	–	80	–
sliced				
in clarified juice	2 slices	–	60	–
in heavy syrup	2 slices	–	90	–
tidbits				
in clarified juice	½ cup	–	60	–
in heavy syrup	½ cup	–	90	–
in light syrup	½ cup	–	80	–
(Empress)				
chunks	½ cup	–	70	–
crushed	½ cup	–	70	–
sliced	½ cup	–	70	–
(S&W) Hawaiian..sliced				
in syrup	2 slices	–	90	–
CANDIED				
(S&W) glace				
slices..all types	1 piece	–	180	–
wedges..all types	5 pieces	–	80	–
DRIED				
(Sun-Maid)..tropical trio				
w/ pineapple..papaya..mango	1.4 oz	–	130	–
FRESH				
(Chiquita)	1 cup	1.0	90	10%
(Del Monte)	½ cup	–	52	–
	2 slices	–	70	–
(Dole)	2 slices	0.5	60	8%
PINEAPPLE JUICE/JUICE BLEND/JUICE DRINK (*See also* FRUIT PUNCH)				
BOTTLED..BOXED. CANNED				
(Del Monte)				
from concentrate	6 fl oz	–	80	–
	8 fl oz	–	130	–
not from concentrate	8 fl oz	–	110	–
(Dole)				
bottled				
pineapple orange	10 fl oz	–	150	–
pineapple orange banana	10 fl oz	–	160	–
pineapple passion banana	10 fl oz	–	160	–
canned				
pineapple				
from concentrate	8 fl oz	–	120	–
not from concentrate	8 fl oz	–	110	–
pineapple grapefruit	6 fl oz	–	100	–
pineapple orange	6 fl oz	–	100	–
pineapple orange banana	6 fl oz	–	100	–
Juice Cooler	8.45 fl oz	–	130	–

Food and Description	Amount	Fat Grams	Total Calories	% Fat Calories
100% juice				
refrigerated				
pineapple	8 fl oz	–	130	–
pineapple mango	8 fl oz	–	120	–
pineapple orange	8 fl oz	–	120	–
pineapple orange banana	4 fl oz	–	70	–
	8 fl oz	–	130	–
pineapple orange berry	8 fl oz	–	130	–
pineapple orange guava	8 fl oz	–	120	–
(Kern's)				
Nectar				
pineapple mango	8 fl oz	–	150	–
(R.W. Knudsen)				
pineapple coconut	8 fl oz	1.0	130	7%
pineapple nectar	8 fl oz	–	150	–
(S&W)	6 fl oz	–	90	–
	8 fl oz	–	110	–
individual serving	12 fl oz	–	180	–
(Welch's)				
pineapple orange..juice cocktail	11.5 oz	–	150	–
FROZEN				
(Dole) prepared				
100% pineapple juice	8 fl oz	–	130	–
pineapple grapefruit	8 fl oz	–	130	–
pineapple orange	8 fl oz	–	120	–
pineapple orange banana	8 fl oz	–	130	–
pineapple orange guava	8 fl oz	–	120	–
pineapple orange strawberry	8 fl oz	–	130	–
pineapple passion banana	8 fl oz	–	120	–
pineapple strawberry	8 fl oz	–	130	–
PINK BEAN				
CANNED				
(Goya)..habichuelas rosadas				
Spanish-style	½ cup	0.5	80	9%
original	½ cup	0.5	80	9%
DRIED				
boiled	½ cup	0.5	125	4%
raw	½ cup	1.0	360	3%
PIÑON/PINYON (*See* **PINE NUT**)				
PINTO BEAN				
CANNED				
(Bush's)				
original	½ cup	0.5	110	4%
w/bacon	½ cup	1.0	110	8%
w/bacon & jalapeños	½ cup	1.5	110	12%
w/pork	½ cup	2.5	120	19%
(Eden)..Organic				
original	½ cup	–	100	–
refried	½ cup	1.0	90	–

Food and Description	Amount	Fat Grams	Total Calories	% Fat Calories
refried..spicy				
w/jalapeño & red peppers	½ cup	1.0	90	–
(Goya) Spanish-style	½ cup	0.5	110	4%
(Luck's) seasoned w/pork				
regular	7 oz	3.0	200	14%
	½ cup	4.0	140	26%
w/Great Northern beans	½ cup	2.0	130	14%
w/onions	½ cup	3.0	150	18%
(Trappey's)..w/bacon				
jalapinto	½ cup	1.0	120	10%
original	½ cup	1.0	120	10%
DRIED..raw				
(Arrowhead Mills)	¼ cup	0.5	150	3%
(Bean Cuisine)	¼ cup	1.0	115	8%
SPROUTED..mature seeds				
boiled-drained	½ cup	0.5	25	18%
raw	½ cup	1.0	65	14%
PINYON/PIÑON (*See* PINE NUT)				
PISTACHIO				
(Alma)..all types	1 oz	14.0	160	79%
(Ann's House of Nuts)..natural	1 oz	14.0	160	79%
(Blue Diamond)..raw	1 oz	15.0	200	68%
(Dole) dry-roasted				
shelled	1 oz	14.0	160	79%
unshelled	1 oz	7.0	90	70%
(Fisher) red	1 oz	15.0	170	79%
(Lance)				
roasted in shell..1.125-oz pkg	1 pkg	7.0	90	70%
	¼ cup	7.0	100	63%
	2 oz pkg	9.0	120	68%
(Planters) dry-roasted				
shelled				
Munch 'n' Go	2 oz	29.0	330	79%
regular	1 oz	14.0	160	79%
unshelled				
red..salted	1 oz	14.0	160	79%
uncolored	½ cup	14.0	160	79%
	1 oz	14.0	160	79%
	2.25 oz	16.0	190	76%
PITANGA/BRAZILIAN CHERRY/SURINAM CHERRY				
fresh	2 pieces	<1.0	5	11%
	1 cup	0.7	57	11%
	1 lb	1.6	132	11%
PIZZA (*See also* FROZEN ENTRÉE/DINNER; VEGETARIAN FOODS; individual FAST FOOD listings.)				
■ (Atkins)				
Quick Cuisine				
pepperoni	1 pkg	25.0	440	51%
smokehouse	1 pkg	23.0	420	49%
Supreme	1 pkg	19.0	360	48%

Food and Description	Amount	Fat Grams	Total Calories	% Fat Calories
■ (Boca)				
meatless pizza				
pepperoni	⅓ pizza	8.0	240	30%
pepperoni..tomato & herb	⅓ pizza	8.0	240	30%
Supreme..meatless				
pepperoni & sausage	⅓ pizza	8.0	260	28%
■ (California Pizza Kitchen)				
3-pieces pizza				
BBQ chicken recipe	⅓ pizza	9.0	280	29%
5-cheese & tomato	⅓ pizza	15.0	320	42%
Jamaican Jerk	⅓ pizza	9.0	270	30%
Thai chicken recipe	⅓ pizza	10.0	290	31%
6-pieces pizza				
BBQ recipe chicken	⅙ pizza	9.0	320	26%
5-cheese & tomato	⅙ pizza	15.0	350	39%
Thai chicken recipe	⅓ pizza	11.0	310	32%
■ (Celeste)				
Pizza for One				
cheese	1 pizza	20.0	420	43%
4-cheese				
original	1 pizza	26.0	470	49%
zesty	1 pizza	25.0	470	48%
deluxe	1 pizza	25.0	470	48%
pepperoni	1 pizza	27.0	470	52%
sausage	1 pizza	26.0	480	49%
sausage & pepperoni	1 pizza	34.0	560	55%
Supreme	1 pizza	29.0	530	49%
vegetable	1 pizza	22.0	430	46%
Zesty Chicken Supreme	1 pizza	19.0	380	45%
Pizza//Large				
cheese	¼ pizza	13.0	300	39%
deluxe	¼ pizza	17.0	340	45%
pepperoni	¼ pizza	17.0	350	44%
Pizza..Rising Crust..fresh-baked				
4-cheese	⅙ pizza	11.0	320	31%
pepperoni	⅙ pizza	13.0	330	35%
Supreme	⅙ pizza	15.0	360	38%
3-meat	⅙ pizza	13.0	340	34%
■ (Di Giorno)				
Rising Crust				
8-inch				
chicken Supreme	⅓ pizza	9.0	270	30%
4-cheese	⅓ pizza	9.0	260	31%
Italian sausage	⅓ pizza	13.0	310	38%
pepperoni	⅓ pizza	14.0	310	41%
sausage & pepperoni	⅓ pizza	14.0	320	39%
spinach..mushroon	⅓ pizza	8.0	260	28%
Supreme	⅓ pizza	14.0	320	39%
3-meat	⅓ pizza	14.0	320	39%
vegetable	⅓ pizza	8.0	260	27%

Food and Description	Amount	Fat Grams	Total Calories	% Fat Calories
12-inch				
cheese-stuffed	⅙ pizza	19.0	390	44%
4-cheese	⅙ pizza	11.0	320	31%
Italian sausage	⅙ pizza	14.0	350	36%
pepperoni	⅙ pizza	16.0	370	39%
sausage & pepperoni	⅙ pizza	16.0	360	40%
spinach..mushroom	⅙ pizza	9.0	300	27%
Supreme	⅙ pizza	15.0	370	36%
3-meat	⅙ pizza	16.0	360	40%
vegetable	⅙ pizza	9.0	300	27%
deep dish				
pepperoni	⅛ pizza	22.0	390	51%
Supreme	⅛ pizza	17.0	310	49%
Rising Crust..Half & Half				
pepperoni & cheese	⅙ pizza	18.0	390	42%
Supreme	⅙ pizza	17.0	380	40%
■ (Dining In)				
3-pieces..Rising Crust Pizza				
pepperoni..6-cheese	⅓ pizza	12.0	290	37%
portabello mushroom & 5-cheese	⅓ pizza	8.0	250	29%
Supreme..6-cheese	⅓ pizza	13.0	310	38%
3-meat..6-cheese	⅓ pizza	11.0	280	35%
tomato..w/basil & 6-cheeses	⅓ pizza	8.0	250	29%
6-pieces..Rising Crust..6-cheese Pizza				
cheese	⅙ pizza	8.0	290	25%
pepperoni	⅙ pizza	12.0	340	32%
Supreme	⅙ pizza	13.0	350	33%
3-meat	⅙ pizza	12.0	340	32%
Half & Half Pizza				
pepperoni/cheese..6-cheese	⅓ pizza	15.0	370	36%
other pizza				
BBQ recipe chicken	⅓ pizza	10.0	300	30%
roasted vegetable & 5-cheese	⅓ pizza	8.0	240	30%
■ (Freschetta)				
8-inch				
4-cheese	½ pizza	16.0	410	35%
garlic chicken	⅓ pizza	9.0	260	31%
mozzarella & basil margherita	½ pizza	15.0	370	36%
pepperoni	½ pizza	21.0	450	42%
roasted garlic chicken	½ pizza	12.0	370	29%
Southwest-style	½ pizza	12.0	360	30%
Supreme	½ pizza	21.0	460	41%
12-inch				
4-meat	⅙ pizza	15.0	350	39%
4-cheese	⅙ pizza	15.0	390	34%
pepperoni	⅙ pizza	16.0	360	40%
sausage	⅙ pizza	16.0	360	40%
sausage & pepperoni	⅙ pizza	16.0	370	39%
Special Deluxe	⅙ pizza	15.0	350	39%

Food and Description	Amount	Fat Grams	Total Calories	% Fat Calories
Supreme	⅙ pizza	16.0	360	40%
vegetable primavera	⅕ pizza	13.0	360	33%
brick oven..fire-baked crust				
cheese & bacon	¼ pizza	14.0	320	39%
Classic Supreme	¼ pizza	17.0	370	41%
5-Italian cheese	¼ pizza	14.0	330	38%
Italian-style pepperoni	¼ pizza	22.0	410	48%
portabello mushroom & spinach	¼ pizza	10.0	290	31%
Southwest-style chicken	¼ pizza	14.0	340	37%
stuffed crust				
4-cheese	⅕ pizza	12.0	340	32%
pepperoni	⅕ pizza	16.0	370	39%
sausage & pepperoni				
25 oz	⅕ pizza	15.0	370	36%
28.9 oz	⅙ pizza	16.0	360	40%
Supreme..w/grilled vegetables	⅙ pizza	13.0	310	38%
vegetable medley	⅕ pizza	9.0	310	26%
■ (Jack's)				
Great Combinations/9-inch				
double cheese	½ pizza	21.0	430	44%
pepperoni & sausage	½ pizza	18.0	380	43%
Great Combinations..12-inch				
bacon cheeseburger	¼ pizza	18.0	360	45%
double cheese	¼ pizza	19.0	380	45%
pepperoni	¼ pizza	19.0	410	42%
pepperoni & mushroom	¼ pizza	16.0	340	42%
sausage	¼ pizza	18.0	390	42%
sausage & mushroom	¼ pizza	15.0	310	44%
sausage & pepperoni	¼ pizza	19.0	350	49%
Supreme	¼ pizza	18.0	350	46%
Original Pizza...12-inch				
Canadian-style bacon	¼ pizza	10.0	280	32%
cheese	¼ pizza	13.0	350	33%
hamburger	¼ pizza	14.0	300	42%
pepperoni	¼ pizza	15.0	330	41%
sausage	¼ pizza	14.0	300	42%
spicy Italian sausage	¼ pizza	13.0	290	40%
Pizza Bursts..7 oz box				
combination sausage & pepperoni	½ pkg	13.0	250	47%
pepperoni	½ pkg	15.0	260	52%
sausage	½ pkg	12.0	250	43%
SuperCheese	½ pkg	13.0	250	47%
Supreme	½ pkg	14.0	260	48%
■ (Jenos)				
Crisp 'n' Tasty Pizza				
Canadian-style bacon	1 pizza	19.0	440	39%
cheese	1 pizza	21.0	460	41%
combination	1 pizza	26.0	500	47%
hamburger	1 pizza	25.0	500	45%

Food and Description	Amount	Fat Grams	Total Calories	% Fat Calories
pepperoni	1 pizza	27.0	510	48%
sausage	1 pizza	24.0	480	45%
Supreme	1 pizza	26.0	500	47%
3-meat	1 pizza	25.0	490	46%
■ LEAN CUISINE				
deluxe	1 pizza	9.0	370	22%
4-cheese	1 pizza	7.0	380	17%
pepperoni	1 pizza	9.0	380	21%
roasted vegetable	1 pizza	4.5	330	12%
■ (Mama Rosa's)				
Bite My Slice				
double pepperoni	½ pizza	8.0	140	30%
nacho beef	½ pizza	8.0	240	30%
Deluxe..2-count	4.7 oz	13.0	310	38%
Mini Mama's..4-count				
cheeseburger	¼ pkg	9.0	270	30%
combo	¼ pkg	13.0	320	37%
party	¼ pkg	12.0	320	34%
pepperoni	¼ pkg	14.0	340	37%
party cheese..2-count	⅛ pkg	11.0	280	35%
pepperoni..34 oz	⅛ pizza	14.0	340	37%
pepperoni..2-pack	4.7 oz	13.0	310	38%
pepperoni..dessert style..2-pack	8 oz	13.0	310	38%
■ (Red Baron)				
Deep-Dish Breakfast..5-inch				
bacon scramble	½ pizza	22.0	400	50%
ham scramble	½ pizza	15.0	330	41%
sausage & gravy	½ pizza	18.0	360	45%
sausage scramble	½ pizza	18.0	350	46%
Western scramble	½ pizza	22.0	400	50%
Deep-Dish Mini Pizzas..8-count				
cheese	½ pkg	15.0	380	36%
pepperoni	½ pkg	20.0	400	45%
sausage & pepperoni	½ pkg	15.0	310	44%
Supreme	½ pkg	17.0	320	48%
Deep-Dish Pan-style				
4-cheese	⅓ pizza	17.0	370	41%
meat trio	⅓ pizza	20.0	390	46%
pepperoni	⅓ pizza	21.0	400	47%
Supreme	⅓ pizza	21.0	410	46%
Deep-Dish Singles				
4-cheese	1 pizza	23.0	440	47%
cheese	1 pizza	21.0	420	45%
meat trio	1 pizza	21.0	420	45%
pepperoni	1 pizza	25.0	460	49%
sausage	1 pizza	28.0	480	53%
special deluxe	1 pizza	24.0	430	50%
Supreme	1 pizza	27.0	470	52%
Vegetable Supreme	1 pizza	19.0	400	43%
Original..Classic Pizza				
Canadian bacon	¼ pizza	19.0	380	45%

Food and Description	Amount	Fat Grams	Total Calories	% Fat Calories
4-cheese	¼ pizza	23.0	420	49%
hamburger	⅕ pizza	18.0	330	55%
Mexican-style	⅕ pizza	21.0	360	53%
pepperoni	¼ pizza	26.0	440	51%
pepperoni deluxe	⅕ pizza	18.0	350	46%
sausage	⅕ pizza	16.0	330	44%
sausage & mushroom	⅕ pizza	18.0	350	46%
sausage & pepperoni	⅕ pizza	21.0	330	57%
special deluxe	⅕ pizza	19.0	340	50%
Supreme	⅕ pizza	20.0	350	51%
Pizza Pouches..2-count				
meat trio	½ pkg	14.0	320	39%
pepperoni	½ pkg	16.0	340	42%
sausage & pepperoni	½ pkg	16.0	340	42%
Supreme	½ pkg	14.0	320	39%
Pizza Slices..stuffed..2-count				
Italian sausage	½ pkg	16.0	340	42%
Italian sausage & pepperoni	½ pkg	18.0	360	45%
pepperoni	½ pkg	19.0	370	46%
roasted garlic chicken	½ pkg	10.0	290	31%
Supreme	½ pkg	16.0	340	42%
Pizzeria-style				
4-cheese	⅙ pizza	13.0	360	33%
meat trio	⅙ pizza	15.0	370	36%
pepperoni	⅙ pizza	16.0	370	39%
sausage	⅙ pizza	15.0	370	38%
special deluxe	⅙ pizza	17.0	390	39%
Supreme	⅙ pizza	21.0	360	53%
■ **(San Francisco Foods)**				
calzones				
bacon, egg & cheese	½ calzone	20.0	370	49%
5-cheese	½ calzone	11.0	280	35%
ham & cheddar	½ calzone	14.0	340	37%
ham & Swiss	½ calzone	13.0	330	35%
pepperoni	½ calzone	13.0	300	39%
sausage, egg & cheese	½ calzone	17.0	350	44%
spinach & feta	½ calzone	10.0	280	32%
Supreme	½ calzone	16.0	310	46%
Western omelette	½ calzone	12.0	300	36%
stuffed pizza				
5-cheese	¼ pizza	15.0	420	32%
meat combo	¼ pizza	16.0	430	33%
pepperoni	¼ pizza	16.0	410	35%
spinach & feta	¼ pizza	16.0	400	36%
Supreme	¼ pizza	17.0	400	38%
Western chicken	¼ pizza	12.0	310	35%
■ **(Schwan's)**				
deep-dish mini				
cheese	4 pizzas	22.0	430	46%
pepperoni	4 pizzas	27.0	470	52%

Food and Description	Amount	Fat Grams	Total Calories	% Fat Calories
deep-dish single-serve pizza				
4-cheese	⅙ pizza	18.0	410	40%
pepperoni	⅙ pizza	19.0	380	45%
Supreme	⅙ pizza	18.0	380	43%
self-rising				
cheese	⅙ pizza	18.0	410	40%
pepperoni	⅙ pizza	19.0	380	45%
Supreme	⅙ pizza	18.0	380	43%
Special Recipe Pizza				
Canadian bacon	¼ pizza	23.0	430	48%
4-cheese	⅓ pizza	23.0	400	52%
pepperoni	¼ pizza	29.0	460	57%
sausage	¼ pizza	24.0	370	58%
sausage & pepperoni	¼ pizza	24.0	380	57%
Supreme	¼ pizza	23.0	360	58%
stuffed pizza slice				
pepperoni	1 piece	27.0	470	52%
Supreme	1 piece	16.0	340	42%
■ **(Stouffer's)..French Bread Pizza** (*See* FROZEN ENTRÉE/DINNER)				
■ **(Tombstone)**				
deep-dish				
cheese	1 pizza	21.0	460	41%
Pepperoni..Cheese Supreme	1 pizza	25.0	500	45%
Supreme	1 pizza	16.0	310	46%
double-top pizza				
pepperoni w/double cheese	⅙ pizza	20.0	350	51%
sausage & pepperoni	⅙ pizza	20.0	360	50%
sausage w/double cheese	⅙ pizza	19.0	350	49%
half & half				
pepperoni..cheese				
cheese portion	¼ pizza	15.0	340	40%
pepperoni portion	¼ pizza	23.0	430	48%
Mexican-style				
fajita	¼ pizza	14.0	300	42%
nacho grande	¼ pizza	19.0	380	45%
Supreme	¼ pizza	17.0	360	43%
original				
cheese & pepperoni	¼ pizza	21.0	400	47%
extra cheese	¼ pizza	15.0	340	40%
Supreme	⅕ pizza	16.0	310	46%
oven-rising crust				
pepperoni	⅙ pizza	20.0	380	47%
3-cheese	⅙ pizza	11.0	300	33%
stuffed crust				
cheese	⅕ pizza	19.0	390	44%
■ **(Tony's)**				
deep-dish				
cheese				
5.5 oz	⅙ pizza	17.0	360	43%
33 oz	1 pizza	22.0	410	48%

Food and Description	Amount	Fat Grams	Total Calories	% Fat Calories
pepperoni				
6.27 oz	⅙ pizza	26.0	460	51%
37.5 oz	1 pizza	30.0	510	53%
sausage..6.33 oz	1 pizza	29.0	490	53%
Supreme				
6.5 oz	⅙ pizza	24.0	440	49%
39 oz	1 pizza	27.0	470	52%
Mini Pizza for One				
Canadian bacon	1 pizza	28.0	510	49%
cheese	1 pizza	30.0	550	49%
pepperoni	1 pizza	37.0	620	54%
sausage	1 pizza	36.0	620	52%
sausage & pepperoni	1 pizza	37.0	620	54%
Supreme	1 pizza	38.0	640	53%
Original..w/Italian-style Pastry Crust				
Canadian bacon	⅓ pizza	22.0	390	51%
cheese	⅓ pizza	22.0	390	51%
4-cheese	⅓ pizza	23.0	390	53%
hamburger	⅓ pizza	25.0	420	54%
meat trio	¼ pizza	22.0	350	57%
Mexican..fiesta-style	¼ pizza	22.0	340	58%
pepperoni	⅓ pizza	28.0	440	57%
sausage	⅓ pizza	27.0	440	55%
sausage & mushroom	¼ pizza	21.0	340	56%
sausage & pepperoni	⅓ pizza	29.0	450	58%
Supreme	¼ pizza	16.0	310	46%
vegetable	⅓ pizza	23.0	400	52%
Super Rise				
4-cheese	¼ pizza	13.0	340	34%
meat trio	¼ pizza	17.0	380	40%
pepperoni	¼ pizza	20.0	410	44%
sausage	¼ pizza	18.0	390	42%
Supreme	⅙ pizza	16.0	330	44%
Thin Crust				
cheese	⅓ pizza	14.0	310	41%
pepperoni	⅓ pizza	16.0	330	44%
sausage	⅓ pizza	17.0	340	45%
Supreme	⅓ pizza	18.0	350	46%
■ (Totino's)				
Family-Size				
cheese	⅓ pizza	16.0	370	39%
combination	¼ pizza	17.0	310	49%
pepperoni	⅓ pizza	23.0	420	49%
sausage	¼ pizza	16.0	300	48%
Party Pizza..crisp crust				
bacon burger	½ pizza	21.0	390	48%
Canadian-style bacon	½ pizza	15.0	330	41%
cheese	½ pizza	14.0	320	39%
combination	½ pizza	22.0	390	51%
hamburger	½ pizza	19.0	370	46%

Food and Description	Amount	Fat Grams	Total Calories	% Fat Calories
Mexican-style	½ pizza	16.0	320	45%
pepperoni	½ pizza	22.0	380	52%
sausage & mushroom	½ pizza	19.0	360	48%
sausage & sliced pepperoni	½ pizza	21.0	390	48%
sliced pepperoni	½ pizza	21.0	380	50%
Supreme	½ pizza	21.0	380	50%
3-cheese	½ pizza	15.0	330	41%
3-meat	½ pizza	19.0	360	48%
Zesty Italiano	½ pizza	21.0	390	48%
Pizza Rolls				
cheese	6 rolls	7.0	200	32%
cheesy taco	6 rolls	10.0	210	43%
combination	6 rolls	12.0	230	47%
hamburger	6 rolls	9.0	210	39%
pepperoni	6 rolls	11.0	230	43%
Pepperoni Supreme	6 rolls	10.0	220	41%
sausage	6 rolls	11.0	230	43%
spicy pepperoni	6 rolls	11.0	230	43%
Supreme	6 rolls	10.0	220	41%
3-meat	6 rolls	10.0	220	41%
■ **(Weight Watchers)**				
Bistro Selections				
BBQ-style chicken	1 pizza	7.0	380	17%
4-cheese	1 pizza	7.0	400	16%
pepperoni	1 pizza	9.0	400	20%
spicy sausage	1 pizza	10.0	390	23%
veggie..Ultimate Crust	1 pizza	5.0	400	11%
■ **(Wolfgang Puck)**				
rising crust				
cheeseless	⅓ pizza	2.0	150	12%
4-cheese	½ pizza	11.0	270	37%
mushroom & spinach	⅓ pizza	8.0	230	31%
pepperoni & mushrooms	⅓ pizza	13.0	310	38%
sausage & herb	⅓ pizza	13.0	350	33%
spicy chicken	⅓ pizza	11.0	270	37%
sourdough crust				
pepperoni				
8"	½ pizza	15.0	390	35%
12"	¼ pizza	13.0	370	32%
vegetable..12"	¼ pizza	15.0	360	38%
whole wheat crust				
4-cheese	½ pizza	15.0	360	38%
PIZZA CRUST				
(Better Pizza Crusts)				
Ready-to-Eat	½ crust	2.0	80	23%
(Betty Crocker)				
prepared...9"	⅛ crust	8.0	110	65%
(Boboli)..Italian bread shell..				
prebaked..ready to use				
Italian..8 oz pkg	¼ shell	3.0	150	18%

Food and Description	Amount	Fat Grams	Total Calories	% Fat Calories
Italian original..14 oz	⅛ shell	2.5	140	16%
Italian personal size..10 oz	¼ shell	5.0	200	23%
Italian thin..10-oz pkg	⅕ shell	3.5	170	19%
(Jiffy) prepared	¼ crust	3.0	180	15%
(Mama Mary's)..fresh baked gourmet				
7" dia	⅛ slice	5.0	200	23%
12" dia				
deep-dish	1/12 slice	5.0	200	23%
original	1/12 slice	5.0	200	23%
(Martha White) mix/crust only				
crispy crust	1 slice	1.0	160	6%
deep pan	1 slice	1.0	140	6%
(Pet Ritz)..frozen				
deep-dish crust	⅛ crust	5.0	90	50%
all-vegetable	⅛ crust	5.0	90	50%
extra-large	⅛ crust	6.0	110	49%
regular crust	⅛ crust	4.0	80	45%
all-vegetable	⅛ crust	4.5	80	51%
(Pillsbury)				
refrigerated..all ready	⅛ crust	7.0	120	53%
(Ragu)..Pizza Quick..mix only	½ cup	1.0	130	7%
(Robin Hood)..mix..prepared	¼ crust	2.0	160	11%
PIZZA SAUCE (*See* SAUCE)				
PLANTAIN/BAKING BANANA/COOKING BANANA				
cooked..sliced	1 cup	<1.0	180	3%
raw				
sliced	½ cup	<1.0	90	3%
whole	1 medium	1.0	220	4%
PLUM				
canned				
(S&W) whole..peeled				
purple..in heavy syrup	½ cup	–	130	–
(Stokely)..in light syrup	½ cup	–	100	–
dried				
(Sunsweet)				
w/pits	3 large	–	100	–
without pits	7 pieces	–	100	–
fresh..raw				
(Dole)	2 medium	1.0	80	11%
sliced	½ cup	–	90	–
POI	½ cup	–	135	–
POKEBERRY/fresh				
cooked	½ cup	–	16	–
raw	½ cup	–	20	–
POLENTA				
chilled				
(Frieda's)	4 oz	–	100	–
(Melissa's)	4 oz	–	100	–
mix				
(Fantastic Foods)	¼ cup	5.0	260	17%

Food and Description	Amount	Fat Grams	Total Calories	% Fat Calories
POLISH SAUSAGE (*See* SAUSAGE)				
POLLACK/POLLOCK (*See also* SEAFOOD ENTRÉE/DINNER)				
Alaskan/walleye				
cooked—dry heat	3 oz	1.0	100	9%
raw	3 oz	0.7	70	9%
Atlantic/raw	3 oz	1.0	80	10%
POMEGRANATE				
fresh	1 medium	0.5	104	4%
(Dole)	1 medium	–	104	–
(Frieda's)	5 oz	–	100	–
POMEGRANATE JUICE				
(R. W. Knudsen)	8 fl oz	–	150	–
PANO/Florida				
breaded & fried	3 oz	17.0	270	57%
cooked—dry heat	3 oz	10.0	180	50%
raw	3 oz	8.0	140	51%
POP (*See* COCKTAIL MIXER; SOFT DRINK; SPORTS DRINK)				
POP-TART (*See* PASTRY, TOASTER)				
POPCORN (*See also* POPCORN BARS & CAKES)				
(NOTE: Unless stated otherwise, data are for popped corn.)				
(ACTII)..microwave				
butter	⅓ pkg	10.0	160	56%
light	½ pkg	4.5	110	37%
mini bags	⅙ pkg	14.0	210	60%
classic white	⅓ pkg	14.0	180	70%
kettle corn				
buttery	⅓ pkg	12.0	170	64%
94% fat-free	⅓ pkg	2.5	130	12%
original	⅓ pkg	12.0	170	64%
movie theater..butter	⅓ pkg	12.0	170	64%
sweet corn on the cob	⅓ pkg	13.0	180	65%
xtreme butter	⅓ pkg	13.0	180	65%
(Bearitos)..ready-to-eat				
buttery	2½ cups	12.0	170	64%
buttery..lite	3½ cups	6.0	140	39%
caramel..fat-free	1 cup	–	120	–
cheddar..white	2⅓ cups	11.0	170	58%
no oil	5 cups	1.5	110	12%
no oil..no salt	~5 cups	1.5	120	11%
(Betty Crocker)..Pop Secret..unpopped				
94% fat-free..3 Tbs unpopped				
butter..popped	6 cups	12.0	180	60%
Butter..3 Tbs unpopped				
popped				
extra	4 cups	13.0	180	65%
Jumbo Pop	3½ cups	11.0	170	58%
movie theater	3½ cups	11.0	170	58%
light	4 cups	6.0	140	39%
movie theater	4 cups	13.0	180	65%

Food and Description	Amount	Fat Grams	Total Calories	% Fat Calories
toffee butter	4 cups	13.0	190	62%
home-style..3 Tbs unpopped popped	4 cups	12.0	170	64%
honey butter..3 Tbs unpopped popped	4 cups	13.0	190	62%
kettle corn..3 Tbs unpopped popped	4 cups	13.0	190	62%
(Blue Heaven)..microwavable				
blue corn	2 cups	8.0	130	55%
(Cape Cod)				
cheese-flavored	3 cups	13.0	200	59%
old-fashioned butter	3 cups	12.0	170	64%
Flamin' Hot	2½ cups	11.0	170	58%
(Chester's)				
microwave				
butter	5 cups	12.0	200	54%
natural	5 cups	12.0	200	54%
prepopped				
butter	3 cups	12.0	160	68%
cheddar cheese	3 cups	13.0	190	68%
(Cracker Jack)				
butter toffee	½ cup	4.0	140	26%
caramel	½ cup	4.0	140	26%
crispy clusters marshmallow				
crispy rice treats	18 pieces	3.0	120	23%
Nothing but Nuts				
butter toffee	4 Tbs	15.0	200	68%
original	3 Tbs	12.0	170	64%
(Crunch & Munch)..buttery popcorn				
Almond Supreme	1 oz	5.0	140	32%
caramel	1 oz	7.0	160	39%
toffee				
buttery	1 oz	6.0	150	36%
fat-free	1 oz	–	110	–
(Fiddle Faddle)..ready-to-eat				
regular	⅔ cup	2.5	130	17%
w/Heath toffee bits	½ cup	1.5	100	14%
w/Planters peanuts	⅔ cup	3.0	130	21%
(Jiffy Pop)				
bag				
butter	5 cups	14.0	180	70%
butter-flavored	5 cups	7.0	140	45%
natural/light	5 cups	7.0	140	45%
white cheddar cheese	5 cups	11.0	170	58%
microwavable				
butter	3 cups	7.0	140	45%
regular	3 cups	7.0	140	45%
(Jolly Time)				
jar..American's Best				
white	1 oz	0.5	100	5%

Food and Description	Amount	Fat Grams	Total Calories	% Fat Calories
yellow	1 oz	1.0	100	9%
microwavable				
Big Cheez Ultimate				
cheddar cheese	⅓ pkg	9.0	140	58%
Blast 'O Butter Theatre Style	1.16 oz	11.0	150	66%
butter				
American's best				
butter/94% fat-free	1 oz	2.0	90	20%
Butter-licious	1.16 oz	9.0	140	58%
Crispy 'n White/natural				
light	3 cups	5.0	120	38%
regular	3 cups	10.0	150	60%
Healthy Pop..94% fat-free butter	3 cups	2.0	90	20%
(Louise's)..fat-free..ready-to-eat				
apple cinnamon	1 oz	–	100	–
buttery toffee	1 oz	–	100	–
caramel	1 oz	–	100	–
(Michael Seasons) Gourmet Sensations..ready-to-eat				
butter toffee w/pecans & almonds	¾ cup	6.0	130	42%
chocolate-covered butter toffee	¾ cup	7.0	140	45%
(Newman's Own)..Old-style Picture Show				
microwave				
butter				
Butter Boom	3½ cups	11.0	170	58%
fat-free	3½ cups	1.5	110	12%
light	3½ cups	3.0	110	25%
regular	3½ cups	11.0	170	58%
natural				
light	3½ cups	3.0	110	25%
no salt	3½ cups	11.0	170	
original	3½ cups	11.0	170	58%
white cheddar..genius food	3½ cups	10.0	190	47%
(Orville Redenbacher's)..unpopped, unless otherwise specified				
bag...popcorn..original	1.42 oz	1.5	120	11%
butter toffee popcorn clusters/bag	1 oz	2.5	130	17%
cheddar cheese	2 Tbs	9.0	145	43%
Cinnabon	⅓ pkg	14.0	180	70%
Drizzlers				
milk chocolate	2.8 oz	6.0	150	36%
white fudge	2.8 oz	6.0	150	36%
gourmet popcorn				
buttery toffee clusters	⅓ pkg	5.0	130	35%
w/almonds & cashews	⅓ pkg	4.5	130	31%
home-style	2 Tbs	11.0	170	58%
honey butter	⅓ pkg	12.0	180	60%
microwavable				
butter				
light	2 Tbs	5.0	110	41%
Movie Theater	⅓ pkg	12.0	170	64%
mini bags	1.5 oz bag	15.0	210	64%

Food and Description	Amount	Fat Grams	Total Calories	% Fat Calories
no salt added	2 Tbs	12.0	160	68%
old-fashioned	2 Tbs	11.0	160	62%
Pour Over Movie Theater	⅛ pkg	14.0	170	74%
regular	2 Tbs	12.0	160	68%
Smart Pop..94% fat-free	2 Tbs	2.0	110	16%
Sweet 'n Buttery	⅓ pkg	14.0	180	70%
Movie Theater..light	2 Tbs	5.0	110	41%
natural				
light	2 Tbs	5.0	110	41%
no salt added	2 Tbs	12.0	175	62%
regular	2 Tbs	11.0	15	60%
regular popcorn kernels..unpopped				
original	2 Tbs	1.5	90	15%
white	2 Tbs	1.5	90	15%
Smart Pop				
butter..94% fat-free	⅛ pkg	2.0	110	16%
mini bags	1 bag	2.0	110	16%
Kettle Korn	⅛ pkg	12.0	170	64%
Movie Theater	⅛ pkg	2.0	120	15%
Tender white	⅛ pkg	13.0	180	65%
(Pop Secret) (*See* Betty Crocker in this section)				
(Poppycock) ready-to-eat				
popcorn, pecans & almonds	½ cup	10.0	180	50%
(Smartfood)..reduced-fat				
white cheddar cheese	3 cups	6.0	140	39%
regular..white cheddar cheese	1¾ cups	10.0	160	56%
(Vic's)..Corn Popper..ready-to-eat				
butter				
low-fat	3 cups	1.5	120	11%
regular	2½ cups	7.0	150	42%
caramel				
fat-free	1 cup	–	110	–
light	1 cup	2.0	110	16%
regular	¾ cup	4.0	130	28%
cheese				
white				
light	2½ cups	6.0	130	42%
regular	2 cups	13.0	180	65%
yellow				
light	2½ cups	7.0	140	45%
regular	1½ cups	14.0	190	66%
white				
light				
full salt	2¾ cups	3.0	130	21%
½ salt	2¾ cups	3.0	130	21%
low-fat	3½ cups	1.0	110	8%
regular				
full salt	2½ cups	6.0	150	36%
½ salt	2½ cups	6.0	150	36%

Food and Description	Amount	Fat Grams	Total Calories	% Fat Calories
(Weight Watchers)				
microwavable	1 pouch	1.0	100	9%
ready-to-eat				
butter	0.66 oz	3.0	90	30%
butter-free	0.9 oz	2.5	110	20%
butter toffee	0.9 oz	3.0	110	25%
caramel	0.9 oz	1.0	100	9%
white cheddar	0.66 oz	4.0	90	40%
(Wise)..ready-to-eat				
buttery cheddar	1 oz	11.0	160	62%
hot cheese-flavored	1 oz	9.0	150	54%
light butter	1 oz	5.0	140	32%
original butter	1 oz	10.0	150	60%
white cheddar cheese	1 oz	11.0	160	62%
POPCORN BARS & CAKES (*See also* RICE CAKES)				
(Hain)				
butter				
mini	7 cakes	1.0	50	18%
regular	1 cake	–	50	–
caramel..mini	6 cakes	–	50	–
lightly salted..mini	8 cakes	–	50	–
mild cheddar..mini	6 cakes	1.0	50	18%
plain..regular	1 cake	–	35	–
white cheddar..regular	1 cake	1.0	50	18%
(Mother's)				
butter-flavored	1 cake	–	35	–
unsalted	1 cake	–	35	–
(Orville Redenbacher's)				
butter				
mini	8 cakes	1.0	60	15%
regular	2 cakes	1.0	60	15%
caramel				
mini	6 cakes	–	60	–
regular	2 cakes	–	40	–
chocolate peanut crunch				
mini	6 cakes	0.5	60	8%
regular	1 cake	–	45	–
peanut caramel crunch				
mini	6 cakes	0.5	60	8%
sour cream & onion				
mini	8 cakes	1.0	60	15%
white cheddar				
regular	2 cakes	1.0	60	15%
(Quaker)				
butter				
mini	6 cakes	1.0	50	18%
regular	1 cake	–	35	–
caramel				
mini	5 cakes	1.0	50	18%

Food and Description	Amount	Fat Grams	Total Calories	% Fat Calories
regular	1 cake	–	50	–
cheddar cheese/mini	6 cakes	1.0	50	18%
Monterey Jack				
mini	6 cakes	1.0	50	18%
regular	1 cake	–	40	–
strawberry crunch	1 cake	–	50	–
white cheddar				
mini	6 cakes	1.0	50	18%
regular	1 cake	–	40	–
POPCORN OIL (See OIL)				
POPPY SEED (See also POPPY SEED FILLING)				
	1 tsp	1.0	15	60%
	1 Tbs	4.0	50	72%
POPPY SEED FILLING				
(Solo)	2 Tbs	4.0	140	26%
POPSICLE (See FRUIT ICES, BARS & POPS; ICE CREAM BARS, SANDWICHES & FROZEN NOVELTIES)				
PORGY				
beaded & fried	3 oz	13.0	246	48%
cooked—dry heat	3 oz	8.7	172	46%

PORK (See also BACON; HAM; LUNCHEON MEAT; PORK ENTRÉE; SAUSAGE)
(NOTE: The information listed under Today's Leaner Pork was provided by the National Pork, Livestock, and Meat Board. Following this is nutritional information provided by the United States Department of Agriculture. "Lean" means pork trimmed of separable fat before cooking, "Lean & fat" means untrimmed and cooked or eaten as purchased. Prime cuts have the most fat; choice cuts less; and select cuts the least. In most cases, 4 ounces of raw pork yields approximately 3 ounces cooked. Serving amounts do not include bone.)

■ **TODAY'S LEANER PORK**
(Note: Unless otherwise stated, meat has been trimmed of all separable fat and roasted.)

Food and Description	Amount	Fat Grams	Total Calories	% Fat Calories
blade steak	3 oz	10.7	193	50%
center loin chop	3 oz	6.9	165	38%
center rib chop	3 oz	8.3	179	43%
loin chop	3 oz	6.6	173	34%
loin roast	3 oz	6.0	165	33%
rib chop	3 oz	8.3	186	41%
rib roast	3 oz	8.6	182	43%
ribs (country-style)	3 oz	12.6	210	54%
sirloin chop	3 oz	5.7	164	31%
sirloin roast	3 oz	8.7	184	43%
tenderloin	3 oz	4.0	139	26%
top loin chop	3 oz	6.6	165	36%
■ **PORK CUTS/FRESH**				
backfat/raw	1 oz	24.0	230	94%
	3.5 oz	84.5	812	94%
backribs/lean & fat/roasted	3 oz	23.0	315	66%
	7.7 oz	58.5	815	65%

Food and Description	Amount	Fat Grams	Total Calories	% Fat Calories
belly/raw	1 oz	14.0	150	84%
	1 lb	225.5	2,350	86%
center loin/bone in				
chop				
lean				
braised	3 oz	6.5	175	33%
broiled	3 oz	6.0	170	32%
pan-fried	3 oz	8.0	200	36%
lean & fat				
braised	3 oz	11.0	210	47%
broiled	3 oz	10.0	205	44%
pan-fried	3 oz	13.0	235	50%
roast/roasted				
lean	3 oz	7.0	170	36%
lean & fat	3 oz	10.5	200	47%
ground				
cooked	3 oz	16.0	250	58%
	1 lb	59.0	930	57%
raw	4 oz	22.0	300	66%
leg				
rump half				
lean				
roasted	3 oz	6.5	175	33%
roasted/chopped or diced	1 cup	10.0	280	32%
lean & fat				
roasted	3 oz	11.0	215	46%
roasted/chopped or diced	1 cup	17.5	340	46%
shank half				
lean				
roasted	3 oz	8.0	185	39%
roasted/chopped or diced	1 cup	13.0	290	40%
lean & fat				
roasted	3 oz	15.5	245	57%
roasted/chopped or diced	1 cup	24.5	390	57%
whole				
lean				
roasted	3 oz	7.5	180	37%
roasted/chopped or diced	1 cup	11.5	285	36%
lean & fat				
roasted	3 oz	13.5	230	53%
roasted/chopped or diced	1 cup	21.5	370	52%
loin				
blade/bone-in/chop				
lean				
braised	3 oz	10.0	190	47%
broiled	3 oz	10.5	200	47%
pan-fried	3 oz	11.5	205	50%
roasted	3 oz	11.0	210	47%
lean & fat				
braised	3 oz	19.5	275	64%

Food and Description	Amount	Fat Grams	Total Calories	% Fat Calories
broiled	3 oz	19.0	275	62%
pan-fried	3 oz	21.0	290	65%
roasted	3 oz	19.0	275	62%
center rib				
chop/bone-in				
lean				
braised	3 oz	7.5	175	39%
broiled	3 oz	7.0	190	33%
pan-fried	3 oz	9.0	185	44%
lean & fat				
braised	3 oz	12.0	215	50%
broiled	3 oz	12.0	225	48%
pan-fried	3 oz	13.5	225	54%
chop/boneless				
lean				
braised	3 oz	8.0	180	40%
broiled	3 oz	7.5	185	36%
pan-fried	3 oz	9.5	190	45%
lean & fat				
braised	3 oz	12.5	215	52%
broiled	3 oz	12.0	220	49%
pan-fried	3 oz	14.0	235	54%
roast/bone-in				
lean/roasted	3 oz	9.0	190	43%
lean & fat/roasted	3 oz	12.0	220	49%
roast/boneless				
lean/roasted	3 oz	7.5	185	36%
lean & fat/roasted	3 oz	11.5	215	48%
ribs/country-style				
lean				
braised	3 oz	10.0	200	45%
roasted	3 oz	11.0	210	47%
whole				
lean				
braised	3 oz	7.0	175	36%
broiled	3 oz	7.5	180	38%
roasted	3 oz	7.0	180	35%
shoulder				
arm picnic				
lean				
braised	3 oz	9.5	215	40%
braised/chopped or diced	1 cup	22.0	490	40%
roasted	3 oz	10.0	195	45%
roasted/chopped or diced	1 cup	22.0	435	46%
Boston blade				
roast				
lean				
raw	1 lb	30.5	555	49%
roasted	3 oz	11.0	200	50%
steak				

Food and Description	Amount	Fat Grams	Total Calories	% Fat Calories
lean				
braised	3 oz	12.0	235	47%
broiled	3 oz	9.5	195	44%
whole				
lean				
roasted	3 oz	10.5	200	47%
roasted/chopped or diced	1 cup	16.5	315	47%
sirloin				
chop/bone-in				
lean				
braised	3 oz	7.0	170	37%
broiled	3 oz	7.5	180	37%
chop/boneless				
lean				
braised	3 oz	5.0	150	30%
broiled	3 oz	5.0	165	27%
roast/bone-in				
lean				
raw	1 lb	19.0	450	38%
roasted	3 oz	8.0	185	39%
roast/boneless	3 oz	5.5	165	30%
lean				
raw	1 lb	22.5	610	33%
roasted	3 oz	6.0	170	32%
spareribs/lean & fat				
braised	3 oz	23.5	340	62%
raw	1 lb	48.5	700	62%
tenderloin				
lean				
broiled	3 oz	4.5	160	25%
raw	1 lb	13.5	545	22%
roasted	3 oz	3.5	140	23%
lean & fat				
broiled	3 oz	6.0	170	32%
roasted	3 oz	4.5	150	27%
top loin				
chop/boneless				
lean				
braised	3 oz	6.5	170	34%
broiled	3 oz	6.0	175	31%
pan-fried	3 oz	8.0	190	38%
lean & fat				
braised	3 oz	10.0	200	45%
broiled	3 oz	8.5	195	41%
pan-fried	3 oz	11.5	220	47%
roast/boneless				
lean/roasted	3 oz	5.5	165	30%
lean & fat				
raw	1 lb	31.0	690	40%
roasted	3 oz	9.0	195	42%

Food and Description	Amount	Fat Grams	Total Calories	% Fat Calories
■ **PORK CUTS, ORGAN & OTHER/FRESH**				
brain..braised	3 oz	4.5	120	33%
	13.5 oz	18.0	530	31%
chitterlings..chitlins..simmered	3 oz	23.0	260	80%
	6 oz	46.0	520	80%
ear..simmered	1 ear	–	185	–
	15 oz	–	700	–
feet..simmered	2.5 oz	8.0	140	51%
	5 oz	16.0	275	52%
heart				
braised	1 heart	5.0	190	24%
braised..chopped or diced	1 cup	5.5	215	23%
jowl..raw	4 oz	75.0	740	91%
kidney				
braised	3 oz	3.0	130	21%
braised..chopped or diced	1 cup	5.0	215	22%
liver..braised	3 oz	2.5	140	16%
lung..braised	3 oz	2.0	85	21%
pancreas..braised	3 oz	–	190	–
salt pork..cured..raw				
(Country Creek)	2 oz	25.0	260	87%
generic	1 oz	22.0	215	92%
	8 oz	174.0	1700	92%
spleen/braised	3 oz	2.0	130	14%
stomach/raw	4 oz	–	180	–
tail				
raw	4 oz	35.0	430	73%
simmered	3 oz	28.0	340	74%
tongue..braised	3 oz	14.5	230	57%
PORK CUTS/FRESH by BRAND				
(Hormel)..Always Tender				
seasoned				
garlic pork tenderloin	4 oz	5.0	130	35%
honey mustard pork				
loin fillet	4 oz	5.0	140	32%
mesquite pork tenderloin	4 oz	5.0	130	35%
mojo pork loin fillet	4 oz	5.0	140	32%
onion garlic pork				
shoulder roast	4 oz	11.0	180	55%
peppercorn pork				
tenderloin	4 oz	4.0	140	26%
teriyaki tenderloin	4 oz	4.0	140	26%
PORK & BEANS (*See* BEANS, BAKED & VARIETY)				
PORK ENTRÉE (*See also* ASIAN FOOD; FROZEN ENTRÉE/DINNER)				
(Betty Crocker)..prepared				
Pork Helper...box mix				
breaded pork chops				
& mashed potatoes	⅕ box	18.0	340	48%
pork chops & stuffing	⅕ pkg	14.0	320	39%
pork fried rice	⅕ pkg	15.0	340	40%
(Bob Evans)..frozen				

Food and Description	Amount	Fat Grams	Total Calories	% Fat Calories
pulled pork.. w/wildfire BBQ sauce	2 oz	6.0	150	36%
(Bryan)..frozen..pre-cooked				
baby back ribs	3 oz	17.0	310	49%
Boston butt	3 oz	9.0	110	65%
St. Louis–style ribs	3 oz	19.0	240	71%
(Castleberry's)..BBQ pork in				
hickory-smoked sauce	2.2 oz	12.0	160	68%
(Delores)				
pickled pork rinds	2 oz	3.0	60	30%
pig's feet	2 oz	6.0	90	60%
(Hillshire Farm)..frozen				
BBQ ribs..St. Louis–style..w/sauce				
cooked..frozen	5 oz	26.0	350	67%
boneless cooked pork roast	3 oz	11.0	170	58%
premier roast of pork loin	3 oz	8.0	170	42%
(Hormel)				
fully cooked entrées				
pork roast	5 oz	7.0	180	35%
pork chops..w/gravy	5 oz	5.0	160	28%
pulled BBQ pork	2 oz	2.5	90	25%
sliced BBQ pork	5 oz	4.5	200	20%
Southwestern pork carnitas	2 oz	2.0	60	30%
pickled				
pig's feet	2 oz	6.0	80	68%
pork hocks	2 oz	8.0	110	65%
pork tidbits	2 oz	8.0	100	72%
(Plumrose)..ready-to-eat				
baby back ribs..BBQ sauce	5 oz	11.0	280	35%
(Schwan's)				
BBQ baby back ribs	5 oz	22.0	370	54%
center-cut pork loin chops	6.0 oz	12.0	240	45%
pork loin chop..boneless	6 oz	12.0	250	43%
pork roast..herb & garlic				
oven-roasted	4 oz	5.0	130	35%

PORK FAT (See LARD)
PORK RINDS (See PORK ENTRÉE; SNACKS)
PORK SAUSAGE (See SAUSAGE)
POTPIE (See BEEF DISH/ENTRÉE; CHICKEN ENTRÉE/DINNER; FROZEN ENTRÉE/DINNER; TURKEY ENTRÉE/DINNER; VEGETARIAN FOODS)
POTATO (See also POTATO DISH/ENTRÉE; SWEET POTATO; YAM)
CANNED

(Bush's Best)..all types	½ cup	–	40	–
(Del Monte)				
new				
diced	½ cup	–	45	–
sliced	⅔ cup	–	60	–
whole..new w/liquid	~2 medium	–	60	–
Savory Sides..potatoes				
au gratin	½ cup	2.5	80	28%

Food and Description	Amount	Fat Grams	Total Calories	% Fat Calories
(S&W)..new				
small..whole	½ cup	–	60	–
(The Allen's Butterfield)				
new				
diced	6 oz	–	100	–
sliced	6 oz	–	100	–
whole	6 oz	–	90	–
sticks				
shoestring	1 oz	9.0	150	54%
	1.7 oz	15.0	250	54%
FLAKES..GRANULES				
(Betty Crocker) Potato Buds				
original..mix only	⅓ cup	–	80	–
(Idaho) mashed potatoes/prepared w/2% milk and margarine				
flakes	½ cup	6.0	150	36%
granules	½ cup	7.0	160	39%
(Idahoan) mix only				
cheddar/spicy	⅙ pkg	1.0	90	10%
real	⅓ cup	1.0	80	11%
FRESH				
baked				
in microwave				
w/skin	1 large	–	212	–
w/o skin	1 large	–	156	–
in oven				
w/skin	~7 oz	–	220	–
w/o skin	~5.5 oz	–	145	–
boiled				
w/skin	½ cup	–	68	–
w/o skin	½ cup	–	67	–
raw				
w/skin	1 medium	–	110	–
w/o skin	1 medium	–	100	–
FROZEN or REFRIGERATED				
(Bob Evans)				
hash browns..original	1 serving	–	70	–
home fries	1 serving	–	80	–
mashed				
garlic	1 serving	6.0	150	36%
original	1 serving	8.0	160	45%
(C&W) whole red	2 large			
	or 3 small	–	60	–
(Inland Valley)				
Crinkle Cuts				
French-fried style	8 oz	5.0	150	30%
Crispy Classics				
French fries	3 oz	7.0	180	15%
Curley QQQ's	1⅓ cups	8.0	180	40%
French fries	3 oz	4.0	180	20%

Food and Description	Amount	Fat Grams	Total Calories	% Fat Calories
hash browns				
O'Brien	1 cup	–	60	–
Simply Shreds	1 cup	–	70	–
Southern-style	3 oz	–	70	–
mashed				
home-style	⅔ cup	6.0	160	34%
Papa's onduladas	8 oz	5.0	180	25%
Potato				
pancakes	1 pancake	8.0	120	60%
stix	3 oz	10.0	170	53%
Seasoned & coated				
criss-cut fries	3 oz	7.0	160	39%
fajita fries	3 oz	8.0	170	42%
Long Branch	3 oz	7.0	160	39%
Santa Fe corn fries	8 oz	9.0	180	45%
tasty QQQ's	1½ cups	9.0	190	43%
Tater Babies	3 oz	5.0	130	35%
shredded..seasoned				
potato patties	1 patty	2.0	130	14%
skins..twice-baked				
gourmet..5 oz	1 skin	12.0	280	39%
sour cream..bacon..				
& cheddar	1 skin	8.0	240	30%
triple-cheese				
5.1 oz	1 skin	10.0	250	36%
triple-cheese..stuffed shell	8 oz	17.0	400	38%
steak fries	3 oz	3.0	110	25%
Stuffed Spudz	8 0z	11.0	210	47%
Tater Puffs	3 oz	7.0	160	39%
(Lamb Weston)				
Colossal Crinkles	4.5 oz	7.0	170	37%
Crinkle Cuts				
slim	4 oz	7.0	170	37%
wedge-cut..skin on	5 oz	7.0	160	39%
MunchSkins				
cheddar..bite-size rounds	4 oz	10.0	180	50%
natural	4 oz	4.0	120	30%
pepper shape	4 oz	10.0	190	47%
Southwest				
cheddar..bite-size				
rounds	4 oz	9.0	180	45%
regular cuts..skin on	4.5 oz	5.0	160	28%
regular cuts..thin..skin on	4 oz	6.0	170	32%
shoestrings	4 oz	8.0	190	38%
steak house fries..skin-on	5 oz	5.0	140	32%
MICROWAVE BOWLS				
(Dinty Moore)				
au gratin potatoes				
w/ham	1 bowl	15.0	310	44%

POTATO CHIPS & SNACKS (*See also* SNACKS)

Food and Description	Amount	Fat Grams	Total Calories	% Fat Calories
(Aunt Lisa's)				
Classic Selects..all styles	1 oz	10.0	150	60%
(Barbara's)				
no salt added	1 oz	10.0	150	60%
regular	1 oz	10.0	150	60%
ripple	1 oz	10.0	150	60%
yogurt & green onion	1 oz	9.0	150	54%
(Borden)				
Calypso/sweet & spicy Caribbean	1 oz	10.0	160	56%
Curlie/plain	1 oz	10.0	150	60%
home fries	1 oz	10.0	150	60%
Krunchers				
jalapeño	1 oz	8.0	140	51%
mesquite BBQ	1 oz	8.0	140	51%
original	1 oz	9.0	150	54%
New York Deli				
jalapeño	1 oz	8.0	140	51%
plain	1 oz	10.0	150	60%
original				
BBQ	1 oz	10.0	160	56%
hot	1 oz	10.0	150	60%
lightly salted	1 oz	10.0	150	60%
onion & garlic	1 oz	10.0	150	60%
salt & vinegar	1 oz	10.0	150	60%
Ranch Fries..all styles	1 oz	10.0	150	60%
Ridgies..all flavors	1 oz	10.0	150	60%
(Cape Cod)				
no salt	1 oz	10.0	150	60%
original	1 oz	8.0	150	48%
sea salt & vinegar	1 oz	8.0	150	48%
select	1 oz	6.0	130	42%
sour cream & chive	1 oz	9.0	150	54%
(Frito-Lay)				
Lay's Baked Potato Crisps				
BBQ	1 oz	3.0	120	23%
original	1 oz	1.5	110	12%
sour cream & onion	1 oz	3.0	120	23%
Lay's Bristo & Gourmet				
applewood BBQ &				
smoked cheddar	1 oz	10.0	150	60%
peppercorn ranch	1 oz	9.0	150	54%
roasted garlic & herb	1 oz	9.0	150	54%
sharp cheddar &				
jalapeño	1 oz	10.0	150	60%
Lay's Deli-Style				
original	1 oz	10.0	150	60%
Lay's Kettle-Cooked				
classic potato	1 oz	8.0	150	48%
jalapeño..extra-crunchy	1 oz	8.0	140	51%
mesquite BBQ	1 oz	8.0	140	51%

Food and Description	Amount	Fat Grams	Total Calories	% Fat Calories
Lay's original potato chips				
Cracker Barrel..sharp				
cheddar cheese	1 oz	10.0	150	60%
deli-style original	1 oz	10.0	150	60%
KC Masterpiece BBQ	1 oz	10.0	150	60%
Limon	1 oz	10.0	150	60%
original	1 oz	10.0	150	60%
Santa Fe ranch	1 oz	9.0	150	54%
sea salt & vinegar	1 oz	10.0	160	60%
sour cream & onion	1 oz	9.0	160	51%
spicy BBQ	1 oz	9.0	150	51%
Taste of America				
California cool dill	1 oz	10.0	160	60%
Memphis BBQ	1 oz	10.0	160	60%
unsalted	1 oz	10.0	160	56%
wavy original	1 oz	10.0	160	56%
Ruffles baked potato chips				
all flavors	1 oz	3.0	120	23%
Ruffles original potato chips				
3 D's				
BBQ	1 oz	7.0	140	45%
maximum cheddar	1 oz	7.0	140	45%
Supreme sour cream	1 oz	8.0	140	51%
buffalo-style	1 oz	10.0	160	56%
Bull's Eye..BBQ	1 oz	10.0	150	60%
cheddar & sour cream	1 oz	10.0	160	56%
Flavor Rush				
big BBQ & cheddar	1 oz	10.0	160	56%
buffalo Wild Wings & ranch	1 oz	10.0	150	60%
zesty sour cream & onion	1 oz	10.0	150	60%
French onion	1 oz	10.0	150	60%
KC Masterpiece BBQ	1 oz	9.0	150	54%
original	1 oz	10.0	160	60%
reduced-fat				
BBQ	1 oz	7.0	140	45%
sea-salted natural	1 oz	6.0	140	39%
sour cream & onion	1 oz	10.0	150	60%
The Works	1 oz	11.0	160	62%
Wow! fat-free potato chips				
Lay's				
mesquite BBQ	1 oz	–	75	–
original	1 oz	–	75	–
sour cream & chive	1 oz	–	80	–
Ruffles				
cheddar & sour cream	1 oz	–	75	–
original	1 oz	–	75	–
(Garden of Eatin')				
onion & garlic	1 oz	8.0	140	51%
original	1 oz	9.0	150	54%
Parmesan garlic	1 oz	9.0	150	54%

Food and Description	Amount	Fat Grams	Total Calories	% Fat Calories
salt & vinegar	1 oz	9.0	150	54%
(Health Valley)..all styles	1 oz	10.0	160	60%
(Kettle Chips) Natural Gourmet				
Krinkle Cut				
dill & sour cream	1 oz	8.0	140	51%
lightly salted	1 oz	9.0	150	54%
salsa..w/mesquite	1 oz	6.0	140	39%
salt & fresh ground pepper	1 oz	9.0	150	54%
Krisps..low-fat..baked				
French onion	1 oz	1.5	110	12%
hickory BBQ	1 oz	1.5	110	12%
lightly salted	1 oz	1.5	110	12%
mustard & honey	1 oz	1.5	110	12%
New York cheddar w/herbs	1 oz	9.0	150	54%
no salt	1 oz	9.0	150	54%
organically grown	1 oz	9.0	150	54%
original				
habañero chili				
w/ginger	1 oz	8.0	140	51%
honey Dijon	1 oz	8.0	150	48%
lightly salted				
krinkle cut	1 oz	9.0	150	54%
regular	1 oz	9.0	150	54%
Parmesan & black pepper	1 oz	9.0	150	54%
salsa w/mesquite				
krinkle cut	1 oz	8.0	140	51%
sea salt & vinegar	1 oz	8.0	150	48%
yogurt & green onion	1 oz	8.0	150	48%
(Krunchers!)				
all-natural	1 oz	9.0	150	54%
jalapeño	1 oz	8.0	140	52%
mesquite	1 oz	8.0	140	52%
(Lance)				
Boomin' Barbecue Rumble	22 chips	8.0	140	51%
Chargin' sour cream & onion				
big bag	1 oz	10.0	160	56%
Howlin' Hot & Spicy Rumble	22 chips	8.0	140	51%
Original Rumble	23 chips	10.0	160	56%
Rumble				
buffalo wing & blue cheese	22 chips	8.0	150	48%
Wild Sour Cream & Onion	22 chips	9.0	150	54%
Stormy Salt & Vinegar Rumble	22 chips	8.0	150	48%
(Lay's) (See (Frito-Lay) in this section)				
(Louise's) potato chips				
Maui onion/fat-free	1 oz	–	110	–
mesquite BBQ				
fat-free	1 oz	–	110	–
"1g"	1 oz	1.0	110	8%
70% less fat	1 oz	3.0	110	25%
no salt/fat-free	1 oz	–	110	–

Food and Description	Amount	Fat Grams	Total Calories	% Fat Calories
original				
fat-free	1 oz	–	110	–
"1g"	1 oz	1.0	110	8%
70% less fat	1 oz	3.0	110	25%
(Michael Season's)				
Kettle-Cooked				
jalapeño & cheese	1 oz	8.0	150	48%
lightly salted	1 oz	8.0	140	51%
mesquite barbecue	1 oz	8.0	140	51%
reduced-fat				
cheddar & sour cream	1 oz	7.0	140	45%
honey BBQ	1 oz	6.0	140	39%
lightly salted				
regular	1 oz	6.0	130	42%
ripple	1 oz	6.7	140	43%
salt & vinegar	1 oz	6.0	130	42%
unsalted	1 oz	6.0	130	42%
yogurt & green onion	1 oz	6.0	130	42%
(Mike-Sell's)				
Groovy Party Size	1 oz	9.0	150	54%
Honey Bar-B-Que	1 oz	9.0	150	48%
old-fashioned family-size	1 oz	8.0	150	48%
original family-size	1 oz	9.0	150	54%
reduced-fat	1 oz	6.7	140	43%
zesty BBQ	1 oz	9.0	150	54%
(Old Vienna)				
Missouri dairy sour cream & onion	1 oz	9.0	150	54%
original/Heartland Pride	1 oz	11.0	180	55%
Ozark hickory	1 oz	10.0	170	53%
Riplets				
grilled steak & onion	1 oz	9.0	150	54%
Heartland Pride	1 oz	10.0	150	60%
red-hot	1 oz	9.0	150	54%
Wisconsin cheddar & sour cream	1 oz	10.0	150	60%
(Pik-Nik)				
shoestring potatoes				
¾ oz can	1 can	18.0	250	65%
50% less salt	⅔ cup	10.0	158	57%
(Poore Brothers)				
BBQ	1 oz	8.0	140	51%
Cajun	1 oz	8.0	140	51%
dill pickle	1 oz	8.0	140	51%
jalapeño	1 oz	8.0	140	51%
original				
regular	1 oz	10.0	150	60%
unsalted	1 oz	8.0	140	51%
Parmesan & garlic	1 oz	8.0	140	51%
salt & vinegar	1 oz	7.0	130	48%
sour cream & onion	1 oz	8.0	140	51%
(Pringle's) potato crisps				

Food and Description	Amount	Fat Grams	Total Calories	% Fat Calories
regular				
BBQ..sweet mesquite				
fat-free	1 oz	–	70	–
regular	1 oz	11.0	160	62%
Right Crisp	1 oz	7.0	140	45%
Cheez-ums/regular	1 oz	11.0	160	62%
original				
fat-free	1 oz	–	70	–
regular	1 oz	11.0	160	62%
Right Crisp	1 oz	7.0	140	45%
Pizza-Licious/regular	1 oz	11.0	160	62%
ranch				
fat-free	1 oz	–	70	–
regular	1 oz	11.0	160	62%
Right Crisp	1 oz	7.0	140	45%
salt & vinegar	1 oz	11.0	160	62%
sour cream 'n' onion				
fat-free	1 oz	–	70	–
regular	1 oz	10.0	160	56%
right	1 oz	7.0	140	45%
(Route 11)				
classic chips				
BBQ	1 oz	7.0	150	42%
Chesapeake Crab	1 oz	7.0	150	42%
dill pickle	1 oz	7.0	150	42%
garlic & herb	1 oz	8.0	150	48%
llightly salted	1 oz	8.0	150	48%
no salt	1 oz	7.0	150	42%
salt 'n' vinegar	1 oz	7.0	150	42%
sour cream 'n' chive	1 oz	7.0	150	42%
specialty chips				
Hayman	1 oz	8.0	150	48%
Mama Zuma's Revenge	1 oz	8.0	150	48%
green chile enchilada	1 oz	8.0	150	48%
Mama Zuma's Revenge				
habañero	1 oz	8.0	150	48%
Route 11				
mixed vegetable	1 oz	8.0	150	48%
sweet potato chips	1 oz	8.0	150	48%
Tabard Farm Yukon golds	1 oz	8.0	150	48%
Taro	1 oz	8.0	150	48%
Ruffles (*See* Frito-Lay in this section)				
(Snyder's)				
regular chips				
BBQ	1 oz	6.0	150	36%
BBQ rib	1 oz	7.0	140	45%
buffalo wing hot	1 oz	7.0	150	42%
cheddar bacon	1 oz	8.0	150	48%
jalapeño	1 oz	6.0	150	36%
kosher dill	1 oz	6.0	140	39%

Food and Description	Amount	Fat Grams	Total Calories	% Fat Calories
no salt	1 oz	10.0	150	60%
original	1 oz	6.0	140	39%
salt & vinegar	1 oz	6.0	140	39%
sausage pizza	1 oz	6.0	150	36%
sour cream & onion	1 oz	7.0	150	42%
unsalted	1 oz	6.0	140	39%
ripple chips..original	1 oz	6.0	140	39%
(T.G.I. Friday's)				
potato skins snack chips				
cheddar & bacon	16 chips	10.0	150	60%
sour cream & onion	16 chips	10.0	150	60%
(Terra) chips				
Blues	1 oz	6.0	140	39%
original	1 oz	7.0	140	45%
potpourri	1 oz	7.0	140	45%
Red Bliss				
olive oil & fine herbs	1 oz	7.0	140	45%
roasted garlic & Parmesan	1 oz	7.0	140	45%
sun-dried tomato				
& balsamic vinegar	1 oz	7.0	140	45%
spiced	1 oz	5.0	130	35%
sticks	1 oz	9.0	150	54%
sweet potato				
Frites				
American	1 oz	8.0	150	48%
aioli	1 oz	8.0	150	48%
malt vinegar	1 oz	8.0	150	48%
seasoned salt	1 oz	8.0	150	48%
Southwestern spices	1 oz	10.0	160	56%
jalapeño	1 oz	7.0	140	45%
mesquite BBQ	1 oz	7.0	140	45%
original..no salt	1 oz	7.0	140	45%
salsa	1 oz	7.0	140	45%
spiced	1 oz	7.0	140	45%
Terra				
Mediterranean	1 oz	7.0	140	45%
original	1 oz	7.0	140	45%
spiced taro chips	1 oz	5.0	130	35%
zesty tomato	1 oz	7.0	140	45%
Yukon Gold..50% less fat				
all flavors	1 oz	5.0	130	35%
(Wise)				
all-natural				
New York deli	1 oz	9.0	150	60%
regular	1 oz	10.0	150	60%
ridged	1 oz	10.0	150	60%
regular				
BBQ	1 oz	10.0	160	56%
cheddar & sour cream	1 oz	10.0	160	56%
cottage fries				

Food and Description	Amount	Fat Grams	Total Calories	% Fat Calories
no salt added	1 oz	10.0	150	60%
honey BBQ	1 oz	10.0	150	60%
original	1 oz	10.0	150	60%
hot	1 oz	11.0	160	62%
lightly salted	1 oz	10.0	150	60%
New York deli jalapeño	1 oz	8.0	140	51%
onion garlic	1 oz	10.0	150	60%
plain	1 oz	10.0	150	60%
salt & vinegar	1 oz	10.0	150	60%
Smoky Mountain BBQ	1 oz	10.0	150	60%
sour cream & onion	1 oz	10.0	150	60%
Ridgies				
all-natural	1 oz	10.0	150	60%
BBQ	1 oz	10.0	150	60%
cheddar & sour cream	1 oz	10.0	160	56%
mesquite	1 oz	10.0	150	60%
original	1 oz	10.0	150	60%
plain	1 oz	10.0	150	60%
sour cream & onion	1 oz	10.0	150	60%
rippled	1 oz	10.0	150	60%

POTATO DISH/ENTRÉE (*See also* FROZEN ENTRÉE/DINNER; SEASONINGS; VEGETARIAN FOODS)

■ CANNED/FRESH/MICROWAVABLE

Food and Description	Amount	Fat Grams	Total Calories	% Fat Calories
(Fantastic)..microwavable..potato cups				
bacon & white cheddar				
stuffed	1 cup	2.5	160	14%
chili bean & cheese	1 cup	2.5	150	15%
creamy butter	1 cup	3.0	140	19%
roasted chicken				
w/vegetables	1 cup	2.0	150	12%
roasted garlic	1 cup	3.0	170	16%
roasted garlic & mushroom	1 cup	3.0	160	17%
sour cream & chives	1 cup	2.0	160	11%
white cheddar & broccoli	1 cup	3.0	170	16%
(Purely Idaho)				
potatoes..heat & serve				
au gratin	¼ pkg	7.0	185	34%
cheddar-crusted	¼ pkg	1.0	120	8%
garlic Parmesan	¼ pkg	0.5	120	4%
hash browns	¼ pkg	–	100	–
herb-roasted	¼ pkg	–	110	–
home-style..mashed	¼ pkg	7.0	170	37%
	⅓ pkg	7.0	150	42%
roasted garlic..mashed	⅓ pkg	7.0	150	42%
roasted onion	¼ pkg	–	110	–
scalloped Southwest-style	¼ pkg	6.0	170	32%
(Read)..canned				
potato salad German-style	½ cup	3.0	120	23%
(Reser's)..fresh				
Potato Express				

Food and Description	Amount	Fat Grams	Total Calories	% Fat Calories
mashed				
caramelized	½ cup	7.0	160	39%
country	½ cup	3.5	130	24%
creamy deluxe	½ cup	8.0	160	45%
garlic	½ cup	6.0	150	34%
low-sodium	½ cup	3.5	130	24%
premium	½ cup	4.0	130	28%
red skin	½ cup	4.5	140	29%
sweet potato	½ cup	5.0	140	32%
potato salad				
deviled egg	½ cup	13.0	230	51%
farm-style	½ cup	10.0	190	47%
mustard	½ cup	8.0	180	40%
red potato	½ cup	19.0	270	63%
regular	½ cup	12.0	230	47%
seasoned potatoes				
chipotle BBQ–seasoned	3 oz	–	80	–
garden herb–seasoned	3 oz	–	90	–
rosemary roasted garlic	3 oz	–	80	–
■ FROZEN OR REFRIGERATED				
(Lamb Weston)				
Lamb's Supreme				
mashed potatoes..prepared				
original recipe	1 serving	3.5	120	26%
redskin	1 serving	4.0	120	30%
roasted garlic	1 serving	5.0	150	30%
seasoned	1 serving	4.5	150	27%
lightly seasoned	1 serving	6.0	160	34%
(Larry's) stuffed potatoes				
bacon & cheese	1 potato	10.0	200	45%
bacon..onion..& tomato	1 potato	9.0	190	42%
broccoli & cheese	1 potato	9.0	190	42%
cheddar cheese	1 potato	10.0	200	45%
creamy ranch	1 potato	8.0	170	42%
old-fashioned butter	1 potato	8.0	190	38%
Parmesan & garlic	1 potato	7.0	170	37%
Parmesan & herb..w/potato skins	1 potato	7.0	170	37%
roasted garlic	1 potato	9.0	200	41%
sour cream & chives	1 potato	9.0	190	42%
toasted onion & cheddar	1 potato	7.0	170	37%
w/classic beef gravy	1 potato	7.0	160	39%
w/classic chicken gravy	1 potato	8.0	170	42%
(Mrs. Ts) pierogies				
potato				
& cheddar	¼ pkg	2.5	180	13%
mini	¼ pkg	1.5	130	10%
& cheese blend	¼ pkg	4.5	160	25%
& onion	¼ pkg	2.0	180	10%
& roasted garlic	4 oz	3.5	190	17%
American cheese	4 oz	3.5	180	18%

Food and Description	Amount	Fat Grams	Total Calories	% Fat Calories
broccoli & cheddar	4 oz	4.5	200	20%
cheddar & bacon..mini	¼ pkg	3.0	140	19%
cheddar & jalapeño	¼ pkg	2.5	180	13%
4-cheese blend	4 oz	7.0	220	29%
jalapeño & cheddar..mini	¼ pkg	2.0	130	14%
sour cream & chive	4 oz	5.0	200	23%
(Ore-Ida)				
baked/topped/broccoli & cheese	10.25 oz	8.0	310	23%
Crispers!				
Texas	3 oz	7.0	150	42%
original	½ pkg	12.0	210	51%
Crispy Crowns	3 oz	9.0	170	48%
French fries				
country-style	3 oz	4.5	120	34%
golden crinkles	3 oz	3.5	120	26%
golden fries	3 oz	3.5	120	26%
golden patties	1 patty	8.0	150	48%
golden twirls	3 oz	7.0	160	39%
hash browns				
country-style shredded	1¼ cups	–	80	–
pixie crinkles	3 oz	4.5	130	31%
shoestrings	3 oz	6.0	150	36%
shredded	1 patty	–	70	–
Southern-style	⅔ cup	–	70	–
steak				
country-style	3 oz	3.5	110	29%
regular	3 oz	3.0	110	25%
toaster	3.5 oz	12.0	220	49%
waffle	3 oz	7.0	150	42%
wedges	3 oz	4.0	120	30%
Hot Bites!				
deep-dish minis				
cheese..sausage & pepperoni	2 bites	10.0	260	35%
pepperoni & cheese	2 bites	12.0	280	39%
3-cheese	2 bites	9.0	240	34%
li'l calzones				
sausage..pepperoni & cheese	3 bites	6.0	200	27%
3-cheese	3 bites	6.0	190	28%
nacho dippers	5 bites	14.0	260	48%
tater dogs	4 bites	18.0	280	58%
mashed potatoes	½ cup	2.0	90	20%
potatoes O'Brien	⅛ pkg	–	60	–
sweet potatoes..candied w/sauce packet	5 oz	–	180	–
Tater Tots				
mini	3.5 oz	18.0	280	58%
seasoned	¹⁄₁₁ pkg	7.0	150	42%
w/onion	9 pieces	8.0	170	42%

Food and Description	Amount	Fat Grams	Total Calories	% Fat Calories
twice-baked				
butter flavor	5 oz	6.0	160	34%
cheddar cheese	5 oz	7.0	180	35%
wedges w/skin on				
country-style	3 oz	3.0	110	25%
regular	3 oz	2.5	110	20%
Zesties!	3 oz	7.0	150	42%
Zesty twirls	3 oz	6.0	150	36%
(Owens)				
mashed potatoes				
garlic	⅕ pkg	6.0	150	36%
original	⅕ pkg	8.0	160	36%
(Simply Potatoes)				
hash browns..shredded				
plain	⅐ pkg	–	70	–
onion	⅙ pkg	–	80	–
Southwestern-style	⅐ pkg	–	70	–
sliced home-fried	⅕ pkg	–	90	–
wedges	⅐ pkg	–	50	–
(T.G.I. Friday's)				
stuffed potatoes				
broccoli & cheddar	⅓ pkg	6.0	140	39%
cheddar & bacon	⅓ pkg	9.0	170	48%
4-cheese pepperoni	⅓ pkg	8.0	160	34%
■ MIX				
(Betty Crocker)..prepared by regular recipe				
specialty potatoes				
au gratin	½ cup	6.0	150	36%
broccoli au gratin	½ cup	4.0	120	30%
butter & herb..mashed	½ cup	7.0	160	39%
cheddar & bacon	½ cup	4.5	130	31%
cheddar & bacon..mashed	½ cup	7.0	150	42%
cheesy scalloped..home-style	½ cup	6.0	150	36%
chicken & herb	½ cup	7.0	150	42%
creamy butter..mashed	½ cup	7.0	160	39%
deluxe cheesy cheddar au gratin	½ cup	9.0	180	45%
4-cheese..mashed	½ cup	7.0	160	39%
hash brown	½ cup	5.0	160	20%
julienne	⅔ cup	3.5	110	29%
mashed				
gravy & hearty beef	½ cup	7.0	170	37%
gravy & roast chicken	¾ cup	7.0	170	37%
roasted garlic	½ cup	8.0	160	30%
roasted garlic & cheddar	½ cup	7.0	160	39%
sour cream 'n' chives	½ cup	7.0	150	42%
ranch	⅔ cup	3.5	130	24%
roasted garlic	½ cup	4.0	120	30%
scalloped	½ cup	4.0	130	28%
sour cream 'n' chives	⅔ cup	4.0	120	30%

Food and Description	Amount	Fat Grams	Total Calories	% Fat Calories
3-cheese	⅔ cup	4.0	130	28%
twice-baked..cheddar & bacon	¾ cup	9.0	180	40%
(Idahoan)..mix only				
au gratin	⅕ box	1.5	110	20%
hash brown				
skillet	⅕ box	0.5	90	5%
mashed				
butter & herb	¼ box	2.5	110	20%
buttery home-style	¼ box	2.5	110	20%
complete	⅛ box	2.0	110	16%
4-cheese	¼ box	2.5	100	23%
loaded baked-flavor	¼ box	2.5	110	23%
original	¼ box	–	80	–
roasted garlic	¼ box	2.5	110	23%
Southwest	¼ box	2.5	110	23%
scalloped	⅕ box	1.5	100	14%
Southwestern	¼ pkg	2.0	110	23%
(Manischewitz)..potato pancake				
mix only	3 Tbs	1.0	80	11%
(Mrs. Manischewitz)..latka				
home-style	2 Tbs	1.0	80	11%
(Panni)..mix only				
Bavarian potato dumpling	⅐ pkg	–	80	–
dumplings..potato..6-count	1 dumpling	–	100	–
Bavarian potato pancake	1/12 pkg	–	50	–
POTATO PANCAKE (*See* POTATO DISH/ENTRÉE)				
POTATO SNACKS (*See* POTATO CHIPS & SNACKS)				
POTATO SOUP (*See* SOUP)				
POTATO STARCH				
(Manischewitz)	1 Tbs	–	30	–
	½ cup	–	285	–
POTTED MEAT (*See* LUNCHEON MEAT; LUNCHEON MEAT SPREAD)				
POULTRY SEASONING (*See* SEASONINGS)				
POUT, OCEAN				
raw	3 oz	1.0	70	13%
PRESERVES (*See* JAM/JELLY/PRESERVES)				
PRETZEL				
(Auntie Anne's)..soft baked..large				
almond	1 pretzel	8.0	400	18%
w/cinnamon sugar	1 pretzel	9.0	450	18%
w/o butter	1 pretzel	1.5	350	4%
Blazin' Raisin	1 pretzel	4.0	510	7%
w/o butter	1 pretzel	0.5	470	1%
cinnamon sugar	1 pretzel	9.0	450	18%
w/o butter	1 pretzel	2.0	350	5%
garlic	1 pretzel	4.5	350	9%
w/o butter	1 pretzel	1.0	320	3%
jalapeño	1 pretzel	4.5	310	13%
w/o butter	1 pretzel	1.0	270	3%
maple crumb	1 pretzel	6.0	550	10%

Food and Description	Amount	Fat Grams	Total Calories	% Fat Calories
w/o butter	1 pretzel	3.0	520	5%
original	1 pretzel	4.0	370	10%
w/o butter	1 pretzel	1.0	340	3%
Parmesan herb	1 pretzel	13.0	440	27%
w/o butter	1 pretzel	5.0	390	12%
pretzel dog	1 dog	16.0	290	50%
sesame	1 pretzel	12.0	410	26%
w/o butter	1 pretzel	6.0	350	15%
Smart Bites	1 bite	0.5	10	45%
	15 bites	7.5	150	45%
sour cream & onion	1 pretzel	5.0	340	13%
w/o butter	1 pretzel	1.0	310	3%
Sticks				
cinnamon sugar	1 stick	6.0	300	18%
w/o butter	1 stick	1.0	233	4%
original	1 stick	3.0	247	11%
w/o butter	1 stick	1.0	227	4%
whole wheat	1 stick	4.5	370	11%
w/o butter	1 stick	1.5	350	4%
(Borden)				
fat-free				
low-fat mini..all flavors	21 pieces	1.5	110	12%
thins	6 pieces	–	100	–
ultra-thin	8 pieces	–	100	–
(Combos)				
cheddar cheese				
family bag	⅓ cup	4.5	130	31%
single bag	1.8 oz	8.0	240	30%
nacho cheese				
family bag	⅓ cup	4.5	130	31%
single bag	1.8 oz	8.0	240	30%
pizzeria				
family bag	⅓ cup	4.5	130	31%
single bag	1.8 oz	8.0	230	31%
(Michael Season's) O.G.'s Organic				
honey mustard nuggets	1 oz	<1.0	120	3%
lightly salted..all shapes	1 oz	<1.0	110	3%
sesame garlic nuggets	1 oz	1.0	120	8%
unsalted..all shapes	1 oz	<1.0	110	3%
(Mike Sell's)				
Dutch oven-baked	1 oz	2.0	130	14%
pretzel				
nuggets..fat-free sourdough	1 oz	0.5	110	5%
thins..fat-free	1 oz	–	110	–
twists..mini	1 oz	1.5	110	12%
(Mrs. Manischewitz) bagel pretzel				
all styles	4 pretzels	–	110	–
(Newman's Own)..Organic				
Bavarian sourdough	1 pretzel	–	90	–
hi-protein	1 oz	1.5	120	11%

Food and Description	Amount	Fat Grams	Total Calories	% Fat Calories
nuggets	1 oz	1.5	120	11%
rods	1 oz	1.5	120	11%
rounds				
regular	1 oz	1.0	110	8%
unsalted	1 oz	1.0	110	8%
salt & pepper	1 oz	1.0	100	9%
spelt	1 oz	1.0	120	8%
thins				
regular	1 oz	1.0	110	8%
unsalted	1 oz	1.0	110	8%
salt & pepper	1 oz	1.0	120	8%
sticks	1 oz	1.0	110	8%
(Planters) twists	1 oz	0.5	100	5%
	1.5 oz	1.0	160	6%
(Pocket Pretzels) peanut butter–filled	1 oz	4.0	126	29%
(Quinlan)				
beer	1 oz	1.0	110	8%
logs	1 oz	1.5	110	12%
mini				
fat-free	1 oz	–	100	–
logs	1 oz	1.5	110	12%
low-fat	1 oz	1.0	110	8%
regular	1 oz	1.0	110	8%
nuggets	1 oz	1.0	110	8%
rods	1 oz	2.0	110	16%
sourdough..hard				
sticks	1 oz	1.0	110	8%
thins				
party	1 oz	1.0	110	8%
plain	1 oz	1.0	110	8%
sourdough	1 oz	–	100	–
tiny thins..all types	1 oz	1.0	110	8%
ultra thins..fat-free	1 oz	–	110	–
(Rokeach)				
Dutch	1 oz	–	110	–
no salt	1 oz	–	110	–
party canister	1 oz	1.0	110	8%
(Rold Gold)				
Cracker Barrel..sharp				
cheddar cheese	1 oz	1.0	110	8%
fat-free				
thins	1 oz	–	110	–
tiny twists	1 oz	–	100	–
regular				
classic				
cheddar cheese				
tiny twists	1 oz	1.0	110	8%
honey mustard				
tiny twists	1 oz	1.0	110	8%
natural	1 oz	0.5	110	4%

Food and Description	Amount	Fat Grams	Total Calories	% Fat Calories
sticks	1 oz	–	120	–
thins twists	1 oz	1.0	120	8%
tiny twists	1 oz	1.0	110	8%
hard sourdough	1 oz	0.5	100	5%
honey mustard	1 oz	1.0	130	7%
Parmesan herb	1 oz	5.0	130	35%
rods	1 oz	1.0	110	8%
snack mix				
Colossal Cheddar	¾ cup	8.0	160	45%
Munchies	¾ cup	6.0	140	39%
original	¾ cup	8.0	160	45%
sourdough nuggets	1 oz	–	100	–
sourdough special	1 oz	0.5	110	4%
(Snyder's)				
Nibblers				
Cheddar PB-Zels	1 oz	6.0	130	42%
garlic bread	1 oz	3.0	130	21%
honey mustard & onion	1 oz	3.0	130	21%
honey-roasted PB-Zels	1 oz	6.0	140	39%
no salt..fat-free	1 pz	–	120	–
oat bran	1 oz	1.0	110	8%
sourdough				
fat-free	1 oz	–	120	–
original..savory	1 oz	3.0	130	21%
old-fashioned hard	1 oz	–	110	–
Old Tyme				
regular	1 oz	–	118	–
unsalted	1 oz	–	110	–
pieces				
apple cinnamon rounds	1 oz	7.0	140	45%
buttermilk ranch	1 oz	6.0	140	39%
cheddar cheese	1 oz	6.0	130	42%
creamy caramel	1 oz	6.0	140	39%
honey BBQ	1 oz	5.0	130	35%
honey mustard & onion	1 oz	7.0	140	45%
jalapeño	1 oz	5.0	140	32%
pepperoni pizza	1 oz	8.0	150	48%
pretzels				
butter snaps	1 oz	1.0	120	8%
chocolate				
milk..mini dips	1 oz	6.0	130	42%
white..mini dips	1 oz	6.0	130	42%
golden cheese nibbler	1 oz	2.0	130	14%
hard				
sourdough	1 oz	–	100	–
unsalted	1 oz	–	100	–
home-style	1 oz	1.0	120	8%
honey wheat nibbler	1 oz	2.0	100	18%
log	1 oz	1.0	110	8%
mini	1 oz	–	110	–

Food and Description	Amount	Fat Grams	Total Calories	% Fat Calories
unsalted	1 oz	–	110	–
nibbler	1 oz	–	120	–
oat bran	1 oz	1.0	110	8%
old-fashioned dipping sticks	1 oz	–	100	–
Olde Tyme	1 oz	1.0	120	8%
rod	1 oz	1.0	120	8%
snaps	1 oz	1.0	120	8%
sourdough..hard	1 oz	–	100	–
specials	1 oz	1.0	120	8%
sticks	1 oz	1.0	110	8%
honey wheat	1 oz	2.0	120	15%
thin	1 oz	–	110	–
tiny butter sticks	1 oz	–	120	–
(SuperPretzel) soft-baked..frozen pretzels				
bites	5 bites	0.5	140	3%
original				
6-count box	1 pretzel	1.0	180	5%
25-count box	1 pretzel	1.0	190	5%
Pretzel Fils				
onion veggie	2 sticks	4.0	140	26%
pepper Jack	2 sticks	3.5	140	23%
pizza	2 sticks	3.0	140	19%
Softstix cheddar	2 stix	3.5	140	23%
PRICKLY PEAR	1 medium	0.5	42	11%
PROSCIUTTO (See SAUSAGE)				
PRUNE				
CANNED				
(Best Yet)				
large..whole	1.33 oz	–	110	–
(Oregon Fruit Products)..pitted Italian ..whole in heavy syrup	4.25 oz	0.5	130	3%
(S&W)..in heavy syrup	8 pieces	–	210	–
DRIED				
(Del Monte) uncooked				
pitted	2 oz	–	140	–
unpitted	2 oz	–	120	–
(Dole) pitted	¼ cup	–	110	–
(Mariani)				
large	¼ cup	1.0	140	6%
pitted	¼ cup	1.0	140	6%
(Sunsweet)				
bite-size breakfast	¼ cup	–	140	–
medium	¼ cup	–	140	–
orange essence/pitted	6 medium	–	100	–
pitted	¼ cup	–	140	–
(Sun-Maid)				
California				
pitted plums	1 oz	–	110	–
PRUNE JUICE/bottled or canned				

Food and Description	Amount	Fat Grams	Total Calories	% Fat Calories
(Del Monte)..unsweetened	8 fl oz	–	170	–
(Langer's)	8 fl oz	–	180	–
(Seneca)	8 fl oz	–	180	–
(Sunsweet)				
regular	8 fl oz	–	180	–
w/prune pulp	8 fl oz	–	170	–

PUDDING & MOUSSE (*See also* CUSTARD; PIE FILLING)

■ **MIX** (Note: Unless stated otherwise, 1 serving of mix = the amount in ½ cup prepared.)

Food and Description	Amount	Fat Grams	Total Calories	% Fat Calories
(Crosse & Blackwell)				
plum pudding	⅓ pkg	10.0	460	20%
(Jell-O) pudding & pie filling				
Americana pudding & custard				
Custard..prepared w/2% milk	½ cup	2.5	140	16%
rice pudding prepared w/skim milk	½ cup	–	140	–
tapioca pudding prepared w/skim	½ cup	–	130	–
cook & serve..mix only				
fat-free				
prepared w/skim milk				
chocolate	½ cup	–	130	–
vanilla	½ cup	–	130	–
instant..mix only				
chocolate				
fat & sugar-free	¼ pkg	–	35	–
regular	¼ pkg	–	100	–
Oreo cookies 'n' cream				
w/cookie pieces	¼ pkg	1.0	120	8%
original..mix only				
chocolate	¼ pkg	–	150	–
vanilla	¼ pkg	–	140	–
vanilla				
fat & sugar-free	⅛ pkg	–	25	–
regular	¼ pkg	–	90	–
(Kraft)..Kraft Minute..pudding				
rice..mix only	¼ pkg	–	90	–
(Royal) mix only (the amount of mix in 1 serving prepared)				
cook & serve				
banana cream	1 serving	–	80	–
butterscotch	1 serving	–	90	–
chocolate	1 serving	–	90	–
dark 'n' sweet chocolate	1 serving	–	90	–
vanilla	1 serving	–	80	–
regular				
banana cream	1 serving	–	90	–
butterscotch	1 serving	–	90	–
cherry vanilla	1 serving	–	90	–
chocolate	1 serving	–	100	–
chocolate almond	1 serving	1.0	120	8%
chocolate chocolate chip	1 serving	1.0	110	8%
chocolate peanut butter	1 serving	1.0	110	8%

Food and Description	Amount	Fat Grams	Total Calories	% Fat Calories
dark 'n' sweet	1 serving	–	110	–
lemon	1 serving	–	90	–
pistachio	1 serving	1.0	90	10%
strawberry	1 serving	–	100	–
toasted coconut	1 serving	2.0	100	18%
vanilla	1 serving	–	90	–
vanilla chocolate chip	1 serving	1.0	90	10%
(Uncle Ben's)..dry mix				
cinnamon & raisins				
rice pudding	⅓ pkg	1.0	160	6%
French vanilla				
rice pudding	⅓ pkg	–	120	–
■ READY-TO-SERVE				
(Hunt's)				
Snack Pack				
banana cream pie	1 snack	5.0	140	32%
butterscotch	1 snack	4.5	130	31%
chocolate caramel swirl	1 snack	5.0	140	32%
chocolate fudge	1 snack	5.0	150	30%
chocolate marshmallow	1 snack	5.0	130	35%
chocolate mud pie	1 snack	5.0	140	32%
chocolate peanut butter pie	1 snack	5.0	140	32%
chocolate vanilla	1 snack	4.5	130	31%
dulce de leche	1 snack	5.0	140	32%
lemon	1 snack	3.0	120	23%
lemon meringue pie	1 snack	5.0	140	32%
milk chocolate swirl	1 snack	5.0	140	32%
s'mores swirl	1 snack	5.0	140	32%
tapioca	1 snack	4.5	130	31%
Snack Pack..fat-free				
chocolate	1 snack	–	90	–
vanilla	1 snack	–	80	–
tapioca	1 snack	–	80	–
Squeez 'n' Go portable pudding				
chocolate	1 snack	3.0	90	30%
chocolate brownie	1 snack	4.5	120	34%
chocolate fudge	1 snack	3.5	100	32%
creamy strawberry & banana	1 snack	3.0	90	30%
vanilla nut	1 snack	3.0	90	30%
(Jell-O)				
Kraft..Handi-Snacks				
banana	1 snack	3.5	120	26%
butterscotch	1 snack	3.5	120	26%
chocolate				
fat-free	1 snack	–	90	–
Mega Cup	1 snack	6.0	170	32%
regular	1 snack	3.5	130	24%
chocolate chip cookie	1 snack	1.0	120	8%
pudding doubles				
chocolate vanilla	1 snack	3.5	120	26%

Food and Description	Amount	Fat Grams	Total Calories	% Fat Calories
rice	1 snack	6.0	140	39%
tapioca	1 snack	3.5	120	26%
vanilla				
fat-free	1 snack	–	90	–
regular	1 snack	3.5	120	26%
pudding..chocolate..canister	½ cup	5.0	190	24%
Pudding Snacks				
chocolate	1 snack	4.0	140	26%
chocolate fudge sundaes	1 snack	3.5	140	23%
chocolate vanilla swirls	1 snack	4.0	140	26%
Oreo	1 snack	4.0	140	26%
tapioca	1 snack	3.0	130	21%
vanilla	1 snack	3.5	130	24%
X-treme cotton candy				
& bubble gum	1 snack	3.5	140	23%
pudding snacks..Crème Savers				
chocolate & caramel				
crème swirled	1 snack	5.0	160	28%
pudding snacks..fat-free				
chocolate	1 snack	–	100	–
chocolate vanilla swirls	1 snack	–	100	–
devil's food	1 snack	–	100	–
tapioca	1 snack	–	100	–
vanilla & chocolate	1 snack	–	100	–
vanilla caramel sundaes	1 snack	–	100	–
(Kozy Shack) cups				
banana	4 oz	3.0	130	21%
chocolate	4 oz	3.5	140	23%
rice	4 oz	3.0	130	21%
tapioca	4 oz	3.0	140	19%
vanilla	4 oz	3.0	130	21%
(Swiss Miss)				
pudding snacks				
butterscotch	1 snack	6.0	160	34%
chocolate				
fat-free	1 snack	–	90	–
regular	1 snack	5.0	160	28%
chocolate cream pie	1 snack	7.0	170	37%
chocolate fudge				
light	1 snack	1.0	100	9%
regular	1 snack	6.0	220	25%
chocolate sundae	1 snack	7.0	220	29%
chocolate vanilla parfait	1 snack	6.0	165	33%
chocolate vanilla swirl	1 snack	6.0	160	34%
lemon meringue pie	1 snack	3.0	150	18%
milk chocolate fudge parfait	1 snack	6.0	165	33%
Pie Lover's Pudding				
chocolate cream pie	1 snack	6.0	150	36%
tapioca				
fat-free	1 snack	–	90	–
regular	1 snack	5.0	160	28%

vanilla				
light	1 snack	1.0	100	9%
regular	1 snack	7.0	190	33%
vanilla chocolate parfait				
light	1 snack	1.0	100	9%
regular	1 snack	6.0	180	30%
vanilla sundae	1 snack	7.0	200	32%
PUMMELO/POMELO				
fresh				
sections	1 cup	–	70	–
whole	1 medium	–	230	–
PUMPKIN				
canned				
(Comstock)	½ cup	–	50	–
(Libby's)				
pumpkin easy pie mix	½ cup	0.5	90	5%
pure pumpkin	½ cup	0.5	60	8%
(Stokely)	½ cup	–	50	–
fresh				
boiled mashed	1 cup	–	48	–
raw/cubed	1 cup	–	30	–
PUMPKIN FLOWER				
cooked	½ cup	<1.0	10	45%
raw	½ cup	<1.0	5	90%
PUMPKIN LEAVES/cooked	½ cup	<1.0	7	64%
PUMPKIN PIE SPICE (See SEASONINGS)				
PUMPKIN SEEDS				
dried/hulled	1 oz	13.0	155	75%
kernels/roasted				
(David)	1 oz	13.0	160	73%
single bag	2.25 oz	23.0	280	74%
	¼ cup	13.0	160	73%
whole/roasted	1 oz	5.5	127	39%
PUNCH (See FRUIT PUNCH; SOFT DRINK; SOFT DRINK MIX)				
PURPLE HULL PEA				
canned				
(Allens Fresh)	½ cup	0.5	100	5%
frozen				
(Birds Eye)				
southern	½ cup	0.5	110	4%
(Frosty Acres)	3.3 oz	–	130	–
PURSLANE				
boiled	½ cup	–	10	–
raw	1 cup	–	7	–

Q

Food and Description	Amount	Fat Grams	Total Calories	% Fat Calories
QUAIL/raw				
breast meat only	~2 oz	1.7	69	22%
meat & skin—raw	~4 oz	13.0	210	56%
meat only	~3 oz	4.0	123	29%
QUICHE (See also EGG DISH/MEAL)				
(Nancy's) frozen				
broccoli	1 quiche	26.0	430	61%
cheese trio	1 quiche	28.0	450	56%
Florentine	1 quiche	26.0	440	53%
Lorraine	1 quiche	29.0	480	54%
QUINCE/fresh	1 medium	–	53	–
QUINOA (See also FLOUR; PASTA; QUINOA SEED)				
whole-grain/dry				
(Eden)	¼ cup	3.5	180	18%
(Quinoa Corporation)				
dry	¼ cup	3.0	166	16%
QUINOA SEED				
(Arrowhead Mills)	¼ cup	2.0	140	13%

R

Food and Description	Amount	Fat Grams	Total Calories	% Fat Calories
RABBIT				
domesticated/meat only				
roasted	3 oz	5.5	130	38%
roasted/chopped or diced	1 cup	9.0	220	37%
stewed	3 oz	7.0	175	36%
stewed/chopped or diced	1 cup	12.0	290	37%
wild/meat only				
stewed	3 oz	3.0	150	18%
stewed/chopped or diced	1 cup	5.0	245	18%

Food and Description	Amount	Fat Grams	Total Calories	% Fat Calories
RACCOON/meat only				
roasted	3 oz	12.5	220	51%
RADICCHIO/raw/shredded	½ cup	–	5	–
RADISH				
dried				
Chinese	¼ cup	–	75	–
daikon	¼ cup	–	75	–
fresh				
black	1 oz	–	5	–
Chinese				
cooked/drained/sliced	½ cup	–	15	–
raw..whole	1 medium	–	60	–
daikon				
cooked/drained/sliced	½ cup	–	15	–
raw..whole	1 medium	–	60	–
red/raw	10 pieces	–	7	–
(Dole)	7 medium	–	20	–
white icicle/raw..whole	1 medium	–	2	–
RADISH SPROUTS	½ cup	0.5	8	56%
RAISIN (*See also* SNACKS)				
(Del Monte)				
golden	¼ cup	–	130	–
natural	¼ cup	–	120	–
	1.5-oz box	–	140	–
	1-oz box	–	90	–
yogurt raisin snack bag				
strawberry	0.9 oz	3.0	110	25%
vanilla yogurt	0.9 oz	3.0	110	25%
(Dole)				
California/seedless	¼ cup	–	130	–
dark/seedless	½ cup	–	250	–
golden	¼ cup	–	130	–
	½ cup	–	250	–
(S&W)				
dark/seedless	¼ cup	–	130	–
golden/seedless	¼ cup	–	130	–
(Sun-Maid)				
baking	¼ cup	–	120	–
dark/seedless				
regular	¼ cup	–	130	–
golden	1.42 oz	–	130	–
& cherries	1.5 oz	–	130	–
w/seeds	½ cup	–	250	–
muscat	½ cup	1.0	270	3%
snack box	1.5 oz	–	130	–
yogurt raisins				
chocolate	1 oz	4.0	123	29%
vanilla	1 oz	5.0	130	35%

Food and Description	Amount	Fat Grams	Total Calories	% Fat Calories
RASPBERRY				
canned				
(Oregon)				
in heavy syrup	½ cup	–	120	–
fresh				
black	1 cup	2.0	100	18%
red	1 cup	0.7	61	10%
(Dole)	1 cup	–	45	–
frozen				
(Big Valley)	⅔ cup	–	150	–
(Birds Eye)..red/in light syrup	4.5 oz	–	90	–
(Cascadian Farms)	1 cup	0.5	60	10%
(C&W) red/sweetened	1 cup	–	50	–
RASPBERRY JUICE/JUICE BLEND/JUICE DRINK (*See* also FRUIT PUNCH; LEMONADE/LEMONADE-FLAVORED DRINK; SOFT DRINK; SOFT DRINK MIX)				
bottled, boxed, or canned				
(Dole) country raspberry 100% juice blend				
bottled	8 fl oz	–	140	–
	10 fl oz	–	180	–
refrigerated	4 fl oz	–	70	–
	8 fl oz	–	140	–
(Knudsen)				
raspberry peach	8 fl oz	–	150	–
razzleberry	8 fl oz	–	133	–
red raspberry..spritzer	12 fl oz	–	170	–
(Walnut Acres)				
raspberry juice	8 fl oz	–	130	–
(Welch's) wild raspberry	8 fl oz	–	140	–
fresh..black	4 fl oz	–	50	–
frozen..prepared				
(Dole) country raspberry 100% juice blend				
	8 fl oz	–	140	–
RAVIOLI (*See* BEEF DISH/ENTRÉE; FROZEN ENTRÉE/DINNER; PASTA ENTRÉE/DINNER; VEGETARIAN FOODS)				
RED BEAN (*See also* BEANS, BAKED & VARIETY; RICE DISH)				
canned				
(Eden)				
small red	½ cup	0.5	100	5%
(Joan of Arc) dry beans in brine	½ cup	0.5	100	5%
(Knorr)				
refried	½ cup	2.0	120	15%
(Red Gold)	½ cup	0.5	110	4%
(S&W)				
Louisiana-style w/tomato..onions & Cajun sauce	½ cup	–	80	–
(Van Camp's)	1 cup	1.0	195	5%
dry				
(Bean Cuisine)	½ cup	1.0	115	8%

Food and Description	Amount	Fat Grams	Total Calories	% Fat Calories
RED BEAN SOUP (*See* SOUP)				
REFRIED BEANS (*See* MEXICAN FOOD)				
RELISH (*See* CHUTNEY; CORN DISH; PICKLE RELISH)				
RENNIN PRODUCTS	1 tablet	–	1	–
	1 pkg	–	12	–
RHUBARB				
fresh				
cooked/sweetened	1 cup	–	280	–
raw/diced	½ cup	–	13	–
RICE (*See also* ASIAN FOOD; RICE DISH)				
(A Taste of Thai)..dry (unless otherwise noted)				
rice				
brown jasmine	½ cup	–	220	–
soft jasmine	¼ cup	–	160	–
rice noodles				
extra-thin	2 oz	–	200	–
extra-wide	2 oz	–	200	–
original	2 oz	–	200	–
(Arrowhead Mills) dry				
basmati..long-grain	¼ cup	1.0	150	6%
brown				
long-grain	¼ cup	1.0	150	6%
medium-grain	¼ cup	1.0	160	6%
short-grain	¼ cup	1.0	170	6%
(Carolina)..dry				
brown rice				
gold..parboiled	¼ cup	1.0	150	6%
jasmine Thai	¾ cup	–	160	–
white rice..extra-long-grain	¼ cup	–	150	–
(Fantastic Foods)..Elegant Grains..dry				
arborio	¼ cup	–	160	–
basmati				
brown	¼ cup	1.5	160	8%
white	¼ cup	–	160	–
jasmine				
brown	¼ cup	1.5	160	8%
white	¼ cup	–	160	–
organic				
couscous	¼ cup	1.0	190	5%
whole wheat couscous	¼ cup	1.0	210	4%
(Gourmet House)..wild..dry				
blends				
brown & wild	¼ cup	0.5	160	3%
garden	¼ cup	0.5	190	3%
long-grain & wild	¼ cup	–	170	–
cultivated..Minnesota	¼ cup	–	170	–
hand-harvested				
Minnesota lake & river	¼ cup	–	170	–
machine-harvested				
Canadian lake & river	¼ cup	–	170	–

Food and Description	Amount	Fat Grams	Total Calories	% Fat Calories
other				
Minnesota-cultivated				
cracked	¼ cup	–	170	–
quick-cooking	¼ cup	–	170	–
(Kraft)..dry				
boil-in-bag				
long-grain white..enriched	1.5 oz	–	180	–
Instant				
long-grain..white	1.5 oz	–	160	–
long-grain rice				
enriched	1.5 oz	–	160	–
long-grain..white				
premium..enriched	1.5 oz	–	160	–
whole-grain...brown	1.5 oz	–	169	–
(Lundberg Family Farms)				
Lundberg Wehani				
brown	1.5 oz	1.5	170	8%
Lundberg Wild Blend				
gourmet blend..wild				
& brown	1.5 oz	1.5	150	9%
organic black japonica				
gourmet black				
& mahogany	1.5 oz	2.0	170	11%
(Mahatma)..dry				
basmati..Indian fragrance	1.5 oz	–	160	–
brown	1.5 oz	–	160	–
instant	1.5 oz	–	160	–
Valencia short-grain	1.5 oz	–	160	–
white..long-grain	1.5 oz	–	150	–
(Minute)..(See (Kraft) within this category)				
(MJB) brown				
quick/cooked	½ cup	1.0	110	8%
(Patak's Original)				
basmati	1 pouch	5.0	430	10%
coconut	1 pouch	12.0	500	22%
garlic & cilantro	1 pouch	4.5	420	10%
yellow rice	1 pkg	5.0	440	10%
(Riceland)				
brown..natural..extra				
long-grain	1.67 oz	1.0	150	6%
enriched				
extra-long-grain	1.67 oz	–	160	–
medium-grain plum & tender	1.67 oz	–	170	–
gold parboiled..long-grain	1.67 oz	–	170	–
gold perfected parboiled				
long-grain	1.5 oz	–	170	–
(Rivana)..dry				
brown..natural whole-grain				
boil-in-bag	1.5 oz	1.0	150	6%
jasmine..long-grain	1 oz	–	160	–

Food and Description	Amount	Fat Grams	Total Calories	% Fat Calories
natural..long-grain				
boil-in-bag	2 oz	–	190	–
white	¼ cup	–	150	–
(S&W)..dry				
regular				
brown..natural				
long-grain	¼ cup	1.0	150	6%
quick	½ cup	1.0	150	6%
Indian basmati	¼ cup	–	160	–
Italian arborio	¼ cup	–	150	–
Thai jasmine	¼ cup	–	160	–
white..long-grain	¼ cup	–	100	–
white..long-grain..premium	¼ cup	–	150	–
white..long-grain				
& wild	¼ cup	–	140	–
wild	½ cup	1.0	110	8%
organic..all types	¼ cup	1.0	150	6%
(Success)..dry				
brown				
boil-in-bag..prepared	½ cup	1.0	150	6%
10-minute..prepared	½ cup	1.0	190	5%
brown & wild/dry	½ cup	1.0	190	5%
white..natural long-grain				
precooked..prepared	½ cup	–	190	–
(Texmati)..dry				
basmati				
brown	¼ cup	1.0	170	5%
white	¼ cup	0.5	150	3%
brown	¼ cup	1.0	170	5%
jasmati	¼ cup	–	150	–
kasmati	¼ cup	0.5	150	3%
light brown	¼ cup	1.0	170	5%
risotto	¼ cup	–	150	–
Royal Blend	¼ cup	0.5	160	3%
white/long-grain	¼ cup	0.5	150	3%
(Tony Chachere's)..Creole				
dirty rice dinner..mix only	⅛ box	–	160	–
red beans & rice				
dinner..mix only	¼ box	–	100	–
(Uncle Ben's)..dry mix, unless otherwise noted				
brown				
instant	½ cup	1.5	190	7%
original	¼ cup	1.5	170	8%
white				
aromatic/cooked	½ cup	–	100	–
boil-in-bag	⅓ cup	0.5	19	2%
converted	¼ cup	–	170	–
Rice-in-an-Instant	½ cup	0.5	190	2%
wild/combinations/fast-cooking				
brown & wild	1 serving	1.0	120	8%

Food and Description	Amount	Fat Grams	Total Calories	% Fat Calories
RICE BRAN (See also CEREAL)				
crude	½ cup	8.5	130	59%
RICE BRAN OIL				
(Hollywood)	1 Tbs	14.0	120	100%
RICE CAKES (See also POPCORN BARS & CAKES)				
(Hain)				
mini				
apple cinnamon	6 cakes	–	60	–
honey nut	6 cakes	–	60	–
plain				
original	6 cakes	–	60	–
no salt added	6 cakes	–	60	–
ranch	6 cakes	3.5	70	45%
regular				
apple cinnamon	1 cake	–	50	–
honey nut	1 cake	–	50	–
plain..all types	1 cake	–	40	–
(Lundberg)				
classic cakes.. Nutra-Farmed				
all types	1 cake	–	70	–
organic..all types	1 cake	–	70	–
Savory Cakes				
Nutra-Farmed				
sesame tamari	1 cake	0.5	70	6%
toasted sesame	1 cake	–	70	–
organic				
Koku				
seaweed	1 cake	–	80	–
sesame	1 cake	0.5	80	6%
sesame tamari	1 cake	0.5	70	6%
tamari seaweed	1 cake	–	70	–
Sweet Cakes...all types	1 cake	0.5	80	6%
(Mother's)				
mini				
apple	5 cakes	–	50	–
caramel	5 cakes	–	50	–
cinnamon	5 cakes	–	50	–
plain/unsalted	7 cakes	–	60	–
regular..all types	1 cake	–	35	–
(Quaker)				
Crisp'ums..all types	1 pouch	5.0	150	30%
mini rice snacks				
apple cinnamon	8 cakes	–	60	–
BBQ	10 cakes	2.0	70	26%
caramel corn	7 cakes	–	60	–
cheddar cheese	9 cakes	2.5	70	32%
chocolate crunch	7 cakes	1.0	60	15%
creamy ranch	10 cakes	2.5	70	32%
nacho	9 cakes	2.5	70	32%

Food and Description	Amount	Fat Grams	Total Calories	% Fat Calories
sour cream & onion	10 cakes	2.5	70	32%
Quaker Rice Snacks				
apple cinnamon	8 pieces	–	60	–
BBQ	10 pieces	2.5	70	32%
caramel corn	7 pieces	–	60	–
cheddar cheese	9 pieces	2.5	70	32%
chocolate crunch	7 pieces	1.0	60	15%
creamy ranch	10 pieces	2.5	70	32%
nacho	9 pieces	2.5	70	32%
sour cream & onion	10 pieces	2.5	70	32%
regular..large rice cakes				
apple cinnamon	1 cake	–	50	–
banana nut crunch	1 cake	–	50	–
buttered popcorn	1 cake	–	35	–
caramel apple	1 cake	0.5	60	8%
caramel chocolate chip	1 cake	1.0	60	15%
caramel corn	1 cake	–	50	–
chocolate crunch	1 cake	1.0	60	15%
cinnamon streusel	1 cake	1.0	60	15%
peanut butter	1 cake	1.0	60	15%
plain...all types	1 cake	–	35	–
strawberry crunch	1 cake	–	50	–
white cheddar corn	1 cake	0.5	45	10%
(Roman Meal) mini cakes	8 cakes	–	50	–
(Westbrae Natural)				
rice cakes..all types	2 cakes	–	50	–

RICE DISH (*See also* ASIAN FOOD; FROZEN ENTRÉE/DINNER; MEXICAN FOOD)

■ CANNED

(Old El Paso) Spanish rice	1 cup	1.0	130	7%
(Van Camp's) Spanish rice	1 cup	4.0	160	23%

■ FROZEN

(Uncle Ben's) Rice Bowls				
BBQ beef	1 bowl	4.5	430	9%
Cajun-style				
chicken & sausage	1 bowl	7.0	350	18%
chicken Bombay	1 bowl	5.0	440	10%
chicken fried rice	1 bowl	7.0	410	15%
chicken vegetable	1 bowl	5.0	360	13%
chili..w/beans & rice	1 bowl	7.0	360	18%
honey Dijon chicken	1 bowl	3.5	400	8%
Mexican-style				
beef fajita	1 bowl	4.5	300	14%
chicken fajita	1 bowl	5.0	330	14%
Santa Fe chicken	1 bowl	6.0	350	15%
Southwestern-style black beans	1 bowl	4.5	360	11%
spicy beef & broccoli	1 bowl	4.5	370	11%
sweet & sour chicken	1 bowl	3.0	360	8%
teriyaki stir-fry w/vegetables	1 bowl	4.0	360	10%
turkey..wild rice				
& cranberries	1 bowl	4.0	360	10%

Food and Description	Amount	Fat Grams	Total Calories	% Fat Calories
■ MIX				
(A Taste of Thai)				
coconut ginger..prepared	¾ cup	–	190	–
garlic basil..prepared	¾ cup	–	160	–
golden..prepared	¾ cup	1.5	180	8%
(Casbah).. pilaf/prepared				
nutted	1 cup	3.0	220	12%
original	1 cup	1.0	200	5%
Spanish	1 cup	1.0	200	2%
(Carolina)..dry mix				
authentic Spanish	1 serving	0.5	180	3%
black beans & rice	1 serving	1.5	200	7%
chicken & rice	1 serving	–	190	–
classic pilaf	1 serving	–	190	–
long-grain & wild	1 serving	0.5	190	2%
red beans & rice	1 serving	1.0	190	5%
saffron yellow	1 serving	–	190	–
spicy yellow	1 serving	0.5	180	3%
(Fantastic Foods)				
Carb'Tastic..ready meals				
ginger shiitake				
w/rice noodles	1 meal	10.0	340	26%
pad Thai..w/rice noodles	1 meal	11.0	400	25%
Spanish paella	1 meal	5.0	280	16%
Thai lemongrass	1 meal	10.0	340	15%
Tuscany mushroom risotto	1 meal	1.5	310	4%
pilaf..dry mix only				
basmati	¼ cup	0.5	150	3%
4-grain	½ cup	1.0	160	6%
Hacienda Spanish	¼ cup	1.0	150	6%
organic	¼ cup	–	160	–
vegetarian chicken	¼ cup	0.5	180	3%
rice & beans..dry mix only				
Bombay curry/cup	½ pkg	1.5	190	7%
Cajun/cup	½ pkg.	1.5	180	8%
Jamaican				
side dish	⅓ cup	1.5	140	10%
spicy w/black beans/cup	½ pkg	1.0	190	5%
New Orleans	⅓ cup	1.5	130	10%
Tex-Mex/cup	½ pkg	3.0	190	14%
risotto..dry mix only				
Classico	¼ cup	1.0	160	6%
Tuscany mushroom	¼ cup	0.5	180	3%
(Golden Grain) prepared according to pkg directions				
Rice-A-Roni				
beef & mushroom	1 cup	7.0	290	22%
beef flavor	1 cup	9.0	310	26%
broccoli	1 cup	10.0	280	32%
broccoli au gratin	1 cup	10.0	270	33%
⅓ less salt	1 cup	11.0	320	31%

Food and Description	Amount	Fat Grams	Total Calories	% Fat Calories
regular	1 cup	17.0	370	41%
chicken & broccoli	1 cup	5.0	230	20%
chicken..Cajun	1 cup	8.0	250	29%
chicken & garlic	1 cup	8.0	260	28%
chicken & mushroom	1 cup	14.0	360	35%
chicken & vegetables	1 cup	7.0	290	22%
chicken flavor				
low-fat	1 cup	3.0	210	9%
⅓ less salt	1 cup	5.0	280	16%
original	1 cup	9.0	310	26%
chicken teriyaki	1 cup	8.0	260	28%
4-cheese	1 cup	12.0	280	39%
fried rice				
⅓ less salt	1 cup	3.5	260	12%
regular	1 cup	11.0	320	31%
garden vegetable	1 cup	6.0	240	23%
herb & butter	1 cup	9.0	320	25%
herb-roasted chicken	1 cup	8.0	260	28%
long-grain & wild rice				
original	1 cup	6.0	240	23%
long-grain & wild rice pilaf	1 cup	6.0	240	23%
long-grain & wild rice chicken				
w/almonds	1 cup	8.0	300	24%
Mexican-style	1 cup	8.0	250	29%
Oriental stir-fry	1 cup	6.0	290	19%
rice pilaf	1 cup	9.0	310	26%
savory chicken				
vegetable..low-fat	1 cup	2.5	210	11%
Spanish rice	1 cup	8.0	300	24%
Stroganoff	1 cup	15.0	360	38%
white cheddar & herbs	1 cup	14.0	340	37%
(Health Valley)				
Rice Cups..low-fat				
Cantonese	½ cup	1.0	140	6%
chicken-flavored	½ cup	1.0	140	6%
rice primavera	½ cup	1.5	140	10%
shiitake	½ cup	1.5	140	10%
Thai	½ cup	1.5	140	10%
(Kashi) 7 whole grain & sesame				
pilaf/cooked	½ cup	3.0	170	26%
(Knorr) dry mix only				
Italian risotto Milanese				
arborio-style	2.55 oz	1.0	260	3%
lemon herb pilaf	2.55 oz	2.0	260	7%
Mexican-style	1.95 oz	1.0	200	5%
rice & black beans	2.28 oz	1.0	220	4%
rice & pinto beans	2.28 oz	1.0	230	4%
Spanish-style	¼ box	1.0	200	5%
yellow	2.28 oz	0.5	230	2%

Food and Description	Amount	Fat Grams	Total Calories	% Fat Calories
(Konriko) wild pecan rice	⅕ box	1.0	160	6%
(Kraft)				
New Meals..mix only				
cheesy broccoli	¼ bag	2.0	210	9%
teriyaki stir-fry	¼ bag	–	210	–
(Lipton) mix only				
Asian side dishes				
chicken fried rice	½ cup	2.0	240	8%
teriyaki rice	½ cup	1.0	240	4%
rice & sauce				
Alfredo broccoli	½ pkg	5.0	240	19%
beef	½ pkg	1.5	220	6%
beef broccoli	½ pkg	1.5	220	6%
Cajun-style	½ pkg	1.5	220	6%
dirty rice	½ cup	1.5	250	5%
garlic butter	½ cup	4.0	260	14%
New Orleans–style chicken	½ cup	1.0	240	4%
w/rice and beans	½ cup	1.5	290	5%
Fiesta sides				
Mexican rice	½ cup	1.0	250	4%
smoked chipotle	½ cup	1.5	260	5%
Spanish	½ cup	1.0	240	4%
taco	½ cup	1.0	250	4%
rice sides				
beef	½ cup	2.0	240	8%
cheddar broccoli	½ cup	2.5	260	9%
chicken				
broccoli	½ cup	2.0	240	8%
creamy	½ cup	5.0	270	17%
flavored	½ cup	3.0	250	11%
& Parmesan risotto	½ cup	2.5	220	10%
herb & butter	½ cup	4.0	250	14%
long-grain & wild rice				
mushroom & herb	½ cup	1.0	240	4%
medley	½ cup	2.0	230	8%
pilaf	½ cup	1.0	220	4%
(Luzianne) dinner kit/mix only				
"dirty" rice	⅕ box	1.0	160	6%
étouffee	¼ box	1.0	200	5%
gumbo	⅕ box	1.0	160	6%
jambalaya	⅕ box	1.0	200	5%
shrimp Creole	⅕ box	1.0	150	6%
(Mahatma) dry mix only				
black bean	⅓ pkg	1.5	200	7%
broccoli & cheese	⅓ pkg	3.0	200	14%
chicken & rice	½ pkg	–	190	–
jambalaya	⅙ pkg	0.5	190	2%
nacho cheese	¼ pkg	3.0	250	11%
pilaf..classic	½ pkg	–	190	–

Food and Description	Amount	Fat Grams	Total Calories	% Fat Calories
red beans & rice	⅓ pkg	1.0	190	5%
Spanish..authentic yellow	½ pkg	0.5	180	3%
saffron	⅓ pkg	–	190	–
spicy	¼ pkg	0.5	180	3%
(Marrakesh Express)..box mix				
rice				
pilaf..cheddar & broccoli	⅓ pkg	2.0	200	9%
risotto				
arborio rice..plain	⅛ pkg	1.0	260	3%
Parmesan cheese	⅓ pkg	1.0	200	5%
roasted red pepper	⅓ pkg	1.0	200	5%
sun-dried tomato & herb	⅓ pkg	–	190	–
wild mushroom	⅓ pkg	1.0	200	5%
(MJB) prepared				
fried rice Oriental	½ cup	1.0	110	8%
herb & butter	½ cup	1.0	100	9%
Mexican-style	½ cup	–	120	–
rice pilaf	½ cup	1.0	110	8%
savory beef	½ cup	1.0	100	9%
savory chicken	½ cup	1.0	100	9%
(Near East)				
Creative Grains..rice mixes..prepared				
chicken & herb	1 cup	6.0	270	20%
creamy Parmesan	1 cup	8.0	280	26%
roasted garlic	1 cup	5.0	220	20%
roasted pecan & garlic	1 cup	9.0	240	34%
rice pilaf..prepared				
brown rice	1 cup	4.0	210	17%
chicken flavor	1 cup	4.0	220	16%
curry pilaf	1 cup	3.5	220	14%
garlic & herb	1 cup	3.5	220	14%
lentil	1 cup	2.5	200	11%
long-grain & wild rice	1 cup	4.0	220	16%
Mediterranean black bean & rice	1 cup	5.0	270	17%
Mediterranean chicken w/wild rice	1 cup	3.0	210	13%
red beans & rice	1 cup	3.5	220	14%
rice pilaf	1 cup	3.5	220	12%
roasted chicken & garlic pilaf	1 cup	3.0	220	12%
Spanish rice pilaf	1 cup	8.0	310	23%
toasted almond	1 cup	6.0	230	23%
wheat pilaf	1 cup	4.0	220	16%
wild mushroom & herb	1 cup	3.5	220	14%
(Patak's Original)				
microwavable				
vegetable curry				
rich creamy coconut mild	1 pkg	18.0	400	41%

Food and Description	Amount	Fat Grams	Total Calories	% Fat Calories
rich tomato & onion				
w/rice..mild	1 pkg	6.0	290	19%
tangy lemon & cilantro				
medium	1 pkg	7.0	300	21%
yellow rice	1 pkg	5.0	440	10%
Rice-A-Roni (*See* (Golden Grain) in this section)				
(Spice Hunter)				
Risotto Cups				
spinach & garlic	1 cup	2.0	230	8%
3-cheese	1 cup	3.0	240	11%
wild mushroom	1 cup	1.5	220	6%
(Success)..as packaged				
boil-in-bag				
broccoli & cheese	1 serving	4.5	210	19%
brown & wild	1 serving	1.0	190	5%
cheesy rice	1 serving	4.5	220	18%
chicken..classic	1 serving	4.5	220	18%
grilled chicken				
& broccoli	1 serving	1.0	190	5%
long-grain & wild	1 serving	–	190	–
pilaf	1 serving	–	200	–
red beans & rice	1 serving	1.0	240	4%
Spanish	1 serving	0.5	190	2%
yellow	1 serving	–	150	–
(Uncle Ben's)				
brown & wild rice..prepared				
mushroom recipe	1 cup	1.5	190	7%
Country Inn..prepared				
broccoli rice au gratin	1 cup	2.0	200	9%
chicken				
& broccoli	1 cup	1.0	190	5%
& vegetable	1 cup	1.5	190	7%
& wild rice	1 cup	0.5	200	2%
flavored	1 cup	1.0	200	5%
Mexican fiesta rice	1 cup	1.0	200	5%
Oriental fried	1 cup	0.5	200	2%
rice pilaf	1 cup	0.5	200	2%
3-cheese	1 cup	2.5	200	11%
Flavorful Rice				
chicken herb	1 cup	1.0	200	5%
garlic & butter	1 cup	0.5	200	2%
lemon & herb	1 cup	0.5	190	2%
Parmesan & butter	1 cup	1.0	200	5%
roasted chicken	1 cup	1.0	200	5%
Spanish rice	1 cup	0.5	200	2%
tomato & herb	1 cup	0.5	190	2%
long-grain & wild rice..prepared				
butter & herb	1 cup	2.0	190	9%
original recipe	1 cup	0.5	190	2%
roasted garlic	1 cup	1.0	190	5%

Food and Description	Amount	Fat Grams	Total Calories	% Fat Calories
vegetable & herb	1 cup	1.5	210	6%
Ready Rice				
long-grain & wild	4.4 oz	2.5	180	13%
original long-grain	4.4 oz	2.5	190	12%
roasted chicken	4.4 oz	2.0	190	9%
Spanish-style	4.4 oz	4.0	190	19%
whole-grain..brown	4.4 oz	2.5	190	12%
(Vigo) dry mix only				
black beans & rice	⅓ cup	0.5	190	2%
pinto beans & rice	⅛ cup	2.0	200	9%
red beans & rice	⅓ cup	–	190	–
Santa Fe beans & rice	⅓ cup	2.0	200	9%
yellow rice	⅓ cup	1.0	190	5%
(Zatarain's)..prepared				
gumbo w/rice	1 cup	–	150	–
New Orleans jambalaya	1 cup	–	130	–
red beans & rice..New Orleans-style	1 cup	–	90	–
■ RICE DRINK				
(Lundberg Family Farms)..lactose-free drink..rice				
original..non-dairy	8 fl oz	2.5	120	19%
vanilla	8 fl oz	2.5	120	19%
(Rice Dream)				
carob	8 fl oz	2.5	150	15%
chocolate	8 fl oz	3.0	170	21%
enriched	8 fl oz	2.0	120	15%
original	8 fl oz	2.0	120	15%
vanilla	8 fl oz	2.0	130	14%
Heartwise	8 fl oz	2.0	130	14%
original	8 fl oz	2.0	130	14%
vanilla	8 fl oz	2.0	140	13%
(Westbrae)..rice beverage				
plain	1 cup	2.5	100	18%
vanilla	1 cup	2.5	120	19%
RICE FLOUR (See FLOUR)				
RICE FROZEN DESSERT				
(Rice Dream)				
Dream Bar				
chocolate/chocolate	1 bar	15.0	270	50%
chocolate nutty	1 bar	18.0	270	60%
strawberry	1 bar	13.0	250	47%
vanilla	1 bar	14.0	270	47%
vanilla nutty	1 bar	18.0	260	62%
non-dairy frozen dessert				
cappuccino	½ cup	6.0	150	36%
carob	½ cup	6.0	150	36%
carob almond	½ cup	8.0	170	40%
carob chip	½ cup	6.0	150	36%
cherry vanilla	½ cup	6.0	150	36%
chocolate	½ cup	7.0	150	42%

Food and Description	Amount	Fat Grams	Total Calories	% Fat Calories
chocolate chip	½ cup	8.0	170	42%
cocoa marble fudge	½ cup	6.0	150	36%
Cookies 'n' Dream	½ cup	7.0	170	37%
mint carob chip	½ cup	8.0	170	42%
mint chocolate chip	½ cup	8.0	170	42%
Neapolitan	½ cup	6.0	150	36%
orange vanilla swirl	½ cup	6.0	150	36%
strawberry	½ cup	5.0	140	32%
vanilla	½ cup	6.0	150	36%
vanilla Swiss almond	½ cup	8.0	180	40%
Rice Dream non-dairy pies				
mint	1 pie	18.0	320	51%
other flavors	1 pie	17.0	320	48%
Rice Dream Supreme				
Pralines 'n' Dream	½ cup	9.0	180	45%
RICE NOODLE (*See* ASIAN FOOD)				
RICE POLISH/stirred & spooned into cup	1 cup	13.0	278	42%
RICE PUDDING (*See* PUDDING & MOUSSE)				
RICE SYRUP (*See also* PANCAKE & WAFFLE SYRUP)				
(Lundberg) Sweet Dreams	1 Tbs	<1.0	40	7%
RIGATONI (*See* PASTA; PASTA ENTRÉE/DINNER)				
ROAST BEEF (*See* BEEF, LUNCHEON MEAT)				
ROAST BEEF HASH (*See* BEEF DISH/ENTRÉE)				
ROCKFISH				
Pacific/mixed species				
cooked	3 oz	2.0	110	16%
raw	3 oz	1.0	80	11%
ROLL (*See also* CROISSANT; PASTRY; SCONE)				
■ **BROWN & SERVE**				
(Arnold)				
Francisco				
French	1 roll	2.0	190	9%
sourdough	1 roll	1.0	100	10%
(Bread De Jour)				
honey wheat	1 roll	1.0	90	10%
Italian rolls	1 roll	0.5	90	5%
(Fisherman's Wharf)				
sour French bread	½" slice	0.5	120	4%
(Pepperidge Farm)				
bakery..French	½ roll	2.0	180	10%
European Bake Shoppe				
club	1 roll	1.5	130	10%
(San Francisco)				
French	1 roll	0.5	140	3%
sourdough	⅛ loaf	0.5	80	6%
	1 roll	0.5	80	6%
8-pack	1 roll	0.5	110	4%
(Wonder) Rolls				
du jour				
cracked wheat	1 roll	1.0	100	9%
crusty Italian	1 roll	0.5	90	5%

Food and Description	Amount	Fat Grams	Total Calories	% Fat Calories
sourdough	1 roll	0.5	90	5%
w/buttermilk	1 roll	2.0	80	23%
Wonder				
sourdough	1 roll	1.5	70	13%
wheat	1 roll	1.5	80	17%
white	1 roll	0.5	80	6%
■ FROZEN				
(Cole's)				
garlic	1 roll	5.0	100	45%
(Mama Bella) garlic dinner	1 roll	4.0	130	28%
(Pepperidge Farm)				
garlic & cheese	1 roll	5.0	130	35%
(Rhodes) bread dough, baked				
cinnamon roll	1 roll	10.0	240	38%
cracked wheat	1 roll	3.0	140	19%
fat-free	1 roll	–	85	–
Rhodes Anytime!				
crusty rolls..large				
heat & serve	1 roll	0.5	100	5%
Texas dinner				
wheat	1 roll	3.0	140	19%
white	1 roll	3.0	150	18%
white dinner	1 roll	2.0	95	19%
(Rich's)				
home-style roll dough	2 rolls	3.0	150	18%
(Sara Lee) ..soft				
butterfly	1 roll	3.0	90	30%
cloverleaf	1 roll	3.0	90	30%
crescent	1 roll	5.0	100	5%
finger	3 rolls	5.0	170	27%
Parker House	3 rolls	5.0	170	27%
sesame seed	1 roll	3.0	70	39%
white	1 roll	2.0	90	20%
■ HEAT & SERVE				
(Pepperidge Farm) Brown 'n' Serve				
butter crescent	1 roll	6.0	110	49%
golden twist	1 roll	5.0	110	41%
(Sister Schubert's)..yeast rolls				
cheddar	1 roll	5.0	110	41%
cinnamon	1 roll	6.0	190	28%
Parker House–style	1 roll	6.0	190	28%
■ MIX				
(Pillsbury)..Specialty..mix only				
hot roll	¼ cup	1.5	110	12%
■ READY TO SERVE				
(Arnold)				
Arnold				
dinner				
country white				
12 per pkg	1 roll	1.0	50	18%
24 per pkg	1 roll	1.5	110	12%

Food and Description	Amount	Fat Grams	Total Calories	% Fat Calories
enriched 24 per pkg	1 roll	2.5	120	19%
w/sesame seeds	2 rolls	1.0	50	18%
hamburger				
8 per pkg	1 roll	2.0	130	14%
12 per pkg	1 roll	2.0	120	15%
hot dog				
New England–style	1 roll	2.0	110	16%
regular				
8 per 11-oz pkg	1 roll	2.0	100	18%
8 per 12-oz pkg	1 roll	2.0	110	16%
12 per pkg	1 roll	2.0	110	16%
kaiser sandwich				
w/sesame seeds	1 roll	3.5	140	23%
onion				
premium	1 roll	1.0	180	5%
soft	1 roll	–	140	–
potato				
dinner	1 roll	1.5	110	12%
hot dog	1 roll	2.0	120	15%
Italian	1 roll	3.5	280	11%
plain	1 roll	2.0	140	13%
sandwich/soft				
Dutch sesame/8 per pkg	1 roll	3.0	170	16%
original/12 per pkg	1 roll	3.0	130	21%
plain	1 roll	2.0	150	12%
Francisco				
French				
6" roll	1 roll	3.0	210	13%
mini	1 roll	2.0	130	14%
kaiser	1 roll	1.0	180	5%
sourdough	1 roll	1.0	100	9%
steak	1 roll	2.0	170	11%
(Awrey's)				
dinner	1 roll	1.0	60	15%
cracked wheat	2 rolls	1.5	120	11%
crusty	2 rolls	1.5	130	10%
plain	2 rolls	1.5	130	10%
hoagie	1 roll	2.0	230	8%
(Better Bakery)				
Better				
dinner rolls	½ roll	1.0	44	20%
hamburger buns				
onion	½ bun	2.0	84	21%
plain	½ bun	2.0	84	21%
sesame	½ bun	2.0	84	21%
hot dog buns	½ bun	3.5	134	24%
(Brownberry)				
Brownberry hot dog sliced	1 roll	2.0	110	16%
wheat	1 roll	2.0	120	15%

Food and Description	Amount	Fat Grams	Total Calories	% Fat Calories
sandwich				
potato	1 roll	2.5	150	15%
wheat	1 roll	2.0	150	12%
white	1 roll	2.5	140	16%
Francisco International				
dinner	1 roll	1.0	120	8%
French/6" roll	1 roll	1.0	170	5%
kaiser	1 roll	1.0	170	5%
(Ciabatta)				
dinner rolls	1 roll	0.5	90	5%
sandwich	1 roll	1.0	180	5%
(King's Hawaiian)				
honey wheat	1 roll	2.0	90	20%
multigrain	1 roll	3.0	100	27%
regular	1 roll	2.0	90	20%
(Martin's)				
Big Marty				
dinner	1 roll	1.0	90	30%
poppy	1 roll	2.0	170	11%
sesame	1 roll	3.0	170	15%
hoagie				
plain	1 roll	3.0	240	11%
sesame	1 roll	4.0	250	14%
potato				
dinner	1 roll	1.0	100	9%
long	1 roll	2.0	140	13%
party	3 rolls	2.0	140	13%
potato/sliced	1 roll	1.0	90	30%
sandwich	1 roll	2.0	140	13%
whole wheat	1 roll	1.0	100	9%
(Oroweat)				
health nut	1 roll	3.0	160	17%
master's best/winter wheat	1 roll	4.0	160	23%
(Pepperidge Farm)				
bakery				
country-style..dinner	1 roll	1.5	90	5%
farmhouse				
country wheat	1 roll	4.0	210	17%
golden potato classic	1 roll	4.5	220	18%
hearty white	1 roll	4.5	210	19%
sesame white	1 roll	6.0	230	23%
finger				
w/poppyseeds	3 rolls	4.5	150	27%
w/sesame seeds	3 rolls	4.5	150	27%
frankfurter				
side-sliced	1 roll	2.5	140	16%
top-sliced	1 roll	2.5	140	16%
garlic & cheese	1 roll	5.0	130	35%
hamburger/sliced	1 roll	2.5	120	19%

Food and Description	Amount	Fat Grams	Total Calories	% Fat Calories
hoagie				
deli classic soft	1 roll	4.0	200	18%
multigrain	1 roll	4.0	200	18%
soft	1 roll	5.0	200	23%
Hot & Crusty				
French	1 roll	1.0	100	9%
7-grain French	1 roll	2.0	80	23%
sourdough	1 roll	1.0	100	9%
onion sandwich buns				
w/poppy seeds	1 roll	2.5	150	15%
Parker House	1 roll	2.0	80	23%
party				
round white	3 rolls	4.0	150	24%
sandwich				
multigrain	1 roll	3.0	130	21%
(San Francisco)				
49'ers				
sourdough rolls	1 roll	1.0	100	9%
French rolls				
6 pack	1 roll.	1.0	170	5%
8 pack	1 roll	1.0	90	10%
hamburger buns	1 roll	2.5	230	10%
hoagie rolls	1 roll	1.5	190	7%
sourdough..sliced				
6 pack	1 roll	1.5	170	8%
sourdough dinner				
8 pack	1 roll	1.0	110	8%
sourdough sandwich				
4 pack	1 roll	1.5	240	6%
6 pack	1 roll	1.5	170	8%
sweet French rolls				
6 pack	1 roll	2.5	200	11%
8 pack	1 roll	1.0	90	10%
(Sara Lee)				
Classic				
hamburger buns..white	1 bun	3.0	200	14%
wheat baker buns	1 bun	3.5	200	16%
Gourmet				
hot dog buns	1 bun	1.5	120	11%
(Wenner)				
onion swirl buns	1 bun	2.5	150	15%
salt stick crescent roll	1 roll	1.5	160	8%
(Wonder)				
dinner rolls				
honey rich	1 roll	1.5	100	14%
wheat	2 rolls	3.0	140	19%
white	1 roll	1.0	130	7%
French				
club	1 roll	1.5	120	11%
hoagie	1 roll	2.5	220	10%

Food and Description	Amount	Fat Grams	Total Calories	% Fat Calories
grain				
club	1 roll	1.5	120	11%
hoagie	1 roll	3.0	220	12%
hamburger				
bun	1 bun	2.0	120	15%
light	1 bun	1.0	80	11%
hot dog				
bun	1 roll	2.0	120	15%
light	1 roll	1.0	80	11%
kaiser				
buns	1 bun	3.0	180	15%
hoagie	1 roll	2.5	220	10%
regular	1 roll	1.5	150	9%
potato buns	1 bun	1.0	110	8%
sourdough				
club	1 roll	1.5	120	11%
hoagie	1 roll	2.5	220	10%
steak	1 roll	2.5	190	12%
■ REFRIGERATED				
(Pillsbury)				
crescent				
Grands!	1 roll	15.0	270	50%
original	1 roll	6.0	110	49%
reduced-fat	1 roll	4.5	100	41%
dinner				
home-baked classics				
crusty French	1 roll	1.5	110	12%
traditional				
wheat	1 roll	2.0	110	16%
white	1 roll	2.0	110	16%
ROSE APPLE/fresh	3.5 oz	<1.0	25	11%
ROSELLE/raw	½ cup	–	15	–
ROSEMARY/dried	1 tsp	–	4	–
ROTINI (See PASTA; PASTA ENTRÉE/DINNER)				
ROUGHY (See ORANGE ROUGHY)				
RUTABAGA/fresh				
boiled-drained				
cubed	½ cup	–	30	–
mashed	½ cup	–	40	–
raw	½ cup	–	25	–
RYE (See also FLOUR; CEREAL)				
(Arrowhead Mills)				
flakes..rolled	⅓ cup	0.5	110	4%
whole grain	¼ cup	1.0	160	6%

S

Food and Description	Amount	Fat Grams	Total Calories	% Fat Calories
SABLEFISH				
raw	3 oz	13.0	165	71%
smoked	3 oz	17.0	220	70%
SAFFLOWER MEAL	1 oz	0.7	97	6%
SAFFLOWER OIL (*See* OIL)				
SAFFLOWER SEEDS				
kernels/dried	1 oz	11.0	150	66%
SAFFRON				
dried	1 tsp	–	2	–
SAGE				
ground	1 tsp	–	4	–
SALAD DRESSING (*See also* MAYONNAISE/MAYONNAISE-TYPE DRESSING)				
■ MIX (Note: Unless otherwise stated, mixes were prepared as directed on package.)				
(A Taste of Thai)				
spicy peanut	2 Tbs	1.5	40	34%
(Good Seasons)..mix only (makes 2 Tbs..prepared)				
cheese garlic	⅛ pkt	–	5	–
garlic & herbs	⅛ pkt	–	5	–
gourmet				
Caesar	⅛ pkt	–	15	–
Parmesan Italian	⅛ pkt	–	10	–
Italian				
fat-free	⅛ pkt	–	10	–
mild	⅛ pkt	–	10	–
regular	⅛ pkt	–	5	–
zesty	⅛ pkt	–	5	–
Oriental sesame	⅛ pkt	–	15	–
roasted garlic	⅛ pkt	–	10	–
(Hidden Valley)..ranch..prepared				
bacon	2 Tbs	12.0	120	90%
blue cheese	2 Tbs	12.0	120	90%
honey Dijon	2 Tbs	12.0	120	90%
original..buttermilk	2 Tbs	11.0	110	90%
low-fat	2 Tbs	1.0	30	30%
milk	2 Tbs	12.0	120	90%
reduced-calorie	2 Tbs	6.0	70	77%
ranch Italian	2 Tbs	14.0	140	90%
(Lawry's) mix only				
Caesar	1 pkg	3.0	75	36%

Food and Description	Amount	Fat Grams	Total Calories	% Fat Calories
Italian				
regular	1 pkg	<1.0	45	4%
w/cheese	1 pkg	2.0	75	24%
(Weight Watchers) mix only (Note: 1 serving of mix = the amount in 2 Tbs prepared.)				
blue cheese	1 serving	–	10	–
French	1 serving	–	–	–
Italian				
creamy	1 serving	–	5	–
regular	1 serving	–	–	–
Russian	1 serving	–	–	–
Thousand Island	1 serving	–	–	–
■ **READY-TO-USE**				
(Annie's)..wild herbal organics				
Asian sesame	2 Tbs	14.0	140	90%
balsamic	2 Tbs	10.0	100	90%
buttermilk	2 Tbs			
Caesar	2 Tbs	12.0	120	90%
cilantro & lime	2 Tbs	10.0	100	90%
cowgirl ranch	2 Tbs	11.0	120	83%
French	2 Tbs	9.0	90	90%
garden-style	2 Tbs	12.0	120	90%
gingerly	2 Tbs	10.0	100	90%
goddess	2 Tbs	13.0	130	90%
green garlic	2 Tbs	9.0	90	90%
green goddess	2 Tbs	13.0	130	98%
papaya poppy seed	2 Tbs	11.0	120	83%
pizza pie	2 Tbs	11.0	110	90%
shiltake & sesame	2 Tbs	13.0	120	98%
Thousand Island	2 Tbs	7.0	90	70%
tutti frutti..85% organic	2 Tbs	7.0	80	79%
vinaigrette				
balsamic	2 Tbs	10.0	100	90%
basil & garlic	2 Tbs	14.0	130	97%
ginger & chamomile	2 Tbs	13.0	130	90%
gingerly..low-fat	2 Tbs	2.0	40	45%
honey & turmeric	2 Tbs	15.0	170	79%
honey mustard..low-fat	2 Tbs	2.0	45	40%
raspberry..low-fat	2 Tbs	1.5	35	39%
red wine & olive oil	2 Tbs	17.0	160	96%
roasted red pepper	2 Tbs	6.0	70	77%
sea veggie & sesame	2 Tbs	11.0	110	90%
sesame ginger	2 Tbs	9.0	100	81%
shiitake & sesame	2 Tbs	13.0	120	98%
Tuscany Italian	2 Tbs	7.0	80	79%
yogurt..w/dill				
fat-free	2 Tbs	–	20	–
zoom	2 Tbs	14.0	150	84%
(Ayla's) fat-free				
creamy dill	2 Tbs	–	15	–
French	2 Tbs	–	10	–

Food and Description	Amount	Fat Grams	Total Calories	% Fat Calories
garlic & onion	2 Tbs	–	10	–
Italian				
creamy	2 Tbs	–	15	–
regular	2 Tbs	–	10	–
Russian	2 Tbs	–	10	–
spicy Indonesian	2 Tbs	2.5	35	64%
(Bernstein's)				
fat-free				
cheese & garlic Italian	2 Tbs	–	10	–
Light Fantastic				
Cheese Fantastico	2 Tbs	1.5	25	54%
Classico Italian	2 Tbs	1.5	25	54%
Italian w/cheese	2 Tbs	2.0	25	72%
Oriental	2 Tbs	1.5	60	23%
Parmesan garlic ranch	2 Tbs	2.5	50	45%
Restaurant Ranch	2 Tbs	2.0	45	40%
roasted garlic balsamic	2 Tbs	3.5	45	70%
regular				
balsamic Italian	2 Tbs	11.0	110	90%
Caesar/creamy	2 Tbs	13.0	120	98%
cheese & garlic Italian	2 Tbs	11.0	110	90%
Cheese Fantastico	2 Tbs	10.0	100	90%
Chunky Blue Cheese	2 Tbs	13.0	120	98%
Creamy Roasted Garlic	2 Tbs	15.0	150	90%
French vinaigrette	2 Tbs	10.0	100	90%
herb & garlic Italian	2 Tbs	13.0	130	90%
herb garden French	2 Tbs	11.0	130	76%
Italian dressing & marinade	2 Tbs	12.0	110	98%
olive oil vinaigrette	2 Tbs	9.0	90	90%
Parmesan garlic ranch	2 Tbs	14.0	140	90%
red wine & garlic Italian	2 Tbs	11.0	110	91%
Restaurant Recipe Italian	2 Tbs	12.0	120	90%
Sweet Herb Italian	2 Tbs	11.0	130	90%
Wine Country Italian	2 Tbs	11.0	110	91%
(Brianna's) home-style				
blush wine vinaigrette	2 Tbs	6.0	100	54%
poppy seed	2 Tbs	10.0	130	69%
real French vinaigrette	2 Tbs	10.0	130	69%
(Cardini's)				
Natural				
Caesar	2 Tbs	17.0	160	95%
Parmesan ranch	2 Tbs	15.0	150	90%
roasted red pepper	2 Tbs	11.0	110	90%
Romano cheese Italian	2 Tbs	13.0	130	90%
spicy French	2 Tbs	11.0	130	76%
Original				
aged Parmesan ranch	2 Tbs	15.0	150	90%

Food and Description	Amount	Fat Grams	Total Calories	% Fat Calories
balsamic vinaigrette	2 Tbs	16.0	150	96%
Caesar				
fat-free	2 Tbs	–	40	–
light	2 Tbs	7.0	80	79%
regular	2 Tbs	17.0	160	96%
honey mustard	2 Tbs	14.0	150	84%
Italian				
w/blue cheese crumbles	2 Tbs	13.0	130	90%
kalamata olive				
& Romano cheese	2 Tbs	13.0	120	98%
Parmesan/low-fat	2 Tbs	2.0	45	40%
poppyseed	2 Tbs	1.0	35	26%
w/shallots	2 Tbs	14.0	160	79%
red wine & vinegar	2 Tbs	8.0	90	80%
roasted Asian sesame	2 Tbs	10.0	120	75%
roasted garlic	2 Tbs	14.0	130	97%
southwest Caesar	2 Tbs	14.0	140	90%
white wine	2 Tbs	12.0	110	98%
(Dorothy Lynch)				
fat-free	2 Tbs	–	30	–
home-style	2 Tbs	–	55	–
(Emeril's)				
caesar	2 Tbs	14.0	130	97%
honey mustard	2 Tbs	9.0	100	81%
house herb vinaigrette	2 Tbs	10.0	100	90%
Kicked-Up French	2 Tbs	5.0	80	56%
(Estee)				
Creamy French	2 Tbs	–	10	–
Italian	2 Tbs	–	5	–
(Girard's)				
balsamic vinaigrette				
fat-free	2 Tbs	–	25	–
regular	2 Tbs	9.0	90	90%
blue cheese vinaigrette	2 Tbs	2.0	100	18%
Caesar				
fat-free	2 Tbs	–	40	–
light	2 Tbs	7.0	80	79%
regular	2 Tbs	15.0	150	90%
Champagne				
light	2 Tbs	5.0	60	75%
regular	2 Tbs	16.0	150	96%
French..original	2 Tbs	13.0	120	98%
honey Dijon				
peppercorn	2 Tbs	13.0	140	90%
Greek feta vinaigrette	2 Tbs	11.0	100	99%
Italian				
Olde Venice	2 Tbs	13.0	130	90%
Romano cheese	2 Tbs	13.0	130	90%
Oriental	2 Tbs	11.0	120	83%
Oriental chicken salad	2 Tbs	11.0	120	83%

Food and Description	Amount	Fat Grams	Total Calories	% Fat Calories
Parmesan peppercorn	2 Tbs	17.0	160	96%
raspberry				
fat-free	2 Tbs	–	50	–
regular	2 Tbs	10.0	120	75%
red wine vinaigrette				
fat-free	2 Tbs	–	20	–
shiitake & chardonnay				
vinaigrette	2 Tbs	9.0	100	81%
spinach	2 Tbs	2.0	80	23%
(Hain)				
buttermilk/old-fashioned	1 Tbs	7.0	70	90%
Caesar				
creamy	1 Tbs	6.0	60	90%
low-salt	1 Tbs	6.0	60	90%
Canola				
garden tomato	1 Tbs	6.0	60	90%
Italian	1 Tbs	5.0	50	90%
spicy French mustard	1 Tbs	5.0	50	90%
tangy citrus	1 Tbs	5.0	50	90%
cucumber dill	1 Tbs	7.0	70	90%
French				
creamy	1 Tbs	6.0	60	90%
garlic & sour cream	1 Tbs	7.0	70	90%
honey & sesame	1 Tbs	5.0	60	75%
Italian/creamy				
no salt added	1 Tbs	8.0	80	90%
regular	1 Tbs	8.0	80	90%
traditional	1 Tbs	8.0	80	90%
traditional/no salt added	1 Tbs	8.0	80	90%
Italian cheese vinaigrette	1 Tbs	6.0	55	98%
savory herb/no salt added	1 bs	10.0	90	100%
Thousand Island	2 Tbs	9.0	110	74%
vinaigrette				
raspberry	2 Tbs	–	12	–
white wine	2 Tbs	–	25	–
(Hidden Valley)				
bacon	2 Tbs	15.0	150	90%
blue cheese	2 Tbs	17.0	160	96%
coleslaw	2 Tbs	15.0	150	90%
creamy				
herb Italian	2 Tbs	13.0	140	84%
Parmesan	2 Tbs	15.0	140	96%
fiesta	2 Tbs	14.0	140	90%
French/low-fat	2 Tbs	1.0	35	26%
honey Dijon	2 Tbs	15.0	140	96%
original ranch				
low-fat	2 Tbs	3.0	40	68%
reduced-calorie	2 Tbs	7.0	80	95%
regular	2 Tbs	14.0	140	90%
nacho cheese	2 Tbs	14.0	130	97%

Food and Description	Amount	Fat Grams	Total Calories	% Fat Calories
pizza	2 Tbs	14.0	140	90%
ranch..Italian	2 Tbs	12.0	120	90%
super-creamy	2 Tbs	14.0	140	90%
taco	2 Tbs	13.0	130	90%
Thousand Island	2 Tbs	10.0	110	82%
(Hollywood)				
buttermilk/old-fashioned	1 Tbs	8.0	75	85%
Caesar	1 Tbs	7.0	70	90%
Dijon vinaigrette	1 Tbs	6.0	60	90%
French/creamy	1 Tbs	7.0	70	90%
Italian				
cheese	1 Tbs	8.0	80	90%
creamy	1 Tbs	9.0	90	90%
regular	1 Tbs	9.0	90	90%
Poppyseed Ranchers	1 Tbs	8.0	75	96%
Thousand Island	1 Tbs	6.0	60	90%
(Ken's) Steak House				
fat-free				
honey Dijon	2 Tbs	–	40	–
peppercorn	2 Tbs	–	40	–
raspberry pecan	2 Tbs	–	45	–
sun-dried tomato vinaigrette	2 Tbs	–	60	–
lite				
Caesar w/imported anchovies	2 Tbs	6.0	70	77%
country French	2 Tbs	5.0	90	50%
creamy Parmesan				
w/cracked peppercorn	2 Tbs	9.0	90	90%
honey mustard	2 Tbs	4.0	70	51%
raspberry walnut vinaigrette	2 Tbs	6.0	80	68%
red wine vinegar & olive oil	2 Tbs	5.0	50	90%
(Knott's Berry Farm)				
California fruit	2 Tbs	4.0	70	51%
honey Dijon	2 Tbs	13.0	130	90%
honey poppyseed	2 Tbs	9.0	120	68%
Oriental chicken salad	2 Tbs	11.0	130	76%
raspberry vinaigrette				
low-fat	2 Tbs	2.0	50	36%
roasted garlic	2 Tbs	14.0	140	90%
sun-dried tomato				
vinaigrette	2 Tbs	10.0	100	90%
tropical vinaigrette				
low-fat	2 Tbs	1.0	45	20%
(Kraft)				
Caesar				
classic	2 Tbs	11.0	110	90%
Italian				
fat-free	2 Tbs	–	25	–
original	2 Tbs	10.0	100	90%
ranch	2 Tbs	11.0	110	90%

Food and Description	Amount	Fat Grams	Total Calories	% Fat Calories
CarbWell				
classic Caesar	2 Tbs	11.0	110	90%
Italian	2 Tbs	7.0	70	90%
ranch	2 Tbs	11.0	100	99%
roka blue cheese	2 Tbs	13.0	120	98%
Fat-Free				
Catalina	2 Tbs	–	35	–
honey Dijon	2 Tbs	–	50	–
Italian	2 Tbs	–	15	–
ranch	2 Tbs	–	50	–
Thousand Island	2 Tbs	–	40	—
Light Done Right				
blue cheese..roka	2 Tbs	6.0	70	77%
creamy French	2 Tbs	6.0	90	60%
Italian	2 Tbs	7.0	70	90%
zesty	2 Tbs	1.5	25	54%
ranch	2 Tbs	7.0	80	79%
buttermilk	2 Tbs	16.0	150	96%
Thousand Island	2 Tbs			
regular dressings				
blue cheese..roka	2 Tbs	13.0	130	90%
Caesar				
regular	2 Tbs	11.0	190	52%
w/bacon	2 Tbs			
French..creamy	2 Tbs	15.0	160	84%
honey Dijon	2 Tbs	10.0	110	82%
Italian				
creamy	2 Tbs	11.0	110	90%
zesty	2 Tbs	11.0	110	90%
ranch				
garlic	2 Tbs	19.0	180	95%
regular	2 Tbs	18.0	170	95%
Thousand Island				
regular	2 Tbs	10.0	120	75%
(Lawry's)				
Caesar				
creamy	2 Tbs	14.0	130	97%
regular	2 Tbs	13.0	130	90%
Italian	2 Tbs	14.0	140	90%
red wine vinaigrette	2 Tbs	7.0	90	70%
San Francisco				
w/Romano cheese	2 Tbs	13.0	120	98%
(Life) all-natural				
avocado w/tofu	1 Tbs	7.0	70	90%
creamy egg salad/egg-free	1 Tbs	4.0	40	90%
garlic w/tofu	1 Tbs	7.0	70	90%
tofu	1 Tbs	7.0	75	84%
(Litehouse)				
fat-free				
Caesar	2 Tbs	–	15	–

Food and Description	Amount	Fat Grams	Total Calories	% Fat Calories
ranch	2 Tbs	–	10	–
honey bacon	2 Tbs	–	50	–
honey Dijon	2 Tbs	–	35	–
raspberry vinaigrette	2 Tbs	–	15	–
sesame ginger				
dressing & sauce	2 Tbs	–	35	–
vinaigrette	2 Tbs	–	5	–
wild huckleberry				
vinaigrette..Naturals	2 Tbs	–	20	–
Naturals				
balsamic vinaigrette	2 Tbs	7.0	80	79%
bleu cheese vinaigrette	2 Tbs	13.0	130	90%
chipotle ranch	2 Tbs	6.0	60	90%
cranberry vinaigrette				
fat-free	2 Tbs	–	25	–
creamy garlic Caesar	2 Tbs	8.0	80	90%
roasted red pepper	2 Tbs	5.5	50	99%
wild huckleberry				
vinaigrette..fat-free	2 Tbs	–	20	–
other..jars				
bleu cheese				
Big Bleu	2 Tbs	17.0	160	95%
light	2 Tbs	6.0	70	77%
original	2 Tbs	16.0	150	96%
Caesar	2 Tbs	14.0	140	90%
coleslaw	2 Tbs	7.0	90	70%
country ranch	2 Tbs	13.0	120	98%
Parmesan garlic	2 Tbs	13.0	120	98%
poppyseed	2 Tbs	12.0	130	83%
ranch				
light	2 Tbs	6.0	60	90%
light salsa	2 Tbs	4.5	50	81%
peppercorn	2 Tbs	10.0	100	90%
regular	2 Tbs	12.0	120	90%
Roquefort	2 Tbs	14.0	130	97%
sweet red French	2 Tbs	7.0	110	57%
Thousand Island	2 Tbs	13.0	120	98%
other..dressing & sauce				
Thai peanut	2 Tbs	9.0	100	81%
(Luzinne)				
La Martinique	1 Tbs	11.0	100	99%
Old Dutch sweet & sour	2 Tbs	–	50	–
(Maple Grove Farms)				
fat-free				
balsamic vinaigrette	2 Tbs	–	10	–
cranberry balsamic				
vinaigrette	2 Tbs	–	30	–
honey Dijon	2 Tbs	–	45	–
lime basil vinaigrette	2 Tbs	–	25	–
raspberry vinaigrette	2 Tbs	–	35	–

Food and Description	Amount	Fat Grams	Total Calories	% Fat Calories
low-carb dressings				
bacon vinaigrette	2 Tbs	9.0	90	90%
balsamic vinaigrette	2 Tbs	–	–	–
Dijon..sugar-free	2 Tbs	8.0	80	90%
Italian balsamic				
sugar-free	2 Tbs	9.0	90	90%
raspberry vinaigrette	2 Tbs	–	5	–
other dressings				
Caesar..light	2 Tbs	5.0	70	64%
honey mustard..light	2 Tbs	5.0	80	56%
Romano..light	2 Tbs	3.5	40	79%
Vermont				
honey mustard	2 Tbs	9.0	120	68%
Parmesan				
& cracked pepper	2 Tbs	11.0	120	83%
(Marie's)				
blue cheese				
chunky	2 Tbs	19.0	180	95%
fat-free	2 Tbs	–	30	–
light	2 Tbs	7.0	100	63%
original	2 Tbs	18.0	170	95%
Caesar				
creamy	2 Tbs	18.0	180	90%
cole slaw	2 Tbs	13.0	150	78%
feta cheese & herb	2 Tbs	17.0	170	90%
ranch/creamy	2 Tbs	20.0	190	95%
raspberry vinaigrette/fat-free	2 Tbs	–	35	–
Roquefort classic premium recipe	2 Tbs	20.0	190	95%
(Marzetti) (See (T. Marzetti) in this section)				
(Nasoya) Vegi dressings				
dill/creamy	2 Tbs	7.0	70	90%
Italian/creamy	2 Tbs	6.0	60	90%
sesame garlic	2 Tbs	6.0	60	90%
Thousand Island	2 Tbs	6.0	70	77%
(Naturally Fresh)				
fat-free dressings				
balsamic vinaigrette	2 Tbs	–	5	–
balsamic vinaigrette II	2 Tbs	8.0	80	90%
honey ranch	2 Tbs	–	25	–
lemon vinaigrette	2 Tbs	–	25	–
ranch	2 Tbs	–	20	–
raspberry vinaigrette	2 Tbs	–	25	–
Thousand Island	2 Tbs	–	20	–
light dressings				
honey mustard	2 Tbs	6.0	80	68%
peppercorn ranch	2 Tbs	8.0	80	89%
ranch	2 Tbs	8.0	80	89%
other dressings				
bleu cheese				
classic	2 Tbs	14.0	130	97%

Food and Description	Amount	Fat Grams	Total Calories	% Fat Calories
light	2 Tbs	10.0	100	90%
regular	2 Tbs	18.0	170	95%
roasted garlic	2 Tbs	18.0	170	95%
Caesar				
4 oz	2 Tbs	18.0	170	95%
16 oz	2 Tbs	13.0	120	98%
classic	2 Tbs	18.0	170	95%
grilled	2 Tbs	15.0	140	96%
classic Oriental	2 Tbs	11.0	100	99%
cranberry orange	2 Tbs	–	45	–
cranberry walnut	2 Tbs	10.0	110	82%
French..honey	2 Tbs	11.0	120	83%
French II	2 Tbs	11.0	110	90%
ginger	2 Tbs	7.0	70	90%
honey mustard				
bacon honey mustard	2 Tbs	5.0	70	64%
Dijon honey mustard	2 Tbs	12.0	110	98%
honey mustard II	2 Tbs	10.0	130	69%
Italian				
fat-free	2 Tbs	–	5	–
4-cheese	2 Tbs	10.0	110	82%
herb vinaigrette	2 Tbs	12.0	110	98%
Italian II	2 Tbs	1.0	15	60%
light	2 Tbs	–	5	–
poppyseed	2 Tbs	13.0	140	84%
ranch				
classic	2 Tbs	16.0	150	96%
fat-free	2 Tbs	–	20	–
light	2 Tbs	8.0	80	90%
pesto	2 Tbs	7.0	70	90%
ranch II	2 Tbs	10.0	100	90%
slaw	2 Tbs	10.0	120	75%
Thousand Island				
16 oz	2 Tbs	12.0	120	90%
Thousand Island II	2 Tbs	10.0	120	75%
wine & cheese	2 Tbs	14.0	140	90%
(Newman's Own)				
balsamic vinaigrette				
light	2 Tbs	4.0	45	80%
regular	2 Tbs	9.0	90	90%
Caesar				
creamy	2 Tbs	18.0	170	95%
original	2 Tbs	16.0	150	96%
family recipe				
Italian	2 Tbs	3.0	120	23%
Italian				
light	2 Tbs	6.0	60	90%
original	2 Tbs	16.0	150	96%
olive oil & vinegar	2 Tbs	16.0	150	96%

Food and Description	Amount	Fat Grams	Total Calories	% Fat Calories
Parisienne Dijon lime	2 Tbs	13.0	120	98%
parmegiano Italianio	2 Tbs	14.0	140	90%
Parmesan & roasted garlic	2 Tbs	11.0	110	90%
ranch	2 Tbs	15.0	140	96%
raspberry walnut..light	2 Tbs	5.0	70	64%
red wine vinegar				
& olive oil	2 Tbs	10.0	110	82%
two Thousand Island	2 Tbs	14.0	140	90%
(Ott's)				
buttermilk ranch	2 Tbs	14.0	140	90%
Caesar	2 Tbs	11.0	110	90%
honey mustard	2 Tbs	8.0	100	72%
Italian	2 Tbs	10.0	100	90%
original				
fat-free	2 Tbs	–	35	–
reduced-calorie	2 Tbs	3.0	60	30%
regular	2 Tbs	6.0	80	68%
poppyseed				
fat-free	2 Tbs	–	45	–
regular	2 Tbs	7.0	90	70%
ranch	2 Tbs	16.0	150	96%
Thousand Island	2 Tbs	8.0	100	72%
(Pfeiffer)				
balsamic vinaigrette	2 Tbs	9.0	100	90%
blue cheese	2 Tbs	18.0	170	95%
buttermilk & herb	2 Tbs	20.0	180	100%
Caesar				
house	2 Tbs	16.0	150	96%
light	2 Tbs	1.0	20	45%
original	2 Tbs	13.0	120	98%
coleslaw	2 Tbs	16.0	170	85%
French				
California				
fat-free	2 Tbs	–	40	–
regular	2 Tbs	12.0	140	77%
original				
fat-free	2 Tbs	–	20	–
light	2 Tbs	2.0	40	45%
regular	2 Tbs	13.0	150	78%
garlic..roasted vinaigrette	2 Tbs	10.0	130	69%
honey Dijon	2 Tbs	12.0	140	77%
Italian				
creamy	2 Tbs	17.0	160	96%
garlic	2 Tbs	10.0	100	90%
original				
fat-free	2 Tbs	–	20	–
light	2 Tbs	4.0	50	72%
regular	2 Tbs	10.0	100	90%
Tuscan	2 Tbs	12.0	110	98%
zesty garlic	2 Tbs	10.0	100	90%

Food and Description	Amount	Fat Grams	Total Calories	% Fat Calories
ranch				
California	2 Tbs	12.0	140	77%
Dijon	2 Tbs	18.0	170	95%
garden	2 Tbs	17.0	160	96%
original				
fat-free	2 Tbs	–	25	–
light	2 Tbs	7.0	80	79%
regular	2 Tbs	16.0	150	96%
peppercorn				
fat-free	2 Tbs	–	25	–
(S&W)				
Vintage Lites..fat-free				
Italian balsamic	2 Tbs	–	35	–
raspberry blush	2 Tbs	–	40	–
red wine & herb	2 Tbs	–	40	–
white wine & herb	2 Tbs	–	40	–
(Seven Seas)				
blue cheese/chunky	2 Tbs	13.0	130	90%
Caesar				
classic	2 Tbs	10.0	100	90%
creamy	2 Tbs	15.0	140	96%
Green Goddess	2 Tbs	13.0	130	90%
herb vinaigrette	2 Tbs	15.0	140	96%
herbs & spices	2 Tbs	9.0	90	90%
honey mustard	2 Tbs	10.0	110	82%
Italian				
creamy				
reduced-fat	2 Tbs	–	45	–
regular	2 Tbs	12.0	110	98%
regular/fat-free	2 Tbs	–	10	–
2-cheese	2 Tbs	7.0	70	90%
Viva				
fat-free	2 Tbs	–	15	–
reduced-fat	2 Tbs	4.0	45	80%
regular	2 Tbs	9.0	90	90%
robust	2 Tbs	9.0	90	90%
w/olive oil	2 Tbs	5.0	50	90%
ranch				
fat-free	2 Tbs	–	45	–
reduced-calorie	2 Tbs	9.0	100	90%
regular	2 Tbs	17.0	160	96%
raspberry vinaigrette	2 Tbs	–	30	–
red wine vinegar				
fat-free	2 Tbs	–	15	–
red wine vinegar & oil				
reduced-fat	2 Tbs	4.0	45	80%
regular	2 Tbs	9.0	90	90%
(Simply Delicious) organic				
ginger plum	2 Tbs	10.0	110	82%
herb garlic	2 Tbs	10.0	110	82%

Food and Description	Amount	Fat Grams	Total Calories	% Fat Calories
honey mustard	2 Tbs	10.0	110	82%
miso sesame	2 Tbs	11.0	110	90%
tofu poppyseed	2 Tbs	10.0	110	82%
(T. Marzetti)				
balsamic vinaigrette				
light	2 Tbs	4.0	50	72%
Marzetti	2 Tbs	9.0	100	90%
house	2 Tbs	8.0	90	80%
organic	2 Tbs	9.0	90	90%
regular	2 Tbs	9.0	100	90%
blue cheese				
chunky	2 Tbs	15.0	150	90%
Italian vinaigrette	2 Tbs	9.0	100	81%
light	2 Tbs	8.0	90	80%
organic	2 Tbs	14.0	130	97%
regular	2 Tbs	18.0	170	95%
buttermilk & herb	2 Tbs	20.0	180	100%
Caesar				
creamy	2 Tbs	15.0	150	90%
house	2 Tbs	16.0	150	96%
light	2 Tbs	6.0	70	77%
organic	2 Tbs	16.0	150	96%
original	2 Tbs	13.0	120	98%
coleslaw	2 Tbs	16.0	170	85%
French				
California				
fat-free	2 Tbs	–	40	–
light	2 Tbs	6.0	90	60%
regular	2 Tbs	12.0	160	68%
country..pourable	2 Tbs	15.0	160	84%
honey	2 Tbs	4.0	80	45%
honey..produce	2 Tbs	14.0	170	74%
original				
fat-free	2 Tbs	–	20	–
light	2 Tbs	2.0	40	45%
regular	2 Tbs	13.0	150	78%
garlic				
roasted	2 Tbs	15.0	150	90%
roasted vinaigrette	2 Tbs	10.0	130	69%
vinaigrette	2 Tbs	8.0	90	80%
Greek vinaigrette	2 Tbs	8.0	80	90%
honey Dijon				
fat-free	2 Tbs	–	50	–
regular	2 Tbs	12.0	140	77%
honey French				
blue cheese	2 Tbs	13.0	160	73%
honey mustard				
dip & dressing	2 Tbs	12.0	130	83%
Italian				
creamy	2 Tbs	17.0	160	96%
fat-free	2 Tbs	–	20	–

Food and Description	Amount	Fat Grams	Total Calories	% Fat Calories
garlic	2 Tbs	10.0	100	90%
light	2 Tbs	5.0	60	75%
original				
fat-free	2 Tbs	–	20	–
light	2 Tbs	4.0	50	72%
regular	2 Tbs	10.0	100	90%
romano..pourable	2 Tbs	16.0	150	96%
roasted garlic vinaigrette	2 Tbs	13.0	120	98%
Tuscan..Marzetti	2 Tbs	12.0	110	98%
Parmesan..organic	2 Tbs	14.0	140	90%
peppercorn Parmesan	2 Tbs	17.0	160	96%
peppercorn..cracked				
produce	2 Tbs	16.0	150	96%
poppyseed				
fat-free	2 Tbs	–	60	–
pourable..Marzetti	2 Tbs	13.0	160	73%
regular	2 Tbs	11.0	140	71%
potato salad dressing	2 Tbs	15.0	150	90%
ranch				
bacon..produce	2 Tbs	17.0	160	96%
buttermilk				
light	2 Tbs	9.0	90	90%
regular	2 Tbs	20.0	180	100%
California	2 Tbs	12.0	140	77%
Dijon	2 Tbs	18.0	170	95%
garden	2 Tbs	17.0	160	96%
original				
fat-free	2 Tbs	–	25	–
light	2 Tbs	7.0	80	79%
regular	2 Tbs	16.0	150	96%
peppercorn				
fat-free	2 Tbs	–	30	–
original	2 Tbs	19.0	180	95%
raspberry vinaigrette	2 Tbs	8.0	100	72%
Marzetti..house	2 Tbs	8.0	90	80%
red wine vinaigrette	2 Tbs	9.0	90	90%
Marzetti	2 Tbs	8.0	90	80%
Russian	2 Tbs	14.0	140	90%
sesame oriental				
Marzetti	2 Tbs	9.0	110	74%
slaw				
light	2 Tbs	7.0	100	63%
low-fat	2 Tbs	1.5	60	23%
regular	2 Tbs	16.0	170	85%
southern recipe	2 Tbs	11.0	150	66%
sour cream blue cheese				
dip & dressing	2 Tbs	18.0	170	95%
spinach	2 Tbs	2.0	80	23%
sun-dried tomato				
vinaigrette	2 Tbs	11.0	130	76%

Food and Description	Amount	Fat Grams	Total Calories	% Fat Calories
sweet & sour				
fat-free	2 Tbs	–	50	–
light	2 Tbs	6.0	100	54%
pourable	2 Tbs	13.0	160	73%
regular	2 Tbs	13.0	160	73%
Sweet Italian..produce	2 Tbs	14.0	150	84%
Thousand Island				
fat-free	2 Tbs	–	45	–
light	2 Tbs	5.0	70	64%
original	2 Tbs	14.0	140	90%
produce	2 Tbs	15.0	150	90%
Two Lightful..Marzetti				
blue				
Caesar	2 Tbs	2.0	45	40%
honey				
Dijon	2 Tbs	2.0	60	30%
French	2 Tbs	2.0	50	36%
Italian	2 Tbs	2.0	40	45%
peppercorn ranch	2 Tbs	2.0	60	30%
ranch	2 Tbs	2.0	50	36%
(Toby's)				
chunky feta	2 Tbs	10.0	100	90%
blue cheese	2 Tbs	10.0	100	90%
creamy vinaigrette	2 Tbs	7.0	70	90%
jalapeño ranch	2 Tbs	10.0	100	90%
ranch	2 Tbs	10.0	100	90%
toasted sesame	2 Tbs	4.0	40	90%
(Walden Farms)				
carb-free..sugar-free				
balsamic vinegar	2 Tbs	–	40	–
hot bacon	2 Tbs	–	40	–
Italian	2 Tbs	2.0	20	90%
ranch	2 Tbs	–	–	–
Thousand Island	2 Tbs	–	–	–
fat-free..calorie-free				
carb-free..sugar-free				
all types & flavors	2 Tbs	–	–	–
Organic Dressings				
balsamic vinaigrette	2 Tbs	7.0	80	79%
bleu cheese	2 Tbs	10.0	110	82%
Caesar	2 Tbs	11.0	120	83%
honey Dijon	2 Tbs	8.0	100	72%
ranch	2 Tbs	10.0	110	82%
(Weight Watchers)..fat-free				
Salad Celebrations				
French	2 Tbs	–	40	–
honey Dijon	2 Tbs	–	45	–
Italian				
creamy	2 Tbs	–	30	–

Food and Description	Amount	Fat Grams	Total Calories	% Fat Calories
regular	2 Tbs	–	10	–
ranch	2 Tbs	–	35	–
(Western)				
blue cheese	2 Tbs	12.0	140	77%
French				
creamy	2 Tbs	11.0	140	71%
fat-free	2 Tbs	–	45	–
Just 2 Good!				
low-fat	2 Tbs	2.0	70	26%
regular	2 Tbs	3.0	70	38%
light	2 Tbs	3.0	70	38%
The Original	2 Tbs	12.0	160	67%
w/bacon flavor	2 Tbs	11.0	140	71%
(Wish-Bone)				
balsamic vinaigrette	2 Tbs	5.0	60	75%
Italian	2 Tbs	6.0	70	77%
berry vinaigrette	2 Tbs	5.0	50	90%
blue cheese				
chunky				
fat-free	2 Tbs	–	35	–
regular	2 Tbs	17.0	160	96%
Just 2 Good!	2 Tbs	2.0	45	40%
regular	2 Tbs	17.0	170	90%
Caesar				
citrus splash..vinaigrette	2 Tbs	7.0	90	70%
classic	2 Tbs	10.0	110	82%
creamy	2 Tbs	18.0	170	95%
low-fat	2 Tbs	2.0	40	45%
Just 2 Good!				
classic	2 Tbs	2.0	45	40%
creamy	2 Tbs	2.0	40	45%
creamy roasted garlic				
fat-free	2 Tbs	–	40	–
regular	2 Tbs	13.0	140	84%
French				
deluxe				
low-fat	2 Tbs	2.0	50	36%
regular	2 Tbs	11.0	120	83%
Just 2 Good!				
deluxe	2 Tbs	2.0	50	36%
sweet 'n' spicy	2 Tbs	2.0	50	36%
sweet 'n' spicy				
regular	2 Tbs	12.0	130	83%
honey Dijon				
Just 2 Good!				
low-fat	2 Tbs	2.0	50	36%
vinaigrette	2 Tbs	6.0	80	68%
Italian				
5-cheese	2 Tbs	10.0	120	75%
classic house	2 Tbs	14.0	140	90%

Food and Description	Amount	Fat Grams	Total Calories	% Fat Calories
Country..w/herbs				
low-fat	2 Tbs	2.0	30	60%
creamy				
fat-free	2 Tbs	–	10	–
house	2 Tbs	10.0	100	90%
Parmesan basil				
low-fat	2 Tbs	2.0	45	40%
regular	2 Tbs	10.0	110	82%
Just 2 Good!				
country	2 Tbs	2.0	30	60%
Parmesan basil	2 Tbs	2.0	40	45%
regular	2 Tbs	2.0	35	51%
original				
fat-free	2 Tbs	–	10	–
regular	2 Tbs	8.0	80	90%
robusto	2 Tbs	8.0	90	80%
lemon garlic & herb				
vinaigrette	2 Tbs	5.0	70	64%
olive oil vinaigrette	2 Tbs	5.0	60	75%
Oriental	2 Tbs	5.0	70	64%
Parmesan				
& onion	2 Tbs	10.0	110	82%
peppercorn ranch				
low-fat	2 Tbs	2.0	45	40%
ranch				
classic	2 Tbs	15.0	140	96%
fat-free	2 Tbs	–	40	–
garlic	2 Tbs	15.0	150	90%
Just 2 Good!				
low-fat	2 Tbs	2.0	40	45%
original	2 Tbs	17.0	160	96%
spring onion	2 Tbs	14.0	140	90%
red wine vinaigrette				
fat-free	2 Tbs	–	30	–
regular	2 Tbs	5.0	90	50%
roasted garlic vinaigrette	2 Tbs	6.0	70	77%
Russian	2 Tbs	6.0	110	49%
sun-dried tomato vinaigrette	2 Tbs	5.0	60	75%
sweet & spicy French				
low-fat	2 Tbs	2.0	50	36%
Thousand Island				
Just 2 Good!	2 Tbs	2.0	60	30%
regular	2 Tbs	12.0	130	83%
white wine vinaigrette	2 Tbs	4.5	60	68%
zesty	2 Tbs	15.0	140	96%
SALAD..CANNED..DELI..SERVICE DELI				
(Bumble Bee)..packaged				
with crackers				
chicken salad	3.5 oz	8.0	140	51%
seafood salad..w/crab	3.3 oz	17.0	200	77%

Food and Description	Amount	Fat Grams	Total Calories	% Fat Calories
tuna salad				
fat-free	3.5 oz	–	70	–
regular	3.5 oz	16.0	190	76%
(Giant Foods).. Super G Healthy Ideas				
Gourmet Kitchens				
black beans & rice	½ cup	0.5	140	3%
Cajun lentil & pea				
confetti	½ cup	0.5	140	3%
creamy cole slaw	½ cup	2.5	70	32%
creamy dill potato	1 cup	–	100	–
cucumber vinaigrette	½ cup	–	20	–
curried brown rice				
w/chicken	½ cup	1.0	150	6%
linguini & herbs	1 cup	2.5	240	9%
salmon & penne	1 cup	2.5	210	11%
tropical fruit salad	½ cup	1.0	70	13%
tuna salad..white meat	⅓ cup	18.0	230	70%
Wampler chicken salad	⅓ cup	14.0	200	63%
wild rice..w/smoked				
turkey	½ cup	1.0	130	7%
winter garden Dutch				
potato salad	½ cup	9.0	210	39%
(Read's)				
canned				
4-bean	½ cup	–	110	–
German potato	½ cup	3.0	120	23%
3-bean	½ cup	–	100	–

SALAD TOPPINGS & MIXES (*See also* BACON BITS, CHIPS & PIECES; CROUTONS; SEASONINGS)

Food and Description	Amount	Fat Grams	Total Calories	% Fat Calories
(Betty Crocker)..Prepared				
Suddenly Salad				
Caesar	1 cup	10.0	250	36%
classic pasta	1 cup	7.0	240	26%
creamy Parmesan	1 cup	24.0	360	60%
ranch & bacon	¾ cup	23.0	330	63%
roasted garlic Parmesan	¾ cup	22.0	340	58%
(Fresh Gourmet)				
Almond Toppers				
country ranch	1 Tbs	3.5	40	79%
roasted garlic	1 Tbs	3.5	40	79%
robust Parmesan	1 Tbs	3.5	40	79%
spicy Szechuan	1 Tbs	3.5	40	79%
sun-dried tomato basil	1 Tbs	4.0	45	80%
(Hidden Valley) Salad Crispins				
bacon & onion	1 Tbs	1.0	35	26%
cheddar & onion	1 Tbs	1.0	35	26%
Italian Parmesan	1 Tbs	1.0	35	26%
ranch	1 Tbs	1.0	35	26%
sour cream & herb	1 Tbs	1.0	35	26%

Food and Description	Amount	Fat Grams	Total Calories	% Fat Calories
(McCormick/Schilling)				
Salad Toppin's				
garden vegetable	1⅓ Tbs	1.0	30	30%
Oriental	1⅓ Tbs	2.0	40	45%
original	1⅓ Tbs	1.5	35	39%
SALAMI (*See* LUNCHEON MEAT; SAUSAGE)				
SALMON (*See also* SALMON SPREAD; SEAFOOD ENTRÉE/DINNER)				
canned				
(Black Top)				
chum..Alaska	2.10 oz	4.0	90	40%
pink	2.25 oz	5.0	90	50%
Alaska	2.10 oz	5.0	90	50%
chunk-style..skinless				
boneless	2.4 oz	2.0	60	30%
red				
sockeye				
fancy	2.25 oz	7.0	110	57%
fancy Alaska	2.10 oz	2.0	60	30%
(Bumble Bee)				
blueback..Alaska				
fancy	2.14 oz	7.0	110	57%
Keta..Alaska	2.11 oz	4.0	90	40%
pink				
Alaska	¼ cup	5.0	90	50%
fancy	¼ cup	8.0	160	45%
regular	¼ cup	5.0	90	50%
skinless..boneless	¼ cup	1.0	50	18%
red				
Alaska sockeye	¼ cup	7.0	110	57%
(Chicken of the Sea)				
pink				
chunk-style	2 oz	2.0	60	30%
skinless-boneless				
in spring water	2 oz	2.0	60	30%
	2.8 oz	2.0	80	23%
	1 pouch	3.0	90	30%
traditional	2 oz	5.0	90	50%
red				
chunk				
boneless..skinless	2 oz	2.0	60	30%
traditional	2 oz	7.0	110	57%
(Ducktrap River)				
Atlantic				
Kendall Brook	2 oz	9.0	130	62%
Spruce Point	2 oz	7.0	110	57%
Winter Harbor	2 oz	9.0	130	62%
pastrami-style				
Spruce Point	2 oz	9.0	130	62%
roasted	2 oz	6.0	100	54%

Food and Description	Amount	Fat Grams	Total Calories	% Fat Calories
(Geisha)				
pink				
fresh Alaska	2 oz	5.0	90	50%
traditional	2 oz	4.0	90	40%
red				
fresh Alaska	2 oz	7.0	110	57%
(Lasco)				
sliced..smoked	2 oz	1.0	60	15%
tulp pink	¼ cup	5.0	90	50%
fresh				
Atlantic				
cooked—dry heat	3 oz	7.0	155	41%
raw	3 oz	5.5	120	41%
Chinook/lox				
raw	3 oz	9.0	155	29%
smoked	3 oz	3.7	100	33%
chum/keta/raw	3 oz	3.0	100	27%
coho				
cooked—moist heat	3 oz	6.5	160	36%
raw	3 oz	5.0	125	36%
pink				
cooked—dry heat	3 oz	4.0	130	27%
raw	3 oz	3.0	100	27%
red/sockeye				
cooked—dry heat	3 oz	9.0	185	44%
raw	3 oz	7.0	143	44%
smoked				
Chinook	3 oz	3.7	100	33%
(Duck Trap River)..pâté	¼ cup	14.0	150	84%
SALMON CAVIAR (See also CAVIAR)				
(Crown Prince)..Alaskan coho salmon	1 Tbs	1.5	30	45%
SALMON SPREAD..(Vita)	¼ cup	5.0	180	25%
SALSA (See MEXICAN FOOD; SAUCE)				
SALSIFY				
fresh/sliced				
cooked-drained	½ cup	–	46	–
raw	½ cup	–	55	–
SALT (See also SEASONINGS)				
(Durkee)..all types	½ tsp	–	–	–
(Hain) sea salt...all types	1 tsp	–	–	–
SALT PORK (See PORK)				
SALT SUBSTITUTE (See also SEASONINGS)				
(Durkee) seasoned	½ tsp	–	–	–
(Estee) Salt It	⅛ tsp	–	–	–
(Featherweight)..all types	¼ tsp	–	–	–
(Lawry's)				
plain	1 tsp	–	10	–
seasoned	1 tsp	–	3	–
(McCormick) Salt-Less	¼ tsp	–	–	–
SANDWICH SPREAD (See also LUNCHEON MEAT SPREAD)				

Food and Description	Amount	Fat Grams	Total Calories	% Fat Calories
(Hellmann's)	1 Tbs	5.0	50	90%
Sandwich Spread				
original	1 Tbs	4.0	50	72%
reduced-fat	1 Tbs	2.5	35	64%
(Kraft)	1 Tbs	4.0	50	72%
(Loma Linda)	¼ cup	4.5	80	51%
(McCormick Hispanic)..Mayonesa				
w/chipotle peppers	1 Tbs	6.0	60	90%
w/jalapeño peppers	1 Tbs	4.0	50	72%
SAPODILLO				
tropical American	1 medium	1.9	140	12%
	1 cup	2.0	178	10%
SAPOTE/fresh	1 medium	1.5	300	5%
SARDINE				
(Chicken of the Sea)				
Fancy Brisling				
in chili sauce	2 oz	5.0	90	50%
in hot sauce	2 oz	3.0	70	39%
in mustard sauce	2 oz	4.0	80	45%
in oil	1 can	16.0	210	69%
in water	⅓ cup	3.0	80	34%
tall sardines in water	2 oz	3.0	80	34%
(Crown Prince)				
1-layer Brisling				
in water..2.9 oz	1 can	17.0	210	73%.
2-layer brisling				
in mustard..3.79 oz	1 can	16.0	210	69%
in olive oil..2.9 oz	1 can	16.0	210	69%
skinless..boneless				
in olive oil..3.5 oz	1 can	15.0	230	59%
in water..3.2 oz	1 can			
(Empress) Norway/boneless & skinless				
in olive oil	3.8 oz	38.0	420	81%
in soy oil	4.4 oz	45.0	500	81%
(Goya)				
in				
lemon sauce	¼ cup	9.0	120	68%
tomato sauce	¼ cup	9.0	130	62%
spiced	¼ cup	9.0	120	68%
(King Oscar)				
in				
olive oil				
cross-pack	3.75 oz	11.0	150	66%
one layer	3.75 oz	10.0	150	60%
pure spring water	3.75 oz	13.0	173	68%
two layers	3.75 oz	11.0	150	66%
(Underwood)				
in mustard sauce	3.73 oz	12.0	180	60%
in soybean oil	2.96 oz	16.0	220	65%
in tomato sauce	3.73 oz	11.0	180	55%

Food and Description	Amount	Fat Grams	Total Calories	% Fat Calories
(Viking's Delight)..Brisling..in olive oil				
drained	3.75 oz	20.0	260	69%
undrained	3.75 oz	42.0	460	82%
SAUCE (*See also* ASIAN FOOD; BARBECUE SAUCE; GRAVY; MARINADE; MEXICAN FOOD; PASTA ENTRÉE/DINNER; SEASONINGS; SOUP, TOMATO; TOMATO SAUCE)				
■ MIX				
(A Taste of Thai)..mix only				
chicken & rice	¼ pkt	–	15	–
fish	1 Tbs	–	15	–
garlic pepper	1 tsp	–	10	–
pad Thai	2 Tbs	1.0	90	10%
peanut sauce	¼ pkg	1.5	45	30%
satay sauce	2 Tbs	4.5	80	51%
spicy Thai peanut	¼ pkg	1.5	45	30%
sweet red chili	1 tsp	–	10	–
tangy hot sweet & sour sauce	¼ envelope	–	45	–
(Durkee)				
dry mix only				
chicken				
cacciatore	⅒ pkg	–	10	–
Mexican salsa	⅒ pkg	–	10	–
mushroom	⅛ pkg	–	15	–
sweet & sour	⅑ pkg	–	20	–
enchilada	⅛ pkg	–	10	–
fish				
lemon pepper dill	⅙ pkg	0.5	20	23%
tomato basil	⅐ pkg	–	15	–
sloppy joe	⅙ pkg	–	20	–
spaghetti	⅕ pkg	–	15	–
American-style	⅙ pkg	–	15	–
family-style	⅒ pkg	–	20	–
w/mushrooms	⅛ pkg	–	15	–
white	¼ pkg	0.5	20	23%
zesty	⅕ pkg	–	20	–
prepared according to pkg directions				
à la king	1 cup	4.0	60	60%
cheese				
nacho	2 Tbs	2.0	25	72%
original	¼ cup	2.0	25	72%
hollandaise	2 Tbs	–	10	–
white	¼ cup	1.0	20	45%
(Knorr)				
as packaged				
Classic Sauce				
béarnaise	⅒ pkg	–	10	–
hollandaise	⅒ pkg	–	10	–
hot sauce	⅒ pkg	–	10	–
lemon dill	⅕ pkg	1.0	30	30%

Food and Description	Amount	Fat Grams	Total Calories	% Fat Calories
meat sauce	⅛ pkg	–	30	–
Mexican	⅛ pkg	–	25	–
mushroom	⅛ pkg	1.0	20	45%
Newburg	⅛ pkg	1.0	35	26%
peppercorn	⅛ pkg	1.0	25	36%
white	⅛ pkg	1.0	25	36%
Knorr sauce				
made from vegetables				
& spices	2 Tbs	–	25	–
Mexican cooking sauces				
adobo	½ cup	1.5	50	27%
chipotle	½ cup	0.5	60	8%
guajillo	½ cup	0.5	50	9%
mole	½ cup	5.0	130	35%
pasilla	½ cup	1.0	40	23%
pipan	½ cup	5.0	120	38%
seasoned tomato	½ cup	1.5	45	30%
pasta sauce				
Alfredo	⅓ pkg	3.0	60	45%
carbonara	⅙ pkg	3.0	70	39%
creamy cheddar	⅓ pkg	3.0	60	45%
4-cheese	⅙ pkg	3.0	60	45%
garlic herb	⅓ pkg	3.5	70	45%
parma rosa	½ oz	2.5	60	38%
pesto				
creamy	⅙ pkg	1.0	25	36%
original	⅓ pkg	–	15	–
red bell pepper	¼ pkg	0.5	25	18%
sun-dried tomato	¼ pkg	0.5	35	13%
tomato basil	⅓ pkg	1.0	70	13%
(Lawry's)..mix only				
chicken sauté/garlic Italian				
w/roasted garlic & basil	2 Tbs	2.0	30	60%
pasta sauce				
Alfredo	1 pkg	13.0	225	52%
pesto	2 tsp	2.0	20	90%
rich & thick	1 pkg	2.0	145	12%
w/mushrooms	1 pkg	1.5	145	9%
Stroganoff	1 pkg	<1.0	125	2%
Weekday Gourmet Sauce				
chicken				
Dijon	⅓ pkg	3.0	80	34%
fajitas	⅛ pkg	0.5	20	23%
teriyaki	¼ pkg	–	40	–
peppercorn steak				
w/green peppercorns	⅛ pkg	3.0	40	68%
teriyaki steak	1 Tbs	1.0	25	36%
(McCormick)				
Chicken Sauce Blends				
dry mix only				
Dijon	¼ pkg	1.5	40	34%

Food and Description	Amount	Fat Grams	Total Calories	% Fat Calories
Italian	⅙ pkg	–	20	–
lemon herb	¼ pkt	–	30	–
mesquite	⅙ pkg	–	20	–
piccata	1⅓ Tbs	–	25	–
stir-fry	⅙ pkg	–	20	–
teriyaki	¼ pkg	1.0	40	23%
McCormick Collection				
dry mix only				
béarnaise	⅒ pkt	1.0	10	9%
country Dijon	¼ cup	2.0	45	40%
hollandaise	⅒ pkt	–	15	–
hunter	¼ pkt	–	25	–
lemon & dill	¼ cup	2.5	45	50%
pepper medley	¼ cup	1.5	30	45%
pesto	¼ pkt	–	10	–
white				
sauces..dry mix only				
beef Stroganoff	⅙ pkg	–	15	–
enchilada	⅙ pkt	–	15	—
hollandaise	⅒ pkg	–	15	–
spaghetti				
thick & zesty	⅙ pkt	–	25	–
w/mushroom	⅕ pkg	–	25	–
seafood sauce				
for shrimp				
scampi	⅛ pkt	25.0	240	94%
lemon butter dill	⅙ pkt	10.0	120	75%
(Old Bay) mix only				
crab classic	1 Tbs	1.0	30	30%
Dash o' Lemon	¼ tsp	–	–	–
Salmon Classic	5 tsp	1.5	40	34%
Seas'n Easy				
garlic & herb	1 Tbs	–	25	–
lemon dill	1 Tbs	–	30	–
seafood marinara	1 Tbs	–	25	–
tuna classic	1 Tbs	1.0	30	30%
■ READY-TO-USE				
(A.1.) steak sauce				
bold & spicy	1 Tbs	–	20	–
Chicago steak house	1 Tbs	–	20	—
original	1 Tbs	–	15	–
steak sauce				
regular	1 Tbs	–	15	–
w/Tabasco	2 Tbs	–	10	–
thick & hearty	1 Tbs	–	25	–
(A Taste of Thai)				
chili sauce				
green	1 tsp	–	10	–
red	1 tsp	–	10	–
garlic chili pepper	1 tsp	–	–	–
mole fiesta	1 Tbs	1.5	35	39%

Food and Description	Amount	Fat Grams	Total Calories	% Fat Calories
peanut (satay)	2 Tbs	3.0	50	54%
seasoning fish	1 Tbs	–	15	–
tomatillo chile	1 tsp	–	2	–
(Angostura)				
salsa-flavored steak sauce				
low-sodium	1 Tbs	–	8	–
soy sauce				
light	1 Tbs	–	10	–
steak sauce	1 Tbs	–	12	–
teriyaki sauce				
light	1 Tbs	–	10	–
Worcestershire sauce				
low-sodium	1 tsp	–	5	–
(Atkins)				
Quick Quisine				
regular sauce				
& marinade	1 Tbs	–	5	–
teriyaki sauce				
& marinade	1 Tbs	1.0	10	9%
(Aunt Nellie's)				
Old-Style Sauce	1 Tbs	6.0	70	77%
(Barilla)..pasta sauce				
green & black olive	½ cup	3.5	80	39%
lasagna	½ cup	3.0	210	13%
marinara	½ cup	3.5	80	39%
mushroom & garlic	½ cup	3.5	80	39%
roasted garlic & onion	½ cup	3.5	80	39%
spicy pepper	½ cup	3.5	80	39%
sweet peppers & garlic	½ cup	3.5	80	39%
tomato & basil	½ cup	3.5	80	39%
(Bella Vita)..pasta sauce				
low-carb				
meat flavor	½ cup	5.0	70	64%
roasted garlic	½ cup	5.0	70	64%
spicy tomato	½ cup	5.0	70	64%
tomato basil	½ cup	5.0	70	64%
(Bennett's)				
cocktail sauce	¼ cup	2.0	80	23%
horseradish sauce	1 Tbs	5.0	50	90%
hot seafood sauce	2 Tbs	–	50	–
(Bertolli Lucca)..pasta sauce				
pasta sauces				
creamy				
Alfredo	¼ cup	10.0	110	82%
garlic Alfredo	¼ cup	10.0	100	90%
mushroom				
w/white wine	¼ cup	7.0	80	90%
5-cheese..w/Asiago				
& fontina cheeses	½ cup	3.0	90	30%
marinara..w/Burgundy				

Food and Description	Amount	Fat Grams	Total Calories	% Fat Calories
wine	½ cup	3.0	80	34%
Mediterranean olive				
w/sun-dried tomatoes	½ cup	4.0	100	36%
olive oil & garlic				
w/fresh tomatoes	½ cup	4.0	90	40%
mushroom				
& roasted garlic	½ cup	3.0	80	34%
w/white wine	½ cup	7.0	80	79%
roasted red pepper				
w/Italian herbs	½ cup	3.0	80	34%
summer vegetable				
w/bell pepper & onion	½ cup	3.0	80	34%
tomato & basil				
w/fresh tomatoes	½ cup	2.5	80	28%
traditional basil..w/extra-				
virgin olive oil	½ cup	7.0	270	23%
Vidalia onion				
w/roasted garlic	¼ cup	2.5	80	28%
vodka	½ cup	10.0	140	64%
w/Italian sausage, garlic				
& Romano	½ cup	4.0	90	40%
(Best Foods)				
Dippin' Sauce				
Honey Mustard Madness				
Squeeze	1 Tbs	3.0	40	68%
Rockin' Ranch..squeeze	1 Tbs	6.0	60	90%
Totally BBQ..squeeze	1 Tbs	1.0	30	30%
tartar sauce				
low-fat	2 Tbs	1.0	40	23%
original	2 Tbs	7.0	80	79%
(Boar's Head)				
cooking sauce				
brown sugar & spice				
ham glaze	2 Tbs	–	120	–
Horseradish sauce				
pub-style	1 tsp	1.5	15	90%
sweet Vidalia onions				
& sauce	1 Tbs	–	10	–
(Buitoni)..pasta sauce..refrigerated				
Alfredo				
light	¼ cup	5.0	80	56%
regular	¼ cup	16.0	180	80%
marinara	½ cup	4.0	80	45%
roasted garlic	½ cup	2.0	60	30%
pesto..w/basil				
reduced-fat	¼ cup	18.0	230	70%
regular	¼ cup	24.0	290	74%
(Chef Paul)				
Magic Sauce & Marinades				
pepper sauce	1 tsp	–	–	–

Food and Description	Amount	Fat Grams	Total Calories	% Fat Calories
sauce & marinades				
California sun-dried				
tomato	1 Tbs	–	17	–
Louisiana red pepper	1 Tbs	–	16	–
Southwest chipotle	1 Tbs	–	16	–
(China Bowl)				
chili paste				
w/garlic	2 Tbs	–	15	–
hoisin	1 tsp	–	10	–
oyster	½ tsp	–	5	–
(Classico)..pasta sauce				
Alfredo				
regular	¼ cup	11.0	100	99%
roasted garlic	¼ cup	9.0	100	81%
sun-dried tomato	¼ cup	10.0	120	75%
cabernet marinara				
w/herbs	½ cup	2.0	60	30%
fire-roasted tomato				
& garlic	½ cup	0.5	50	9%
Florentine spinach				
& cheese	½ cup	5.0	80	56%
4-cheese	½ cup	5.0	90	50%
garden vegetable				
primavera	½ cup	1.0	60	15%
Italian sausage				
w/peppers & onions	½ cup	2.0	90	20%
mushrooms & ripe olives	½ cup	1.0	60	15%
roasted chicken..w/Parmesan				
& garlic	½ cup	2.0	90	20%
spicy red pepper				
& pesto	½ cup	4.0	90	40%
sweet basil marinara	½ cup	1.0	70	13%
tomato & basil	½ cup	1.0	60	15%
triple mushroom	½ cup	2.0	80	23%
(Comida Sabrosa)				
hot sauce				
salsa roja habañera				
extremely hot	1 tsp	–	–	–
salsa verde habañera				
extremely hot	1 tsp	–	–	–
w/lime	1 tsp	–	–	—
(Contadina)				
pizza sauce				
flavored w/pepperoni	¼ cup	1.0	35	26%
4-cheese	¼ cup	0.5	30	15%
original	¼ cup	–	30	–
squeeze bottle	¼ cup	–	30	–
sweet & sour sauce				
w/pineapple..can	1 Tbs	1.0	40	23%
(Crosse & Blackwell) sauce				
brandied hard	2 Tbs	8.0	180	40%

Food and Description	Amount	Fat Grams	Total Calories	% Fat Calories
mint	1 Tbs	–	5	–
seafood cocktail	¼ cup	–	110	–
shrimp..zesty	¼ cup	–	110	–
steak	1 Tbs	–	30	–
Worcestershire	1 Tbs	–	5	–
(Crystal)				
cayenne sauce				
garlic	1 tsp	–	–	–
original	1 tsp	–	–	–
chicken wing sauce				
hot	1 oz	–	25	–
habañero sauce	1 tsp	–	–	–
hot sauce				
extra-hot	1 tsp	–	–	–
for wings	1 tsp	–	–	–
Louisiana's pure	1 tsp	–	–	–
soy sauce				
original	1 Tbs	–	20	–
steak sauce				
bold	1 tsp	–	5	–
original	1 Tbs	–	15	–
sweet & sour sauce	2 Tbs	–	60	–
wing sauce				
BBQ	2 Tbs	–	45	–
extra-hot	2 Tbs	–	25	–
hot barbecue	2 Tbs	–	45	–
original	2 Tbs	–	25	–
Worcestershire sauce	1 tsp	–	5	–
(Del Monte)				
chili sauce	1 Tbs	–	20	–
seafood cocktail sauce	¼ cup	–	100	–
sloppy joe sauce				
hickory flavor	¼ cup	–	60	–
original recipe	¼ cup	–	60	–
spaghetti sauce				
4-cheese	½ cup	1.5	70	19%
garlic & herb/chunky	½ cup	1.5	60	27%
Italian herb/chunky	½ cup	1.0	60	15%
w/garlic & onion	½ cup	1.0	80	11%
w/green peppers & mushrooms	½ cup	1.0	80	11%
w/meat	½ cup	1.0	60	15%
w/mushrooms	½ cup	0.5	60	8%
tomato & basil	½ cup	1.0	70	13%
traditional	½ cup	0.5	60	8%
(Di Giorno)..pasta sauce..refrigerated				
Alfredo				
light	¼ cup	9.0	140	51%
regular	¼ cup	18.0	180	90%
basil pesto	¼ cup	31.0	320	87%
4-cheese	¼ cup	15.0	160	84%

Food and Description	Amount	Fat Grams	Total Calories	% Fat Calories
garlic pesto	¼ cup	33.0	340	87%
marinara	½ cup	–	70	–
plum tomato & mushroom	½ cup	–	60	–
plum tomato cream sauce	½ cup	13.0	160	73%
roasted red bell pepper cream	¼ cup	10.0	140	64%
traditional meat	½ cup	6.0	120	45%
(Eden)				
pasta sauce	½ cup	2.5	80	28%
soy sauce..shoyu				
imported				
organic	1 Tbs	–	15	–
traditional	1 Tbs	–	15	–
reduced-sodium	1 Tbs	–	10	–
tamari				
domestic	1 Tbs	–	15	–
imported	1 Tbs	–	10	–
(Emeril's)				
marinade				
& grilling sauce				
ginger teriyaki	1 tsp	0.5	25	18%
pasta sauces				
kicked-up tomato	½ cup	3.0	70	39%
puttanesca	½ cup	5.0	80	56%
roasted garlic	½ cup	3.0	70	39%
vodka	½ cup	8.0	130	55%
(Enrico's)				
Alfredo sauce				
original	¼ cup	2.5	80	28%
w/olives	¼ cup	2.5	80	28%
pasta sauces				
all-natural sauces				
garlic marinara	½ cup	2.0	65	28%
garlic & sun-dried tomato	½ cup	2.0	60	30%
Italian-style				
no salt added	½ cup	1.5	60	23%
traditional	½ cup	1.5	60	23%
mushrooms	½ cup	<1.0	55	8%
peppers & mushrooms	½ cup	1.5	70	19%
Sicilian	½ cup	2.5	80	28%
tomato basil	½ cup	2.0	65	28%
traditional				
fat-free				
no salt	½ cup	–	45	–
no salt added	½ cup	1.5	60	23%
original	½ cup	1.5	60	23%
regular	½ cup	–	45	–
vodka	½ cup	7.0	120	53%
Modei cuisine sauces				
garlic marinara	½ cup	4.0	75	48%
herbed marinara	½ cup	4.0	75	48%

Food and Description	Amount	Fat Grams	Total Calories	% Fat Calories
organic marinara	½ cup	4.0	75	48%
tomato walnut	½ cup	5.0	80	56%
organic sauces				
bountiful basil	½ cup	–	50	–
garlic lover's	½ cup	–	50	–
mushroom madness	½ cup	–	60	–
traditional	½ cup	–	45	–
original sauces				
marinara-style	½ cup	1.0	60	15%
meat flavor	½ cup	1.0	60	15%
mushrooms	½ cup	1.0	60	15%
sausage flavor	½ cup	1.0	60	15%
traditional	½ cup	1.0	60	15%
pizza sauces				
regular	¼ cup	–	30	–
roasted garlic	¼ cup	1.0	40	23%
(Five Brothers) pasta sauce				
Alfredo				
creamy	¼ cup	9.0	100	90%
tomato	¼ cup	4.0	70	51%
w/mushrooms	¼ cup	7.0	80	79%
4-cheese/quattro fromaggio	¼ cup	9.0	90	90%
5-cheese	½ cup	3.0	90	90%
grilled				
eggplant	½ cup	3.0	100	27%
summer vegetable	½ cup	5.0	80	56%
marinara w/Burgundy wine	½ cup	3.0	80	34%
Mediterranean tomato & olive	½ cup	4.0	80	45%
mushroom & garlic	½ cup	3.0	90	30%
oven-roasted garlic & onion	½ cup	1.5	70	19%
pesto, creamy	¼ cup	9.0	100	90%
spicy pepper trio	½ cup	3.0	80	34%
(Girard's) Seafood Shop				
cocktail	2 Tbs	1.0	90	10%
tartar sauce	2 Tbs	15.0	140	96%
(Golden Dipt)				
cocktail sauce				
extra-hot	¼ cup	–	100	–
seafood	¼ cup	–	100	–
serving jar	¼ cup	–	100	–
seafood sauce				
for shrimp..scampi	1 Tbs	25.0	240	94%
lemon butter				
dill	2 Tbs	10.0	120	75%
fat-free	2 Tbs	–	35	–
tartar sauce				
fat-free	2 Tbs	–	35	–
regular	2 Tbs	15.0	160	84%
(Gordon's)				
cocktail..Chesapeake	¼ cup	0.5	50	9%

Food and Description	Amount	Fat Grams	Total Calories	% Fat Calories
pasta sauce				
red				
w/crabmeat	¼ cup	0.5	25	18%
white				
w/crabmeat	¼ cup	1.0	25	36%
(Great Impressions)				
horseradish	2 Tbs	14.0	140	90%
seafood				
Creole	1 Tbs	–	20	–
dipping	1 Tbs	–	17	–
Polynesian	1 Tbs	<1.0	40	11%
(Healthy Choice) pasta sauce				
flavored w/meat	½ cup	1.0	50	18%
garlic & herbs	½ cup	–	60	–
mushroom & sweet				
peppers..super-chunky	½ cup	–	45	–
super-chunky vegetables	½ cup	–	50	–
super-tomato..mushroom				
& garlic	½ cup	–	45	–
traditional	½ cup	–	60	–
(Heinz)				
chili sauce	1 Tbs	–	15	–
Heinz 57 steak sauce				
hickory smoke	1 Tbs	–	10	–
regular	1 Tbs	–	10	–
horseradish	1 Tbs	7.0	75	84%
seafood	¼ cup	–	60	–
Worcestershire	1 tsp	–	–	–
(Hellmann's)				
Dippin' Sauce				
Honey Mustard Madness				
Squeeze	1 Tbs	3.0	40	68%
Rockin' Ranch..squeeze	1 Tbs	6.0	60	90%
Totally BBQ..squeeze	1 Tbs	1.0	30	30%
tartar sauce				
low-fat	2 Tbs	1.0	40	23%
original	2 Tbs	7.0	80	79%
(Hoffman House)				
chili sauce	1 Tbs	–	10	–
shrimp & seafood	1 Tbs	4.5	110	35%
tartar	2 Tbs	7.0	90	70%
(Hormel)..Not-So-Sloppy Joe	¼ cup	–	60	–
(House of Tsang) (See ASIAN FOOD)				
(Hunt's)				
Family Favorites sauce mixes				
chili sauce	2 oz	–	25	–
lasagna	2 oz	–	30	–
meat loaf	2 oz	–	30	–
pizza sauce	2 oz	–	25	–
Manwich				
BBQ	¼ cup	–	50	–

Food and Description	Amount	Fat Grams	Total Calories	% Fat Calories
bold	¼ cup	5.0	60	90%
original	¼ cup	–	30	–
spaghetti sauce				
cheese & garlic	½ cup	1.0	50	18%
chunky vegetable	½ cup	1.0	50	18%
4-cheese	½ cup			
garlic & herb	½ cup			
Italian sausage	½ cup	1.5	60	23%
light	½ cup	–	45	–
meat	½ cup	1.0	60	15%
mushroom	½ cup	1.0	50	18%
no salt added	½ cup	1.0	45	20%
roasted garlic & onion	½ cup	1.0	50	18%
traditional				
steak sauce	1 Tbs	–	10	–
(Jack Daniel's)				
grilling sauces				
honey	2 Tbs	–	50	–
original	2 Tbs	–	50	–
spicy	2 Tbs	–	50	–
Tennessee hickory	2 Tbs	–	50	–
(Jake's) World-Famous				
cocktail	¼ cup	0.5	45	10%
tartar sauce	2 Tbs	15.0	140	96%
(Kaukauna)..cheese sauce				
Micro Melts..squeeze				
Real Cheddar	1 oz	7.0	90	70%
Real Cheddar Jalapeño	1 oz	7.0	90	70%
Squeeze..nacho cheese	1 oz	6.0	80	68%
(Kikkoman)				
all-purpose seasoning sauce	1 Tbs	–	10	–
dipping sauce				
plum sauce	1 oz	0.5	80	6%
restaurant series				
sweet & sour	1 Tbs	–	35	–
soy sauce				
lite	1 Tbs	–	10	–
milder	1 Tbs	–	10	–
regular	1 Tbs	–	10	–
sushi & sashimi	1 Tbs	–	15	–
soy sauce & dressing				
ponzu citrus	1 Tbs	–	10	–
steak sauce	1 Tbs	–	20	–
stir-fry & marinade				
black bean sauce				
w/garlic	2 Tbs	1.0	50	18%
hoisin	2 Tbs	1.5	80	16%
Thai-style chili	2 Tbs	1.0	70	13%
	1 Tbs	–	20	–
sweet & sour	1 Tbs	–	20	–

Food and Description	Amount	Fat Grams	Total Calories	% Fat Calories
teriyaki baste & glaze				
regular	2 Tbs	–	50	–
w/honey & pineapple	2 Tbs	–	80	–
Tonkatsu sauce	1 Tbs	–	20	–
(Kiss the Cook)..pasta sauce				
bolognese	½ cup	6.0	130	42%
mushroom & wine	½ cup	3.5	90	35%
puttanesca	½ cup	4.5	100	41%
(Kitchen Bouquet)..seasoning sauce	1 tsp	–	15	–
(Knorr)..grilling & broiling sauce				
spicy plum	⅛ bottle	–	60	–
(Kraft)				
Kraft				
sandwich spread & burger sauce				
reduced-fat	1 Tbs	2.5	35	64%
regular	1 Tbs	4.0	50	72%
Sauceworks				
cocktail				
hot & spicy	¼ cup	0.5	60	9%
regular	¼ cup	0.5	60	9%
horseradish	1 tsp	1.5	20	68%
sweet 'n' sour	2 Tbs	–	60	–
tartar sauce				
fat-free	2 Tbs	–	25	–
hot & spicy	2 Tbs	6.0	70	77%
lemon & herb	2 Tbs	16.0	150	96%
natural lemon & herb flavor	2 Tbs	16.0	150	96%
original	2 Tbs	6.0	70	77%
(La Choy)				
bead molasses	1 Tbs	–	50	–
brown gravy	¼ cup	–	275	–
plum	1 Tbs	–	25	–
soy sauce/light	1 Tbs	–	15	–
stir-fry				
mandarin soy sauce	½ cup	–	70	–
sweet & sour	½ cup	–	140	–
Szechuan	½ cup	–	80	–
teriyaki	½ cup	–	95	–
sweet & sour..all types	2 Tbs	–	60	–
teriyaki				
light	1 Tbs	–	18	–
original	1 Tbs	–	16	–
(Lea & Perrins)				
steak				
garlic peppercorn	1 Tbs	–	25	–
private label	1 Tbs	–	15	–
sweet & spicy	1 Tbs	–	25	–
Worcestershire				
for chicken	1 tsp	–	5	–
hot pepper				
sweet 'n' spicy kick	1 Tbs	–	25	–

Food and Description	Amount	Fat Grams	Total Calories	% Fat Calories
original	1 tsp	–	5	–
pure blend	1 Tbs	–	17	–
thick & tangy	1 Tbs	–	18	–
white wine	1 tsp	–	–	–
(Litehouse)				
dressing & sauce				
sesame ginger				
fat-free	1 Tbs	–	18	–
Thai peanut	1 Tbs	4.4	48	83%
(Luna Rossa's)..Pasta sauce				
fire-roasted garlic	½ cup	5.0	80	56%
Chianti mushroom	½ cup	4.5	70	58%
Italian garden				
Vegetable	½ cup	3.5	120	26%
Romano pomodoro	½ cup	5.0	90	50%
(Luzianne)				
TryMe				
Bullfighter				
steak & burger sauce	1 Tbs	–	15	–
Cajun Sunshine				
hot pepper sauce	1 tsp	–	–	–
Caribbean Clipper				
oyster & shrimp sauce	1 tsp	–	10	–
Dragon Sauce	1 tsp	–	5	–
liquid smoke	1 tsp	–	–	–
Tennessee Sunshine				
hot pepper sauce	1 tsp	–	–	–
Tiger Sauce	1 tsp	–	10	–
wine & pepper				
Worcestershire sauce	1 tsp	–	–	–
Yucatan Sunshine				
habañero pepper sauce	1 tsp	–	–	–
Woody's				
cookin' sauce	2 Tbs	4.0	50	72%
Sweet'n BBQ Sour Sauce	2 Tbs	–	70	–
(Maple Grove Farms) marinade & grilling sauces				
marinade & basting sauces..sugar-free				
Dijon..low-carb	1 Tbs	5.0	50	90%
hickory..low-carb	1 Tbs	–	20	–
lemon rosemary..low-carb	1 Tbs	–	40	–
sweet & sour..low-carb	1 Tbs	–	40	–
teriyaki..low-carb	1 Tbs	–	–	–
(Maull's) steak..all types	1 Tbs	–	20	–
(McCormick)				
grilling sauces				
hickory BBQ	2 Tbs	0.5	80	6%
honey mustard	2 Tbs	0.5	70	6%
mesquite	2 Tbs	0.5	60	8%
roasted garlic & herb	2 Tbs	–	35	–
teriyaki	2 Tbs	1.0	60	15%

Food and Description	Amount	Fat Grams	Total Calories	% Fat Calories
(Monterey Pasta Co.)				
pasta sauces				
Carb-Smart sauce				
4-cheese	½ cup	15.0	190	71%
pesto sauce..w/basil				
pine nuts & cheese	1 Tbs	28.0	280	90%
regular sauces				
Alfredo..w/Asiago				
& Parmesan cheese	½ cup			
roasted vegetable chunky				
w/Italian seasonings	½ cup	3.5	50	63%
(Muir Glen)				
organic..low-fat pasta sauce				
balsamic roasted onion	½ cup	0.5	50	9%
cabernet marinara	½ cup	0.5	50	9%
chunky tomato–style	½ cup	0.5	50	9%
garden vegetable	½ cup	1.0	50	18%
garlic & onion	½ cup	0.5	55	8%
garlic roasted garlic	½ cup	0.5	55	8%
green olive	½ cup	1.5	60	23%
Italian herb	½ cup	0.5	55	8%
mushroom marinara	½ cup	–	45	–
portabello mushroom	½ cup	–	50	–
roasted red pepper	½ cup	1.5	60	23%
sun-dried tomato	½ cup	1.0	55	16%
tomato basil	½ cup	1.0	50	18%
(Naturally Fresh)				
cocktail sauce				
seafood				
jar	2 Tbs	–	25	–
square tub	2 Tbs	–	25	–
seafood II..4 oz	2 Tbs	0.5	30	15%
hot sauce II	1 tsp	2.0	30	60%
seafood dipping sauce	2 Tbs	15.0	140	96%
sweet & sour sauce	2 Tbs	2.0	70	26%
tartar sauce				
jar	2 Tbs	14.0	130	97%
square tub	2 Tbs	14.0	130	97%
tartar sauce II				
4 oz	2 Tbs	15.0	140	96%
(Nestlé) (*See* (Contadina) in this section)				
(Newman's Own)..pasta sauce				
Bombolina tomato				
& fresh basil	½ cup	4.0	100	45%
5-cheese	½ cup	3.0	90	30%
Fra Diavolo				
hot & spicy	½ cup	3.0	70	39%
marinara	¼ cup	2.0	60	30%
mushroom marinara	½ cup	2.0	60	30%

Food and Description	Amount	Fat Grams	Total Calories	% Fat Calories
roasted garlic & peppers	½ cup	2.5	70	32%
Sockarooni	½ cup	2.0	60	30%
tomato & roasted garlic	½ cup	2.5	70	32%
vodka sauce	½ cup	5.0	110	41%
(Old Bay)				
cocktail	¼ cup	0.5	110	4%
tartar sauce	2 Tbs	12.0	130	83%
(Patak's)..Original				
Cooking sauces				
rich creamy coconut				
mild	½ can	17.0	210	73%
tangy lemon & cilantro	¼ jar	9.0	120	68%
marinade & grill sauce				
spicy ginger & garlic				
mild	⅒ jar	1.0	35	26%
(Prego) pasta sauce				
Pasta Bakes				
hearty meat	⅛ jar	6.0	60	90%
Italian sausage	⅛ jar	4.5	100	41%
tomato, garlic & basil	⅛ jar	3.5	80	39%
pasta sauce				
beef & mushroom..Hearty				
Meat..meat sauce	½ cup	6.0	130	42%
diced onion & garlic	½ cup	4.5	120	34%
flavored w/meat	½ cup	5.0	140	32%
fresh mushroom				
jar	½ cup	3.5	120	26%
plastic container	½ cup	4.5	140	29%
garden combination	½ cup	2.0	90	30%
Garlic Supreme	½ cup	4.5	120	11%
Itallan sausage				
& garlic	½ cup	5.0	120	38%
Italian sausage.. Hearty				
Meat..meat sauce	½ cup	7.0	150	42%
marinara	½ cup	5.0	90	50%
meatball Parmesan				
Hearty Meat..meat sauce	½ cup	8.0	160	45%
mini meatball	½ cup	6.0	150	36%
mushroom & garlic	½ cup	2.0	110	16%
mushroom & green pepper				
chunky garden	½ cup	3.5	100	32%
mushroom Parmesan	½ cup	3.5	130	24%
Mushroom Supreme	½ cup	4.5	130	31%
Mushroom Supreme				
chunky garden	½ cup	5.0	130	35%
ricotta Parmesan	½ cup	3.5	120	26%
roasted garlic				
& herb	½ cup	4.0	110	33%
Parmesan	½ cup	2.0	110	16%

Food and Description	Amount	Fat Grams	Total Calories	% Fat Calories
roasted red pepper & garlic				
chunky garden	½ cup	4.0	120	30%
3-cheese	½ cup	2.0	90	20%
tomato..basil..garlic	½ cup	2.0	90	20%
tomato..onion & garlic				
chunky garden-style	½ cup	3.5	110	29%
Tomato Supreme	½ cup	4.0	130	28%
traditional				
jar	½ cup	3.0	110	25%
plastic container	½ cup	4.5	120	34%
Zesty Mushroom	½ cup	3.5	110	29%
(Premier Japan)..wheat-free				
ginger tamari	1 Tbs	–	5	–
hoisin sauce	1 Tbs	–	15	–
sesame garlic	1 Tbs	0.5	10	45%
teriyaki sauce	1 Tbs	–	15	–
wasabi tamari	1 Tbs	–	5	–
(Pritikin) pasta sauce..all types	½ cup	–	30	–
(Progresso)..pasta sauce				
Alfredo/authentic	½ cup	15.0	200	68%
creamy clam	½ cup	6.0	110	49%
lobster	½ cup	7.0	100	63%
red clam	½ cup	1.0	60	15%
white clam	½ cup	10.0	140	64%
(Ragu)..pasta sauce				
Alfredo				
classic	¼ cup	10.0	110	82%
light	¼ cup	6.0	80	68%
Carb Options Pasta				
Alfredo	¼ cup	10.0	120	75%
double cheddar	½ cup	8.0	90	80%
garden-style	½ cup	4.5	80	51%
Cheese Creations				
double cheddar	¼ cup	10.0	110	82%
4-cheese	¼ cup	11.0	120	83%
roasted garlic Parmesan	¼ cup	11.0	120	83%
spicy cheddar				
& tomato	¼ cup	2.0	150	12%
light				
tomato & basil				
no sugar added	½ cup	1.5	60	23%
regular	½ cup	–	50	–
Old World-style				
spaghetti sauce				
beef	½ cup	4.0	80	45%
marinara	½ cup	5.0	80	56%
mushroom	½ cup	–	70	–
traditional	½ cup	3.0	70	34%
pasta sauce..chunky garden-style				
garden combination				
sweet bell pepper	½ cup	3.5	110	29%

Food and Description	Amount	Fat Grams	Total Calories	% Fat Calories
mushroom				
super	½ cup	3.0	80	34%
super chunky	½ cup	3.0	80	34%
mushroom & green pepper	½ cup	3.5	110	29%
mushroom & onion	½ cup	3.5	120	26%
roasted red pepper				
& onion	½ cup	3.5	120	26%
super garlic	½ cup	2.0	90	30%
tomato				
garlic & onion	½ cup	3.5	120	26%
spinach & cheese	½ cup	3.5	120	26%
vegetable primavera	½ cup	3.5	110	29%
Rich & Meaty				
beef..onion & garlic	½ cup	5.0	100	45%
classic Italian	½ cup	8.0	130	55%
Mama's meat sauce	½ cup	5.0	110	41%
sausage..peppers				
& onion	½ cup	11.0	160	62%
Robustol				
beef w/mushroom	½ cup	3.0	70	39%
chopped tomato..olive				
oil & garlic	½ cup	5.0	100	45%
classic Italian meat	½ cup	4.0	90	30%
flavored				
w/sautéed beef	½ cup	4.0	120	30%
Parmesan & Romano	½ cup	3.5	120	26%
red wine & herbs	½ cup	3.0	100	27%
roasted garlic	½ cup	3.0	120	23%
sautéed beef..onion				
& garlic	½ cup	4.0	120	30%
sautéed onion				
& garlic	½ cup	4.0	90	40%
sautéed onion				
& mushroom	½ cup	3.5	110	29%
7-herb tomato	½ cup	3.0	110	25%
6-cheese	½ cup	3.0	80	34%
spicy red pepper	½ cup	4.0	90	40%
sweet Italian sausage				
& cheese	½ cup	4.5	90	45%
sauce..Pizza Quick				
cheesy mushroom	¼ cup	1.5	40	34%
garlic & basil	¼ cup	2.0	40	45%
pepperoni snack	¼ cup	2.0	50	36%
traditional	¼ cup	2.0	45	40%
(S&W)				
cocktail sauce..seafood	1 Tbs	–	20	–
cooking sauce & marinade				
mesquite steakhouse	1 Tbs	–	10	–

Food and Description	Amount	Fat Grams	Total Calories	% Fat Calories
Oriental stir-fry	1 Tbs	–	25	–
Southwestern fajitas	1 Tbs	–	10	–
teriyaki				
lite	1 Tbs	–	25	–
restaurant recipe	1 Tbs	–	25	–
steakhouse chili	1 Tbs	–	15	–
(Sagawa's)..sauces				
Polynesian BBQ	1 Tbs	–	60	–
stir-fry	1 Tbs	–	25	–
sweet & sassy	1 Tbs	–	60	–
sweet & sour	1 Tbs	–	50	–
teriyaki	1 Tbs	–	30	–
Sauceworks (See (Kraft) in this section)				
(Snow's)				
Newburg w/sherry	⅓ cup	8.0	120	60%
Welsh rarebit cheese	½ cup	11.0	170	58%
(Tabasco)				
habañero	1 tsp	–	5	–
other sauces	1 tsp	–	–	–
(Texas Best)				
grilling sauces				
Cajun BBQ	2 Tbs	–	50	–
mesquite BBQ	2 Tbs	–	50	–
original rib sauce	2 Tbs	–	50	–
hot sauce	1 tsp	–	–	–
steak sauce	1 Tbs	–	15	–
(The Wizard's)..all types	1 tsp	–	–	–
Hot Stuff sauce	1 tsp	–	–	–
(Troy's)..Wheat-free				
Rainforest..organic				
ginger curry sauce	1 Tbs	1.0	15	60%
ginger sauce	1 Tbs	–	10	–
mango sauce	1 Tbs	–	15	–
papaya pepper sauce	1 tsp	–	–	–
peanut sauce	1 Tbs	1.5	25	54%
(Tuttorosso)..pasta sauce				
marinara	½ cup	3.5	100	32%
mushroom	½ cup	3.0	100	27%
3-cheese	½ cup	2.0	90	20%
tomato basil	½ cup	2.0	80	23%
tomato garlic & onion				
w/extra-virgin olive oil	½ cup	2.0	90	20%
traditional	½ cup	3.0	100	27%
w/meat	½ cup	2.5	90	25%
(Walden Farms)				
cocktail sauce	1 Tbs	–	–	–
pasta sauces..all flavors	⅓ cup	–	–	–
(Walnut Acres)				
organic sauces				
garlic-garlic	½ cup	1.0	50	18%

Food and Description	Amount	Fat Grams	Total Calories	% Fat Calories
marinara				
& herbs	½ cup	1.0	50	18%
& zinfandel	½ cup	1.0	50	18%
roasted garlic	½ cup	1.0	60	15%
sweet pepper				
& onion	½ cup	1.0	50	18%
tomato basil				
low-sodium	½ cup	–	40	–
regular	½ cup	1.0	50	18%
tomato & mushroom	½ cup	1.0	50	18%
zesty basil	½ cup	1.0	50	18%
(Walnut Farm)				
BBQ Sauce..all flavors	2 Tbs	–	–	–
marinara sauce..calorie-free	⅓ cup	–	–	–
SAUERKRAUT				
can..jar..bag				
(B&G)				
sauerkraut	1 oz	–	6	–
(Boar's Head)				
sauerkraut	2 Tbs	–	5	–
(Bush's Best)				
Bavarian kraut	1 oz	–	15	–
shredded	1 oz	–	5	–
(Cascadian Farm)..all types	1 oz	–	5	–
(Claussen)				
sauerkraut	1 oz	–	5	–
(Eden)	½ cup	–	25	–
(Farman's)..barrel-cured	1 oz	–	5	–
(Hebrew National)				
gallon kraut	½ cup	–	25	–
regular	2 Tbs	–	50	–
(Krrrrisp Kraut)				
barrel-cured	1 oz	–	5	–
Bavarian-style..barrel-cured	1 oz	–	10	–
(Libby's)				
Bavarian-style	2 Tbs	–	10	–
crispy	2 Tbs	–	5	–
(S&W)..red cabbage	2 Tbs	–	5	–
(Silver Floss)				
bag				
barrel-cured	1 oz	–	5	–
Bavarian-style barrel	1 oz	–	10	–
can				
barrel-cured	4 oz	–	20	–
Bavarian-style barrel	4 oz	–	40	–
(Stokely's)				
Bavarian..traditional				
w/mild caraway seeds	½ cup	–	35	–
traditional shredded				
& chopped	¼ cup	–	5	–

Food and Description	Amount	Fat Grams	Total Calories	% Fat Calories
(Vlasic)				
old-fashioned	1 oz	–	4	–
SAUERKRAUT JUICE/canned				
(Bush's Best)	1 cup	–	15	–
(S&W)	10 fl oz	–	35	–
SAUSAGE (See also FRANKFURTER; LUNCHEON MEAT; SAUSAGE DISH; SAUSAGE STICK)				
■ (Aidell's)				
sausage links..3.5 oz, unless noted otherwise				
beef				
chorizo..raw	1 link	37.0	400	83%
chicken				
& apple..fresh	1 link	7.0	100	63%
& apple..smoked	1 link	16.0	210	69%
cocktail..2 oz	6 links	8.0	100	72%
lemon..smoked	1 link	16.0	210	69%
teriyaki..raw	1 link	15.0	210	64%
& turkey..artichoke				
smoked	1 link	14.0	180	70%
& turkey..habañero				
3.2 oz	1 link	10.0	160	56%
& turkey..curry				
smoked Burmese	1 link	15.0	220	61%
& turkey..New Mexico				
smoked	1 link	16.0	210	69%
& turkey..pesto				
smoked	1 link	16.0	220	65%
& turkey..smoked				
& turkey/Thai				
fresh..raw	1 link	16.0	200	72%
smoked	1 link	16.0	220	65%
& turkey..w/sun-dried				
tomatoes & basil..raw	1 link	15.0	200	68%
fresh	1 link	15.0	200	68%
smoked	1 link	15.0	200	68%
duck				
& turkey..smoked	1 link	16.0	220	65%
lamb & beef				
w/rosemary..fresh	1 link	16.0	220	65%
pork				
& veal..smoked	1 link	19.0	240	71%
Italian..raw	1 link	18.0	230	70%
smoked..andouille				
Cajun	1 link	17.0	220	70%
whiskey fennel	1 link	17.0	220	70%
turkey..cranberry				
smoked	1 link	16.0	210	69%
w/scallions & herbs				
fresh	1 link	12.0	200	54%

Food and Description	Amount	Fat Grams	Total Calories	% Fat Calories
■ (Amour)				
Vienna sausage..canned				
BBQ	2 oz	13.0	150	78%
chicken	2 oz	9.0	110	74%
hot & spicy	2 oz	13.0	150	78%
jalapeño	2 oz	16.0	170	77%
lite..50% less fat	2 oz	7.0	90	70%
in sauce	2 oz	14.0	150	84%
smoked	2 oz	14.0	150	84%
■ (Ball Park)..bun-size				
smoked sausage	2 oz	17.0	180	85%
■ (Big Mama)				
pickled sausage				
1.4 oz..57-oz jar	1 sausage	10.0	110	82%
2.4 oz				
16-count jar	1 sausage	14.0	180	70%
■ (Bilinski's)				
sausage links				
3.5 oz, unless otherwise noted				
chicken				
andouille..Cajun-style				
2 oz	1 link	4.0	80	45%
apple & chardonnay	1 link	5.5	70	71%
cilantro	1 link	3.5	70	45%
Italian..w/peppers				
& onions..2 oz				
hot	1 link	4.0	70	51%
mild	1 link	3.5	70	45%
jalapeño	1 link	4.0	70	51%
pesto	1 link	5.0	90	50%
spinach	1 link	3.5	70	45%
sun-dried tomato	1 link	3.5	70	45%
■ (Bob Evans)				
Express sausage links				
light	2 links	5.0	80	56%
maple	2 links	10.0	120	75%
original	2 links	14.0	160	79%
roll sausage..chub				
Italian	2 oz	19.0	210	81%
original recipe	2 oz	19.0	210	81%
special seasonings	2 oz	21.0	230	82%
sausage..other				
chub..maple log cabin	2 oz	17.0	200	77%
links				
Italian-style				
5-count pkg	1 link	21.0	270	70%
maple..14-count pkg	3 links	14.0	170	74%
patties..original				
9-count pkg				
18-count pkg	2 patties	19.0	210	81%

Food and Description	Amount	Fat Grams	Total Calories	% Fat Calories
■ **(Boca)**				
vegetarian				
soy protein sausage				
bratwurst..60% less				
fat..4-count pkg	1 brat	7.0	140	45%
sausage				
ground	2 oz	0.5	60	8%
links				
Italian..65% less fat				
4-count pkg	1 link	6.0	130	42%
smoked..70% less fat				
4-count pkg	1 link	6.0	130	42%
■ **(Butterball)**				
turkey sausage				
Italian				
hot	1 link	10.0	170	53%
sweet	1 link	10.0	170	53%
lean..extra tender				
smoked..2-count	1 link	6.0	100	54%
lean..hot fresh				
Italian links..1-count	1 link	10.0	170	53%
lean..sweet fresh				
Italian links..1-count	1 link	10.0	170	53%
original	3 links	9.0	120	68%
Polish	1 link	10.0	170	53%
salami	1 oz	4.0	60	60%
■ **(Eckrich)**				
sausage				
country..chub	2.6 oz	22.0	230	86%
smoked..2-count pkg	2.6 oz	15.0	170	79%
smoked..beef				
2-count pkg	2 oz	16.0	180	80%
smoked..grillers				
8-count pkg	2 oz	16.0	180	80%
■ **(Fire Cracker)**				
pickled sausage..red hot				
The Original				
15-count pkg	1 link	7.0	100	63%
The Original Giant				
15-count pkg	1 link	10.0	140	64%
■ **(Galileo)**				
cappacola..hot	2 oz	11.0	140	71%
mortadella	2 oz	14.0	160	79%
pepperoni..pizza-size	9 slices	13.0	140	84%
salami				
cotto..jumbo	2 oz	14.0	170	74%
Genoa	2 oz	14.0	170	74%
hard	1 oz	11.0	120	49%
Italian dry				
light	5 slices	4.0	60	60%

Food and Description	Amount	Fat Grams	Total Calories	% Fat Calories
no burn..sliced	8 slices	11.0	120	83%
thin-sliced	5 slices	8.0	110	65%
whole..2x2	1 oz	10.0	120	75%
summer..smoked	2 oz	16.0	190	76%
■ (Healthy Choice)				
frozen				
breakfast sausage links				
8-count pkg	3 links	3.0	70	39%
low-fat..smoked				
links..2-count pkg	2 oz	2.5	80	28%
patties	3 patties	3.0	70	39%
refrigerated				
breakfast sausage				
links	3 links	3.0	70	39%
patties	3 patties	3.0	70	39%
Polska kielbasa	2 oz	6.0	80	68%
smoked sausage	2 oz	6.0	80	68%
beef	2 oz	6.0	80	68%
■ (Hebrew National)				
knockwurst				
4-count pkg	3 oz	24.0	260	83%
salami..beef				
lean				
chub	1 oz	2.5	45	50%
sliced	1 oz	2.5	45	50%
regular				
midget chub	2 oz	14.0	170	74%
sliced	1 oz	7.0	80	79%
■ (Hillshire Farm)				
sausage..natural-casing				
bratwurst				
cooked				
2.8 oz	1 link	23.0	260	80%
4 oz	1 link	28.0	330	76%
smoked..2.7 oz	1 link	23.0	250	83%
Cheddar Wurst..5.5"	2.8 oz	24.0	270	80%
country-style				
mettwurst 7" link	2 oz	17.0	190	81%
Italian..brown & serve	4 oz	33.0	360	83%
hot	4 oz	28.0	330	76%
Italian sausage				
mild..raw	2.7 oz	22.0	270	73%
sweet				
6-count pkg	1 link	20.0	250	72%
casing	3.25 oz	25.0	280	80%
knockwurst..2.7 oz	1 link	22.0	240	83%
Polish sausage				
2.7 oz	1 link	23.0	250	83%
4 oz	1 link	34.0	380	81%
sausage..skinless				

Food and Description	Amount	Fat Grams	Total Calories	% Fat Calories
Big Red smokey	3.25 oz	26.0	280	84%
bratwurst...brown & serve	3.25 oz	23.0	270	77%
Cheddar Wurst				
2 oz	1 link	17.0	190	81%
3.25 oz	1 link	27.0	300	81%
Endless beef sausage rope..smoked	2 oz	17.0	190	81%
Lickety Split..smoked	2.8 oz	23.0	250	83%
Lit'l Polskas	2 oz	16.0	180	80%
Lit'l Smokies				
beef	2 oz	15.0	170	79%
cocktail	6 links	18.0	200	81%
pepper smoked..6"	1 link	23.0	250	83%
pepperjack cheese smoked..6"	1 link	26.0	290	81%
Polish				
3.25 oz	1 link	26.0	280	84%
4 oz	1 link	32.0	350	82%
■ (Hormel)				
Breakfast..Little Sizzlers..cooked				
brown 'n' serve				
links				
hot & spicy flavored w/Tabasco	3 links	22.0	230	86%
maple-flavored	3 links	20.0	220	82%
original	3 links	20.0	210	86%
pepperoni				
chunk..6 oz pkg	1 oz	13.0	140	84%
mild	15 slices	13.0	140	84%
pillow pack				
regular	14 slices	13.0	140	84%
turkey	17 slices	4.0	80	45%
Rosa Grande	1 oz	13.0	140	84%
sliced..3.5 oz pkg	15 slices	13.0	140	84%
twin..5-oz pkg	1 oz	13.0	140	84%
sausage..smoked turkey..packed in vinegar	2 oz	11.0	140	71%
summer..cervelat	2 oz	9.0	120	68%
summer..Old Smokehouse	2 oz	18.0	200	81%
■ (Jenny-O Turkey Store)				
turkey sausage				
breakfast links				
maple	2 oz	11.0	140	71%
original	2 oz	11.0	140	71%
Breakfast Lover's skinless	2 oz	11.0	130	76%
breakfast patties	2 patties	12.0	150	72%
smoked..lean				

Food and Description	Amount	Fat Grams	Total Calories	% Fat Calories
95% fat-free	2 oz	3.0	70	39%
sweet..lean				
Italian..5-count pkg	1 link	10.0	160	56%
■ (Jimmy Dean)				
breakfast sausage..cooked				
formed patty				
.6 oz each	3 patties	14.0	160	79%
1.5 oz	1 patty	11.0	130	76%
2 oz	1 patty	22.0	230	86%
mild	2 oz	15.0	170	79%
Patty Master				
.8 oz each	3 patties	27.0	280	87%
1.5 oz	1 patty	13.0	300	39%
sage	1.5 oz	11.0	130	76%
turkey	1 patty	9.0	140	58%
stuffed & sliced..thick				
sausage patty				
1.6 oz	2 patties	15.0	240	56%
2.5 oz	2 patties	18.0	190	85%
breakfast sausage..cooked				
links				
maple	1.22 oz	5.0	100	41%
mild	2 oz	15.0	170	79%
skinless				
1.3 oz	2 links	13.0	160	73%
2 oz	2 links	27.0	270	90%
Trim Breakfast links				
	1.6 oz	18.0	180	90%
	1.8 oz	22.0	230	86%
turkey				
1.35 oz	2 links	7.0	110	57%
Breakfast Sausage–Flavored				
Pork Crumbles	2 oz	17.0	180	85%
■ (Johnsonville)				
(Note: All portions are cooked unless stated otherwise.)				
bratwurst..fresh varieties				
beef				
bratwurst patty..3.3 oz				
pan-fried	1 pattie	21.0	240	79%
grilling chorizo	1 link	32.0	370	78%
other brat links..all types	1 link	25.0	300	75%
breakfast sausage..pan-fried				
brown sugar & honey				
pan-fried	3 links	15.0	190	71%
hickory-smoked breakfast	3 links	17.0	200	77%
maple breakfast patties				
pan-fried				
9 oz	2 patties	17.0	210	73%
12 oz	2 patties	15.0	180	75%
original	3 links	16.0	190	76%

Food and Description	Amount	Fat Grams	Total Calories	% Fat Calories
link..pan-fried	3 links	16.0	190	76%
original breakfast patty				
9 oz	2 patties	17.0	210	73%
12 oz	2 patties	15.0	180	75%
Heat & Serve products				
bratwurst	1 link	23.0	260	80%
Italian sausage	1 link	23.0	260	80%
maple breakfast	3 links	20.0	230	78%
original breakfast	3 links	20.0	230	78%
hot links..all types	1 link	20.0	230	78%
Vermont maple syrup				
pan-fried				
link	3 links	16.0	190	76%
patty	2 patties	15.0	180	75%
Italian sausage				
hot	1 link	25.0	300	75%
Italian..ground..raw				
1 portion	2.5 oz	18.0	210	77%
Italian patty..raw	1 patty	29.0	340	77%
mild	1 link	25.0	300	75%
Italian..ground..raw				
1 portion	2.5 oz	18.0	210	77%
patty..pan-fried	3.3 oz	21.0	240	79%
perri..raw				
all links	1 link	20.0	230	78%
sweet Italian patty	1 patty	29.0	340	77%
simply Italian				
hot..raw	1 link	23.0	270	77%
mild..raw	1 link	23.0	270	77%
sweet rope..1 portion	2.5 oz	18.0	210	77%
sweet sausage..raw	1 link	23.0	170	77%
sausages..cooked				
bratwurst	1 link	22.0	240	83%
cooked Beer'N Bratwurst	1 link	22.0	240	83%
mild Italian	1 link	22.0	240	83%
stadium-style bratwurst	1 link	22.0	240	83%
semi-dry sausage..summer sausage				
beef	2 oz	15.0	180	75%
beef summer sticks	1 stick	11.0	120	83%
garlic	2 oz	15.0	180	75%
Old World	2 oz	16.0	190	76%
original	2 oz	15.0	180	75%
■ **(Jones Dairy Farm)**				
all natural				
brown & serve				
light	1 link	4.0	60	60%
maple	2 links	18.0	190	85%
golden brown	1 patty	14.0	150	84%
beef	1 link	6.0	75	72%
mild	2 links	18.0	190	85%

Food and Description	Amount	Fat Grams	Total Calories	% Fat Calories
pork/light	1 link	4.0	55	65%
spicy	2 links	18.0	190	85%
flavored sausages				
links..maple..skinless	2 links	8.0	90	80%
patty				
hot & zesty	2 patties	16.0	170	85%
maple	2 patties	16.0	170	85%
Golden Brown Pork sausages				
links..casing				
.8 oz	3 links	8.0	80	90%
1.6 oz	1 link	15.0	160	84%
links..skinless				
.74 oz	3 links	9.0	90	90%
.95 oz	2 links	12.0	120	90%
1.63 oz	2 links	20.0	210	86%
patties				
.72 oz	2 patties	8.0	80	90%
.95 oz	2 patties	11.0	120	83%
1.3 oz	1 patty	14.0	150	84%
1.43 oz	2 patties	16.0	170	85%
Italian				
link..skinless..2.15 oz	1 link	13.0	160	73%
patty..2.68 oz	1 patty	17.0	210	73%
light sausages				
sausage				
& rice link	1 link	7.0	90	70%
& rice patty	1 patty	7.0	100	63%
poultry sausages				
turkey				
link	2 links	1.5	30	45%
patty	1 patty	3.0	60	45%
Roller Grillers				
Italian links	1 link	18.0	210	77%
scrapple	1.5 oz	6.0	90	60%
■ (Kahn's)				
bratwurst	1 sausage	17.0	190	81%
kielbasa				
bun-size Polska	1 sausage	17.0	190	81%
salami				
beef..8-oz pkg	1 slice	6.0	70	77%
smoked sausage..Big Red				
Smokey's sausage	1 link	16.0	180	80%
■ (Libby's)				
Vienna sausages				
in chicken broth	3 links	8.0	100	72%
w/chicken & pork				
in BBQ sauce	3 links	12.0	140	77%
in chicken broth	3 links	14.0	150	84%
meat/regular or w/BBQ sauce	3 links	12.0	130	83%

Food and Description	Amount	Fat Grams	Total Calories	% Fat Calories
■ **(Louis Rich)..Turkey sausage**				
original	2 oz	8.0	120	60%
smoked	2.5 oz	5.0	90	50%
■ **(Old Wisconsin)**				
beef sausage				
snack bites				
8-oz pkg	1 oz	9.0	110	74%
11-oz pkg	1 oz	9.0	110	74%
Snack Stick	½ oz	5.0	60	75%
summer sausage				
Snack Slices	2 oz	8.0	210	34%
bratwurst				
light..6-count pkg	1 link	5.0	110	41%
Premium Festival				
6-count pkg	1 link	23.0	250	83%
Italian..festival				
6-count pkg	1 link	23.0	210	99%
Polish sausage				
premium smoked	4.66 oz	21.0	240	79%
6-count pkg	1 link	25.0	260	87%
smoked sausage				
Premium Real Wisconsin				
Cheddar Links	2.66 oz	21.0	250	76%
■ **(Owens)**				
bratwurst/cooked				
beer	1 link	21.0	270	70%
Italian	1 link	21.0	270	70%
original	1 link	21.0	270	70%
fresh pork sausage..chubs				
country-style				
extra-mild	2 oz	15.0	180	75%
hot picante				
36-count pkg	2 oz	19.0	210	81%
48-count pkg	2 oz	19.0	210	81%
maple	2 oz	15.0	180	75%
mild	2 oz	18.0	210	77%
Italian	2 oz	15.0	180	75%
regular	2 oz	15.0	180	75%
8-count pkg	3 oz	21.0	240	79%
36-count pkg	3 oz	19.0	210	81%
smoked	2 oz	16.0	170	85%
special seasoning	2 oz	15.0	180	75%
pork sausage				
patties				
hot picante				
36-count pkg	2 oz	19.0	210	81%
regular				
8-count pkg	2 patties	21.0	240	79%
36-count pkg	2 oz	19.0	210	81%

Food and Description	Amount	Fat Grams	Total Calories	% Fat Calories
■ **(Perdue)**				
turkey sausage				
breakfast links				
2.3 oz..fully cooked	3 links	14.0	170	74%
hot Italian links				
2.8 oz..fully cooked	1 link	9.0	150	54%
Polish sausages				
fully cooked				
3.2 oz	1 link	15.0	190	71%
3.3 oz	1 link	15.0	190	71%
sausage links..mild				
2 oz fully cooked	1 link	8.0	120	60%
2 oz ready-to-cook	2 links	3.5	140	23%
sausage patties..fully cooked				
mild				
2 oz	1 patty	12.0	150	72%
2 oz	2 patties	8.0	110	65%
sausage patties..ready-to-cook..mild				
2 oz	1 patty	8.0	120	60%
3 oz	2 patties	16.0	210	69%
sweet Italian links				
2.4 oz..cooked	1 link	9.0	150	54%
2.7 oz..raw	1 link	9.0	150	54%
3 oz..roasted	1 link	9.0	150	54%
■ **(Purnell's Old Folks)**				
sausage				
country				
flame-broiled				
patties..24-count pkg	2 patties	19.0	220	78%
skinless links..medium	2 oz	19.0	210	81%
Italian sausage				
6-count pkg	1 link	17.0	210	73%
pork links..fresh				
12-count pkg	2 links	13.0	150	18%
turkey sausage..patties				
16-count pkg	2 oz	5.0	180	25%
whole				
beef sausage	2.67 oz	15.0	194	70%
whole hog sausage				
chorizo	2 oz	1.0	190	81%
country				
medium	2 oz	19.0	220	78%
spicy..medium	2 oz	19.0	220	78%
Italian sausage	2 oz	19.0	220	78%
patties				
country				
hot	2 patties	19.0	220	78%
spicy	2 patties	19.0	220	78%
spicy..medium				

Food and Description	Amount	Fat Grams	Total Calories	% Fat Calories
30-count pkg	2 oz	19.0	220	78%
smoky flavor	2 patties	18.0	190	85%
■ (Rudy's Farm)				
breakfast sausage patty				
cooked..1.5 oz	1 patty	14.0	150	84%
rolled mild breakfast				
sausage..cooked	2 oz	21.0	210	90%
Whole Hog..stuffed &				
sliced breakfast				
sausage patty				
1.5 oz each	2 patties	28.0	300	84%
2 oz	1 patty	19.0	220	78%
Whole Hog..stuffed & sliced				
breakfast patty				
hot				
2.4 oz	2 patties	27.0	300	81%
mild				
1.5 oz	1 patty	15.0	170	79%
2 oz	1 patty	22.0	240	83%
Whole Hog breakfast..cooked				
sausage casing				
link..mild..2.2 oz	3 links	23.0	240	86%
■ (Schwan's)				
bratwurst				
fresh	1 link	22.0	250	79%
Italian sausage	2 oz	12.0	160	68%
Old World..smoked	2 oz	12.0	140	77%
Polish sausage	1 link	19.0	220	78%
pork..fully cooked..premium				
links	2 links	17.0	200	76%
country sausage patties	1 patty	22.0	230	86%
sausage links..fully cooked	2 links	24.0	250	86%
sausage patties..country	1 patty	22.0	230	86%
summer sausage	2 oz	13.0	160	73%
■ (Shelton's)				
turkey sausage				
Italian links	1 link	16.0	160	90%
original				
links	1 link	14.0	140	90%
patties..2 oz	1 patty	11.0	140	71%
■ (The Turkey Store)				
turkey sausage				
breakfast links..all flavors	2 oz	9.0	140	51%
breakfast patties				
apple cinnamon	2.3 oz	12.0	160	68%
hot	2.3 oz	12.0	150	72%
maple syrup	2.3 oz	11.0	140	71%
mild	2 oz	11.0	140	71%
	2.3 oz	10.0	160	56%
w/smoked bacon	2.3 oz	12.0	150	72%

Food and Description	Amount	Fat Grams	Total Calories	% Fat Calories
lean..Italian...Polish				
links..all types	3 oz	8.0	140	51%
rope..all types	2.5 oz	7.0	110	57%
smoked seasoned	3 oz	8.0	140	51%
SAUSAGE DISH (See also BREAKFAST SANDWICH; FROZEN ENTRÉE/DINNER; SAUSAGE)				
(Mary Kitchen)..sausage hash	1 cup	27.0	410	59%
SAUSAGE STICK (See MEAT SNACK)				
SAUSAGE SUBSTITUTE (See VEGETARIAN FOODS)				
SAVORY/ground	1 tsp	–	4	–
SCALLION/GREEN ONION/SPRING ONION (See also ONION)				
fresh				
chopped	½ cup	–	15	–
(Dole)	1 Tbs	–	2	–
w/tops	5 large	–	10	–
SCALLOP (See also SEAFOOD ENTRÉE/DINNER)				
fresh				
breaded & fried ½ oz each	2 scallops	3.0	67	40%
raw	3 oz	0.6	75	7%
frozen				
(Contessa)	4 oz	–	90	–
(Crystal Isle)	3 oz	1.0	150	6%
imitation				
(Louis Kemp)				
Scallop Delights				
bay-style	13 pieces	–	80	–
smoked				
(Ducktrap River)				
smoked	¼ cup	1.0	60	15%
SCONE (See also ROLL)				
(Awrey's)				
thaw & serve				
cinnamon chip..w/icing	1 scone	19.0	470	36%
classic raisin English	1 scone	5.0	270	17%
cranberry orange	1 scone	15.0	390	35%
maple pecan cluster..w/icing	1 scone	19.0	470	36%
wild blueberry	1 scone	17.0	400	38%
wild blueberry English	1 scone	6.0	250	22%
(Krusteaz)..mix..prepared				
blueberry	1 scone	13.0	280	42%
carrot raisin spice	1 scone	13.0	300	39%
cranberry orange	1 scone	13.0	280	42%
scone & shortcake	1 scone	9.0	180	45%
(Otis Spunkmeyer)				
cinnamon chip	3.75 oz	16.0	380	38%
maple pecan	3.75 oz	14.0	370	34%
wild blueberry	3.5 oz	13.0	330	35%
(Wolferman's)				
apple cranberry	1 scone	14.0	330	38%
chocolate chunk	1 scone	17.0	360	43%

Food and Description	Amount	Fat Grams	Total Calories	% Fat Calories
cinnamon chip	1 scone	16.0	370	39%
classic currant	1 scone	13.0	320	37%
cranberry orange	1 scone	14.0	330	38%
wild blueberry	1 scone	14.0	330	38%
SCOTCH (See LIQUOR, DISTILLED)				
SCOTCH BROTH (See SOUP)				
SCRAPPLE				
(Jones Dairy Farm)..country	1.5 oz	6.0	90	60%
	2 oz	8.0	120	60%
SCROD (See SEAFOOD ENTRÉE/DINNER)				
SCUP/raw	3 oz	2.0	90	20%
SEA BASS (See also SEAFOOD ENTRÉE/DINNER)				
fresh				
breaded & fried	3 oz	7.0	176	36%
cooked—dry heat	3 oz	2.0	105	17%
raw	3 oz	1.7	82	19%
SEA SALT	1 tsp	–	–	–
SEA TROUT/raw	3 oz	3.0	88	31%
SEA VEGETABLE (See SEAWEED)				
SEAFOOD CHOWDER (See SOUP)				
SEAFOOD ENTRÉE/DINNER (See also FROZEN ENTRÉE/DINNER; PASTA ENTRÉE/DINNER; individual listings)				
■ **CANNED**				
(Chicken of the Sea)				
Oysters				
smoked	3 oz	11.0	190	52%
whole	4 oz	3.0	70	39%
(Crown Prince)				
clams..boiled..baby	2 oz	–	40	–
kipper snacks	3.2 oz	13.0	190	62%
oysters..smoked	3 oz	22.0	290	68%
(Gorton's)				
cod cakes	4 oz	0.5	100	5%
crunchy fried clams	3 oz	17.0	260	59%
(Port Clyde)				
fish steaks				
w/Louisiana hot sauce	3.75 oz can	9.0	150	54%
w/mustard sauce	3.75 oz can	7.0	140	45%
w/soybean oil				
drained	3.3 oz can	17.0	220	70%
& hot chilies/drained	3.3 oz can	8.0	155	46%
■ **FROZEN**				
(Avalon Bay)				
fillets				
cod	4 oz	0.5	90	5%
gourmet breaded cod	½ fillet	8.0	210	34%
grouper	4 oz	1.0	100	9%
halibut steaks	3 oz	1.9	93	18%
emperor snapper	4 oz	2.0	110	16%
scallops				
scallop medallions	2 oz	–	40	–

Food and Description	Amount	Fat Grams	Total Calories	% Fat Calories
gourmet breaded scallops	11 scallops	2.0	110	16%
shrimp				
stuffed	3 shrimp	18.0	330	49%
(Captain's Cove)				
fish				
chum salmon fillets	4 oz	4.0	135	27%
cod fillets	4 oz	0.5	90	5%
flounder fillets	4 oz	1.5	100	14%
halibut steaks	4 oz	3.0	130	21%
orange roughy fillets	4 oz	8.0	140	51%
perch fillets	4 oz	2.0	110	16%
swordfish steaks	4 oz	6.0	150	36%
yellowfin tuna steaks	4 oz	1.5	140	10%
scallops				
jumbo	3.2 oz	0.5	70	6%
breaded	3.2 oz	1.0	120	8%
medium				
bacon-wrapped	3.2 oz	19.0	220	78%
shrimp				
cooked..tail on				
low-fat	4 oz	0.5	60	8%
large..cooked ring				
and sauce	4 oz	–	80	–
popcorn	2.85 oz	12.0	210	51%
raw..shell on..low-fat	4 oz	0.5	70	6%
shell on..low-fat				
51- to 60-count pkg	4 oz	0.5	70	6%
(Contessa)				
shrimp				
cooked				
shell on	3 oz	–	60	–
shelled	3 oz	–	40	–
uncooked	4 oz	–	80	–
shrimp & linguini	2 cups	3.0	300	9%
shrimp stir-fry	2¼ cup	–	150	–
(Fisher Boy)				
crab cakes..premium				
lightly breaded				
6-count pkg	2 oz	4.0	110	33%
fish fillets..crispy battered				
15-count pkg	3 oz	8.0	130	55%
fish portions..crunchy				
4-count pkg	¼ pkg	10.0	200	45%
fish portions..crispy battered				
8-count pkg	⅛ pkg	10.0	170	53%
fish shapes..crunchy	3 oz	9.0	210	39%
fish sticks..crunchy	3 oz	11.0	190	52%
fish tenders..crunchy	2.62 oz	12.0	220	49%
Qwikstix..crunchy..minced	3 oz	10.0	200	45%
school o' fish..crunchy..minced	3 oz	9.0	190	43%

Food and Description	Amount	Fat Grams	Total Calories	% Fat Calories
(Gorton's)				
clams	½ pkg	14.0	240	53%
fish fillets				
beer batter..crispy	2 pieces	15.0	250	54%
crispy battered	2 pieces	19.0	270	63%
crunchy golden	2 pieces	15.0	270	50%
garlic & herb..crunchy	2 pieces	16.0	270	53%
grilled Caesar Parmesan	1 piece	3.0	100	27%
grilled Cajun...blackened	1 piece	3.0	100	27%
grilled classic..char-grilled	1 piece	3.0	100	27%
grilled..garlic butter	1 piece	3.0	100	27%
grilled..italian herb	1 piece	3.0	100	27%
grilled..lemon butter	1 piece	3.0	100	27%
grilled..lemon herb				
extra-large	¼ box	7.0	180	35%
grilled..lemon pepper	1 piece	3.0	100	27%
lemon herb..crunchy	2 pieces	13.0	240	49%
lemon pepper..battered	2 pieces	21.0	290	65%
Parmesan..crunchy	2 pieces	15.0	250	54%
premium cod..crunchy				
breaded..extra-large	½ box	12.0	220	49%
premium haddock..crunchy				
breaded..extra-large	½ box	12.0	220	49%
ranch..crunchy breaded	2 pieces	13.0	240	49%
Southern-fried..country-style	2 pieces	13.0	230	51%
tenders..extra-crunchy	4.24 oz	12.0	260	42%
tenders..original batter	4.24 oz	15.0	270	50%
fish portions				
batter-dipped	1 piece	10.0	170	53%
fish sticks				
crunchy golden	6 sticks	14.0	250	50%
garlic & herb	6 sticks	13.0	260	45%
Grilled Fish Fillet Meals				
Alfredo..w/broccoli	1 meal	3.0	160	17%
lemon & herb butter				
w/rice & vegetables	1 meal	3.5	240	13%
popcorn fish..crispy				
golden battered	4 oz	13.0	320	37%
popcorn shrimp				
beer batter..7.2-oz box	½ box	16.0	270	53%
garlic & herb..7.2-oz box	½ box	11.0	250	40%
original..8-oz box	3.2 oz	12.0	240	45%
Shrimp Bowls				
Alfredo fried rice	1 bowl	6.0	270	20%
Alfredo shrimp	1 bowl	6.0	270	20%
butter shrimp	1 bowl	6.0	260	21%
garlic shrimp	1 bowl	6.0	320	17%
primavera shrimp	1 bowl	6.0	270	20%
teriyaki	1 bowl	6.0	320	17%

Food and Description	Amount	Fat Grams	Total Calories	% Fat Calories
(High Liner)				
cod				
fillets				
breaded	3 oz	3.0	110	25%
grilled..w/garlic butter	⅛ pkg	4.0	110	33%
loins..Atlantic	⅛ pk	1.0	90	10%
fish sticks				
crunchy	3 oz	12.0	240	45%
salmon fillets				
in creamy dill sauce	4 oz	3.0	110	25%
stuffed mango & macadamia	¼ pkg	31.0	370	75%
scallops				
roasted garlic & herb	4 oz	2.0	100	18%
sea scallops..breaded	⅙ pkg	9.0	220	37%
unbreaded	⅛ pkg	1.0	100	9%
(Mrs. Paul's)				
cod fillets..breaded	4 oz	12.0	240	45%
crab cakes..deviled	3 oz	8.0	190	38%
fish fillets				
crispy battered				
hearty size..6-count pkg	⅙ pkg	12.0	210	51%
value pack..10-count pkg	⅒ pkg	9.0	150	54%
crispy original				
breaded..97% fat-free	¼ pkg	2.0	130	14%
crunchy..breaded				
6-count pkg	⅓ pkg	15.0	260	52%
fish sticks				
crunchy breaded	⅓ pkg	12.0	230	47%
fish strips..crunchy	4 oz	14.0	270	47%
fish tenders..crispy	4 oz	14.0	260	48%
flounder fillet..breaded	⅓ pkg	9.0	170	48%
fried clams..breaded	3 oz	12.0	250	43%
haddock fillet..breaded	½ pkg	11.0	230	43%
scallops..fried..breaded	3.5 oz	7.0	220	29%
shrimp				
Alfredo	11 oz	9.0	300	9%
fried rice	11 oz	2.0	290	6%
garlic butter	11 oz	3.5	290	11%
marinated..all flavors	5.5 oz	0.5	70	6%
popcorn	4 oz	13.0	290	40%
sour shrimp	11 oz	1.0	310	3%
stir-fry	11 oz	1.0	330	3%
Thai-style peanut	11 oz	6.0	330	16%
tortellini	11 oz	4.0	340	11%
(Phillip's)				
bisque..soup..chowder				
crab soup	7.5 oz	0.5	70	6%
crab & clam chowder	7.5 oz	21.0	290	65%
crab & corn chowder	7.5 oz	21.0	290	65%
crab & shrimp chowder	7.5 oz	10.0	150	60%

Food and Description	Amount	Fat Grams	Total Calories	% Fat Calories
cream of crab	7.5 oz	28.0	340	74%
lobster bisque	7.5 oz	26.0	370	63%
New England clam chowder	7.5 oz	16.0	260	55%
shrimp bisque	7.5 oz	21.0	310	61%
crab				
cocktail crab claws	2 oz	–	45	–
crab cake..minis	3 cakes	9.0	160	51%
crab cakes..boardwalk				
Maryland style..6-count	⅙ pkg	20.0	250	72%
crab meat				
all types	2 oz	–	45	–
crab slammers..jalapeño	2 oz	9.0	160	51%
crab & spinach dip	2 oz	–	45	–
crab-stuffed shrimp	3 pieces	12.0	190	57%
mahimahi				
fillets				
coconut..w/restaurant-style sauce..14-count pkg	¼ pkg	4.0	170	21%
w/Caribbean-style pepper sauce..8-count pkg	⅛ pkg	1.0	100	9%
shrimp				
coconut	5 shrimp	17.0	290	53%
tuna				
yellowfin steak..w/Oriental peanut sauce				
6-count pkg	⅙ pkg	1.0	120	8%
(Schwan's)				
breaded seafood				
blue hake	3 oz	9.0	190	43%
clam strips	½ cup	13.0	270	43%
cod				
Battercrisp	2 oz piece	7.0	120	53%
nuggets	6 nuggets	10.0	200	45%
fantail shrimp	4 oz	2.0	230	8%
haddock				
oven-ready shrimp	3 oz	11.0	240	41%
squares	4 oz	7.0	190	33%
sticks	3 sticks	5.0	140	32%
unbreaded				
black tiger jumbo cooked shrimp	3 oz	1.0	70	13%
Alaskan				
cod fillets	4 oz	0.5	90	5%
halibut fillets	4 oz	4.0	120	30%
perch	4 oz	2.0	90	90%
salmon fillets..bone	4 oz	2.0	100	18%
seafood sampler	4 oz	0.5	90	5%
blue hake loins	4 oz	–	70	–
buttercrisp cod	2 pieces	18.0	280	58%
Caesar Parmesan shrimp	3.3 oz	4.5	110	37%
cod fish nuggets	6 nuggets	10.0	200	45%

Food and Description	Amount	Fat Grams	Total Calories	% Fat Calories
English-style				
fish 'n' chips	¼ bag	30.0	500	54%
(Sea Pak)				
clam strips..oven crunchy	3 oz	14.0	250	50%
crabcakes				
Boardwalk Maryland-style				
6-count pkg	1 cake	20.0	250	72%
Maryland-style	1 cake	12.0	220	49%
6-count pkg	1 cake	9.0	170	48%
minis	4 cakes	9.0	160	56%
oven crunchy	1 cake	15.0	250	54%
popcorn shrimp				
buffalo-style				
oven crunchy	3 oz	11.0	230	43%
jumbo..oven crunchy	3 oz	11.0	240	41%
oven crunchy	3 oz	11.0	240	41%
shrimp				
butterfly..breaded	4 oz	1.0	150	6%
butterfly..jumbo				
oven crunchy	3 oz	9.0	200	41%
butterfly..oven crunchy	4.5 oz	9.0	200	41%
coconut..oven crunchy	3 oz	14.0	250	50%
	3.66 oz	17.0	270	57%
Shrimp Entrées				
Alfredo..w/broccoli	1 entrée	9.0	300	57%
garlic herb	1 entrée	8.0	270	27%
teriyaki..w/rice	1 entrée	8.0	350	21%
shrimp..marinated				
Caesar Parmesan	3.33 oz	4.5	110	37%
garlic herb	3.33 oz	3.0	90	30%
spicy Szechuan	3.33 oz	4.0	110	37%
shrimp scampi				
in Baja lime sauce	4 oz	32.0	350	82%
in Italian Parmesan sauce	4 oz	33.0	350	85%
in traditional garlic sauce	4 oz	32.0	350	82%
(Van de Kamp's)				
battered items				
fillets				
fish	1 fillet	10.0	170	53%
haddock	2 fillets	11.0	220	45%
halibut	3 fillets	10.0	220	41%
ocean perch	2 fillets	13.0	240	49%
fish				
portions	1 portion	9.0	160	51%
tenders	4 pieces	17.0	290	53%
breaded items				
fillets				
fish	2 fillets	17.0	260	59%

Food and Description	Amount	Fat Grams	Total Calories	% Fat Calories
fish sticks				
mini	13 sticks	14.0	250	50%
regular	6 sticks	17.0	290	53%
snack/value	6 sticks	15.0	260	52%
fish strips	4 pieces	14.0	270	47%
Hearty-Size fish fillets	1 fillet	10.0	150	60%
portions	3 portions	24.0	360	60%
Crisp & Healthy/breaded & baked fillets				
garlic & herb	2 fillets	3.0	170	16%
lemon pepper	2 fillets	3.0	170	16%
regular..plain	2 fillets	3.0	170	16%
fish sticks	6 sticks	2.5	170	13%
grilled items/3.75-oz fillets				
garlic butter	1 fillet	6.0	120	45%
lemon butter	1 fillet	6.0	120	45%
lemon pepper	1 fillet	6.0	120	45%
premium breaded Items..fillets				
cod	4-oz fillet	11.0	220	45%
flounder	4-oz fillet	11.0	230	43%
haddock	4-oz fillet	11.0	230	43%
specialty items				
cheese & crab peppers	4 poppers	16.0	320	45%
clams/fried	18 pieces	12.0	250	43%
crab cakes	1 cake	9.0	170	48%
mini	4 cakes	12.0	200	54%
shrimp				
buffalo	20 shrimp	15.0	320	42%
butterfly	7 shrimp	15.0	300	45%
linguine	1½ cups	1.0	180	5%
popcorn	20 shrimp	12.0	270	40%
scampi	16 shrimp	1.0	80	11%
stir-fry	1⅔ cups	0.5	260	2%
stuffed	3 shrimp	13.0	290	40%

■ **MIX** (Note: The amount of fat and calories in dishes prepared from boxed mixes may vary slightly depending on the fat and calorie content of the seafood used in preparation.)

(Betty Crocker) Tuna Helper (Prepared data are for regular recipe only.)

Food and Description	Amount	Fat Grams	Total Calories	% Fat Calories
au gratin	1 cup	12.0	310	35%
cheesy broccoli	1 cup	10.0	300	30%
cheesy pasta	1 cup	11.0	270	37%
classic tuna casserole	1 cup	12.0	280	39%
creamy broccoli	1 cup	13.0	300	39%
creamy pasta	1 cup	13.0	290	40%
fettuccine Alfredo	1 cup	14.0	300	42%
Garden Cheddar	1 cup	11.0	290	34%
tetrazzini	1 cup	12.0	300	36%
tuna melt	1 cup	12.0	280	39%

SEASONINGS (See also ASIAN FOOD; BAKE & FRY MIX; GRAVY; MARINADE; MEXICAN FOOD; SAUCE; individual listings)

Food and Description	Amount	Fat Grams	Total Calories	% Fat Calories
(NOTE: Unless stated otherwise, data are for seasoning or seasoning mix only.)				
(Accent)				
flavor enhancer	⅛ tsp	–	–	–
Sa-son..all types	¼ tsp	–	–	–
(Adolph's)				
chili mix	~1 Tbs	–	60	–
meat..all types	¼ tsp	–	–	–
stir-fry teriyaki	~2 Tbs	–	30	–
(Amazing Taste)..all types	½ tsp	–	<5	–
(Cavender's) All-Purpose Greek	¼ tsp	–	–	–
(Chef Paul)..all types	¼ tsp	–	–	–
(Durkee)				
garlic bread sprinkles	½ tsp	–	–	–
roasting bag				
au jus	⅛ pkg	–	10	–
BBQ chicken	⅙ pkg	–	30	–
beef stew	1/10 pkg	–	15	–
chicken	⅙ pkg	–	20	–
Country Chicken	⅙ pkg	1.5	35	39%
lemon butter fish	¼ pkg	0.5	30	15%
meat loaf	⅛ pkg	–	15	–
onion pot roast	⅙ pkg	–	25	–
pork	⅙ pkg	–	25	–
pot roast	⅙ pkg	–	15	–
spareribs	1/7 pkg	–	25	–
Swiss steak	1/9 pkg	–	10	–
seasoning packet				
beef fajita/"easy"	⅙ pkg	–	15	–
beef stew	1/9 pkg	–	–	–
beef teriyaki/"easy"	⅕ pkg	1.0	30	30%
burrito	1/10 pkg	1.0	35	26%
chicken cacciatore/"easy"	1/10 pkg	–	10	–
chicken mushroom/easy'	⅛ pkg	–	15	–
fried rice	¼ pkg	–	15	–
ground beef	¼ pkg	–	25	–
Italian meatball	⅛ pkg	–	20	–
lemon pepper dill fish/"easy"	⅙ pkg	0.5	20	9%
meat loaf	1/9 pkg	–	20	–
Mexican salsa chicken/"easy"	1/10 pkg	–	10	–
pasta salad	⅙ pkg	–	10	–
sloppy joe	⅙ pkg	–	20	–
Stroganoff	⅛ pkg	–	10	–
sweet & sour chicken/"easy"	1/9 pkg	–	20	–
tomato basil fish/"easy"	1/7 pkg	–	15	–
(French's)				
roasting bag				
au jus	⅛ pkg	<1.0	10	45%
chicken	⅕ pkg	<1.0	25	18%
lemon butter fish	¼ pkg	<1.0	25	18%
meat loaf	⅙ pkg	<1.0	25	18%

Food and Description	Amount	Fat Grams	Total Calories	% Fat Calories
onion pot roast	⅛ pkg	<1.0	18	25%
pork	⅙ pkg	<1.0	25	18%
pot roast	⅛ pkg	<1.0	18	25%
Swiss steak	⅙ pkg	<1.0	20	23%
(Knorr) recipe mix				
beef stew w/wine	⅙ pkg	1.0	40	23%
chicken Dijon	⅙ pkg	1.0	30	30%
goulash beef stew	⅙ pkg	1.0	40	23%
sauerbraten	⅙ pkg	1.0	35	26%
(Lawry's)				
seasoning packets				
bacon onion	1 tsp	–	10	–
beef stew	⅒ pkg	–	10	–
burrito	¼ pkg	–	35	–
chicken & taco	¼ pkg	–	20	–
chili	⅕ pkg	0.5	25	18%
enchilada sauce	⅛ pkt	–	20	–
fajitas	⅛ pkg	–	15	–
chicken	⅛ pkg	–	10	–
garlic pepper	¼ tsp	–	2	–
garlic powder				
w/parsley	1 tsp	–	12	–
garlic salt	1 tsp	–	4	–
guacamole	⅛ pkg	–	15	–
lemon pepper	1 tsp	–	6	–
meat loaf	⅒ pkt	–	35	–
Mexican rice	⅛ pkg	–	15	–
minced onion	1 tsp	–	7	–
pepper/seasoned	1 tsp	–	4	–
pinch of herbs	1 tsp	0.5	9	50%
salsa	⅛ pkg	–	15	–
salt/seasoned				
hot 'n' spicy	1 tsp	–	3	–
light	1 tsp	–	8	–
plain	1 tsp	–	4	–
salt-free	1 tsp	–	3	–
salt-free 17	1 tsp	–	10	–
sloppy joes	⅙ pkg	–	20	–
spaghetti				
extra rich & thick	¼ pkg	1.0	35	26%
traditional	⅕ pkg	–	–	—
taco				
chicken	¼ pkt	–	20	–
hot	⅛ pkg	–	10	–
original				
1-oz pkg	⅙ pkg	–	15	–
2.5-oz pkg	1/12 pkg	–	20	–
seasoning sauces				
stir-fry				
herb & roasted garlic	1 Tbs	–	5	–

Food and Description	Amount	Fat Grams	Total Calories	% Fat Calories
lemon basil	1 Tbs	–	10	–
Oriental style	1 Tbs	–	20	–
sesame ginger	1 Tbs	–	20	–
sweet & spicy	1 Tbs	–	20	–
tenderizing beef marinade (McCormick)	½₂ pkg	–	–	–
Bag 'n' Season				
beef stew	1 tsp	–	15	–
beer batter	1 oz	–	100	–
buffalo wings	1 Tbs	–	30	–
Cajun-style seasoned chicken	⅓ pkg	–	35	–
country	1 Tbs	1.0	25	36%
Italian herb	1 Tbs	–	15	–
Oriental	1 Tbs	–	25	–
original	1 Tbs	–	20	–
chicken..original herbs & spices seasoned	½ pkg	1.0	50	–
home-style seasoned	½ pkg	–	50	–
cracker meal	1 oz	1.0	130	7%
extra-crispy seasoned chicken fry	½ oz	–	60	–
fish fry..lightly seasoned	.769 oz	–	35	–
fish 'n' chips..English-style	1 oz	–	100	–
funnel cake batter	2 Tbs	1.0	120	8%
hot 'n' spicy seasoned chicken	½ oz	–	50	–
hush puppy corn meal mix	1 oz	0.5	130	3%
meat loaf	2 tsp	–	15	–
pork chops	2 tsp	–	15	–
pork tenderloin	2 tsp	–	15	–
onion ring seasoned batter	1 oz	–	100	–
pot roast	1 Tbs	–	10	–
seafood seasoned	½ oz	–	50	–
spareribs	1 Tbs	–	30	–
Swiss steak	1 tsp	–	15	–
tempura Japanese-style batter	1 oz	–	100	–
turkey w/gravy	1 tsp	–	15	–
Grill Mates				
Montreal	¼ tsp	–	–	–
Montreal chicken & fish	¼ tsp	–	–	–
spicy Montreal steak	¼ tsp	–	–	–
International Blends				
Chinese 5-spice	½ tsp	–	–	–
herbes de Provence	½ tsp	–	–	–
Thai	½ tsp	–	–	–
Old Bay...(See (Old Bay) within this category)				
rice seasonings				
Creole	⅔ Tbs	–	20	–

Food and Description	Amount	Fat Grams	Total Calories	% Fat Calories
curry	1 Tbs	1.0	25	36%
Japanese	1½ Tbs	1.5	50	27%
saffron	1 Tbs	–	25	–
Spanish	1½ Tbs	–	45	–
Rotisserie Recipe				
herb & spice	2 tsp	–	15	–
tangy barbecue	2 tsp	–	20	–
salt-free blends..all types	¼ tsp	–	–	–
seasoning blends				
barbecue	¼ tsp	–	<5	–
beef stew	2 tsp	–	15	–
beef Stroganoff	2 tsp	–	15	–
burrito	1 tsp	0.5	25	18%
Cajun	½ tsp	–	–	–
Cajun quick..spicy chicken	¼ tsp	–	<5	–
Caribbean jerk	¼ tsp	–	–	–
celery salt	¼ tsp	–	–	–
cheese sauce	4 tsp	2.0	40	45%
chili				
hot	¼ pkg	1.0	40	23%
mild	¼ pkg	–	30	–
original	¼ pkg	0.5	30	15%
chili powder	¼ tsp	–	–	–
chicken...all types	¼ tsp	–	–	–
citrus pepper	¼ tsp	–	–	–
Creole	¼ tsp	–	–	–
fajita	¼ tsp	–	15	–
garlic season all	¼ tsp	–	–	–
garlic..crushed				
California-style	¼ tsp	–	10	–
garlic..minced-wet				
California-style	1 tsp	0.5	15	30%
garlic & parsley salt	¼ tsp	–	–	–
garlic bread sprinkle	½ tsp	1.0	10	90%
garlic spread				
garlic & herb	½ Tbs	4.5	45	90%
regular	½ Tbs	4.0	45	80%
hamburger	¼ tsp	–	–	–
herb & garlic mix	1 Tbs	–	20	–
herb chicken	¼ tsp	–	–	–
herb classic chicken	¼ tsp	–	–	–
home-style	¼ tsp	–	–	–
imitation butter–flavored salt	¼ tsp	–	–	–
Key West spice blend	¼ tsp	–	–	–
lemon herb	½ tsp	–	–	–
lemon pepper				
California-style	½ tsp	–	5	
meat loaf	1 tsp	–	15	–
mesquite chicken	¼ tsp	–	2	
Monterey spice blend	¼ tsp	–	–	–

Food and Description	Amount	Fat Grams	Total Calories	% Fat Calories
onion salt..California-style	¼ tsp	–	–	–
pesto mix	2 tsp	–	10	–
pizza seasoning..spicy Italian	1 tsp	–	10	–
pork seasoning	½ tsp	–	–	–
primavera mix	1 Tbs	1.0	30	30%
rotisserie chicken	¼ tsp	–	–	–
Salad Supreme Seasoning	¼ tsp	–	–	–
Santa Fe spice blend	¼ tsp	–	–	–
sloppy joe	⅛ pkg	–	15	–
spicy season all	¼ tsp	–	–	–
steak..broiled	¼ tsp	–	<5	–
taco				
40% less sodium	2 tsp	–	20	–
chicken	2 tsp	–	25	–
hot	2 tsp	–	20	–
mild	2 tsp	–	20	–
Thai seasoning	½ tsp	–	–	–
(Mrs. Dash)..all types	1 tsp	–	12	–
(Molly McButter)..all flavors	½ tsp	–	5	–
(NewMenu) Tofumate				
breakfast scramble	¼ pkg	–	15	–
eggless salad	¼ pkg	–	15	–
mandarin stir-fry	¼ pkg	–	30	–
Szechuan stir-fry	¼ pkg	–	25	–
Texas taco	¼ pkg	–	15	–
(Nile Spice)..all types	⅛ tsp	–	–	–
(Old Bay)				
seasoning				
blackened	⅛ tsp	–	–	–
crab cake classic				
original Maryland	⅙ pkg	1.0	30	30%
for seafood				
& poultry salt	⅛ tsp	–	–	–
salmon classic..original	⅓ pkg	1.5	40	34%
seafood..one-step				
crab boil..spicy	Any	–	–	–
tuna classic	⅕ pkg	1.0	30	30%
(Oven Fry)				
extra-crispy				
for chicken	⅛ pkg	1.0	60	15%
for pork	⅛ pkg	1.5	60	23%
fish fry for fish	1 Tbs	0.5	45	10%
home-style for chicken	⅛ pkg	1.5	60	23%
(Phillip's)..seafood..all types	¼ tsp	–	–	–
(Produce Partners)				
onion ring mix	¼ cup	0.5	110	4%
vegetable batter mix	¼ cup	0.5	120	4%
(Shake & Bake)				
French fries				
French fries				
for fresh potatoes	⅙ pkt	–	14	–

Food and Description	Amount	Fat Grams	Total Calories	% Fat Calories
Perfect Potatoes seasoning mix				
crispy cheddar	⅙ pkt	2.0	30	60%
herb & garlic	⅙ pkt	–	20	–
home fries	⅙ pkt	–	20	–
Parmesan peppercorn	⅙ pkt	1.0	25	36%
savory onion	⅙ pkt	–	10	–
zesty cheddar	⅙ pkg	–	25	–
seasoned coating mixture				
buffalo wings	1/10 pkt	1.0	40	23%
country mild recipe	⅛ pouch	2.0	35	51%
for chicken				
crispy chicken nuggets	1/12 pouch	1.0	50	18%
original recipe	⅛ pouch	1.0	40	23%
for chicken or pork				
classic Italian	⅛ pkt	0.5	40	11%
hot & spicy	⅛ pkt	1.0	40	23%
original	⅛ pkt	0.5	45	10%
for fish/original	⅛ pouch	1.5	80	17%
for pork/original recipe	⅛ pouch	0.5	45	10%
garlic & herb	⅛ pkt	0.5	35	13%
hot & spicy	⅛ pkt	1.0	40	23%
Tangy Honey	⅛ pkt	1.0	45	20%
(Taco Bell)..Home Originals..dry mix				
chicken fajita	~1 Tbs	–	25	–
taco	~2 tsp	–	20	–
SEAWEED				
agar				
dried	3 oz	<1.0	260	2%
(Eden)				
bars	1 Tbs	–	10	–
flakes	1 Tbs	–	10	–
raw	3 oz	<1.0	23	20%
arame				
(Eden)	½ cup	–	30	–
hijiki				
(Eden)	½ cup	–	30	–
kelp..raw	3 oz	0.6	37	15%
kombu				
(Eden)..7" sheet	½" sheet	–	10	–
laver/nori				
dried	3 oz	<1.0	30	9%
(Eden)				
sushi nori sea vegetable	1 sheet	–	10	–
raw	3 oz	<1.0	31	15%
spirulina				
dried	3 oz	6.6	249	24%
raw	3 oz	<1.0	22	21%
wakame				
(Eden)..flakes..instant	1 tsp	–	3	–

Food and Description	Amount	Fat Grams	Total Calories	% Fat Calories
SEITAN				
(Lightlife)				
organic				
BBQ	3 oz	1.5	120	11%
teriyaki	3 oz	–	110	–
(White Wave)				
box				
chicken-style				
meat of wheat	3 oz	–	130	–
traditional	3 oz	1.0	140	6%
vegetarian stir-fry strips	3 oz	1.0	100	9%
pack..chicken-style	4.5-oz piece	–	130	–
SELTZER WATER (See SOFT DRINK; WATER)				
SEMOLINA (See also FLOUR)				
enriched	½ cup	0.5	310	1%
unenriched	½ cup	<1.0	110	2%
whole-grain	1 cup	2.0	600	3%
SESAME BUTTER/TAHINI				
(Arrowhead Mills)				
organic				
tahini	2 Tbs	19.0	190	90%
(Erewhon)..all styles	2 Tbs	17.0	190	81%
(Casbah), sauce mix/prepared	¼ cup	13.0	160	73%
(Kettle) Roaster Fresh	2 Tbs	15.0	170	79%
(Peloponnese)				
organic				
tahini..w/ground				
sesame seeds	1 Tbs	8.0	100	72%
(Westbrae)..organic..all styles	2 Tbs	19.0	220	78%
SESAME FLOUR (See FLOUR)				
SESAME SEEDS				
dried/ground	1 tsp	–	5	–
kernels				
(Arrowhead Mills)..hulled	¼ cup	20.0	210	86%
whole				
(Arrowhead Mills)				
brown	¼ cup	20.0	200	90%
(McCormick/Schilling)				
untoasted	¼ tsp	0.4	5	72%
SHAD, AMERICAN				
cooked—dry heat	3 oz	15.0	215	63%
raw	3 oz	12.0	170	63%
SHALLOT				
freeze-dried	1 Tbs	–	3	–
	1 oz	–	100	–
fresh/raw/chopped	1 Tbs	–	7	–
SHARK				
batter-dipped & fried	3 oz	11.8	194	55%

Food and Description	Amount	Fat Grams	Total Calories	% Fat Calories
SHEEPSHEAD				
cooked—dry heat	3 oz	1.0	107	8%
raw	3 oz	2.0	92	20%
SHELLIE BEAN				
canned				
(Stokely's)				
shellie beans	½ cup	–	45	–
sprouted				
(La Choy)	1 cup	–	10	–
SHERBET (*See also* FRUIT ICES, BARS & POPS)				
(Baskin-Robbins)				
blue raspberry	½ cup	1.5	120	11%
orange	½ cup	1.5	120	11%
rainbow	½ cup	1.5	120	11%
tangerine pineapple	½ cup	1.0	120	8%
(Blue Bunny)				
Disney Pixar				
Galactic Buzz Lightyear	½ cup	1.0	80	11%
sherbet cups..all flavors	2.28 oz	1.0	90	10%
sherbet..fat-free..all flavors	½ cup	–	110	–
sherbet..regular..rainbow	½ cup	5.0	110	41%
(Breyers)				
natural				
chocolate rainbow	½ cup	7.0	140	45%
orange	½ cup	1.5	130	10%
rainbow	½ cup	1.5	130	10%
raspberry	½ cup	1.5	130	10%
tropical	½ cup	5.0	140	32%
Take Two! vanilla ice cream				
& orange sherbet	½ cup	5.0	140	32%
(Dreyers)				
berry rainbow	½ cup	1.0	130	7%
lime	½ cup	1.5	130	10%
orange cream	½ cup	2.0	120	15%
raspberry	½ cup	1.0	130	7%
Swiss orange	½ cup	3.0	150	18%
tropical rainbow	½ cup	1.0	130	7%
(Edy's)				
berry rainbow	½ cup	1.0	130	7%
lime	½ cup	1.5	130	10%
orange cream	½ cup	2.0	120	15%
raspberry	½ cup	1.0	130	7%
Swiss orange	½ cup	3.0	150	18%
tropical rainbow	½ cup	1.0	130	7%
(Friendly's)				
ice cream & sherbet roll	½ cup	7.0	200	32%
Sherbet Sensations..orange..lemon				
raspberry	½ cup	1.5	130	10%
Sherbet Watermelon..watermelon..lemon				
& chocolate	½ cup	2.5	170	13%

Food and Description	Amount	Fat Grams	Total Calories	% Fat Calories
(Hiland-Roberts)				
Old Recipe..orange	½ cup	1.0	110	8%
orange	½ cup	1.0	110	8%
(Hood) Fruit Scoops				
lime..orange..lemon	½ cup	1.0	120	8%
(Kemp's)..fat-free..orange	½ cup	–	120	–
(Pet)..sherbet...all flavors	½ cup	1.5	130	10%
(Schwan's)..all flavors	½ cup	1.0	120	8%

SHORTENING, VEGETABLE (*See also* FAT; LARD; OIL; SHORTENING SUBSTITUTE)
(NOTE: All brands of vegetable shortening contain the same amount of calories and fat, just as all types of vegetable oil do. Because of the flexibility manufacturers are given in rounding off nutritional data, it may appear that one product has slightly fewer calories or less fat than another, but don't be fooled: They all get 100% of their calories from fat.)

(Crisco) regular or butter flavor	1 Tbs	12.0	110	100%
	1 cup	205.0	1845	100%
(Swift'ning)	1 Tbs	12.0	110	100%
(Wesson)	1 Tbs	12.0	100	100%

SHORTENING SUBSTITUTE

(PlumLife)..Just Like Shortenin'	1 Tbs	–	70	–
(Smucker's) Baking Healthy	1 Tbs	–	30	–
(Wonderslim)..fat & egg substitute	¼ cup	–	35	–

SHOYU/SOY SAUCE (*See* ASIAN FOOD; SAUCE)

SHRIMP (*See also* ASIAN FOOD; FROZEN ENTRÉE/DINNER; SEAFOOD ENTRÉE/DINNER; SHRIMP PASTE)

canned				
(3 Diamonds)				
shrimp				
small	3.5 oz	1.0	50	18%
tiny..whole	2.0 oz	–	90	.–
(Bumble Bee)				
Bumble Bee..all styles	2 oz	–	40	–
Orleans..all styles	2 oz	–	40	–
(Chicken of the Sea)				
deveined				
medium	2 oz	0.5	45	10%
small	2 oz	0.5	45	10%
medium	2 oz	0.5	45	10%
premium shrimp pouch	2.5 oz	0.5	55	8%
small	2 oz	0.5	45	10%
tiny	2 oz	0.5	45	10%
(Crown Prince)..tiny..peeled	½ can	–	60	–
(Ducktrap River)..smoked	¼ cup	2.0	60	30%
(S&W) deveined	¼ cup	–	45	–
fresh				
breaded & fried	4 large	3.7	73	45%
	3 oz	10.0	206	44%
cooked—moist heat	4 large	–	22	–
	3 oz	0.9	84	10%
raw	3 oz	1.0	90	10%

Food and Description	Amount	Fat Grams	Total Calories	% Fat Calories
SHRIMP PASTE	3 oz	8.0	155	47%
SHRIMP SOUP, CREAM OF (*See* SOUP)				
SIM-SIM (*See* SESAME SEEDS)				
SMELT				
rainbow				
breaded & fried	3 oz	10.6	214	45%
cooked—dry heat	3 oz	2.6	106	22%
SMOKED SALMON (*See* SALMON; SALMON SPREAD; SEAFOOD ENTRÉE/DINNER)				
SMOKED SAUSAGE (*See* SAUSAGE)				
SNACK BAR (*See* CANDY; GRANOLA/GRANOLA-TYPE BAR)				
SNACK CAKE (*See* CAKE, SNACKS; PASTRY; POPCORN BARS & CAKES; RICE CAKES)				
SNACK MIX (*See* SNACKS)				
SNACKS (*See also* FRUIT SNACK; MEXICAN FOOD; NUTS, MIXED; POPCORN; POPCORN BARS & CAKES; POTATO CHIPS & SNACKS; PRETZEL; RICE CAKES; TORTILLA CHIPS/ CORN CHIPS)				
(Air Crisps)				
Cheese Nips	1 oz	4.0	130	28%
Potato Crispy snacks				
BBQ	1 oz	3.5	120	26%
original	1 oz	3.5	120	26%
sour cream & onion	1 oz	3.5	120	26%
Pretzel crispy baked	1 oz	1.0	110	8%
Ritz original	1 oz	5.0	140	32%
Tortilla chips crispy baked				
nacho	1 oz	5.0	130	35%
Wheat Thins crispy baked				
original	1 oz	4.5	130	31%
ranch	1 oz	4.5	130	31%
(Andy Capp)				
fries				
BBQ	1 oz	6.0	140	39%
cheddar	1 oz	8.0	150	48%
hot	1 oz	8.0	150	48%
hot chili cheese steak	1.75 oz	14.0	130	97%
salsa	1 oz	6.0	130	42%
white cheddar	1 oz	15.0	260	52%
(Ann's House of Nuts)				
snack nut mixes				
Cajun	⅓ cup	10.0	170	53%
California	¼ cup	5.0	130	35%
cranberry fruit..nut	3 Tbs	5.0	110	41%
honey nut crunch	3 Tbs	8.0	150	48%
nut 'n' fruit mix	3 Tbs	5.0	120	38%
nut 'n' raisin mix	3 Tbs	6.0	120	45%
Swiss mix	3 Tbs	6.0	130	42%
trail mix..raw	3 Tbs	8.0	130	55%
(Atkins)				
Crunchers snack chips				
BBQ	1 oz	3.0	100	27%
nacho cheese	1 oz	3.0	100	27%

Food and Description	Amount	Fat Grams	Total Calories	% Fat Calories
original	1 oz	3.0	90	30%
sour cream & onion	1 oz	4.0	100	36%
(Baken-ets)				
Fried Pork Skins & Cracklins				
BBQ pork skins	1 oz	5.0	70	64%
hot 'n' spicy cracklins	1 oz	5.0	80	56%
hot 'n' spicy pork skins	1 oz	5.0	80	56%
regular				
Cracklins	1 oz	6.0	80	68%
pork skins	1 oz	5.0	80	56%
sweet 'n' tangy BBQ	1 oz	5.0	80	56%
(Barbara's Bakery)				
natural snacks				
cheese puffs				
jalapeño	1 oz	10.0	150	60%
original	1 oz	10.0	150	62%
cheese puff bakes				
original	1 oz	11.0	160	62%
white cheddar	1 oz	11.0	160	62%
potato chip snacks				
original	1 oz	10.0	150	62%
ripple	1 oz	10.0	150	62%
unsalted	1 oz	10.0	150	62%
yogurt & green onion	1 oz	9.0	150	54%
(Betty Crocker)				
Bugles...all flavors	1⅓ cups	9.0	160	44%
Chex Mix				
Bold Party Blend	½ cup	6.0	140	39%
cheddar cheese	⅔ cup	4.0	130	28%
honey nut	½ cup	4.0	130	28%
hot 'n' spicy	⅔ cup	4.5	130	31%
Nacho Fiesta	⅔ Cup	3.5	120	26%
Peanut Lover's	½ cup	6.0	140	39%
traditional	⅔ cup	4.0	130	28%
trail mix	½ cup	4.5	140	29%
Fruit by the Foot...all flavors	1 roll	1.5	80	17%
Fruit Gushers...all flavors	1 pouch	1.0	90	10%
Fruit Roll-Ups..all flavors	1 roll	1.0	50	18%
(Cheetos)				
Asteroids				
hot	1 oz	9.0	150	54%
regular	1 oz	9.0	150	54%
crunchy	1 oz	10.0	160	56%
curls	1 oz	10.0	150	60%
flamin' hot	1 oz	10.0	160	56%
hot puff rods	1 oz	10.0	160	56%
jumbo puffs	1 oz	10.0	160	56%
puffs	1 oz	10.0	160	56%
natural	1 oz	10.0	170	53%
puffed balls	1 oz	10.0	150	60%

Food and Description	Amount	Fat Grams	Total Calories	% Fat Calories
puffs	1 oz	10.0	160	56%
Wirlz	1 oz	10.0	160	56%
X's & O's	1 oz	11.0	160	62%
Zig Zags	1 oz	11.0	170	58%
(Chex Mix) (*See* (Betty Crocker) in this section)				
(Cornnuts)				
BBQ..crunchy	1.7 oz	8.0	220	33%
chile picante..crunchy	1 oz	4.5	130	31%
	1.7 oz	8.0	210	34%
nacho cheese	1 oz	5.0	130	35%
original..crunchy	1.7 oz	8.0	210	34%
ranch..crunchy	1 oz	5.0	130	35%
	1.7 oz	8.0	220	33%
Salsa Jalisco	1.7 oz	8.0	220	33%
(Cracker Jack) (*See* POPCORN)				
(Crunch & Munch) (*See* POPCORN)				
(David)				
pumpkin seeds				
all-natural	¼ cup	13.0	160	73%
0.75 oz	1 bag	8.0	90	80%
2-oz bag	1 bag	20.0	250	72%
sunflower kernels				
original	¼ cup	17.0	200	77%
1-oz bag	1 bag	27.0	310	78%
1.75-oz bag	1 bag	28.0	330	76%
ranch..1.75-oz bag	1 bag	26.0	310	75%
sizzlin' BBQ	¼ cup	16.0	190	76%
1.75-oz bag	1 bag	27.0	310	78%
sunflower seeds				
BBQ	¼ cup	15.0	190	71%
0.8-oz bag	1 bag	6.0	70	77%
1.75-oz bag	1 bag	13.0	160	73%
jalapeño hot salsa	¼ cup	15.0	190	71%
1.75-oz bag	1 bag	13.0	160	73%
2.5-oz bag	1 bag	18.0	220	74%
nacho cheese	¼ cup	15.0	180	75%
0.8-oz bag	1 bag	5.0	70	64%
1.75-oz bag	1 bag	12.0	150	72%
original	¼ cup	15.0	190	71%
0.9-oz bag	1 bag	7.0	80	75%
1.75-oz bag	1 bag	13.0	160	73%
2.5-oz bag	1 bag	15.0	190	71%
ranch	¼ cup	15.0	190	71%
0.8-oz bag	1 bag	5.0	70	64%
1.75-oz bag	1 bag	13.0	160	73%
2.5-oz bag	1 bag	17.0	220	70%
reduced-sodium	¼ cup	15.0	190	71%
toasted corn snacks				
BBQ	⅓ cup	5.0	140	32%
0.8-oz bag	1 bag	5.0	100	45%

Food and Description	Amount	Fat Grams	Total Calories	% Fat Calories
1.7-oz bag	1 bag	11.0	230	43%
traditional	⅓ cup	6.0	140	39%
0.8-oz bag	1 bag	5.0	100	45%
1.7-oz bag	1 bag	8.0	230	31%
(Edward & Sons)..Brown Rice Snaps				
buckwheat tamari	8 pieces	–	60	–
cheddar	8 pieces	1.0	60	15%
onion garlic	8 pieces	–	60	–
plain	8 pieces	–	50	–
tamari seaweed	8 pieces	–	60	–
tamari sesame	8 pieces	–	60	–
toasted onion	8 pieces	–	60	–
unsalted sesame	8 pieces	–	60	–
vegetable	8 pieces	0.5	60	8%
(Fisher)..snack mixes				
Nuts & Crunchies				
Bayou Blend				
spicy sweet	1 oz	10.0	150	60%
fiesta	1 oz	7.0	140	45%
golden crisp	1 oz	7.0	140	45%
honey crunch	1 oz	6.0	140	39%
nuts & fruits				
California-style	1 oz	8.0	140	51%
honey crunch	1 oz	6.0	140	39%
pineapple banana	1 oz	8.0	140	51%
raisin cranberry	1 oz	9.0	150	48%
snack mix	1 oz	11.0	150	66%
trail-style	1 oz	11.0	150	66%
(Frito-Lay)				
corn nuts				
BBQ..crunchy	1.7 oz	8.0	220	33%
chile picante..crunchy	1 oz	4.5	130	31%
	1.7 oz	8.0	210	34%
nacho cheese	1 oz	5.0	130	35%
original..crunchy	1.7 oz	8.0	210	34%
ranch..crunchy	1 oz	5.0	130	35%
	1.7 oz	8.0	220	33%
Salsa Jilisco	1.7 oz	8.0	220	33%
Doritos..3D's				
corn snacks				
jalapeño cheddar	1 oz	4.0	130	28%
K.C. Masterpiece	1 oz	5.0	140	32%
Nacho Cheesier				
mini	2 oz	11.0	270	37%
regular	1 oz	5.0	130	35%
zesty sour cream & cheddar..mini	2 oz	11.0	270	37%
Flavor Twists				
cheddar ranch	1 oz	9.0	150	54%
honey BBQ	1 oz	10.0	160	56%

Food and Description	Amount	Fat Grams	Total Calories	% Fat Calories
Funyuns onion-flavored rings	1 oz	7.0	140	45%
Munchos	1 oz	10.0	160	56%
Rold Gold				
snack mixes				
Colossal Cheddar	¾ cup	8.0	160	45%
Munchies	¾ cup	6.0	140	39%
original	¾ cup	8.0	160	45%
sunflower seeds				
kernels..original	1 oz	15.0	180	75%
seeds				
BBQ	1 oz	15.0	200	68%
flamin' hot	1 oz	15.0	180	75%
original	1 oz	15.0	180	75%
(Funyuns) (See (Frito-Lay) in this category)				
(Gardetto's)				
deli-style mustard				
pretzel mix	½ cup	2.0	130	14%
Italian cheese blend	½ cup	5.0	140	32%
original recipe	½ cup	7.0	160	39%
reduced-fat	½ cup	5.0	130	35%
sour cream & onion	½ cup	4.0	130	28%
Special Italian Recipe	½ cup	6.0	150	36%
(Genisoy)				
snack bar				
New York–style cheesecake	2.2 oz	4.0	220	16%
Xtreme carrot cake quake	1.6 oz	7.0	190	33%
Soy Crisps				
apple cinnamon crunch	1 oz	2.0	110	16%
creamy ranch..salted	1 oz	2.0	110	16%
deep sea salt	1 oz	2.0	100	18%
nacho cheese	1 oz	2.0	110	18%
rich cheddar	1 oz	2.0	100	18%
roasted garlic	1 oz	2.0	100	18%
tangy salt 'n' vinegar	1 oz	2.0	100	18%
zesty BBQ	1 oz	2.0	110	18%
trail mix				
soy nut happy trails	1.23 oz	6.0	130	42%
soy nut mountain	1.23 oz	6.0	130	42%
soy nut tropical paradise	1.23 oz	4.0	119	30%
(Hain)				
PureSnax..crudités..all types	1 oz	4.0	120	30%
kettle corn..original	½ cup	2.0	120	15%
Soy Munchies				
caramel	7 pieces	–	40	–
ranch	9 pieces	2.0	60	30%
white cheddar	9 pieces	2.5	60	38%
Zoinks corn snacks	3½ cups	4.5	140	29%
(Health Valley) Cheddar Lites	¾ oz	2.0	40	45%
(Keebler)				
Sunshine..Cheez It				
Party Mix..all flavors	½ cup	4.5	130	31%

Food and Description	Amount	Fat Grams	Total Calories	% Fat Calories
original	½ cup	4.5	130	31%
Snack Mix				
Big Crunch	¾ cup	6.0	110	49%
double cheese	¾ cup	5.0	140	32%
Get Nutty	½ cup	8.0	150	48%
original	½ cup	4.5	130	31%
(Lance)				
cheese balls	1 oz	8.0	150	48%
	1¾ oz	14.0	260	48%
crunchy cheese twists	1⅓ oz	14.0	190	66%
hot fries	⅞ oz	10.0	140	64%
onion rings	1 oz	10.0	210	43%
pork skins				
BBQ	1 oz	9.0	140	58%
plain	1 oz	10.0	150	60%
(Lundberg Family Farms)				
bean & rice chips				
BBQ	1 oz	7.0	140	45%
Pico de Gallo	1 oz	7.0	140	45%
sea salt	1 oz	7.0	140	45%
sesame & seaweed	1 oz	6.0	140	39%
(Max Snax) rice curls				
caramel	33 pieces	3.0	135	20%
cheese & tomato	33 pieces	5.0	160	28%
garlic & basil	35 pieces	4.0	130	26%
nacho cheddar	35 pieces	4.0	140	26%
sour cream & onion	35 pieces	5.0	140	32%
white cheddar	35 pieces	5.0	140	32%
(Michael Season's)				
soy protein chips				
original	1 oz	4.5	110	37%
smoky BBQ	1 cup	9.0	110	74%
spicy ranch	1 cup	5.0	110	74%
sweet organic				
cinnamon twists	1 cup	4.5	130	31%
ultimate cheese puffs				
cheddar cheese	1 oz	13.0	180	65%
white cheddar	1 oz	13.0	180	65%
(Munchos) (See (Frito-Lay) in this section)				
(Nabisco)				
Nabisco Fruit Snacks				
Blue's Clues	1 pkg	–	60	–
other..all flavors	1 pkg	–	80	–
Nabisco Teddy Grahams				
graham snacks				
chocolate	1.25 oz	5.0	150	30%
	1 oz	4.5	130	31%
chocolate honey & cinnamon	4 oz	5.0	150	30%
chocolaty chip	1 oz	4.0	130	28%
mini	1 oz	4.5	140	29%

Food and Description	Amount	Fat Grams	Total Calories	% Fat Calories
cinnamon	1.25 oz	5.0	160	28%
cinnamon..honey & chocolate	3 pieces	4.5	150	27%
Clifford The Big Red Dog	1 oz	4.0	130	28%
Clifford The Big Red Dog cinnamon	1 oz	4.0	120	30%
honey..Dora the Explorer	1 oz	4.0	130	28%
honey..fun-size..all flavors	1 oz	3.5	120	26%
Twigs sesame cheese sticks	1 oz	7.0	150	42%
(Old London)				
Bagel snacks				
cinnamon raisin	5 pieces	1.0	60	15%
garlic	5 pieces	3.0	60	45%
original	5 pieces	3.0	60	45%
poppyseed	5 pieces	3.0	60	45%
melba snacks				
bacon	5 pieces	1.5	60	23%
garlic	5 pieces	1.0	60	15%
Mexicali corn	5 pieces	1.5	60	23%
nacho	5 pieces	2.0	70	26%
onion	5 pieces	1.5	60	23%
rye	5 pieces	1.5	60	23%
sesame	5 pieces	3.0	60	45%
white	5 pieces	1.0	60	15%
whole-grain	5 pieces	1.0	60	15%
party snacks				
honey mustard	⅓ cup	3.0	60	45%
zesty	⅓ cup	3.0	60	45%
waffle snacks				
cheddar	3 pieces	4.0	70	51%
Swiss	3 pieces	4.0	70	51%
(Nutcracker)..trail mix				
honey nut & caramel	1 oz	9.0	160	51%
The Ultimate Tropical	1 oz	8.0	160	45%
(Old Dutch)				
cheese curls				
baked	1 oz	12.0	180	60%
cheez	1 oz	12.0	170	64%
crunchy	1 oz	12.0	170	64%
snack mix...classical mixers	1 oz	5.0	140	32%
(Pepperidge Farm) Goldfish cheddar				
snack mix	1 oz	7.0	160	37%
(Planters)				
Cheez Balls	1 oz	10.0	150	60%
Cheez Curls	1 oz	10.0	150	60%
	1.2 oz pkg	12.0	190	57%
Planters CarbWell				
snack bars				
chocolate crunch	1.35 oz	13.0	180	65%

Food and Description	Amount	Fat Grams	Total Calories	% Fat Calories
nut..crunchy	1.35 oz	13.0	180	65%
peanut butter crunch	1.35 oz	12.0	160	68%
trail mix				
fruit & nut mix	1 oz	7.0	130	48%
honey nut & caramel	1 oz	9.0	160	51%
nut & chocolate	1 oz	11.0	170	58%
nuts..cheese nips				
& mini Ritz	1 oz	12.0	160	68%
nuts..seeds				
& raisins	1 oz	12.0	160	68%
spicy nuts &				
Cajun sticks	1 oz	10.0	150	60%
(Poppycock)	½ cup	10.0	180	50%
(Slim-Fast Meal Options)..trail mix				
chewy fruit & nut bar	2 oz	5.0	220	20%
(Snyder's)				
cheese twist	1 oz	12.0	170	64%
Kruncheez cheese fries	1¼ oz	10.0	200	45%
Onion Toasters	1 oz	10.0	180	50%
pork skins..all flavors	1 oz	4.0	80	45%
(Snyder's of Hanover)				
EatSmart				
corn & rice puffs				
cheddars	1 oz	5.0	130	35%
	0.75 oz	3.5	100	32%
veggie crisps				
cheddar & jalapeño	1 oz	7.0	130	45%
regular	1 oz	7.0	140	45%
	1.5 oz	9.0	190	43%
sun-dried tomato				
& pesto	1 oz	7.0	140	45%
Nibblers				
Cheddar..PB-Zels	1 oz	6.0	130	42%
garlic bread	1 oz	3.0	130	21%
honey mustard				
& onion	1 oz	3.0	130	21%
honey roasted				
PB-Zels	1 oz	6.0	140	39%
no salt..fat-free	1 oz	–	120	–
sourdough..fat-free	1 oz	–	120	–
pieces				
apple cinnamon rounds	1 oz	7.0	140	45%
buttermilk ranch pieces	1 oz	6.0	140	39%
cheddar cheese	1 oz	6.0	130	42%
creamy caramel rounds	1 oz	6.0	140	39%
honey BBQ pretzel pieces	1 oz	5.0	130	35%
honey mustard & onion				
pretzel pieces	1 oz	7.0	140	45%
jalapeño pretzel pieces	1 oz	5.0	140	32%
(SunChips)				
French onion	1 oz	7.0	140	45%

Food and Description	Amount	Fat Grams	Total Calories	% Fat Calories
harvest cheddar	1 oz	6.0	140	39%
original	1 oz	6.0	140	39%
(Sunshine) (*See* (Keebler), within this category)				
(Terra Harvest)				
Chips & Nuggets				
sesame chips	1 oz	10.0	150	60%
sesame salad nuggets/bits	1 oz	10.0	160	56%
Mr. Krispies				
gourmet rice chips				
cheddar salsa	1 oz	3.0	120	23%
classic BBQ	1 oz	2.0	120	15%
sea salt				
& cracked pepper	1 oz	1.5	110	12%
sticks				
honey-roasted soy	1 oz	9.0	150	54%
nacho corn	1 oz	7.0	140	45%
poppy & onion	1 oz	10.0	150	60%
salsa corn	1 oz	6.0	130	42%
sesame				
narrow	1 oz	11.0	160	62%
wide	1 oz	11.0	160	62%
sesame oat bran	1 oz	11.0	160	62%
soy	1 oz	7.0	140	45%
unsalted	1 oz	11.0	160	62%
(Weight Watchers)				
Smart Snackers				
cheese curls	½ oz	3.0	70	39%
(Wise)				
corn snacks/cheese-flavored				
Cheese Waffies	1 oz	8.0	140	51%
Cheez Doodles				
crunchy	1 oz	9.0	150	54%
puffed	1 oz	8.0	150	48%
white cheddar	1 oz	10.0	150	60%
Dipsy Doodles	1 oz	10.0	160	56%
Doodle Heads	1 oz	9.0	150	54%
reduced-fat	1 oz	4.0	120	30%
onion-flavored rings	1 oz	6.0	140	39%
pork rinds				
hot & spicy	½ oz	4.5	70	58%
original	½ oz	5.0	80	56%
sweet & mild BBQ	½ oz	6.0	90	60%
SNAIL/ESCARGOT				
canned				
(Reese)				
Maurice precooked	6 pieces	1.0	45	20%
fresh				
cooked—moist heat	3 oz	1.0	230	4%
raw	3 oz	<1.0	117	4%
SNAP BEAN (*See* GREEN BEAN)				

Food and Description	Amount	Fat Grams	Total Calories	% Fat Calories
SNAPPER				
cooked—dry heat	3 oz	1.5	110	12%
raw	3 oz	1.0	85	11%
SNOW PEA				
fresh..raw	–			
(Frieda's)				
snow peas	1 cup	–	35	–
frozen				
(C&W) microwavable box				
all types	⅔ cup	–	40	–
(La Choy)..snow pea pods	½ pkg	–	35	–
SOCKEYE (See SALMON)				
SODA (See COCKTAIL MIXER; SOFT DRINK; SPORTS DRINK)				
SOFT DRINK (See also FRUIT PUNCH; SOFT DRINK MIX; SPORTS DRINK; TEA; individual juice drink listings)				
(A&W)				
cream soda				
diet	12 fl oz	–	–	–
regular	12 fl oz	–	180	–
root beer				
diet	12 fl oz	–	–	–
regular	12 fl oz	–	170	–
(Arizona)..Cowboy Cocktail				
grape kiwi	8 fl oz	–	120	–
kiwi strawberry	8 fl oz	–	120	–
Mucho Mango	8 fl oz	–	100	–
strawberry punch	8 fl oz	–	120	–
(Barq's)				
crème soda				
red				
diet	8 fl oz	–	3.7	–
regular	8 fl oz	–	115	–
vanilla				
diet	8 fl oz	–	1.4	–
regular	8 fl oz	–	112	–
root beer				
diet	8 fl oz	–	1.3	–
regular	12 fl oz	–	160	–
(Blue Sky)				
ginseng..premium				
Citrus Squeeze	12 fl oz	–	170	–
cola	12 fl oz	–	170	–
cranberry raspberry	12 fl oz	–	160	–
crème soda	12 fl oz	–	150	–
ginger ale	12 fl oz	–	150	–
lemon ginger	12 fl oz	–	130	–
orange ginger	12 fl oz	–	150	–
root beer	12 fl oz	–	180	–
Very Berry Crème	12 fl oz	–	150	–

Food and Description	Amount	Fat Grams	Total Calories	% Fat Calories
natural				
black cherry	12 fl oz	–	150	–
cherry cola	12 fl oz	–	140	–
cherry lemon lime	12 fl oz	–	160	–
cherry vanilla creme	12 fl oz	–	180	–
cola	12 fl oz	–	170	–
Dr. Becker	12 fl oz	–	150	–
ginger ale	12 fl oz	–	160	–
grape	12 fl oz	–	140	–
grapefruit	12 fl oz	–	150	–
Jamaican ginger ale	12 fl oz	–	150	–
lemon lime	12 fl oz	–	140	–
New Century cola	12 fl oz	–	160	–
raspberry	12 fl oz	–	180	–
root beer	12 fl oz	–	170	–
truly orange	12 fl oz	–	150	–
(Canada Dry)				
birch beer..all types	8 fl oz	–	110	–
bitter lemon	8 fl oz	–	100	–
Black Cherry Wish	8 fl oz	–	120	–
Cactus Cooler soda	8 fl oz	–	110	–
California strawberry soda	8 fl oz	–	100	–
club soda				
regular	12 fl oz	–	–	–
sodium-free	12 fl oz	–	–	–
Collins mixer	12 fl oz	–	130	–
ginger ale	12 fl oz	–	120	–
cranberry				
diet	12 fl oz	–	5	–
regular	12 fl oz	–	120	–
seltzer	12 fl oz	–	–	–
tonic water	12 fl oz	–	130	–
diet	12 fl oz	–	–	–
(Canfield's)				
cherry fudge soda	12 fl oz	–	–	–
chocolate fudge soda	12 fl oz	–	–	–
(Clearly Canadian)				
apple	8 fl oz	–	80	–
blackberry	8 fl oz	–	100	–
cherry	8 fl oz	–	90	–
cranberry	8 fl oz	–	90	–
loganberry	8 fl oz	–	90	–
peach	8 fl oz	–	90	–
raspberry	8 fl oz	–	80	–
strawberry	8 fl oz	–	80	–
(Coca-Cola)				
Coca-Cola				
cherry				
diet	8 fl oz	–	1	–
regular	8 fl oz	–	125	–

Food and Description	Amount	Fat Grams	Total Calories	% Fat Calories
Citra	8 fl oz	–	91	–
Classic..all types	8 fl oz	–	97	–
Coke 2	8 fl oz	–	105	–
Diet Coke..all types	8 fl oz	–	1	–
Vanilla Coke	12 fl oz	–	–	–
Fanta				
grape	8 fl oz	–	120	–
strawberry	12 fl oz	–	140	–
Fresca	8 fl oz	–	–	–
Mello Yello				
diet	8 fl oz	–	3	–
regular	8 fl oz	–	118	–
Minute Maid				
black cherry soda	8 fl oz	–	110	–
blueberry	8 fl oz	–	110	–
fruit punch..carbonated	8 fl oz	–	113	–
grape soda	8 fl oz	–	113	–
grapefruit soda	8 fl oz	–	108	–
lemonade	8 fl oz	–	106	–
orange soda				
diet	8 fl oz	–	2	–
regular	8 fl oz	–	118	–
Mr. Pibb				
diet	8 fl oz	–	1	–
regular	8 fl oz	–	97	–
Sprite				
diet	8 fl oz	–	3	–
regular	8 fl oz	–	96	–
Surge	8 fl oz	–	116	–
Tab	8 fl oz	–	1	–
(Crush)				
cherry	8 fl oz	–	120	–
fruity red	8 fl oz	–	120	–
grape	8 fl oz	–	120	–
orange				
regular	12 fl oz	–	180	–
peach	8 fl oz	–	120	–
pineapple	8 fl oz	–	120	–
strawberry	8 fl oz	–	110	–
tropical punch	8 fl oz	–	120	–
(Dr Pepper)				
diet..all types	12 fl oz	–	–	–
regular..all types	12 fl oz	–	160	–
(Faygo)				
crème cola				
rock & rye	8 fl oz	–	120	–
vanilla	8 fl oz	–	110	–
Frosh				
diet	12 fl oz	–	–	–
ginger ale	8 fl oz	–	130	–

Food and Description	Amount	Fat Grams	Total Calories	% Fat Calories
grape	12 fl oz	–	200	–
Moon Mist	12 fl oz	–	180	–
orange				
diet	8 fl oz	–	–	–
regular	8 fl oz	–	130	–
root beer				
diet draft style	8 fl oz	–	–	–
regular	12 fl oz	–	170	–
Twist	8 fl oz	–	110	–
(Health Valley)				
ginger ale	12 fl oz	–	160	–
root beer				
old-fashioned	12 fl oz	–	160	–
sarsaparilla	12 fl oz	–	160	–
(Hires)				
cream soda				
diet	8 fl oz	–	–	–
regular	8 fl oz	–	130	–
root beer				
diet	8 fl oz	–	–	–
regular	8 fl oz	–	130	–
(IBC)				
black cherry	12 fl oz	–	160	–
cherry cola	12 fl oz	–	160	–
cream soda				
diet	12 fl oz	–	–	–
regular	12 fl oz	–	190	–
root beer				
diet	12 fl oz	–	–	–
regular	12 fl oz	–	180	–
(Jolt) cola	12 fl oz	–	150	–
(Jones)..soda				
soda				
Naturals				
Bada Bing!	12 fl oz	–	90	–
banana berry	12 fl oz	–	90	–
berry	12 fl oz	–	90	–
berry white	12 fl oz	–	110	–
Bohemian Raspberry	12 fl oz	–	40	–
Dave	12 fl oz	–	80	–
D'peach Mode	12 fl oz	–	90	–
Fu Cran Fu	12 fl oz	–	100	–
limes with orange	12 fl oz	–	110	–
Strawberry Manilow	12 fl oz	–	80	–
regular				
berry lemonade	12 fl oz	–	190	–
blue bubblegum	12 fl oz	–	190	–
cherry	12 fl oz	–	180	–
chocolate fudge	12 fl oz	–	180	–
cream soda	12 fl oz	–	190	–

Food and Description	Amount	Fat Grams	Total Calories	% Fat Calories
crushed melon	12 fl oz	–	190	–
fufu berry	12 fl oz	–	190	–
grape	12 fl oz	–	180	–
green apple	12 fl oz	–	180	–
fruit punch	12 fl oz	–	190	–
lemon drop	12 fl oz	–	190	–
orange & cream	12 fl oz	–	190	–
root beer	12 fl oz	–	180	–
strawberry lime	12 fl oz	–	190	–
vanilla cola	12 fl oz	–	170	–
sugar-free				
black cherry	12 fl oz	–	–	–
cream soda	12 fl oz	–	–	–
ginger ale	12 fl oz	–	–	–
root beer	12 fl oz	–	–	–
(Kool-Aid)				
Bursts..all flavors	6.75 fl oz	–	100	–
Crystal Light/low-calorie	8 fl oz	–	5	–
(Mountain Dew)				
diet				
caffeine-free	8 fl oz	–	–	–
	12 fl oz	–	–	–
regular	8 fl oz	–	–	–
	12 fl oz	–	–	–
regular				
caffeine-free	8 fl oz	–	110	–
	12 fl oz	–	170	–
regular	8 fl oz	–	110	–
	12 fl oz	–	170	–
(Mug)				
cream soda				
diet	8 fl oz	–	–	–
	12 fl oz	–	5	–
regular	8 fl oz	–	120	–
	12 fl oz	–	170	–
root beer				
diet	8 fl oz	–	–	–
	12 fl oz	–	–	–
regular	8 fl oz	–	100	–
	12 fl oz	–	160	–
(Nehi)				
cream	8 fl oz	–	120	–
fruit punch	8 fl oz	–	120	–
ginger ale	8 fl oz	–	90	–
grape	8 fl oz	–	120	–
orange	8 fl oz	–	130	–
peach	8 fl oz	–	130	–
pineapple	8 fl oz	–	130	–
root beer	8 fl oz	–	120	–
strawberry	8 fl oz	–	120	–

Food and Description	Amount	Fat Grams	Total Calories	% Fat Calories
(Pepsi)				
diet				
caffeine-free	8 fl oz	–	–	–
	12 fl oz	–	–	–
regular	8 fl oz	–	–	–
	12 fl oz	–	–	–
Pepsi 1	8 fl oz	–	1	–
	12 fl oz	–	1	–
Pepsi Twist				
diet	8 fl oz	–	–	–
regular	12 fl oz	–	100	–
Pepsi Vanilla				
diet	8 fl oz	–	–	–
regular	8 fl oz	–	110	–
regular Pepsi				
caffeine-free	8 fl oz	–	100	–
	12 fl oz	–	150	–
regular	12 fl oz	–	150	–
wild cherry				
diet	12 fl oz	–	–	–
regular	8 fl oz	–	110	–
	12 fl oz	–	160	–
(R. W. Knudsen)				
Spritzers				
black cherry	12 fl oz	–	170	–
boysenberry	12 fl oz	–	160	–
cherry cola	12 fl oz	–	170	–
cranberry	12 fl oz	–	190	–
ginger ale	12 fl oz	–	160	–
grape	12 fl oz	–	170	–
Jamaican lemonade	12 fl oz	–	170	–
kiwi lime	12 fl oz	–	130	–
lemon lime	12 fl oz	–	170	–
mandarin lime	12 fl oz	–	170	–
Mango Fandango	12 fl oz	–	190	–
orange passionfruit	12 fl oz	–	160	–
peach	12 fl oz	–	160	–
red raspberry	12 fl oz	–	170	–
strawberry	12 fl oz	–	170	–
tangerine	12 fl oz	–	170	–
vanilla crème	12 fl oz	–	160	–
(Royal Crown)				
cherry cola	8 fl oz	–	110	–
cola				
diet..all types	8 fl oz	–	–	–
regular..all types	8 fl oz	–	110	–
(Schweppes)				
bitter lemon	8 fl oz	–	110	–
club soda..all types	8 fl oz	–	–	–
sodium-free	8 fl oz	–	–	–

Food and Description	Amount	Fat Grams	Total Calories	% Fat Calories
Collins mixer	8 fl oz	–	90	–
ginger ale				
plain				
diet	8 fl oz	–	–	–
regular	8 fl oz	–	90	–
raspberry				
diet	8 fl oz	–	–	–
regular	8 fl oz	–	90	–
ginger beer	8 fl oz	–	90	–
grape soda	8 fl oz	–	120	–
grapefruit soda	8 fl oz	–	100	–
lemon sour	8 fl oz	–	100	–
seltzer..all flavors	8 fl oz	–	–	–
tonic water				
diet..all flavors	8 fl oz	–	–	–
regular..all flavors	8 fl oz	–	80	–
(Seagram's)				
club soda	8 fl oz	–	–	–
ginger ale				
diet..all flavors	8 fl oz	–	2	–
regular..all flavors	8 fl oz	–	90	–
seltzer..naturals				
black cherry	8 fl oz	–	2	–
other flavors	8 fl oz	–	1	–
tonic water				
diet	8 fl oz	–	3	–
plain	8 fl oz	–	83	–
w/a twist of lime	8 fl oz	–	93	–
(7-Up)				
cherry				
diet	12 fl oz	–	–	–
regular	12 fl oz	–	160	–
regular				
diet	12 fl oz	–	–	–
regular	12 fl oz	–	140	–
7-Up Plus				
mixed berry	12 fl oz	–	10	–
(Sierra Mist)				
diet	8 fl oz	–	–	–
regular	8 fl oz	–	100	–
(Sioux City) sarsaparilla				
bottled	12 fl oz	–	110	–
canned	16 fl oz	–	170	–
(Slice)				
cherry lime	12 fl oz	–	160	–
cherry spice	12 fl oz	–	150	–
cola				
diet	12 fl oz	–	–	–
regular	12 fl oz	–	160	–
Dr. Slice	12 fl oz	–	140	–

Food and Description	Amount	Fat Grams	Total Calories	% Fat Calories
fruit punch	12 fl oz	–	190	–
grape soda	12 fl oz	–	190	–
lemon lime soda				
diet	12 fl oz	–	–	–
regular	12 fl oz	–	150	–
orange soda				
diet	8 fl oz	–	–	–
	12 fl oz	–	–	–
w/caffeine	8 fl oz	–	130	–
	12 fl oz	–	170	–
w/o caffeine	12 fl oz	–	190	–
pineapple soda	12 fl oz	–	190	–
red	12 fl oz	–	190	–
strawberry soda	12 fl oz	–	170	–
(Snapple) 16-oz sodas				
cherry lime rickey	8 fl oz	–	110	–
creme d'vanilla	8 fl oz	–	–	–
French cherry	8 fl oz	–	120	–
true root beer	8 fl oz	–	110	–
(Squirt)				
original				
diet	8 fl oz	–	–	–
regular	12 fl oz	–	150	–
ruby red				
diet	8 fl oz	–	–	–
regular	8 fl oz	–	110	–
(Stewart's)				
country orange n' cream	12 fl oz	–	190	–
cream ale	12 fl oz	–	180	–
ginger beer	12 fl oz	–	200	–
root beer				
diet	12 fl oz	–	–	–
original	12 fl oz	–	160	–
(Sun Drop)				
cherry	12 fl oz	–	180	–
regular				
diet	12 fl oz	–	20	–
regular	12 fl oz	–	200	–
(Sunkist)				
cherry	8 fl oz	–	130	–
citrus				
diet	8 fl oz	–	–	–
regular	8 fl oz	–	90	–
fruit punch	8 fl oz	–	120	–
grape	8 fl oz	–	130	–
lemonade				
diet sparkling	8 fl oz	–	–	–
regular	8 fl oz	–	120	–
orange				
diet	8 fl oz	–	–	–

Food and Description	Amount	Fat Grams	Total Calories	% Fat Calories
regular	8 fl oz	–	130	–
(Vernor's) ginger soda				
diet	8 fl oz	–	–	–
regular	8 fl oz	–	100	–
	12 fl oz	–	150	–
(Welch's) sparkling sodas				
apple	8 fl oz	–	200	–
fruit punch	8 fl oz	–	210	–
grape	8 fl oz	–	130	–
lemonade	8 fl oz	–	110	–
orange	8 fl oz	–	120	–
peach	8 fl oz	–	130	–
pineapple	8 fl oz	–	130	–
strawberry	8 fl oz	–	120	–
(Yoo-Hoo)				
chocolate	8 fl oz	1.0	130	7%
double fudge	8 fl oz	1.0	140	6%
Dyna-Mocha	8 fl oz	0.5	150	3%
light	8 fl oz	1.0	70	13%
strawberry	8 fl oz	0.5	130	3%
SOFT DRINK MIX (See also FRUIT PUNCH; SOFT DRINK; SPORTS DRINK; individual fruit drink listings)				
(Crystal Light)				
all flavors..prepared	8 fl oz	–	5	–
(Kool-Aid)				
sugar-free/low-calorie				
all flavors	8 fl oz	–	5	–
prepared w/water				
sugar-sweetened..all flavors				
prepared w/water	8 fl oz	–	60	–
unsweetened..all flavors				
prepared w/sugar & water	8 fl oz	–	100	–
SOLE				
baked w/butter	3 oz	6.0	120	45%
cooked—dry heat	3 oz	1.0	105	91%
raw	3 oz	1.0	80	11%
SORBET (See FRUIT ICES, BARS & POPS; SHERBET)				
SORGHUM..whole grain	1 cup	6.0	650	8%
SORGHUM SYRUP				
cane & maple	1 Tbs	–	53	–
	1 cup	–	794	–
regular	1 Tbs	–	53	–
	1 cup	–	848	–
table blend	1 Tbs	–	59	–
	1 cup	–	941	–

SORREL (See DOCK)
SOUP
(NOTE: Unless stated otherwise, condensed soups were prepared as directed with water. If prepared with milk, whole milk was used unless noted otherwise. Ready-to-serve soups were heated as directed with no added liquid.)

Food and Description	Amount	Fat Grams	Total Calories	% Fat Calories
■ **CANNED**				
(Amy's)				
organic..ready-to-serve..unless				
otherwise noted				
alphabet	1 cup	0.5	80	6%
black bean vegetable	1 cup	1.5	130	10%
butternut squash				
low-fat	1 cup	2.5	100	23%
chunky tomato bisque	1 cup	3.5	120	26%
cream of mushroom				
semi-condensed	1 cup	9.0	140	58%
cream of tomato				
low-fat	1 cup	2.0	100	18%
lentil	1 cup	4.5	150	27%
lentil vegetable				
light in sodium	1 cup	4.0	150	24%
regular	1 cup	4.0	150	24%
no chicken noodle..low-fat	1 cup	3.0	90	30%
pasta & 3-bean	1 cup	5.0	130	35%
split pea..low-fat	1 cup	–	100	–
vegetable barley..low-fat	1 cup	1.0	70	13%
(Anderson's)				
split pea..ready-to-serve	1 cup	–	130	–
(Baxter's) ready-to-serve				
asparagus, cream of	1 cup	10.0	150	60%
country garden/99% fat-free	1 cup	0.5	70	6%
lobster bisque	1 cup	6.0	120	45%
minestrone/99% fat-free	1 cup	1.0	80	11%
onion/99% fat-free	1 cup	0.5	70	6%
potato & leek/100% fat-free	1 cup	–	60	–
(Campbell's)				
condensed/unprepared				
Healthy Request				
bean w/ham & bacon	½ cup	2.0	150	11%
chicken, cream of	½ cup	2.0	70	26%
chicken & broccoli, cream of	½ cup	2.5	80	28%
chicken & stars	½ cup	2.0	70	26%
chicken noodle	½ cup	2.0	60	30%
chicken rice	½ cup	2.0	80	23%
chicken vegetable	½ cup	2.0	80	23%
cream of celery	½ cup	2.0	70	26%
cream of chicken	½ cup	2.0	70	26%
cream of chicken & broccoli	½ cup	2.5	70	32%
cream of mushroom	½ cup	2.5	70	32%
hearty chicken				
w/white & wild rice	½ cup	2.0	110	16%
minestrone	½ cup	0.5	80	6%
tomato	½ cup	1.5	90	15%
vegetable	½ cup	1.0	90	10%
vegetable beef	½ cup	1.0	100	9%

Food and Description	Amount	Fat Grams	Total Calories	% Fat Calories
original soups				
98% fat-free..prepared				
broccoli cheese	½ cup	1.5	70	19%
cream of				
broccoli	½ cup	1.0	60	15%
celery	½ cup	3.0	60	45%
chicken	½ cup	2.0	70	26%
mushroom	½ cup	3.0	70	39%
New England				
clam chowder	½ cup	2.0	80	23%
bean w/bacon	½ cup	4.0	170	21%
beef broth..double strength	½ cup	–	15	–
beef consommé	½ cup	–	20	–
beef noodle	½ cup	2.5	70	32%
beef soup w/vegetables				
& barley	½ cup	1.5	90	15%
beefy mushroom	½ cup	2.0	50	36%
black bean	½ cup	2.0	110	16%
broccoli cheese	½ cup	4.5	100	41%
California-style vegetable	½ cup	0.5	70	6%
cheddar cheese	½ cup	4.5	100	41%
chicken alphabet				
w/vegetables	½ cup	2.0	80	23%
chicken & dumplings	½ cup	3.0	80	34%
chicken & stars	½ cup	2.0	80	23%
chicken broth soup	½ cup	1.0	20	45%
chicken gumbo	½ cup	1.0	60	15%
chicken noodle	½ cup	1.5	60	23%
chicken noodle/26-oz can	½ cup	2.0	60	30%
chicken noodle o's	½ cup	2.5	80	28%
chicken w/rice	½ cup	1.5	80	17%
chicken vegetable	½ cup	1.0	80	11%
chicken w/white & wild rice	½ cup	2.0	70	26%
chicken won ton	½ cup	1.0	45	20%
consommé	½ cup	–	25	–
cream of asparagus	½ cup	7.0	100	63%
cream of broccoli	½ cup	3.5	90	35%
cream of celery	½ cup	6.0	100	54%
cream of chicken	½ cup	7.0	120	52%
cream of chicken mushroom	½ cup	8.0	120	60%
cream of chicken w/herbs	½ cup	4.0	90	40%
cream of mushroom	½ cup	7.0	110	57%
cream of mushroom				
w/roasted garlic	½ cup	7.0	100	63%
cream of onion	½ cup	5.0	100	45%
cream of potato	½ cup	3.0	100	27%
cream of shrimp	½ cup	6.0	90	60%
creamy chicken noodle	½ cup	7.0	120	53%
creamy mushroom				
& roasted garlic	½ cup	2.0	70	26%

Food and Description	Amount	Fat Grams	Total Calories	% Fat Calories
curly chicken noodle	½ cup	2.0	80	23%
double noodle	½ cup	2.0	90	20%
fiesta chili beef w/beans	½ cup	5.0	170	26%
fiesta nacho cheese	½ cup	8.0	120	60%
French onion	½ cup	1.5	45	30%
fun shapes	½ cup	1.5	80	17%
golden mushroom	½ cup	3.5	80	39%
Goldfish				
pasta	½ cup	0.5	130	3%
pasta..w/chicken				
in chicken broth	½ cup	1.5	70	19%
green pea	½ cup	3.0	180	15%
hearty vegetable w/pasta	½ cup	0.5	90	5%
home-style chicken noodle	½ cup	2.0	70	26%
Manhattan-style				
clam chowder	½ cup	0.5	70	6%
mega noodle in				
chicken broth	½ cup	1.5	80	17%
minestrone	½ cup	1.0	90	10%
New England clam chowder	½ cup	2.5	90	25%
old-fashioned				
tomato rice	½ cup	2.0	110	16%
vegetable	½ cup	1.5	80	17%
oyster stew	½ cup	6.0	80	68%
pepper pot	½ cup	4.0	90	40%
Scotch broth soup	½ cup	2.0	70	26%
Southwest-style				
chicken vegetable	½ cup	1.0	110	8%
split pea w/ham	½ cup	3.5	180	18%
tomato	½ cup	–	90	–
tomato bisque	½ cup	• 3.5	130	24%
turkey noodle	½ cup	2.0	70	26%
turkey vegetable	½ cup	2.5	80	28%
vegetable	½ cup	0.5	100	5%
vegetable beef	½ cup	1.0	80	23%
vegetarian vegetable	½ cup	0.5	90	5%
ready-to-serve				
chunky				
baked potato				
w/bacon bits & chives	1 cup	5.0	160	28%
baked potato				
w/cheddar & bacon bits	1 cup	8.0	180	40%
baked potato				
w/steak & cheese	1 cup	9.0	210	39%
beef				
w/country vegetables	1 cup	3.0	160	17%
beef				
cheese tortellini				
w/chicken & vegetables	1 cup	2.0	110	16%
w/white & wild rice	1 cup	2.5	150	15%

Food and Description	Amount	Fat Grams	Total Calories	% Fat Calories
chicken & dumplings	1 cup	9.0	190	43%
chicken broccoli				
& cheese potato	1 cup	12.0	190	57%
chicken corn chowder	1 cup	13.0	230	51%
chicken mushroom chowder	1 cup	17.0	230	67%
clam chowder				
Manhattan-style	1 cup	3.5	130	24%
classic chicken noodle	1 cup	2.5	100	23%
grilled chicken				
& sausage gumbo	1 cup	2.5	140	16%
w/vegetables & pasta	1 cup	1.5	110	12%
grilled sirloin steak				
w/hearty vegetables	1 cup	2.0	130	14%
hearty bean 'n' ham	1 cup	2.0	180	10%
hearty chicken				
w/vegetables	1 cup	1.5	100	14%
hearty vegetables				
w/pasta	1 cup	2.0	130	14%
herb-roasted chicken				
w/potatoes & garlic	1 cup	1.5	110	12%
honey-roasted ham				
w/potatoes	1 cup	2.5	130	17%
New England clam chowder	1 cup	14.0	240	53%
old-fashioned potato				
ham chowder	1 cup	11.0	190	52%
old-fashioned				
vegetable beef	1 cup	2.5	130	14%
pepper steak	1 cup	1.5	120	7%
Salisbury steak mushrooms				
& onion	1 cup	4.5	150	27%
savory chicken				
w/rice (white & wild)	1 cup	1.5	120	11%
seasoned rib roast				
w/potatoes & herbs	1 cup	1.0	110	8%
sirloin burger				
w/country vegetables	1 cup	8.0	180	40%
slow-roasted beef				
w/mushrooms	1 cup	1.5	120	11%
split pea 'n' ham	1 cup	2.5	170	11%
steak & potato	1 cup	3.5	150	21%
tomato cheese ravioli				
w/vegetables	1 cup	3.5	150	21%
vegetable	1 cup	3.5	130	12%
Healthy Request				
chicken noodle	½ cup	2.0	60	30%
chicken rice	½ cup	2.0	80	23%
cream				
of celery	½ cup	2.0	70	26%
of chicken	½ cup	2.5	70	32%
of mushroom	½ cup	2.5	70	32%

Food and Description	Amount	Fat Grams	Total Calories	% Fat Calories
hearty				
chicken..w/white				
& wild rice	1 cup	2.0	110	16%
minestrone	1 cup	0.5	80	6%
tomato ravioli	1 cup	1.5	90	10%
vegetable	1 cup	1.0	100	9%
vegetable beef	1 cup	1.0	90	10%
Kitchen Classics				
bean w/bacon	1 cup	4.0	180	20%
chicken noodle	1 cup	1.0	90	10%
chicken w/white				
& wild rice	1 cup	1.0	100	9%
cream of potato	1 cup	8.0	160	45%
creamy tomato	1 cup	3.5	140	19%
lentil	1 cup	0.5	120	4%
minestrone	1 cup	0.5	110	4%
New England clam chowder	1 cup	16.0	240	60%
tomato	1 cup	–	100	–
vegetable	1 cup	0.5	100	5%
Select soup				
98% fat-free				
New England				
clam chowder	1 cup	1.5	110	12%
bean & ham	1 cup	1.0	170	5%
beef w/portabello mushrooms				
and rice	1 cup	1.5	110	12%
beef w/roasted barley	1 cup	1.5	150	9%
chicken & pasta				
w/roasted garlic	1 cup	1.5	110	12%
chicken & rice	1 cup	1.0	100	9%
chicken vegetable	1 cup	0.5	100	5%
chicken w/egg noodles	1 cup	1.5	100	14%
creamy				
chicken Alfredo	1 cup	12.0	220	49%
potato w/roasted garlic	1 cup	9.0	170	37%
fiesta vegetable	1 cup	0.5	120	4%
grilled chicken w/sun-dried				
tomatoes & mushrooms	1 cup	1.0	110	8%
herbed chicken				
w/roasted vegetables	1 cup	0.5	90	5%
honey-roasted chicken				
w/golden potatoes	1 cup	1.0	100	9%
Italian-style wedding soup	1 cup	2.5	120	19%
minestrone	1 cup	–	100	–
New England clam chowder	1 cup	11.0	200	50%
roasted chicken				
w/long-grain & wild rice	1 cup	0.5	100	5%
w/rotini & penne pasta	1 cup	1.0	100	9%
rosemary chicken				
w/roasted potatoes	1 cup	0.5	100	5%

Food and Description	Amount	Fat Grams	Total Calories	% Fat Calories
savory lentil	1 cup	0.5	140	3%
split pea w/ham	1 cup	1.0	160	6%
tomato garden	1 cup	0.5	100	5%
vegetable	1 cup	0.5	100	5%
vegetable beef	1 cup	2.0	110	16%
Soup At Hand				
blended vegetable				
medley	1 pkg	2.0	110	16%
chicken & stars	1 pkg	0.5	60	8%
chicken w/mini noodles	1 pkg	1.5	80	17%
classic tomato	1 pkg	–	120	–
cream of broccoli	1 pkg	8.0	160	45%
creamy				
chicken	1 pkg	4.0	190	19%
tomato	1 pkg	4.0	190	19%
Mexican-style fiesta	1 pkg	4.0	190	19%
New England clam chowder	1 pkg	6.0	130	42%
pizza soup	l pkg	0.5	130	3%
velvety potato	1 pkg	6.0	150	36%
(Doxsee) New England clam chowder/condensed				
prepared w/skim milk	1 cup	2.0	130	14%
(Gold's) ready-to-serve				
borscht				
low-cal	1 cup	–	20	–
original	1 cup	–	100	–
schav	1 cup	–	25	–
(Gorton's)				
New England clam chowder				
condensed/unprepared	½ cup	1.0	70	13%
ready-to-serve	1 cup	6.0	140	39%
(Hain) ready-to-serve				
chicken				
broth				
no salt added	8.75 oz	5.0	60	75%
regular	8.75 oz	6.0	70	77%
noodle				
no salt added	9.5 oz	4.0	120	30%
regular	9.5 oz	4.0	120	30%
creamy mushroom	9.25 oz	4.0	110	33%
Italian vegetable pasta				
low-sodium	9.5 oz	6.0	140	39%
regular	9.5 oz	5.0	160	28%
minestrone				
no salt added	9.5 oz	4.0	160	23%
regular	9.5 oz	2.0	170	11%
mushroom barley	9.5 oz	2.0	100	18%
New England clam chowder	9.5 oz	4.0	180	20%
split pea				
no salt added	9.5 oz	1.0	170	5%
regular	9.5 oz	1.0	170	5%

Food and Description	Amount	Fat Grams	Total Calories	% Fat Calories
turkey rice				
no salt added	9.5 oz	4.0	120	30%
regular	9.5 oz	3.0	100	27%
vegetable broth				
low sodium	9.5 oz	–	40	–
regular	9.5 oz	–	45	–
vegetarian				
lentil				
no salt added	9.5 oz	3.0	160	17%
regular	9.5 oz	3.0	160	17%
original				
no salt added	9.5 oz	5.0	150	30%
regular	9.5 oz	4.0	140	26%
(Hanover)..ready-to-serve				
Maryland crab	1 cup	0.7	70	9%
(Health Valley) ready-to-serve				
broth				
fat-free				
beef	1 cup	–	10	–
beef-flavored	1 cup	–	10	–
chicken	1 cup	–	30	–
mushroom	1 cup	–	10	–
vegetable	1 cup	–	15	–
low-fat chicken	1 cup	1.5	35	39%
no salt added				
beef-flavored..fat-free	1 cup	–	10	–
chicken	1 cup	1.5	35	39%
organic				
beef-flavored	1 cup	–	15	–
chicken	1 cup	1.0	25	36%
vegetable	1 cup	–	15	–
soups				
98% fat-free				
chicken noodle	1 cup	2.0	130	14%
fat-free soup cups				
chicken-flavored noodles				
w/vegetables	½ cup	–	110	–
corn chowder				
w/tomatoes	½ cup	–	100	–
creamy potato w/broccoli	⅓ cup	–	80	–
garden split w/carrots	⅓ cup	–	110	8%
lentil w/couscous	⅓ cup	–	130	–
pasta Italiano	½ cup	–	140	–
spicy black bean				
w/couscous	⅓ cup	–	130	–
zesty black bean w/rice	⅓ cup	–	100	–
soups..fat-free				
5-bean vegetable	1 cup	–	140	–
14-garden vegetable	1 cup	–	80	–
black bean				
& vegetable	1 cup	–	110	–

Food and Description	Amount	Fat Grams	Total Calories	% Fat Calories
corn & vegetable	1 cup	–	70	–
Italian minestrone	1 cup	–	90	–
lentil & carrots	1 cup	–	100	–
pasta				
cacciatore	1 cup	–	100	–
fagioli	1 cup	–	120	–
romano	1 cup	–	100	–
rotini & vegetable	1 cup	–	70	–
split pea & carrots	1 cup	–	110	–
super broccoli carotene	1 cup	–	70	–
tomato vegetable	1 cup	–	80	–
vegetable barley	1 cup	–	90	–
soups..no salt added..organic				
black bean	1 cup	1.0	130	7%
lentil	1 cup	1.0	100	9%
minestrone	1 cup	–	70	–
mushroom barley	1 cup	–	70	–
potato leek	1 cup	–	70	–
split pea	1 cup	–	110	–
tomato	1 cup	–	80	–
vegetable	1 cup	–	80	–
soups..organic				
black bean	1 cup	1.0	130	7%
lentil	1 cup	1.0	100	9%
minestrone	1 cup	–	110	–
mushroom barley	1 cup	–	70	–
potato & leek	1 cup	–	70	–
split pea	1 cup	–	110	–
tomato	1 cup	–	80	–
vegetable	1 cup	–	89	–
(Healthy Choice) Ready-to-Serve				
bean & ham	1 cup	2.5	170	13%
beef & potato	1 cup	1.0	110	8%
chicken				
corn chowder	1 cup	2.0	140	13%
fiesta	1 cup	2.0	100	18%
roasted Italian-style	1 cup	2.0	120	15%
chicken..hearty	1 cup	3.0	130	21%
chicken noodle	1 cup	2.0	120	15%
chicken				
& dumplings	1 cup	2.0	130	14%
& pasta	1 cup	2.0	110	16%
& rice	1 cup	2.0	100	18%
& roasted garlic	1 cup	2.0	120	15%
chili beef	1 cup	2.0	170	11%
clam chowder	1 cup	1.5	110	12%
country vegetable	1 cup	0.5	100	5%
creamy potato	1 cup	2.0	120	15%
creamy tomato	1 cup	1.5	100	14%
fiesta chicken	1 cup	1.0	90	10%
garden vegetable	1 cup	1.0	120	8%

Food and Description	Amount	Fat Grams	Total Calories	% Fat Calories
hearty chicken	1 cup	2.0	120	15%
Italian bean & pasta	1 cup	1.5	100	14%
lentil	1 cup	1.0	145	6%
minestrone	1 cup	1.0	110	8%
mushroom, cream of	1 cup	1.0	80	11%
old-fashioned chicken noodle	1 cup	2.0	110	16%
split pea & ham	1 cup	2.5	170	13%
turkey w/wild rice	1 cup	1.5	90	15%
vegetable				
clam	1 cup	1.0	80	11%
country	1 cup	1.0	105	9%
garden	1 cup	1.0	120	8%
vegetable beef	1 cup	1.0	130	7%
zesty gumbo	1 cup	2.0	100	18%
(Imagine)..organic				
creamy				
broccoli	1 cup	1.5	70	19%
butternut squash	1 cup	2.0	120	90%
portobello mushroom	1 cup	3.0	80	34%
potato leek	1 cup	2.5	90	25%
sweet corn	1 cup	3.0	100	27%
tomato	1 cup	1.5	90	15%
free-range chicken broth	1 cup	0.5	20	23%
no-chicken broth	1 cup	0.5	20	23%
vegetable broth	1 cup	0.5	30	15%
(Mother's)				
ready-to-serve				
borscht				
low-cal	1 cup	–	25	–
old-fashioned	1 cup	–	100	–
matzo balls				
in broth				
15.5-oz can	1 cup			
	w/3 balls	6.0	170	32%
24-oz can	1 cup			
	w/3 balls	5.0	170	26%
(Pepperidge Farm)				
condensed...undiluted				
black bean	⅔ cup	2.5	120	19%
chicken curry	⅔ cup	8.0	170	42%
chicken w/wild rice	⅔ cup	3.5	80	39%
consommé..madrilene	⅔ cup	0.5	50	9%
French onion	⅔ cup	1.0	50	18%
gazpacho	⅔ cup	2.0	70	20%
mushroom shiitake	⅔ cup	3.0	80	34%
New England clam chowder	⅔ cup	8.0	160	45%
watercress	⅔ cup	3.5	80	39%
(Phillips)				
seafood soup				
crab..Maryland-style..tub	1 cup	0.5	70	6%

Food and Description	Amount	Fat Grams	Total Calories	% Fat Calories
cream of crab				
restaurant recipe..tub	1 cup	28.0	340	74%
(Progresso)				
ready-to-serve				
99% fat-free soups				
beef barley	1 cup	2.0	130	14%
chicken noodle	1 cup	1.5	90	15%
minestrone	1 cup	1.0	110	8%
New England				
clam chowder	1 cup	1.5	110	12%
roasted chicken				
w/wild rice	1 cup	1.5	90	15%
vegetable classic lentil	1 cup	1.5	130	10%
white cheddar potato	1 cup	1.5	100	14%
regular soups				
basil rotini tomato	1 cup	1.5	120	11%
bean & ham	1 cup	2.0	160	11%
beef barley	1 cup	4.0	130	28%
beef minestrone	1 cup	3.0	140	19%
cheese & herb				
tortellini tomato	1 cup	3.0	140	19%
chickarina	1 cup	5.0	130	35%
chicken				
barley	1 cup	1.5	110	12%
broth	1 cup	1.5	20	68%
creamy cheddar	1 cup	9.0	210	39%
hearty	10.5 oz	2.5	120	19%
home-style w/vegetables	1 cup	1.5	90	15%
minestrone	1 cup	1.5	110	12%
vegetable	1 cup	1.5	90	15%
chicken & wild rice	1 cup	1.5	100	14%
chicken noodle	1 cup	2.0	90	20%
chicken rice w/vegetables	1 cup	2.0	90	20%
clam chowder				
Manhattan	1 cup	2.0	110	16%
New England	1 cup	13.0	230	51%
creamy				
mushroom	1 cup	14.0	180	70%
tomato garlic	1 cup	6.0	150	36%
escarole in chicken broth	1 cup	1.0	25	36%
French onion	1 cup	1.5	50	27%
hearty				
black bean	1 cup	1.5	170	8%
chicken & rotini	1 cup	1.5	90	15%
penne in chicken broth	1 cup	1.0	80	11%
herb & rotini vegetable	1 cup	1.0	100	9%
herb & shell minestrone	1 cup	1.5	120	11%
lentil	1 cup	2.0	140	13%
macaroni & bean	1 cup	4.0	160	23%
minestrone...beef	1 cup	3.0	140	19%

Food and Description	Amount	Fat Grams	Total Calories	% Fat Calories
oregano penne Italian-style	1 cup	2.0	90	20%
penne in chicken broth	1 cup	1.0	80	11%
peppercorn penne vegetable	1 cup	2.0	110	16%
potato broccoli & cheese chowder	1 cup	6.0	160	34%
potato ham & cheese chowder	1 cup	7.0	170	37%
roasted				
garlic & lentil	1 cup	1.5	120	11%
potato garlic chowder	1 cup	9.0	180	45%
roasted chicken				
garden herb	1 cup	1.5	70	19%
Italiano	1 cup	1.5	80	17%
rotini	1 cup	1.5	80	17%
Southwestern-style corn chowder	1 cup	7.0	200	32%
spicy chicken & penne	1 cup	1.5	110	12%
split pea w/ham	1 cup	4.0	150	24%
tomato basil	1 cup	2.0	100	18%
tomato vegetable Italiano	1 cup	2.0	90	20%
tortellini chicken broth	1 cup	2.0	70	26%
turkey noodle	1 cup	1.5	90	15%
turkey rice w/ vegetables	1 cup	1.0	110	8%
vegetable	1 cup	1.0	90	10%
vegetable Italiano	1 cup	2.0	90	20%
vegetarian vegetable w/barley	1 cup	0.5	100	5%
zesty herb tomato	1 cup	3.5	130	24%
steak soup				
beef				
& baked potato	1 cup	2.0	100	18%
& mushroom	1 cup	1.5	100	14%
& vegetabes	1 cup	2.5	130	17%
beef barley	1 cup	4.5	140	29%
grilled steak	1 cup	3.5	120	26%
tomato soup				
creamy tomato	1 cup	6.0	190	28%
hearty tomato	1 cup	1.0	110	8%
tomato				
basil	1 cup	3.0	160	17%
rotini	1 cup	0.5	140	3%
white meat soup				
chicken				
& wild rice	1 cup	1.5	100	14%
garden herb	1 cup	1.5	70	19%
grilled chicken Italiano	1 cup	2.5	110	20%
hearty chicken & rotini	1 cup	1.5	80	17%
home-style	1 cup	1.5	90	15%
noodle	1 cup	2.0	90	20%
rice w/vegetables	1 cup	1.5	90	15%

Food and Description	Amount	Fat Grams	Total Calories	% Fat Calories
roasted				
Italiano	1 cup	1.5	80	17%
w/rotini	1 cup	1.5	80	17%
vegetable	1 cup	1.5	90	15%
turkey				
noodle	1 cup	1.5	70	19%
rice..w/vegetables	1 cup	1.0	110	8%
(Rokeach)				
condensed/prepared as directed				
mushroom barley	1 cup	–	85	–
split pea w/egg barley	1 cup	0.5	130	3%
(ShariAnn's) organic ready-to-serve				
cream of tomato	1 cup	–	80	–
French green lentil	1 cup	–	130	–
French onion..vegetarian	1 cup	–	60	–
great plains split pea	1 cup	–	150	–
Indian black bean	1 cup	1.0	150	6%
Italian white bean	1 cup	–	170	–
minestrone	1 cup	2.5	120	19%
potato & cheddar	1 cup	2.5	100	23%
spicy Mexican bean	1 cup	–	210	–
tomato w/red bell pepper	1 cup	–	100	–
tomato w/roasted garlic	1 cup	–	50	–
vegetable barley	1 cup	1.5	100	14%
(Snow's)				
New England clam chowder				
condensed	½ cup	1.5	80	11%
ready-to-serve	1 cup	11.0	170	58%
ready-to-serve..New England				
corn chowder	7.5 oz	6.0	150	36%
fish chowder	7.5 oz	6.0	130	42%
seafood chowder	7.5 oz	6.0	130	42%
(Swanson)				
ready-to-serve broth				
beef				
clear	1 cup	0.5	15	30%
reduced-sodium	1 cup	–	15	–
w/onions	1 cup	0.5	20	23%
chicken				
clear	1 cup	0.5	15	30%
Natural Goodness	1 cup	–	15	–
w/Italian herbs	1 cup	1.0	20	45%
w/roasted garlic	1 cup	1.0	10	45%
vegetable..clear	1 cup	1.0	20	45%
ready-to-serve chicken				
chicken				
à la king	1 can	19.0	320	53%
& dumplings	1 cup	9.0	230	35%
(Walnut Acres)				
Autumn Harvest	1 cup	2.0	200	9%

Food and Description	Amount	Fat Grams	Total Calories	% Fat Calories
classic minestrone	1 cup	–	100	–
country corn chowder	1 cup	3.0	150	18%
Cuban black bean	1 cup	1.0	140	6%
4-bean chili	1 cup	1.5	140	10%
ginger carrot	1 cup	1.0	100	9%
Mediterranean lentil	1 cup	–	130	–
savory tomato	1 cup	2.0	120	15%
(Weight Watchers) ready-to-serve				
chicken & rice	10.5 oz	2.0	110	16%
chicken noodle	10.5 oz	2.0	150	12%
minestrone	10.5 oz	2.0	130	14%
vegetable	10.5 oz	1.0	130	7%
(Westbrae)..Soups of the World ready-to-serve				
Alabama black bean	1 cup	–	140	–
Great Plains savory bean	1 cup	–	120	–
Hearty Milano minestrone	1 cup	–	120	–
Louisiana bean stew	1 cup	–	130	–
Mediterranean lentil	1 cup	–	140	–
New York un-chicken noodle	1 cup	1.0	60	15%
Old World split pea	1 cup	–	150	–
Santa Fe vegetable	1 cup	–	160	–
Spicy Southwest vegetable	1 cup	–	130	–
(Wolfgang Puck's)..ready-to-serve				
barley..thick	1 cup	7.0	180	35%
chicken potpie	1 cup	10.0	180	50%
chicken w/pasta	1 cup	5.0	140	
creamy chicken	1 cup	12.0	210	51%
creamy country chicken	1 cup	12.0	210	51%
egg	1 cup	5.0	90	50%
French onion	1 cup	5.0	140	32%
old-fashioned beef barley	1 cup	4.5	140	29%
Old World minestrone	1 cup	7.0	180	35%
roast chicken w/pasta & mushrooms	1 cup	5.0	130	35%
spicy 7-bean w/Italian sausage	1 cup	11.0	230	43%
thick country potato	1 cup	12.0	200	54%
tomato vegetable	1 cup	8.0	150	48%
turkey w/egg noodles	1 cup	6.0	140	39%
(World Classics)..ready-to-serve				
clam chowder				
Manhattan	1 cup	2.0	110	16%
New England	1 cup	7.0	170	37%
corn chowder				
New England sweet	1 cup	6.0	150	36%
lobster bisque				
New England	1 cup	5.0	120	38%
shrimp bisque				
New England	1 cup	7.0	130	48%

Food and Description	Amount	Fat Grams	Total Calories	% Fat Calories
(Wye River)..condensed..prepared w/water				
cream of crab	1 cup	1.0	60	15%
red crab	1 cup	1.0	40	23%
■ DEHYDRATED/(MIX OR CUBE) & MICROWAVABLE				
(A Taste of Thai)				
Tangy coconut ginger				
mix only	2 tsp	1.0	15	60%
(Arrowhead Mills)..mix only				
7 beans & barley..home-style	¼ cup	–	170	–
(Bean Cuisine)..soup mix..prepared				
Island Black Bean	1 cup	–	210	–
Lots of Lentil Soup	1 cup	–	230	–
Santa Fe corn chowder	1 cup	–	160	–
13-bean bouillabaisse	1 cup	–	220	–
white bean provençal	1 cup	1.0	250	6%
(Bear Creek)..mix..prepared				
cheddar broccoli	1 cup	7.0	170	37%
cheddar cheese	1 cup	7.0	190	33%
chicken noodle	1 cup	1.5	120	9%
clam chowder	1 cup	4.0	140	26%
hot & sour	1 cup	1.5	90	15%
navy bean	1 cup	4.5	130	31%
potato..creamy	1 cup	4.0	160	23%
Santa Fe chipotle	1 cup	1.0	110	8%
split pea	1 cup	2.0	110	16%
tortilla	1 cup	1.0	110	8%
wild rice..creamy	1 cup	3.5	140	23%
(Borden)				
beef bouillon...all types	1 cube	–	5	–
	1 tsp	–	5	–
chicken bouillon..all types	1 cube	–	5	–
	1 tsp	–	5	–
home-style chicken-flavored				
noodle	¼ pkt	1.5	70	19%
Ronco natural	⅓ pkg	0.5	90	5%
(Campbell's)				
soup mix/prepared				
chicken noodle	1 cup	1.5	90	15%
noodle	1 cup	1.5	100	14%
onion	1 cup	–	20	–
Soup at Hand				
blended vegetable medley	1 pkg	2.0	110	16%
chicken & stars	1 pkg	0.5	60	8%
chicken w/mini noodles	1 pkg	1.5	80	17%
classic tomato	1 pkg	–	120	–
cream of broccoli	1 pkg	8.0	160	45%
creamy				
chicken	1 pkg	4.0	190	19%
tomato	1 pkg	4.0	190	19%
Mexican-style fiesta	1 pkg	4.0	190	19%

Food and Description	Amount	Fat Grams	Total Calories	% Fat Calories
New England				
clam chowder	1 pkg	6.0	130	42%
pizza soup	1 pkg	0.5	130	3%
velvety potato	1 pkg	6.0	150	36%
(Edward & Sons)				
bouillon cubes				
herb medley	½ cube	0.5	10	45%
vegetable	½ cube	0.5	10	45%
miso-cups..prepared				
delicious golden vegetable	1 cup	1.0	30	30%
reduced sodium	1 cup	1.0	25	36%
savory seaweed	1 cup	1.0	30	30%
traditional..w/tofu				
organic	1 cup	1.0	35	26%
(Fantastic Foods) dry mix only				
Big Soup Noodle Bowls				
hot & sour	½ pkg	2.0	130	14%
Italian tomato noodle	½ pkg	2.0	130	14%
mandarin broccoli	½ pkg	–	110	–
miso w/tofu	½ pkg	1.0	100	9%
sesame miso	½ pkg	1.0	90	10%
spicy Thai	½ pkg	1.0	110	8%
spring vegetable	½ pkg	–	90	–
vegetarian				
beef noodle	½ pkg	–	100	–
chicken noodle	½ pkg	0.5	90	5%
Carb'tastic Soups				
Asian ginger broccoli	1 pkg	1.5	80	17%
broccoli cheddar	1 pkg	3.0	110	25%
hot & sour	1 pkg	2.5	70	32%
shiitake mushroom	1 pkg	2.0	80	23%
sun-dried tomato basil	1 pkg	1.0	70	13%
vegetarian beef				
w/barley	1 pkg	1.0	70	13%
vegetarian				
chicken gumbo	1 pkg	1.5	90	15%
mandarin chicken	1 pkg	1.0	90	10%
creamy soups				
broccoli cheddar	½ pkg	2.5	130	17%
corn & potato chowder	½ pkg	1.0	130	7%
hearty soups				
cha-cha chili..big cup	½ pkg	2.0	220	8%
country lentil..big cup	½ pkg	1.5	180	8%
couscous with lentils				
big cup	½ pkg	1.0	170	5%
small cup	1 pkg	1.5	230	6%
5-bean..big cup	½ pkg	1.5	180	8%
jumpin' black bean..big cup	½ pkg	2.0	230	8%
minestrone..big cup	½ pkg	1.5	140	10%
split pea..big cup	½ pkg	1.0	160	6%
vegetable barley..big cup	½ cup	0.5	120	4%

Food and Description	Amount	Fat Grams	Total Calories	% Fat Calories
Ramen Noodle Cups				
chicken-free..big cup	½ pkg	0.5	100	5%
vegetable				
curry	½ pkg	1.0	110	8%
miso..big cup	½ pkg	1.0	100	9%
simmer soups..prepared				
creamy potato	1 cup	3.0	130	21%
split pea	1 cup	1.0	125	7%
vegetable barley	1 cup	–	120	–
vegetarian chicken noodle	1 cup	0.5	120	4%
(G. Washington)..seasoning & broth..prepared				
brown..all types	1 serving	–	5	–
golden..all types	1 serving	–	5	–
onion	1 serving	–	10	–
vegetable	1 serving	–	10	–
(Goodman's)				
prepared				
matzo ball & soup				
50% less sodium	1 cup	1.0	50	18%
regular	1 cup	1.0	40	23%
Noodleman				
low-sodium	1 cup	1.0	50	18%
regular	1 cup	1.0	45	20%
onion				
low-sodium	1 cup	1.0	30	30%
regular	1 cup	1.0	30	30%
(Hain)				
savory soup mix/prepared				
cheese	¾ cup	16.0	250	58%
lentil	¾ cup	2.0	130	14%
minestrone	¾ cup	1.0	110	8%
mushroom	¾ cup	15.0	210	64%
onion	¾ cup	2.0	50	36%
potato leek	¾ cup	18.0	260	62%
split pea	¾ cup	10.0	310	29%
tomato	¾ cup	14.0	220	57%
vegetable	¾ cup	1.0	80	11%
(Health Valley)				
organic..cups				
black bean	1 cup	1.0	130	7%
lentil	1 cup	1.0	100	9%
minestrone	1 cup	–	110	–
mushroom barley	1 cup	–	70	–
potato & leek	1 cup	–	70	–
split pea	1 cup	–	110	–
tomato	1 cup	–	80	–
vegetable	1 cup	–	89	–
soup cups..fat-free				
chicken-flavored noodles				
w/vegetables	½ cup	–	110	–
corn chowder w/tomatoes	½ cup	–	100	–

Food and Description	Amount	Fat Grams	Total Calories	% Fat Calories
creamy potato w/broccoli	⅓ cup	–	80	–
garden split pea w/carrots	⅓ cup	–	110	–
lentil w/couscous	⅓ cup	–	130	–
pasta				
Italiano	½ cup	–	140	–
marinara	½ cup	–	100	–
Mediterranean	½ cup	–	100	–
Parmesan	½ cup	–	100	–
spicy black bean				
w/couscous	⅓ cup	–	130	–
zesty black bean w/rice	⅓ cup	–	100	–
(Herb-Ox)				
bouillon cube..all flavors	1 cube	–	5	–
instant bouillon..all flavors	1 tsp	–	5	–
instant broth/seasoning				
beef				
low-sodium	1 pkg	–	10	–
regular	1 pkg	–	5	–
chicken				
low-sodium	1 pkg	–	10	–
regular	1 pkg	–	5	–
liquid				
beef	2 tsp	–	20	–
chicken	2 tsp	–	15	–
(Hormel) Micro Cup Soups				
bean & ham	1 cup	4.0	190	19%
beef vegetable	1 cup	1.0	90	10%
broccoli cheese w/ham	1 cup	13.0	170	69%
chicken & rice	1 cup	3.0	110	25%
chicken noodle	1 cup	2.5	110	20%
New England clam chowder	1 cup	5.0	130	35%
potato cheese w/ ham	1 cup	13.0	190	62%
(Imagine) natural/low-fat/prepared				
creamy broccoli	1 cup	1.5	70	19%
creamy butternut squash	1 cup	2.0	120	90%
creamy mushroom	1 cup	3.0	80	34%
creamy potato leek	1 cup	2.5	90	25%
creamy sweet corn	1 cup	3.0	100	27%
creamy tomato	1 cup	1.5	90	15%
no-chicken broth	1 cup	1.0	35	26%
vegetable broth	1 cup	1.0	45	20%
zesty gazpacho	1 cup	–	60	–
(Just Delicious) Gourmet Foods soup mixes/prepared				
barley beef	1 cup	–	120	–
black bean chili	1 cup	–	60	–
black beans & rice	1 cup	–	123	–
broccoli cheese	1 cup	1.0	20	45%
Champagne				
bean	1 cup	–	100	–
red lentil	1 cup	–	110	–

Food and Description	Amount	Fat Grams	Total Calories	% Fat Calories
split pea	1 cup	0.5	150	3%
chicken, rice,				
& curry spice	1 cup	–	60	–
chicken vegetable	1 cup	–	120	–
corn chowder..golden	1 cup	–	45	–
gourmet minestrone	1 cup	–	30	–
Jamaican black bean	1 cup	–	60	–
lentil chili	1 cup	–	110	–
navy bean	1 cup	0.5	120	4%
potato	1 cup	–	25	–
potato cheese	1 cup	1.0	25	36%
red beans & rice	1 cup	–	120	–
seafood chowder	1 cup	–	40	–
sour cream, onion				
& potato	1 cup	–	25	–
spicy chicken vegetable	1 cup	–	120	–
split pea	1 cup	0.5	150	3%
tortilla	1 cup	–	60	–
(Knorr) bouillon cube..½ cube, prepared				
beef				
box	1 cup	1.0	20	45%
jar	1 cup	1.0	15	60%
chicken				
box	1 cup	1.0	15	60%
jar	1 cup	0.5	15	30%
fish	1 cup	1.0	15	60%
pumpkin	1 cup	0.5	5	90%
pumpkin & ham	1 cup	0.5	5	90%
shrimp				
box	1 cup	1.5	20	68%
jar	1 cup	0.5	10	45%
tomato w/chicken	1 cup	1.5	15	90%
tomato w/chicken flavor				
cubes	1 cup	1.0	15	60%
jar	1 cup	0.5	10	45%
vegetarian vegetable	1 cup	1.0	15	60%
concentrated broth				
beef	¹⁄₁₂ container	–	15	–
chicken	¹⁄₁₂ container	–	5	–
powdered packets..chicken	½ pkt	–	10	–
Recipe Classics Mix..for soup..dip..recipes				
French onion	⅓ box	1.0	35	26%
roasted-garlic herb	⅓ box	1.5	80	17%
vegetable	¼ box	0.5	30	15%
Savory Soups/mix only				
chicken noodle	3 Tbs	1.5	70	19%
creamy chicken w/rice	3 Tbs	2.5	90	25%
Mediterranean style	3 Tbs	2.0	100	18%
soup, dip, and recipe mix..mix only				
broccoli, cream of	3 Tbs	2.5	70	32%
French onion	2 Tbs	1.0	35	26%

Food and Description	Amount	Fat Grams	Total Calories	% Fat Calories
chicken rice..hearty	⅛ pkg	0.5	80	6%
hot & sour	2 Tbs	1.5	45	30%
leek	2 Tbs	2.5	70	32%
noodle w/beef broth	⅛ pkg	0.5	45	10%
noodle w/chicken flavor	⅛ pkg	1.0	50	18%
pasta w/chicken	¼ pkg	1.0	80	11%
spaghetti-style pasta	¼ pkg	1.0	80	11%
roasted garlic	3 Tbs	1.5	80	17%
spring vegetable	2 Tbs	–	25	–
tomato beef..oxtail hearty	2 Tbs	2.0	60	30%
vegetable	2 Tbs	0.5	30	15%
Taste Breaks Soup cups..prepared				
beef vegetable	1 cup	2.0	150	12%
black bean	1 cup	0.5	130	3%
chicken				
noodle	1 cup	2.0	100	18%
low-fat	1 cup	2.0	120	15%
packet	1 pkt	2.0	100	18%
w/rice	1 cup	2.0	180	10%
vegetable	1 cup	1.5	120	11%
corn chowder	1 cup	3.0	140	19%
hearty lentil	1 cup	2.0	220	8%
navy bean..low-fat	1 cup	0.5	130	3%
potato leek				
cup	1 cup	3.5	150	21%
packet	1 cup	3.5	170	19%
split pea	1 cup	0.5	160	3%
(Lipton)				
Cup-A-Soup..mix only				
chicken				
cream of	1 pkg	2.0	70	26%
supreme/hearty	1 pkg	4.0	90	40%
chicken noodle				
country-style hearty	1 pkg	1.0	60	15%
w/white meat	1 pkg	1.0	50	18%
green pea	1 pkg	1.0	80	11%
tomato	1 pkg	2.0	90	20%
vegetable/spring	1 pkg	1.0	45	20%
Recipe Secrets..mix only				
herb				
fiesta w/red pepper	1 Tbs	–	30	–
golden, w/lemon	2 Tbs	1.0	35	26%
Italian, w/tomato	2 Tbs	1.0	40	23%
w/garlic/savory	1 Tbs	–	30	–
mushroom..beefy	1½ Tbs	–	35	–
onion				
beefy	1 Tbs	0.5	25	18%
golden	2 Tbs	1.5	60	23%
mushroom	2 Tbs	1.0	35	26%
regular	1 Tbs	–	20	–
ranch	⅛ box	–	30	–

Food and Description	Amount	Fat Grams	Total Calories	% Fat Calories
vegetable	2 Tbs	–	30	–
(Maggi)				
boullion cubes..all flavors	1 cube	–	5	–
boullion..instant..all flavors	1 tsp	–	5	–
(Manischewitz)..mix only				
matzo ball	1 Tbs	0.5	40	11%
minestrone	¼ pkg	1.0	150	6%
split pea	⅛ pkg	–	110	–
vegetable w/mushroom	⅛ pkg	–	120	–
(Marachun) cup/prepared				
Instant Lunch				
beef	1 container	12.0	290	37%
California vegetable	1 container	11.0	260	62%
cheddar cheese	1 container	16.0	340	42%
chicken	1 container	12.0	280	39%
chili piquin & shrimp	1 container	12.0	280	39%
creamy chicken	1 container	13.0	290	40%
creamy pesto	1 container	15.0	340	40%
picante chicken	1 container	12.0	280	39%
pork	1 container	12.0	280	39%
tomato w/vegetables	1 container	12.0	290	37%
shrimp	1 container	12.0	290	37%
Instant Wonton				
chicken	1 container	12.0	200	54%
shrimp	1 container	12.0	200	54%
Ramen Oriental Noodle Soup				
beef	½ pkt	8.0	190	38%
chicken				
picante..hot	½ pkg	8.0	190	38%
w/mushrooms	½ pkt	8.0	190	38%
creamy chicken	½ pkt	9.0	200	41%
pork	½ pkg	8.0	190	38%
roast				
beef	½ pkt	8.0	190	38%
chicken	½ pkt	8.0	190	38%
shrimp	½ pkt	8.0	190	38%
tomato	½ pkt	8.0	200	36%
(MBT) Romanoff				
beef				
low-sodium	1 pkt	–	15	–
regular	1 pkt	–	15	–
chicken				
low-sodium	1 pkt	–	15	–
regular	1 pkt	–	15	–
onion broth & dip	1 pkt	–	15	–
vegetable	1 pkt	–	10	–
(Mrs. Grass).. Mix only				
chicken w/rice	¼ pkg	1.0	80	11%
noodle				
beef-flavored	¼ pkg	1.0	70	13%
chicken-flavored	¼ pkg	1.5	70	19%

Food and Description	Amount	Fat Grams	Total Calories	% Fat Calories
home-style chicken	¼ pkg	1.5	70	19%
onion				
mushroom	⅓ pkg	1.0	60	15%
reduced-sodium	¼ pkg	–	30	–
regular soup & dip	¼ pkg	0.5	50	9%
vegetable soup & dip				
home-style	¼ pkg	–	35	–
(Nile Spice) home-style cup mix/prepared				
black bean	1 container	2.0	190	9%
chicken vegetable	1 container	2.0	120	15%
lentil	1 container	1.0	180	10%
minestrone	1 container	2.0	160	11%
red beans & rice	1 container	2.0	190	9%
split pea	1 container	2.0	200	9%
sweet corn chowder	1 container	3.0	120	23%
(Nissin) mix only				
Cup O'Noodles				
beef				
hot sauce	2.25 oz	14.0	290	43%
onion	2.25 oz	14.0	300	42%
chicken				
creamy	2.25 oz	13.0	300	39%
hot sauce	3 oz	13.0	300	39%
mushroom	2.25 oz	13.0	300	39%
regular	3.oz	14.0	300	42%
spicy	2.25 oz	14.0	300	42%
teriyaki	2.25 oz	14.0	300	42%
pork	2.25 oz	12.0	290	37%
shrimp	2.25 oz	14.0	300	42%
vegetable/garden	2.25 oz	12.0	290	37%
Top Ramen				
beef				
picante	½ pkg	7.0	180	35%
regular				
low-fat	½ pkg	1.0	150	6%
original	½ pkg	7.0	190	33%
chicken				
Cajun	½ pkg	7.0	180	35%
low-fat	½ pkg	1.0	150	6%
mushroom	½ pkg	7.0	190	33%
original	½ pkg	7.0	180	35%
teriyaki	½ pkg	7.0	190	33%
chile	½ pkg	8.0	190	38%
garden vegetable	½ pkg	7.0	190	33%
Oriental				
low-fat	½ pkg	1.0	150	6%
original	½ pkg	7.0	190	33%
pork	½ pkg	7.0	190	33%
shrimp	½ pkg	7.0	190	33%
(Old Bay).. mix only				
crab, cream of	2 Tbs	2.5	70	32%

Food and Description	Amount	Fat Grams	Total Calories	% Fat Calories
Maryland crab	1⅓ Tbs	–	50	–
(Pritikin)				
instant soup cups..prepared				
brown & wild rice				
amandine	1 serving	2.0	180	10%
Cantonese noodle	1 serving	0.5	100	5%
chicken noodle	1 serving	3.0	130	21%
chicken vegetable	1 serving	–	100	–
clam chowder	1 serving	2.5	130	17%
creamy Thai noodle	1 serving	3.0	140	19%
French country lentil	1 serving	1.0	190	5%
Hunan noodle	1 serving	1.0	120	8%
Kasba curry	1 serving	1.0	150	6%
mandarin noodle	1 serving	1.0	110	8%
Moroccan couscous	1 serving	0.5	170	3%
navy bean	1 serving	1.0	160	6%
potato broccoli	1serving	3.0	110	25%
potato leek	1 serving	3.0	150	18%
spicy Thai noodle	1serving	3.0	150	18%
Szechuan noodle	1 serving	1.0	150	6%
vegetarian chili	1 serving	1.0	160	6%
(Swanson) ..broth..mix only				
beef	1 cube	1.0	20	45%
chicken	1 cube	2.0	30	60%
Oriental	1 cube	–	15	–
vegetable	1 cube	1.0	20	45%
(Tyson)..recipe ready				
Chicken cubes				
bouillon				
plastic jar	1 cube	–	5	–
shaker	1 tsp	–	5	–
broth..can..all types	1 oz	0.5	15	30%
roasted chicken	1 oz	0.5	15	30%
(Ultra Slim Fast)..prepared				
beef noodle	6 oz	<1.0	45	10%
chicken noodle	6 oz	<1.0	45	10%
creamy				
broccoli	6 oz	<1.0	75	6%
chicken leek	6 oz	<1.0	50	9%
potato leek	6 oz	<1.0	80	6%
tomato	6 oz	<1.0	60	8%
(Union Foods)				
Noodles/block..all flavors	½ pkg	8.0	190	38%
Smack cup Ramen				
all flavors	1 pkg	17.0	320	48%
(Weight Watchers) broth				
beef broth	1 pkt	–	10	–
chicken broth	1 pkt	–	10	–
(Westbrae) mix only				
brown rice	½ pkg	0.5	140	3%
buckwheat	½ pkg	0.5	140	3%

Food and Description	Amount	Fat Grams	Total Calories	% Fat Calories
carrot	⅓ pkg	1.0	100	9%
curry	½ pkg	0.5	140	3%
5-spice	½ pkg	0.5	140	3%
green tea	½ pkg	1.0	140	6%
miso	½ pkg	0.5	140	3%
mushroom	½ pkg	0.5	140	3%
seaweed	½ pkg	0.5	140	3%
spinach	½ pkg	0.5	140	3%
(Wyler's)				
bouillon cubes..all flavors	1 cube	–	5	–
instant bouillon/Shakers				
all flavors	1 tsp	–	5	–
very low-sodium	1 tsp	–	10	–
instant broth..all flavors	1 pkt	–	15	–
Soup Starter..mix only				
beef vegetable	⅛ pkg		90	5%
chicken				
noodle	⅛ pkg	1.0	80	11%
vegetable	⅐ pkg	0.5	70	6%
w/white & wild rice	⅛ pkg	0.5	70	6%
chili..3-bean	⅙ pkg	1.0	150	6%
potato	⅙ pkg	3.5	130	24%
vegetable	⅛ pkg	0.5	100	5%
Stew Starter..mix only..beef	⅛ pkg	–	70	–
(Zatarain's).. gumbo base..mix only				
New Orleans–style	1 Tbs	–	45	–
■ **FROZEN OR REFRIGERATED**				
(Stock Pot)				
clam chowder/concentrated				
prepared w/whole milk	1 cup	9.5	200	43%
unprepared	⅓ cup	4.0	100	36%
seafood gumbo	1 cup	5.0	130	35%
(Tabatchnick)				
barley mushroom				
no salt	7.5 oz	–	70	–
regular	7.5 oz	–	70	–
broccoli, cream of	7.5 oz	4.0	90	40%
cabbage	7.5 oz	–	60	–
chicken				
New York	7.5 oz	–	35	–
w/dumplings	7.5 oz	2.0	70	26%
corn chowder	7.5 oz	6.0	150	36%
lentil	7.5 oz	–	140	–
minestrone	7.5 oz	1.0	150	6%
mushroom				
cream of..no salt	7.5 oz	–	70	–
regular	7.5 oz	6.0	110	49%
onion	7.5 oz	–	50	–
pea				
no salt	7.5 oz	1.5	180	8%
regular	7.5 oz	1.5	180	8%

Food and Description	Amount	Fat Grams	Total Calories	% Fat Calories
potato				
New England	7.5 oz	6.0	150	36%
old-fashioned	7.5 oz	–	70	–
spinach, cream of	7.5 oz	4.0	90	40%
tomato rice	7.5 oz	1.5	60	23%
vegetable				
no salt	7.5 oz	1.0	110	8%
regular	7.5 oz	1.0	110	8%
Yankee bean	7.5 oz	1.5	160	8%
SOUR CREAM (See also DIP; SAUCE; SEASONINGS; SOUR CREAM SUBSTITUTE)				
(Blue Bunny)				
sour cream..all types				
light	2 Tbs	2.0	35	51%
regular	2 Tbs	6.0	60	90%
ranch dill	2 Tbs	6.0	60	90%
unflavored				
light	2 Tbs	2.0	35	51%
regular	2 Tbs	6.0	60	90%
(Breakstone)				
sour cream				
fat-free	2 Tbs	–	35	–
original	2 Tbs	5.0	60	75%
reduced-fat	2 Tbs	3.5	45	70%
sour half-and-half	2 Tbs	3.5	45	70%
(Heluva Good Cheese)				
sour cream				
fat-free	2 Tbs	–	20	–
light	2 Tbs	3.0	40	68%
original	2 Tbs	5.0	60	75%
(Hood)				
all-natural	2 Tbs	5.0	60	75%
fat-free	2 Tbs	–	25	–
low-fat	2 Tbs	1.5	35	39%
squeezable	2 Tbs	5.0	60	75%
(Kemp's)				
sour cream				
cultured	1 oz	5.0	60	75%
easy-to-squeeze	1 oz	5.0	60	75%
light	1 oz	2.0	30	6%
regular	1 cup	42.0	450	84%
w/chives	1 oz	5.0	60	75%
Tater Topper/light	1 oz	2.0	30	6%
(Knudsen)				
fat-free	2 Tbs	–	35	–
Hampshire	2 Tbs	6.0	60	90%
light	2 Tbs	2.5	40	56%
(Land O'Lakes)				
sour cream				
fat-free	2 Tbs	–	30	–
light				
plain	2 Tbs	2.0	35	51%

Food and Description	Amount	Fat Grams	Total Calories	% Fat Calories
w/chives	2 Tbs	2.0	40	45%
regular	1 Tbs	3.0	30	90%
	2 Tbs	6.0	60	90%
sour half-and-half	1 Tbs	2.0	25	72%
SOUR CREAM SUBSTITUTE (*See also* SEASONINGS)				
(Chivo)	2 Tbs	5.0	50	90%
(Dean's) Sour Delight	2 Tbs	5.0	50	90%
(Formagg) fat-free sour cream alternative	2 Tbs	–	30	–
generic				
non-butterfat	1 oz	4.0	42	86%
	1 cup	39.0	417	84%
non-dairy	1 oz	6.0	60	90%
	1 cup	45.0	480	84%
(IMO)				
fat-free	2 Tbs	–	20	–
original	2 Tbs	5.0	50	90%
(Land O'Lakes) light dairy blend	1 Tbs	1.0	20	45%
(Soymage) sour cream alternative	2 Tbs	3.0	40	68%
(Tofutti) Sour Supreme/Better Than Sour Cream				
all flavors	2 Tbs	5.0	50	90%
SOURSOP/fresh				
pieces	1 cup	1.0	150	6%
whole	1 medium	2.0	420	4%
SOY CHEESE (*See* CHEESE ALTERNATIVE/IMITATION)				
SOY FLOUR (*See* FLOUR)				
SOY NUTS (*See* SOYBEAN)				
SOY PROTEIN				
concentrate	1 oz	–	92	–
isolate				
w/potassium	1 oz	1.0	96	9%
w/sodium	1 oz	1.0	96	9%
SOY SAUCE (*See* ASIAN FOOD/SAUCES & SEASONINGS; SAUCE)				
SOYBEAN				
canned				
(Eden)				
black soybeans	½ cup	6.0	120	45%
(Westbrae)				
organic..soybeans	½ cup	7.0	150	42%
dried				
(Arrowhead Mills)	¼ cup	8.0	170	42%
(Nature's Select) dry-roasted	¾ oz	4.0	90	40%
frozen				
(C&W)				
soybeans/edamame in the pod	½ cup	0.5	60	8%
sweet soybeans	½ cup	1.0	100	9%
green				
boiled/drained	½ cup	6.0	130	42%
raw				
shelled	½ cup	9.0	190	43%
unshelled	4 oz	4.0	90	40%

Food and Description	Amount	Fat Grams	Total Calories	% Fat Calories
kernels/whole/roasted & toasted	1 oz	7.0	130	48%
	1 cup	26.0	490	48%
sprouted				
raw	10 sprouts	0.5	15	30%
	½ cup	2.3	45	46%
steamed	½ cup	2.0	40	45%
stir-fried in vegetable oil	3 oz	6.0	105	51%

SOYBEAN CURD (See TOFU; TOFU FROZEN DESSERT; VEGETARIAN FOODS)
SOYBEAN OIL (See OIL)
SOYBEAN PASTE (See MISO)
SOY MILK

Food and Description	Amount	Fat Grams	Total Calories	% Fat Calories
dry				
(Loma Linda) Soyagen/prepared				
all types	¼ cup	6.0	130	42%
(MLO)				
milk & egg protein drink				
dry mix only				
canister				
16 oz	1.4 oz	1.5	105	13%
34 oz	1 oz	1.5	110	12%
chocolate	1.2 oz	–	120	–
natural	1.1 oz	–	100	
strawberry banana	1.2 oz	–	120	–
vanilla	1.2 oz	–	130	–
Ultra XT..packets				
chocolate	1.2 oz	–	120	–
natural	1.3 oz	–	100	–
vanilla	1.4 oz	–	120	–
(Worthington) Soyamel	1 oz	7.0	130	49%
liquid				
(8th Continent)				
soy milk				
chocolate	8 fl oz	3.0	80	34%
original	8 fl oz	3.0	90	30%
vanilla	8 fl oz	3.0	140	19%
(Blue Diamond)..Almond Breeze				
non-dairy, soy-flavored				
mix..prepared				
chocolate	8 fl oz	4.5	140	29%
original	8 fl oz	4.5	90	45%
vanilla	8 fl oz	4.5	120	34%
soft drinks				
chocolate	8 fl oz	3.0	110	25%
original	8 fl oz	2.5	60	38%
vanilla	8 fl oz	2.5	90	25%
(Eden)				
organic soy milk				
Edenblend/original	8 fl oz	3.0	120	23%
Edensoy				
carob	8 fl oz	4.0	170	21%
chocolate	8 fl oz	4.0	175	21%

Food and Description	Amount	Fat Grams	Total Calories	% Fat Calories
original				
extra	8 fl oz	4.0	130	28%
light	8 fl oz	2.0	100	18%
regular	8 fl oz	5.0	145	31%
unsweetened	8 fl oz	6.0	120	45%
vanilla				
extra	8 fl oz	3.0	150	18%
light	8 fl oz	2.0	120	15%
regular	8 fl oz	3.0	150	18%
(Health Valley) Soy Moo	1 cup	6.0	120	45%
(Imagine)				
Power Dream				
natural soy energy drink				
Java Jolt	11 fl oz	4.5	240	17%
Mango Passion	11 Fl Oz	4.5	320	13%
Sky High Chai	11 Fl Oz	5.0	250	18%
Vanilla Blast	11 fl oz	5.0	240	19%
X-Treme Chocolate	11 fl oz	5.0	260	17%
(Kikkoman Pearl)..soy milk..organic				
all types	8 fl oz	3.5	110	29%
(Vitasoy)				
soy drink				
chocolate				
light	8 fl oz	2.0	100	18%
green tea	8 fl oz	4.0	120	30%
vanilla..light	8 fl oz	2.0	70	26%
soy milk				
chocolate				
rich	8 fl oz	4.0	160	23%
rich..light	8 fl oz	2.0	100	18%
original				
classic	8 fl oz	4.5	120	34%
creamy smooth	8 fl oz	4.0	100	36%
unsweetened	8 fl oz	4.0	80	45%
vanilla				
Delight	8 fl oz	4.0	120	30%
smooth	8 fl oz	4.0	110	33%
(Westsoy)				
organic soy milk				
chai	8 fl oz	3.0	130	21%
light				
chocolate	8 fl oz	1.5	130	10%
plain	8 fl oz	1.5	90	10%
vanilla	8 fl oz	1.5	110	12%
low-fat				
plain	8 fl oz	1.5	90	15%
vanilla	8 fl oz	1.5	120	11%
non-fat				
plain	8 fl oz	–	70	–
vanilla	8 fl oz	–	80	–
original	8 fl oz	3.5	130	24%

Food and Description	Amount	Fat Grams	Total Calories	% Fat Calories
unsweetened				
chocolate	8 fl oz	4.5	100	40%
plain	8 fl oz	4.5	90	45%
vanilla	8 fl oz	4.5	100	40%
rice drink..natural				
plain	8 fl oz	2.5	110	20%
vanilla	8 fl oz	a2.5	110	20%
Soy Slender				
cappuccino	8 fl oz	3.0	70	39%
chocolate	8 fl oz	3.0	70	39%
vanilla	8 fl oz	3.0	70	39%
Vigoraid..individual container				
chocolate	1	5.0	260	17%
vanilla	1	5.0	230	20%
Westsoy Plus				
plain	8 fl oz	3.0	130	21%
vanilla	8 fl oz	3.0	130	21%
(White Wave)..Silk...cultured soy milk individual containers				
all flavors	1	2.0	160	11%
Silk..soy milk				
chai	1 cup	4.0	140	26%
chocolate..Aseptic Prisma	1 cup	3.5	140	23%
creamer				
French vanilla cream	1 Tbs	1.0	20	45%
hazelnut	1 Tbs	1.0	20	45%
non-flavored	1 Tbs	1.0	15	60%
enhanced	1 cup	5.0	110	41%
nog	½ cup	2.0	90	20%
plain				
single-serve	11 oz	6.0	140	39%
twin pack	1 cup	4.0	100	36%
Soylatte coffee..all flavors	11 fl oz	5.0	230	20%
Starbucks..formula	1 cup	4.0	120	30%
unsweetened	1 cup	4.0	90	40%
vanilla	1 cup	3.5	130	32%
Very Vanilla..Aseptic Prisma	8.25 oz	3.5	130	24%

SPAGHETTI SAUCE (*See* SAUCE)

SPANISH FOOD (*See* FROZEN ENTRÉE/DINNER; MEXICAN FOOD; RICE; RICE DISH; VEGETARIAN FOODS)

SPICES (*See* SEASONINGS; individual listings)

SPINACH

canned				
(Del Monte)..all styles	½ cup	–	30	–
(S&W)..all styles	½ cup	–	30	–
(Stokely)..all styles	½ cup	–	30	–
fresh				
boiled	½ cup	–	21	–
raw				
chopped	½ cup	–	6	–

Food and Description	Amount	Fat Grams	Total Calories	% Fat Calories
(Dole)	3 oz	–	10	–
frozen				
(Birds Eye) all types	1 cup	–	20	–
(C&W) all types	⅓ cup	–	20	–
(Cascadian Farm) chopped	⅓ cup	–	20	–
(Freshlike) cut	3.3 oz	–	20	–
(Pictsweet) leaf	½ cup	–	30	–
SPINACH, NEW ZEALAND/fresh				
boiled	½ cup	–	12	–
raw	1 lb	1.0	86	11%
SPIRULINA (*See* SEAWEED)				
SPLIT PEA (*See* PEA)				
SPOONBREAD (*See* BREAD)				
SPORTS DRINK				
bottled or canned				
(All Sport)..all flavors	8 fl oz	–	70	–
(Gatorade)				
Gator X-Factor..all flavors	8 fl oz	–	50	–
Thirst Quencher..all flavors	8 fl oz	–	50	–
sports bottle	8 fl oz	–	50	–
XO energy drink..all flavors	8 fl oz	–	50	–
(Powerade)..all flavors	8 fl oz	–	73	–
(PowerBar)				
PowerGel energy drink				
chocolate	1 pack	1.5	120	11%
other flavors..all	1 pack	–	110	–
(SoBe)				
energy drink				
Lizard line				
Liz Blizz	8 fl oz	–	120	–
Liz Fuel	8 fl oz	–	130	–
Lizard Lava	8 fl oz	–	120	–
Lizard Lightning	8 fl oz	–	130	–
Love Bus Brew..chocolate milk				
energy drink	8 fl oz	1.0	140	6%
SoBe Adrenalin.. can	8.3 fl oz	–	140	–
SoBe Lean..all flavors	8 fl oz	–	5	–
SoBe Special Recipes	8 fl oz	–	120	–
SoBe Sports System	20 fl oz	–	175	–
SoBe Synergy..all flavors	11.5 oz	–	120	–
(10-K)..all flavors	8 fl oz	–	60	–
SPOT FISH/fresh				
cooked, dry heat	3 oz	4.0	134	27%
raw	2.25-oz fillet	2.5	80	28%
	3 oz	3.0	105	26%
SQUAB/PIGEON				
raw				
breast meat only	~4 oz	4.6	135	30%
meat & skin	~7 oz	47.5	590	72%
meat only	~6 oz	12.6	239	47%

Food and Description	Amount	Fat Grams	Total Calories	% Fat Calories
SQUASH				
acorn/fresh				
baked	½ cup	–	57	–
boiled-mashed	½ cup	–	41	–
banana/fresh/baked	8 oz	1.0	145	6%
butternut				
fresh				
baked	½ cup	–	41	–
boiled/mashed	½ cup	–	50	–
cocozelle				
fresh				
boiled/drained	½ cup	–	14	–
raw/sliced	½ cup	–	9	–
crookneck				
fresh				
boiled/drained	½ cup	–	18	–
raw/sliced	½ cup	–	12	–
hubbard/fresh				
baked/cubed	½ cup	0.6	51	11%
boiled/mashed	½ cup	0.5	37	12%
scallop/fresh				
boiled/drained	½ cup	–	14	–
boiled/drained/mashed	½ cup	–	19	–
raw/sliced	½ cup	–	12	–
spaghetti/fresh				
boiled or baked	½ cup	–	23	–
summer/all varieties/fresh				
boiled/sliced	½ cup	–	18	–
raw				
medium	½ squash	–	20	–
sliced	½ cup	–	13	–
winter/all varieties				
fresh				
baked/cubed	½ cup	0.6	39	14%
boiled/mashed	½ cup	0.6	39	14%
zucchini				
canned				
(Del Monte)				
w/Italian-style				
tomato sauce	½ cup	–	30	–
(Progresso) Italian-style	½ cup	2.0	40	45%
fresh				
boiled/drained	½ cup	–	14	–
raw	½ cup	–	9	–
frozen				
(Big Valley) sliced	3.5 oz	–	12	–
(C&W) sliced	⅔ cup	–	16	–
(Southland) sliced	3.2 oz	–	15	–
SQUASH SEEDS				
dried/hulled	1 oz	13.0	155	75%

Food and Description	Amount	Fat Grams	Total Calories	% Fat Calories
kernels/roasted	1 oz	12.0	148	73%
whole/roasted	1 oz	5.5	127	39%
SQUID				
dried	3 oz	4.6	260	16%
fresh				
breaded & fried	3 oz	6.0	149	36%
raw	3 oz	1.0	78	12%
frozen				
(Fiesta Del Mar) raw calamari	4 oz	2.0	110	16%
pickled	1 oz	–	23	–
SQUIRREL				
roasted	3 oz	3.0	115	23%
roasted/chopped or diced	½ cup	5.0	190	24%
STAR FRUIT/CARAMBOLA				
fresh				
cubed	½ cup	–	25	–
whole	1 medium	0.5	45	10%
STRAWBERRY				
dried				
(Frieda's)	½ cup	–	150	–
fresh				
(Dole)	8 berries	–	45	–
whole	1 cup	0.5	45	9%
	1 pint	1.0	97	9%
frozen				
(Big Valley)	3.5 oz	–	35	–
(Birds Eye)				
halves				
in light syrup	10 oz	–	120	–
in regular syrup	4.8 oz	–	120	–
whole/in light syrup	½ cup	–	100	–
(C&W)..whole	⅔ cup	–	50	–
(Lowes Foods)				
freshly frozen sliced..w/sugar	⅔ cup	–	150	–
whole..unsweetened	⅔ cup	–	50	–
STRAWBERRY JUICE/JUICE BLEND/JUICE DRINK (*See also* FRUIT PUNCH; SOFT DRINK MIX)				
bottled, boxed, or canned				
(Chiquita)				
Calypso breeze				
strawberry kiwi	8 fl oz	–	120	–
	8.45 fl oz	–	130	–
light strawberry guava	8 fl oz	–	35	–
(Dole)..strawberry banana	8 fl oz	–	120	–
(Kern's)				
strawberry	8 fl oz	–	120	–
strawberry banana nectar	12 fl oz	–	220	–
strawberry guava juice blend	8 fl oz	–	105	–
(Knudsen)				
Celebratory				
sparkling..100% juice	8 fl oz	–	110	–

Food and Description	Amount	Fat Grams	Total Calories	% Fat Calories
spritzer	12 fl oz	–	170	–
strawberry juice	8 fl oz	–	140	–
(Libby's)				
Juicy Juice				
strawberry pouch	4.23 fl oz	–	60	–
	8 fl oz	–	120	–
nectar	11.5 fl oz	–	210	–
(Odwalla)				
strawberry banana	8 fl oz	–	120	–
(Snapple)				
juice drink				
kiwi strawberry				
diet	8 fl oz	–	10	–
regular	8 fl oz	–	110	–
(V8 Splash)				
juice drink				
strawberry banana	8 fl oz	–	110	–
strawberry kiwi	8 fl oz	–	110	–
juice drink..diet				
strawberry kiwi	8 fl oz	–	10	–
smoothie				
strawberry banana	8 fl oz	–	130	–
STUFFING/DRESSING				
(Arnold)..dry				
cornbread	¾ cup	2.0	140	13%
other flavers...All	¾ cup	1.5	140	13%
(Brownberry)..dry				
corn bread	½ cup	2.0	130	14%
herb-seasoned..all types	½ cup	1.5	130	10%
home-style for chicken	1 oz	6.0	130	42%
home-style for turkey	1 oz	4.5	120	34%
traditional sage & onion	¾ cup	1.5	140	13%
unseasoned bread cubes	¾ cup	1.5	140	10%
(Butterball)..One-Step/prepared				
corn bread	½ cup	3.0	150	18%
seasoned	½ cup	3.5	160	20%
(Chatam Village)..all types	1 cup	–	130	–
(Golden Grains) prepared				
chicken	½ cup	9.0	180	40%
corn bread	½ cup	9.0	180	40%
herb & butter	½ cup	9.0	180	40%
w/wild rice	½ cup	9.0	180	40%
(Kellogg's) Croutettes mix	1 cup	–	120	–
(Pepperidge Farms) dry mix only				
corn bread	¾ cup	2.0	170	11%
cube				
country-style	¾ cup	1.5	140	10%
original	¾ cup	1.5	140	10%
seasoned w/herbs	½ cup	1.5	170	8%
One Step				
chicken	½ cup	6.0	110	49%

Food and Description	Amount	Fat Grams	Total Calories	% Fat Calories
cornbread	½ cup	6.0	170	32%
garden herb	½ cup	3.0	90	30%
turkey	½ cup	3.0	90	30%
sage & onion	¾ cup	1.0	140	6%
(Stove Top)				
New Meals				
beef	½ cup	9.0	180	45%
chicken				
box				
lower-sodium	⅙ pkg	1.0	110	8%
regular	⅙ cup	1.0	110	`8%
cornbread				
box	⅙ pkg	1.0	110	8%
can	1 oz	3.0	120	23%
home-style herb	⅙ pkg	2.5	110	20%
long grain & wild rice	½ cup	9.0	180	45%
mushroom & onion	½ cup	9.0	180	45%
original	1 oz			
pork	1 oz	1.0	110	8%
San Francisco–style	½ cup	9.0	170	48%
savory herbs	½ cup	9.0	170	48%
traditional sage flavor	½ cup	9.0	180	45%
turkey	⅙ pkg	1.0	110	8%
STURGEON				
cooked—dry heat	3 oz	4.0	115	31%
smoked	3 oz	3.7	147	23%
steamed	3 oz	4.8	135	32%
SUCCOTASH (*See also* VEGETABLES, MIXED)				
canned				
(Blue Boy) whole kernel	½ cup	–	90	–
(Libby)..w/whole kernel corn	½ cup	0.5	90	5%
(S & W) country	½ cup	1.0	80	11%
frozen				
(Hanover)	½ cup	–	80	–
(Pictsweet)	3.3 oz	1.0	100	9%
SUGAR				
brown				
firmly packed	1 tsp	–	18	–
	1 Tbs	–	52	–
	1 cup	–	821	–
loosely packed	1 cup	–	541	–
brown				
(C&H)..all types	1 tsp	–	15	–
(Crystal)..all types	1 tsp	–	15	–
(Domino)				
Brownulated	1 tsp	–	10	–
other types..all	1 tsp	–	15	–
(Hain)	1 tsp	–	15	–
maple	1 Tbs	–	52	–
organic	1 tsp	–	10	–

Food and Description	Amount	Fat Grams	Total Calories	% Fat Calories
raw				
(Sugar in the Raw) from natural cane	1 tsp	–	15	–
regular sugar				
(C&H)..all types	1 pkt	–	15	–
(Domino)	1 tsp	–	15	–
(Hain)	¼ cup	–	140	–
turbinado				
(Hain)	1 Tbs	–	50	–
white				
cube..(C&H)	1 cube	–	15	–
granulated	1 tsp	–	15	–
	1 Tbs	–	46	–
	1 cup	–	770	–
powdered 10X confectioners'				
(C&H)..all types	1 oz	–	120	–
(Domino)..all types	¼ cup	–	110	–
SUGAR APPLE/SWEETSOP				
fresh				
pulp	1 cup	0.8	235	3%
whole	1 medium	0.5	145	3%
SUGAR SUBSTITUTE				
(Equal)	1 pkt	–	–	–
	¼ tsp	–	–	–
(Estee) fructose	1 pkt	–	10	–
	1 tsp	–	15	–
(NutraSweet)	1 tsp	–	–	–
	1 pkt	–	4	–
(Splenda)				
canister	1 tsp	–	<5	–
individual packets	1 tsp	–	<5	–
(Sucaryl)	1 tsp	–	–	–
(Sugar Twin)				
brown sugar	1 tsp	–	2	–
regular	1 tsp	–	2	–
	1 pkt	–	3	–
(Sweet*10)	⅛ tsp	–	–	–
(SweetLite)	1 tsp	–	12	–
(Sweet'n Low)				
granulated				
brown	¼ tsp	–	–	–
white	¼ tsp	–	–	–
liquid	10 drops	–	–	–
powder				
brown sugar	⅒ tsp	–	2	–
regular	1 packet	–	–	–
	1 tsp	–	12	–
tablet	1 tablet	–	–	–
(Weight Watchers) sweetener	1 gm	–	5	–
SUNFISH/PUMPKINSEED				
fresh				
cooked—dry heat	3 oz	0.5	97	5%

Food and Description	Amount	Fat Grams	Total Calories	% Fat Calories
raw	3 oz	0.5	76	6%
SUNFLOWER SEED BUTTER				
(Erewhon)	2 Tbs	18.0	200	81%
(Hain)	2 Tbs	15.0	180	75%
(Kettle)..roaster fresh	2 Tbs	14.0	160	79%
SUNFLOWER SEED FLOUR (*See* FLOUR)				
SUNFLOWER SEEDS/NUTS				
(Arrowhead Mills) hulled	¼ cup	15.0	180	75%
(David)				
sunflower seeds				
BBQ	¼ cup	15.0	190	71%
1.75-oz bag	1 bag	13.0	160	73%
2.5-oz bag	1 bag	18.0	220	74%
jalapeño hot salsa	¼ cup	15.0	190	71%
1.75-oz bag	1 bag	13.0	160	73%
2.5-oz bag	1 bag	18.0	220	74%
nacho cheese	¼ cup	15.0	180	75%
0.8-oz bag	1 bag	5.0	70	64%
1.75-oz bag	1 bag	12.0	150	72%
original	¼ cup	15.0	190	71%
1.75-oz bag	1 bag	13.0	160	73%
2.5-oz bag	1 bag	15.0	190	71%
ranch	¼ cup	15.0	190	71%
1.75-oz bag	1 bag	13.0	160	73%
2.5-oz bag	1 bag	17.0	220	70%
reduced sodium	¼ cup	15.0	190	71%
sunflower kernels				
original	¼ cup	17.0	200	77%
1-oz bag	1 bag	27.0	310	78%
1.75-oz bag	1 bag	28.0	330	76%
ranch..1.75-oz bag	1 bag	26.0	310	75%
Sizzlin' BBQ	¼ cup	16.0	190	76%
1.75-oz bag	1 bag	27.0	310	78%
(Fisher)				
dry-roasted	1 oz	14.0	170	74%
oil-roasted	1 oz	15.0	170	79%
salted in shell				
shelled kernels	1 oz	14.0	160	79%
unshelled seeds	1 oz	15.0	170	79%
(Frito-Lay)				
kernels..original	1 oz	15.0	180	75%
seeds				
BBQ	1 oz	15.0	200	68%
Flamin' Hot	1 oz	15.0	180	75%
original	1 oz	15.0	180	75%
(Lance) shelled kernels/roasted	1⅛ oz	16.0	190	76%
	¼ cup	14.0	170	74%
unshelled seeds	½ cup	11.0	140	71%
	1⅞ oz	14.0	170	74%

Food and Description	Amount	Fat Grams	Total Calories	% Fat Calories
(Planters)				
dry-roasted				
shelled kernels	¼ cup	17.0	190	81%
unshelled seeds				
original	¾ cup	15.0	160	84%
plain				
Munch 'n' Go	0.75 oz	11.0	120	83%
regular	3.25 oz	20.0	230	78%
honey-roasted/shelled kernels	1.7 oz	22.0	280	71%
oil-roasted/shelled kernels				
salted/shelled kernels	1 oz	14.0	170	74%
SURIMI	3 oz	0.8	84	9%
SUSHI (See ASIAN FOOD)				
SWAMP CABBAGE				
fresh/boiled	½ cup	–	10	–
SWEET & SOUR SAUCE (See ASIAN FOOD; SAUCES & SEASONINGS; SAUCE)				
SWEET POTATO (See also YAM)				
can or bag				
(Bruce's) cut				
yams in syrup	⅔ cup	0.5	150	3%
yams in heavy syrup	⅔ cup	–	190	–
(McCain) Roasters				
oven-roasted	½ cup	4.0	120	30%
(Princella)				
candied	½ cup	–	240	–
in heavy syrup	½ cup	–	130	–
in light syrup	⅔ cup	0.5	160	3%
in pineapple orange sauce	½ cup	–	210	–
in water	½ cup	–	90	–
mashed	⅔ cup	1.0	120	8%
(Royal Prince)				
candied	½ cup	–	210	–
in heavy syrup	6.3 oz	0.5	200	2%
in light syrup	½ cup	–	100	–
orange/pineapple	½ cup	–	210	–
(Trappey's) golden sweet..whole yams				
in heavy syrup	6.3 oz	0.5	200	2%
sugary Sam golden mashed yams	⅔ cup	–	120	–
sugary Sam golden				
cut yams in syrup	⅔ cup	–	160	–
fresh				
baked/mashed	½ cup	<1.0	103	4%
boiled/mashed/no skin	½ cup	0.5	172	3%
raw whole/5" long/~2" dia	1 potato	<1.0	135	3%
SWEET POTATO DISH				
frozen				
(Mrs. Paul's)				
candied sweet potatoes	5 oz	1.0	300	3%
candied sweets 'n' apples	1¼ cups	–	270	–

Food and Description	Amount	Fat Grams	Total Calories	% Fat Calories
SWEET ROLL (See PASTRY)				
SWEETBREADS (See individual meat listings)				
SWEETENER, ARTIFICIAL (See SUGAR SUBSTITUTE)				
SWORDFISH				
fresh				
breaded & fried	3 oz	12.0	207	52%
cooked—dry heat	3 oz	4.0	132	27%
raw	3 oz	3.0	103	26%
SYRUP (See also CORN SYRUP; ICE CREAM TOPPING; MAPLE SYRUP; PANCAKE & WAFFLE SYRUP; RICE SYRUP; SORGHUM SYRUP)				
Syrup Flavoring				
(Atkins) sugar-free–all types	1 Tbs	–	–	–
(Da Vinci).. gourmet..sugar all flavors	1 Tbs	–	–	–

T

Food and Description	Amount	Fat Grams	Total Calories	% Fat Calories
TABASCO SAUCE (See SAUCE)				
TABOULI/TABOULE/TABOULY				
(Casbah).. mix/prepared	⅔ cup	<1.0	90	5%
(CedarLane)..tabouli salad	2 Tbs	1.0	30	30%
(Fantastic Foods)..tabouli salad mix only	2 Tbs	–	70	–
(Near East) wheat salad mix prepared	⅔ cup	3.0	120	23%
TACO SAUCE (See SAUCE)				
TAHINI (See SESAME BUTTER)				
TAMALE (See MEXICAN FOOD; FROZEN ENTRÉE/DINNER)				
TAMARIND/fresh	1 medium	–	5	–
TANGELO/fresh	1 medium	–	39	–
TANGERINE (See also MANDARIN ORANGE)				
fresh/whole	1 medium	–	37	–
(Dole)	1 medium	0.5	50	9%
TANGERINE JUICE/JUICE DRINK				
bottled or canned				
(After the Fall)..tangerine spritzer 77% juice	12 fl oz	–	180	–
(R. W. Knudsen)..spritzer	12 fl oz	–	170	–
fresh	8 fl oz	–	108	–
frozen concentrate				
(Minute Maid)..prepared	8 fl oz	–	120	–

Food and Description	Amount	Fat Grams	Total Calories	% Fat Calories
TAPIOCA (*See* PUDDING)				
TARO				
chips (*See also* POTATO CHIPS & SNACKS)	10 chips	6.0	110	49%
leaves				
raw	½ cup	–	12	–
steamed	½ cup	<1.0	17	27%
root/fresh/sliced				
cooked	½ cup	–	94	–
raw	½ cup	–	56	–
shoots/fresh/sliced				
cooked	½ cup	–	10	–
raw	½ cup	–	5	–
Tahitian/fresh/sliced				
cooked	½ cup	<1.0	30	15%
raw	½ cup	1.0	25	36%
TARRAGON/ground	1 tsp	–	5	–
TARTAR SAUCE (*See* SAUCE)				
TEA				
bags				
(Bigelow) all types & flavors	1 bag	–	–	–
(Celestial Seasonings)				
all types & flavors	1 bag	–	–	–
(Good Earth) original herb & tea				
caffeine-free	1 bag	–	5	–
regular	1 bag	–	–	–
(Luzianne)				
decaffeinated	1 bag	–	–	–
regular	1 bag	–	–	–
(Tetley)				
decaffeinated	1 bag	–	–	–
regular	1 bag	–	–	–
bottled, boxed, or canned				
(Arizona)..canned tea				
black tea				
diet..all flavors	8 fl oz	–	–	–
regular..all flavors	8 fl oz	–	90	–
unsweetened	8 fl oz	–	–	–
botanicals..caffeine-free				
black	8 fl oz	–	70	–
green	8 fl oz	–	60	–
red	8 fl oz	–	60	–
green tea				
diet				
green tea	8 fl oz	–	–	–
regular..all flavors	8 fl oz	–	70	–
herbal tea				
* denotes caffeine-free				
RX Energy	8 fl oz	–	120	–
RX Health *	8 fl oz	–	70	–
RX Memory *	8 fl oz	–	80	–

Food and Description	Amount	Fat Grams	Total Calories	% Fat Calories
RX Stress *	8 fl oz	–	60	–
low-carb..all flavors	8 fl oz	–	5	–
no-carb..all flavors	8 fl oz	–	5	–
Palmer's half & half	8 fl oz	–	50	–
(Cool)				
diet	8 fl oz	–	1	–
lemonade tea	8 fl oz	–	90	–
Peach Frrreezer	8 fl oz	–	85	–
Raspbrrry Cooler	8 fl oz	–	90	–
(Le*Nature's) ice tea				
diet..all flavors	8 fl oz	–	–	–
regular..all flavors	8 fl oz	–	80	–
(Lipton)				
ready-to-drink				
green tea	8 fl oz	–	70	–
lemon				
diet	8 fl oz	–	–	–
regular	8 fl oz	–	90	–
peach	8 fl oz	–	110	–
raspberry	8 fl oz	–	110	–
regular				
sweetened	8 fl oz	–	70	–
unsweetened	8 fl oz	–	–	–
sweet tea				
w/lemon	8 fl oz	–	110	–
w/o lemon	8 fl oz	–	100	–
sweet tea..extra sweet	8 fl oz	–	120	–
(Nescafé)				
decaffeinated sweetened	8 fl oz	–	60	–
lemon..natural..sweetened	8 fl oz	–	90	–
peach..natural..sweetened	8 fl oz	–	90	–
(Nestea)				
lemon				
diet	8 fl oz	–	2	–
honey green	8 fl oz	–	80	–
sweet	8 fl oz	–	75	–
raspberry	8 fl oz	–	80	–
sweetened				
decaffeinated	8 fl oz	–	65	–
regular	8 fl oz	–	65	–
unsweetened	8 fl oz	–	2	–
(Snapple)				
caffeine-free	8 fl oz	–	100	–
cranberry raspberry..				
diet	8 fl oz	–	10	–
just plain tea				
cactus tea				
unsweetened	8 fl oz	–	100	–
kiwi strawberry..diet	8 fl oz	–	10	–
Kiwi Teawi	8 fl oz	–	100	–
lemon				

Food and Description	Amount	Fat Grams	Total Calories	% Fat Calories
decaffeinated	8 fl oz	–	100	–
diet	8 fl oz	–	10	–
	11.5 fl oz	–	5	–
regular	8 fl oz	–	110	–
	11.5 fl oz	–	140	–
lemonade iced tea	8 fl oz	–	110	–
lime green				
diet	8 fl oz	–	–	–
regular	8 fl oz	–	100	–
mango	8 fl oz	–	110	–
mint	8 fl oz	–	110	–
moon–green tea	8 fl oz	–	90	–
orange	8 fl oz	–	110	–
passionfruit	8 fl oz	–	110	–
peach				
diet	8 fl oz	–	10	–
regular	8 fl oz	–	100	–
	11.5 fl oz	–	150	–
raspberry				
diet	8 fl oz	–	10	–
regular	8 fl oz	–	100	–
	11.5 fl oz	–	150	–
Snapple apple..diet	8 fl oz	–	15	–
strawberry	8 fl oz	–	100	–
sun tea				
diet	8 fl oz	–	–	–
regular	8 fl oz	–	90	–
sweet tea	8 fl oz	–	120	–
Very Cherry	8 fl oz	–	200	–
(SoBe).. black tea..all natural				
w/ginseng	8 fl oz	–	100	–
(Tradewinds)				
extra sweet tea	8 fl oz	–	120	–
green tea				
diet	8 fl oz	–	–	–
regular	8 fl oz	–	80	–
w/honey	8 fl oz	–	80	–
honey	8 fl oz	–	80	–
lemon	8 fl oz	–	90	–
lemon lime	8 fl oz	–	90	–
mango green tea	8 fl oz	–	80	–
peach	8 fl oz	–	95	–
raspberry				
diet	8 fl oz	–	80	–
regular	8 fl oz	–	90	–
(Tropicana) fruit tea				
lemon				
diet	8 fl oz	–	15	–
regular	8 fl oz	–	100	–
peach	10 fl oz	–	140	–
	11.5 fl oz	–	160	–

Food and Description	Amount	Fat Grams	Total Calories	% Fat Calories
raspberry				
diet	8 fl oz	–	15	–
regular	8 fl oz	–	120	–
brewed				
Russian tea	8 fl oz	–	110	–
loose				
(Lipton)	1 tsp	–	–	–
mix...instant				
(Arizona)				
powder...diet..all types				
mix	⅛ tub	–	–	–
prepared	8 fl oz	–	–	–
(Crystal Light) mix only				
all types	⅛ tub	–	5	–
(General Foods) prepared				
all types & flavors	8 fl oz	2.0	70	26%
(Lipton)..iced tea mix				
green tea w/honey	8 fl oz	–	70	–
lemon				
diet	8 fl oz	–	5	–
regular	8 fl oz	–	70	–
peach				
diet	8 fl oz	–	–	–
regular..sweetened	8 fl oz	–	80	–
raspberry				
sugar-sweetened	8 fl oz	–	80	–
strawberry kiwi				
sugar-sweetened	8 fl oz	–	80	–
sweetened w/sugar				
decaf..w/lemon	8 fl oz	–	70	–
regular..w/lemon	8 fl oz	–	70	–
unsweetened				
no lemon	8 fl oz	–	–	–
(Maxwell House) prepared				
concentrate				
sweetened	8 fl oz	–	80	–
unsweetened	8 fl oz	–	2	–
powder	6 fl oz	–	2	–
(Natural Touch)				
Kaffree Roma beverage	1 tsp	–	10	–
(Nescafe)				
100% tea..decaf				
unsweetened mix	1 tsp	–	–	–
green tea..w/honey				
liquid concentrate	1 oz	–	80	–
lemon liquid concentrate	1 oz	–	80	–
raspberry liquid				
concentrate	1 oz	–	90	–
unsweetened liquid				
concentrate	1 oz	–	–	–
(Nestea)				

Food and Description	Amount	Fat Grams	Total Calories	% Fat Calories
Ice Teasers..all flavors	8 fl oz	–	5	–
regular				
100%				
decaffeinated	8 fl oz	–	–	–
regular	8 fl oz	–	2	–
lemon & sugar	8 fl oz	–	80	–
sugar-free lemon	8 fl oz	–	2	–
(Oregon Chai)				
chai tea latte				
concentrate				
Java chai	4 oz	–	42	–
Kashmir green tea	4 oz	–	81	–
original				
caffeine-free	4 oz	–	78	–
organic	4 oz	–	79	–
regular	4 oz	–	78	–
slightly sweet	4 oz	–	21	–
lemon..w/chai spices	4 oz	–	110	–
nog	4 oz	–	90	–
peach..w/chai spices	4 oz	–	110	–
raspberry	4 oz	–	110	–
Rooibos..w/chai spices				
caffeine-free	4 oz	–	100	–
mix				
caffeine-free				
4-count pkg	1 pkt	3.5	150	21%
decaf original				
4-count pkg	1 pkt	3.5	150	21%
8-count pkg	1 pkt	1.0	100	9%
original				
8-count pkg	1 pkt	1.0	130	7%
spiced original				
8-count pkg	⅓ pkg	1.0	100	9%
vanilla..8-count pkg	⅓ pkg	1.5	120	11%
(Tetley)				
canister				
sugar & natural lemon	1 Tbs	–	80	–
TEMPEH				
(White Wave)				
5-grain	⅓ block	7.0	180	35%
other styles..all	⅓ block	8.0	180	40%
TEMPURA BATTER (See BAKE & FRY MIX)				
TEQUILA (See LIQUOR, DISTILLED)				
TERIYAKI SAUCE (See SAUCE)				
TERRAPIN/baked	¾ cup	4.0	161	22%
THYME/ground	1 tsp	–	4	–
TILEFISH				
cooked—dry heat	3 oz	3.0	125	22%
raw	3 oz	2.0	80	23%
TOASTER PASTRY (See PASTRY, TOASTER)				
TOFU (See also VEGETARIAN FOODS)				

Food and Description	Amount	Fat Grams	Total Calories	% Fat Calories
(Azumaya)				
tofu				
extra-fine				
light	2.8 oz	2.0	60	30%
regular	2.8 oz	4.0	170	51%
firm	2.8 oz	5.0	90	50%
silken				
light	3.2 oz	1.0	40	23%
regular	3.2 oz	2.0	40	45%
tofu..seasoned..all types	3 oz	5.0	90	50%
(Hinoichi)				
Chinese	4 oz	3.0	70	39%
Japanese	4 oz	2.0	60	30%
kinugoshi	4 oz	2.0	50	36%
(Mori-Nu) silken				
extra-firm				
light	1" slice	0.5	35	13%
regular	1" slice	1.5	45	30%
firm				
light	1" slice	0.5	30	15%
regular	1" slice	1.5	45	30%
silken	1" slice	2.5	50	45%
(Nasoya)				
tofu				
extra-firm	⅕ pkg	4.0	80	45%
firm	⅕ pkg	3.0	70	39%
light	⅕ pkg	1.5	40	34%
garlic onion	¼ pkg	5.0	90	50%
silken	⅕ pkg	2.5	45	50%
light	⅕ pkg	1.0	30	30%
soft	⅕ pkg	3.0	60	45%
tofu..marinated cubes				
ginger sesame	5.5 oz	6.0	210	26%
sweet & sour	5.5 oz	4.0	190	19%
Thai peanut tofu	5.5 oz	9.0	240	34%
teriyaki	5.5 oz	9.0	240	34%
Tofu Mate seasoning mix				
breakfast scramble	¼ pkt	–	15	–
eggless salad	¼ pkt	–	15	–
mandarin stir-fry	¼ pkt	–	25	–
Mediterranean herb	¼ pkt	–	15	–
Szechuan stir-fry	¼ pkt	–	25	–
Texas taco	¼ pkt	–	15	–
(Tree of Life)				
ground..all flavors	3 oz	4.0	60	60%
smoked				
hot 'n' spicy	3 oz	5.0	120	38%
original	3 oz	6.0	120	45%
(Vitasoy) (*See* (Azumaya) *within this category*)				
(White Wave)				
flavored	2 oz	6.0	120	45%

Food and Description	Amount	Fat Grams	Total Calories	% Fat Calories
unflavored				
extra-firm style..all types	¼ pkg	6.0	110	49%
organic				
firm..all types	⅕ box	6.0	90	60%
water-packed	⅕ pkg	6.0	110	49%
reduced-fat	⅕ pkg	4.0	90	40%
TOFU DAIRY YOGURT				
(White Wave)				
Silk..cultured soy				
plain & vanilla	1 container	2.0	120	15%
other flavors..all	1 container	2.0	160	11%
TOFU DISH (*See* VEGETARIAN FOODS)				
TOFU FROZEN DESSERT				
(Tofutti)				
TOFU FROZEN DESSERT				
CHEESECAKE SUPREME				
cheesecake..all flavors	½ cup	12.0	200	54%
LOW-FAT SUPREME				
chocolate fudge	½ cup	4.0	145	25%
coffee marshmallow swirl	½ cup	3.0	120	23%
vanilla fudge	½ cup	4.0	130	28%
no sugar added..all flavors	½ cup	5.0	115	39%
premium				
better pecan	½ cup	13.0	210	56%
chocolate cookie crunch	½ cup	11.0	210	47%
chocolate supreme	½ cup	11.0	180	55%
mint chocolate chip	½ cup	13.0	210	56%
vanilla	½ cup	11.0	190	52%
vanilla almond bark	½ cup	13.0	210	56%
vanilla fudge	½ cup	9.0	190	43%
wild berry supreme	½ cup	9.0	190	43%
super soy supreme				
Bella Vanilla	½ cup	8.0	160	45%
Cool Cappuccino	½ cup	9.0	170	48%
Plum Crazy	½ cup	8.0	160	45%
New York, New York chocolate	½ cup	9.0	170	48%
TOFU NOVELTIES				
bars				
Hooray Hooray	1 bar	9.0	150	54%
Marry Me	1 bar	8.0	168	43%
Monkey...peanut butter	1 bar	13.0	220	53%
sandwiches..Cuties				
Blueberry Wave	1 sdw	6.0	140	39%
chocolate	1 sdw	5.0	130	35%
Chocolate Wave	1 sdw	6.0	140	39%
Coffee Break	1 sdw	5.0	130	35%
cookies 'n' cream	1 sdw	6.0	120	45%
Jazzy	1 sdw	5.0	120	38%
mint chocolate chip	1 sdw	5.0	120	38%
peanut butter	1 sdw	8.0	165	44%
Strawberry Wave	1 sdw	6.0	140	39%

Food and Description	Amount	Fat Grams	Total Calories	% Fat Calories
Totally Vanilla	1 sdw	5.0	120	38%
vanilla	1 sdw	5.0	120	38%
no sugar added	1 sdw	5.0	100	45%
wild berry	1 sdw	6.0	140	39%
TOFU PÂTÉ				
(Toby's)				
jalapeño	2 Tbs	7.0	70	90%
original	2 Tbs	7.0	70	90%
light..all flavors	2 Tbs	2.0	30	60%
TOMATO				
canned or jarred				
(Claussen)				
halves	1 oz	–	5	–
(Contadina)				
crushed				
Recipe Ready..all types	¼ cup	–	20	–
diced				
marinara	½ cup	1.5	30	45%
original	½ cup	–	30	–
primavera	½ cup	–	60	–
w/Italian herbs	½ cup	–	45	–
w/roasted garlic	½ cup	–	45	–
w/roasted red pepper	½ cup	–	60	–
w/sautéed onions	½ cup	–	40	–
stewed..all types	½ cup	–	35	–
whole/peeled	½ cup	–	25	–
(Del Monte)				
crushed				
Italian recipe	½ cup	–	45	–
original recipe	½ cup	–	45	–
w/garlic	½ cup	–	50	–
diced				
no salt added	½ cup	–	25	–
original	½ cup	–	25	–
pasta-style	½ cup	–	45	–
w/basil, garlic & oregano	½ cup	–	50	–
w/garlic & onion	½ cup	–	40	–
w/green chili peppers	½ cup	–	30	–
w/green pepper & onion	½ cup	–	40	–
w/jalapeños	½ cup	–	30	–
w/mushroom & garlic	½ cup	–	30	–
zesty chili–style	½ cup	–	30	–
zesty mild				
green chilies	½ cup	–	30	–
chunky				
chili-style	½ cup	–	30	–
pasta-style	½ cup	–	45	–
stewed				
Cajun recipe	½ cup	–	35	–
Italian recipe	½ cup	–	30	–
Mexican recipe	½ cup	–	35	–

Food and Description	Amount	Fat Grams	Total Calories	% Fat Calories
original no salt added	½ cup	–	35	–
regular	½ cup	–	35	–
whole..all styles	½ cup	–	25	–
(Furmano's)				
crushed				
chunky	¼ cup	–	18	–
original	¼ cup	–	20	–
w/garlic & oregano	¼ cup	–	15	–
diced				
Italian-style..w/juice	½ cup	–	40	–
original	½ cup	–	40	–
petite				
w/cilantro & lime	½ cup	–	30	–
w/green chilies	½ cup	–	25	–
w/juice	½ cup	–	25	–
w/green peppers				
& onions	½ cup	0.5	30	–
w/purée	½ cup	–	25	–
plum	½ cup	–	25	–
stewed				
Italian-style	½ cup	–	40	–
original	½ cup	–	45	–
whole peeled	½ cup	–	25	–
(Hebrew National) pickled	1 oz	–	5	–
(Hunt's)				
choice..crushed..all styles	½ cup	–	30	–
diced				
in sauce	½ cup	–	30	–
original	½ cup	–	20	–
w/balsamic vinegar	½ cup	3.0	60	45%
w/basil..garlic				
& oregano	½ cup	–	25	–
w/green pepper..celery				
& onions	½ cup	–	45	–
w/roasted garlic	½ cup	–	30	–
w/sweet onions	½ cup	–	45	–
w/Italian herbs	½ cup	–	24	–
pear-shaped	½ cup	–	20	–
stewed..all styles	½ cup	–	30	–
whole..all styles	2 tomatoes	–	20	–
(Muir Glen) organic				
crushed..w/basil	¼ cup	–	25	–
diced..all styles	½ cup	–	25	–
fire-roasted				
crushed	¼ cup	–	20	–
diced..all styles	½ cup	–	30	–
whole	½ cup	–	30	–
ground..peeled	¼ cup	–	10	–
stewed..all styles	½ cup	–	30	–
whole peeled..all styles	½ cup	–	30	–
(Progresso)				

Food and Description	Amount	Fat Grams	Total Calories	% Fat Calories
peeled..all styles	½ cup	–	30	–
recipe ready..crushed	¼ cup	–	20	–
garlic & olive oil	½ cup	–	45	–
(Rosoff's)				
pickled..half sour	1 oz	–	5	–
(Ro*Tel)..diced				
chunky..w/green chiles	½ cup	–	20	–
extra-hot	½ cup	–	25	–
Mexican fiesta	½ cup	–	30	–
Italian harvest	½ cup	–	30	–
w/green chiles	½ cup	–	20	–
bold Italian	½ cup	–	30	–
chili fixin's..seasoned	½ cup	–	30	–
w/fewer green chiles	½ cup	–	20	–
w/lime juice & cilantro	½ cup	–	20	–
(S&W)				
crushed	½ cup	–	20	–
Italian style..pear	½ cup	–	25	–
no salt	½ cup	–	35	–
petite diced..medium hot w/roasted garlic & sweet onions	½ cup	–	45	–
w/jalapeños	½ cup	–	30	–
ready-cut..diced				
caramelized	½ cup	–	35	–
fire-roasted	½ cup	–	35	–
Italian recipe	½ cup	–	25	–
Mexican recipe	½ cup	–	35	–
no salt	½ cup	–	25	–
original	½ cup	–	25	–
peeled	½ cup	–	25	–
roasted garlic	½ cup	0.5	30	15%
stewed..all flavors	½ cup	–	35	–
(Schorr's)				
pickled	1 oz	–	4	–
stewed	½ cup	–	35	–
(Tuttorosso)				
peeled..crushed..in thick purée				
w/basil	¼ cup	–	10	–
crushed w/basil	¼ cup	–	10	–
plum-shaped				
in tomato juice	½ cup	–	30	–
w/basil	½ cup	–	30	–
fresh				
green	1 medium	–	30	–
red				
chopped or diced	1 cup	–	35	–
whole	1 medium	–	24	–
frozen				
(C&W)..vine-ripened..diced	¾ cup	–	20	–
sun-dried				
(Sonoma)				

Food and Description	Amount	Fat Grams	Total Calories	% Fat Calories
bits	2-3 tsp	–	15	–
halves	2-3 halves	–	15	–
marinated in oil				
halves	2-3 pieces	2.5	35	51%
julienne	7-9 pieces	2.5	35	51%
julienne..roasted				
in garlic	7-9 pieces	3.0	40	68%
pickled spice medley				
oil-drained	1 Tbs	4.0	50	72%
TOMATO ASPIC/canned				
(S&W) supreme	½ cup	–	50	–
TOMATO JUICE/JUICE BLEND				
(Campbell's)				
Healthy Request..all types	8 fl oz	–	50	–
original	8 fl oz	–	50	–
	11.5 fl oz	–	70	–
(Del Monte)				
Snap-E-Tom..tomato & chile cocktail				
from concentrate	8 fl oz	–	50	–
individual can	11.5 fl oz	–	70	–
(Full Circle) organic tomato juice	8 fl oz	–	35	–
(Knudsen)..all types	8 fl oz	–	60	–
(Mott's)				
Beefamato	8 fl oz	–	80	–
Clamato	8 fl oz	–	100	–
Clamato Caesar	8 fl oz	–	100	–
(Muir Glen)..organic tomato juice	5.5 fl oz	–	40	–
(S&W)	5.5 fl oz	–	30	–
	8 fl oz	–	40	–
(V8 Splash)				
100% vegetable juice				
calcium enriched	8 fl oz	–	50	–
lightly tangy	8 fl oz	–	60	–
low sodium	8 fl oz	–	50	–
picante	8 fl oz	–	50	–
spicy hot	8 fl oz	–	50	–
TOMATO PASTE/canned				
(Contadina)				
100% tomatoes	2 Tbs	–	30	–
Italian..all flavors	2 Tbs	0.5	35	13%
(Del Monte)	2 Tbs	–	30	–
(Hunt's)				
basil garlic	2 Tbs	–	25	–
Italian-style	2 Tbs	–	30	–
no salt added	2 Tbs	–	30	–
original	2 Tbs	–	25	–
(Muir Glen)..organic	2 Tbs	–	30	–
(Progresso)	2 Tbs	–	30	–
(S&W)	6 oz	–	150	–
TOMATO PURÉE/canned				
(Contadina)	¼ cup	–	20	–

Food and Description	Amount	Fat Grams	Total Calories	% Fat Calories
(Hunt's)	¼ cup	–	20	–
(Muir Glen)..organic	¼ cup	–	20	–
(Progresso)				
original	¼ cup	–	25	–
thick-style	¼ cup	–	20	–
(S&W)				
original	4 oz	–	60	–
w/diced tomatoes	4 oz	–	35	–
TOMATO SAUCE (*See also* MEXICAN FOOD; SAUCE)				
canned				
(Contadina)				
garlic & onion	¼ cup	–	20	–
Italian	¼ cup	–	15	–
original	¼ cup	–	15	–
thick & zesty	¼ cup	–	20	–
(Del Monte)..all styles	¼ cup	–	20	–
(Hunt's)				
ready sauce				
chunky chili	¼ cup	–	20	–
chunky Italian	¼ cup	–	20	–
chunky Mexican	¼ cup	–	20	–
chunky special	¼ cup	–	20	–
chunky tomato	¼ cup	–	15	–
country herb	¼ cup	–	30	–
garlic	¼ cup	–	30	–
garlic & herb	¼ cup	–	25	–
meat loaf fixin's	¼ cup	–	25	–
original Italian	¼ cup	–	30	–
regular				
basil..garlic.. & oregano	¼ cup	–	15	–
no salt added	¼ cup	–	30	–
original	¼ cup	–	15	–
roasted garlic	¼ cup	–	15	–
(Muir Glen) organic..all styles	¼ cup	–	20	–
(Red Gold)				
original	¼ cup	–	20	–
thick 'n' rich..hot w/garlic..onion & jalapeños	¼ cup	–	15	–
w/garlic..onion & green pepper	¼ cup	–	20	–
(S&W)				
Italian herb	¼ cup	–	35	–
other styles..all	¼ cup	–	20	–
TONIC WATER (*See* COCKTAIL MIXER)				
TORTILLA (*See* MEXICAN FOOD)				
TORTILLA CHIPS/CORN CHIPS				
(Arizona)				
original	1 oz	6.0	140	39%
restaurant-style	1 oz	7.0	140	45%
(Azteca)..Buenitos	1 oz	7.0	140	45%

Food and Description	Amount	Fat Grams	Total Calories	% Fat Calories
(Barbara's)				
blue corn chips				
no salt added	1 oz	7.0	140	45%
regular	1 oz	7.0	140	45%
pita chips/salsa	1 oz	6.0	130	42%
(Borden)				
corn chips	1 oz	10.0	160	56%
Dipsy Doodles				
mesquite barbecue	1 oz	10.0	160	56%
rippled	1 oz	10.0	160	56%
Doodle Twisters				
nacho cheese	1 oz	10.0	160	56%
nacho chips/thinner crispier	1 oz	8.0	150	48%
white tortilla chips				
crispy rounds	1 oz	8.0	150	48%
quarter rounds				
restaurant-style	1 oz	8.0	150	48%
yellow tortilla chips..all styles	1 oz	8.0	150	48%
(Bugles)				
most flavors	1⅓ cups	9.0	160	45%
smokin' BBQ	1⅓ cups	8.0	150	48%
(Doritos)				
cooler ranch				
3D's	2 oz	11.0	270	37%
K.C. Masterpiece BBQ	1 oz	5.0	140	32%
Nacho Cheesier	1 oz	5.0	130	35%
WOW..Nacho Cheesier	1 oz	1.0	90	10%
zesty ranch	2 oz	11.0	270	37%
original	1 oz	7.0	140	45%
EXTREME				
bold BBQ	1 oz	7.0	140	45%
zesty sour cream				
& cheddar	1 oz	7.0	140	45%
flamin' hot	1 oz	7.0	140	45%
4-cheese-flavored	1 oz	8.0	140	51%
nacho cheesier				
3D's	1 oz	7.0	140	45%
baked	1 oz	3.5	120	26%
original	1 oz	7.0	140	45%
salsa verde	1 oz	7.0	140	45%
smokey red BBQ	1 oz	7.0	150	48%
spicier nacho	1 oz	7.0	140	45%
taco	1 oz	7.0	140	45%
toasted corn	1 oz	7.0	140	45%
zesty salsa	1 oz	7.0	140	45%
(Fritos)				
Bar-B-Q	1 oz	10.0	150	60%
cheddar & sour cream	1 oz	10.0	160	56%
chili cheese	1 oz	10.0	160	56%
choice	1 oz	10.0	160	56%
flamin' hot	1 oz	10.0	160	56%

Food and Description	Amount	Fat Grams	Total Calories	% Fat Calories
flavor twists				
cheddar ranch	1 oz	9.0	150	54%
honey BBQ	1 oz	10.0	160	56%
Racerz...all flavors	1 oz	11.0	160	62%
Sabrositas				
flamin' hot	1 oz	10.0	160	56%
lime'n chili	1 oz	9.0	150	54%
Scoops!	1 oz	10.0	160	56%
(Garden of Eatin')				
blue corn				
little soy blues	1 oz	7.0	140	45%
no salt	1 oz	7.0	140	45%
original	1 oz	7.0	140	45%
red hot blues	1 oz	7.0	140	45%
sesame blues	1 oz	8.0	150	48%
sunny blues	1 oz	8.0	150	48%
guacamole chips	1 oz	6.0	140	39%
jalapeño..all flavors	1 oz	7.0	140	45%
mini corn tortilla chips				
yellow rounds	1 oz	7.0	140	45%
white..all styles	1 oz	6.0	140	39%
nacho cheese chips	1 oz	6.0	140	39%
red corn tortilla chips..all styles	1 oz	7.0	140	45%
white corn tortilla chips				
chili lime	1 oz	7.0	140	45%
guacamole	1 oz	6.0	140	39%
pico de gallo	1 oz	7.0	140	45%
tamari	1 oz	7.0	140	45%
white chips	1 oz	6.0	140	39%
yellow corn tortilla chips				
black bean	1 oz	7.0	140	45%
chili	1 oz	7.0	140	45%
garden grains	1 oz	7.0	140	45%
nacho cheese	1 oz	6.0	140	39%
yellow chips	1 oz	7.0	140	45%
(Genisoy)				
low-carb chips..all flavors	1 oz	8.0	140	51%
low-carb assortment	1 oz	8.0	140	51%
(Guiltless Gourmet)..baked				
all flavors	1 oz	2.0	110	16%
no salt	1 oa	1.0	110	8%
(Kettle)				
blue corn	1 oz	6.0	140	39%
5-grain yellow	1 oz	6.0	140	39%
5-grain yellow corn	1 oz	6.0	140	39%
Little Dippers	1 oz	6.0	140	39%
Sesame Blue Moons	1 oz	8.0	150	48%
sesame rye				
w/caraway	1 oz	6.0	140	39%
sweet brown rice				
& black bean	1 oz	6.0	120	45%

Food and Description	Amount	Fat Grams	Total Calories	% Fat Calories
yellow corn	1 oz	6.0	140	39%
(Lance)				
corn chips				
BBQ	1¼ oz	14.0	210	60%
plain	1 oz	10.0	160	56%
	1¼ oz	13.0	200	59%
	1½ oz	15.0	240	56%
tortilla chips				
nacho chips	1 oz	7.0	140	45%
nacho triangles	1 oz	7.0	140	45%
white corn round	1¼ oz	10.0	190	47%
(Mi Ranchito)				
restaurant-style	1 oz	7.0	140	45%
traditional	1 oz	7.0	140	45%
white corn	1 oz	6.0	140	39%
(Michael Season's) organic				
blue corn				
hot & spicy	1 oz	7.0	140	45%
sesame	1 oz	9.0	150	54%
mini yellow	1 oz	6.0	140	39%
salsa/yellow corn	1 oz	6.0	140	39%
white corn/slightly salted	1 oz	6.0	140	39%
(Mission) authentic Mexican tortilla				
chips..all styles & flavors	1 oz	7.0	140	45%
(Old Dutch)				
Arriba nacho cheese	1 oz	7.0	140	45%
bite-size				
restaurant-style	1 oz	8.0	150	48%
restaurant..original	1 oz	7.0	140	45%
(Old El Paso)				
Nachips	9 chips	8.0	150	48%
white corn	11 chips	8.0	140	51%
(Pringles)..all types	1 oz	7.0	140	45%
(Rancho California)				
guacamole	1 oz	7.0	155	41%
Macho Nacho	1 oz	7.0	150	42%
(Santitas)..all styles	1 oz	6.0	130	42%
(Snyder's of Hanover)				
corn chips				
BBQ	1½ oz	14.0	230	55%
original	1½ oz	15.0	230	54%
EatSmart..organic..all styles	1 oz	6.0	140	39%
tortilla chips				
nacho	1 oz	3.5	130	24%
white corn	1 oz	4.5	140	29%
yellow corn				
mini	1 oz	6.0	140	39%
regular	1 oz	4.5	140	29%
unsalted	1 oz	3.0	120	23%
(Torengos)				
pinch of pepper Jack cheese	13 chips	9.0	150	54%

Food and Description	Amount	Fat Grams	Total Calories	% Fat Calories
regular	13 chips	9.0	140	58%
splash of salsa	13 chips	9.0	150	54%
(Tostitos)				
Baked				
bite-size				
cheddar quesadilla	1 oz	3.0	120	23%
original	1 oz	1.0	110	8%
salsa & cream cheese	1 oz	3.0	120	23%
cool ranch	1 oz	3.0	120	23%
original	1 oz	1.0	110	8%
unsalted	1 oz	1.0	110	8%
white	1 oz	1.0	110	8%
original				
100% white corn	1 oz	8.0	140	51%
blue corn..natural				
restaurant-style	1 oz	6.0	140	39%
crispy rounds	1 oz	7.0	140	45%
restaurant-style				
hint of lime	1 oz	6.0	140	39%
white corn	1 oz	6.0	140	39%
Santa Fe gold	1 oz	6.0	140	39%
spicy quesadilla				
bite-size round	1 oz	9.0	150	54%
WOW! restaurant-style	1 oz	1.0	90	9%
yellow corn..natural	1 oz	6.0	140	39%
(Wise) Bravos				
all styles & flavors	1 oz	8.0	150	48%
(WOW!)				
Doritos nacho cheesier	1 oz	1.0	90	10%
Tostitos original	1 oz	1.0	90	10%
TRAIL MIX (*See* CEREAL; FRUIT SNACK; NUTS, MIXED; SNACK MIX)				
TREACLE (*See* MOLASSES)				
TRITICALE (*See also* FLOUR)				
whole-grain	1 oz	0.5	95	5%
	1 cup	4.0	645	6%
TROUT				
mixed species				
cooked—dry heat	3 oz	6.5	165	35%
rainbow				
farmed				
cooked—dry heat	3 oz	5.5	145	34%
wild				
cooked—dry heat	3 oz	4.5	130	31%
smoked	3 oz	3.0	153	18%
sea/mixed species				
cooked—dry heat	3 oz	3.0	115	23%
TUNA (*See also* SEAFOOD ENTRÉE/DINNER; TUNA DISH; VEGETARIAN FOODS)				
canned/drained				
(3 Diamonds)				
chunk				
light..in soybean oil	2 oz	6.0	110	40%

Food and Description	Amount	Fat Grams	Total Calories	% Fat Calories
light..in water	2 oz	0.5	60	8%
light..touch of lemon in water	2 oz	0.5	60	8%
white..in water albacore	2 oz	1.0	60	15%
solid				
white..in soybean oil	2 oz	3.0	90	30%
white..in water				
fancy albacore	2 oz	–	90	–
premium albacore	2 oz	0.5	70	6%
prime fillet in water	2 oz	1.0	70	13%
tonno in olive oil	2 oz	6.0	120	45%
(Bumble Bee)				
chunk light				
in oil/drained	2 oz	6.0	110	40%
in water	2 oz	0.5	60	8%
chunk white				
in oil/drained	2 oz	12.0	160	68%
in water	2 oz	2.0	70	26%
solid white				
in oil/drained	2 oz	8.0	130	55%
in water	2 oz	1.0	60	15%
(Chicken of the Sea)				
chunk light				
in canola oil	2 oz	6.0	110	49%
	2.8 oz	8.0	140	41%
in spring water				
50% less salt	2 oz	0.5	60	8%
low sodium	2 oz	0.5	60	8%
premium				
can	2 oz	0.5	60	8%
pouch	1 pouch	1.0	90	10
regular	2 oz	0.5	60	8%
	2.8 oz	1.0	90	10%
chunk white				
albacore..in spring water	2 oz	1.0	60	15%
low sodium	2.8 oz	1.0	90	10%
very low sodium				
in spring water	2 oz	0.5	60	15%
solid light Genova tonno	2 oz	8.0	130	55%
in olive oil	2.9 oz	12.0	130	83%
solid white				
in canola oil	2 oz	3.0	90	30%
in spring water	2 oz	1.0	70	13%
	2.9 oz	1.0	100	9%
tongol chunk light..in water	2 oz	0.5	60	8%
yellowfin chunk light				
in spring water	2 oz	0.5	60	8%
yellowfin solid light				
in spring water	2 oz	1.0	70	13%
(Crown Prince)				

Food and Description	Amount	Fat Grams	Total Calories	% Fat Calories
chunk				
light tongol				
no salt added	¼ cup	–	70	–
regular	¼ cup	–	60	–
solid white				
albacore				
no salt added	¼ cup	–	60	–
regular	¼ cup	–	60	–
yellowfin				
in olive oil	¼ cup	5.0	110	41%
(StarKist)				
chunk light				
in oil	2 oz	6.0	110	49%
	2.7 oz	8.0	140	51%
in water..drained	2 oz	0.5	60	8%
	2.7 oz	1.0	80	11%
chunk white				
low-salt, low-fat				
in distilled water	2 oz	0.5	60	8%
	2.7 oz	0.5	80	9%
in spring water	2 oz	0.5	60	8%
	2.7 oz	0.5	70	6%
regular..in water	2 oz	1.0	60	15%
	2.8 oz	1.0	80	11%
Lunch-to-Go..pouch				
chunk light	4.5 oz	9.0	210	39%
solid light				
hickory smoke/in water	2 oz	1.0	60	15%
Gourmet's Choice..drained				
in olive oil	2 oz	12.0	160	68%
in spring water	2 oz	1.0	60	15%
Prime Catch..in water	2 oz	1.0	60	15%
	2.8 oz	1.0	80	11%
solid white				
albacore..in water				
drained	2 oz	1.0	70	13%
hickory smoked				
in water	2 oz	1.0	60	15%
regular				
in oil	2 oz	3.0	90	30%
	2.8 oz	5.0	130	35%
in water	2 oz	1.0	70	13%
	2.8 oz	1.0	100	9%
Starkist Select				
Yellowfin..chunk light	2 oz	1.0	60	15%
Tuna Creations				
hickory-smoked	2 oz	1.0	60	15%
fresh				
bluefin				
cooked—dry heat	3 oz	5.0	157	29%
raw	3 oz	4.0	122	30%

Food and Description	Amount	Fat Grams	Total Calories	% Fat Calories
skipjack				
cooked—dry heat	3 oz	1.0	112	8%
raw	3 oz	1.0	88	10%
yellowfin				
cooked—dry heat	3 oz	1.0	118	8%
raw	3 oz	1.0	90	10%
TUNA DISH (*See also* FROZEN ENTRÉE/DINNER; SEAFOOD ENTRÉE/DINNER)				
canned				
(Libby's) The Spreadables tuna salad	⅓ cup	8.0	130	55%
mix/kit				
(Bumble Bee)				
original				
crackers	1 pkg	4.5	90	45%
tuna salad	1 can	16.0	190	76%
Tuna Salad w/crackers				
Crackers..fat-free	1 pkg	1.5	90	15%
tuna salad	1 can	–	70	–
Tuna Salad Kit..w/mayo & crackers				
crackers	1 pkg	4.5	90	45%
tuna salad & mayo	1 can	1.0	70	13%
(Betty Crocker) Tuna Helper (prepared, as directed)				
au gratin	1 cup	12.0	310	35%
cheesy broccoli	1 cup	10.0	300	30%
cheesy pasta	1 cup	11.0	270	37%
creamy broccoli	1 cup	13.0	300	39%
creamy pasta	1 cup	13.0	290	40%
classic tuna casserole	1 cup	12.0	280	39%
fettuccine Alfredo	1 cup	14.0	300	42%
garden cheddar	1 cup	11.0	290	34%
tetrazzini	1 cup	12.0	300	36%
tuna melt	1 cup	12.0	280	39%
TURBINADO SUGAR (*See* SUGAR)				
TURBOT				
cooked—dry heat	3 oz	3.0	104	26%
raw	3 oz	2.5	81	28%
TURKEY (*See also* FRANKFURTER; LUNCHEON MEAT; SAUSAGE)				
■ **TURKEY & TURKEY PARTS/FRESH**				
all classes				
dark meat only..roasted				
w/skin	~2 lb	93.0	1789	47%
w/o skin	~5 oz	10.0	262	34%
chopped/diced	1 cup	9.0	223	36%
giblets	~5 oz	7.0	243	26%
giblets & organs..simmered				
gizzard	~5 oz	5.6	236	21%
heart	~5 oz	8.0	257	28%
liver	~5 oz	8.0	237	30%
light meat only				
w/skin	2¼ lb	87.0	206	38%
w/o skin	~5 oz	4.5	219	19%
chopped/diced	1 cup	4.0	194	19%

Food and Description	Amount	Fat Grams	Total Calories	% Fat Calories
meat & skin..dark & light/no giblets	~4 lb	180.6	3857	42%
or neck	~5 oz	7.0	238	26%
fryer..roaster..roasted				
back				
w/skin	4 oz	11.5	230	45%
w/o skin	4 oz	6.5	195	30%
breast				
w/skin	4 oz	3.6	175	19%
w/o skin	4 oz	1.0	155	6%
dark meat				
w/skin	4 oz	8.0	206	35%
w/o skin	4 oz	5.0	185	24%
chopped..diced	1 cup	6.0	227	24%
leg				
w/skin	4 oz	6.0	193	28%
w/o skin	4 oz	4.3	180	22%
light meat				
w/skin	4 oz	5.0	185	24%
w/o skin	4 oz	1.3	159	7%
chopped..diced	1 cup	1.7	195	8%
wing				
w/skin	4 oz	11.2	235	43%
w/o skin	4 oz	3.9	185	19%
young hen..roasted				
back w/skin	4 oz	17.7	288	55%
breast w/skin	4 oz	9.0	220	37%
dark meat				
w/skin	4 oz	14.5	265	49%
w/o skin	4 oz	9.0	220	37%
leg w/skin	4 oz	12.0	245	40%
light meat				
w/skin	4 oz	10.7	235	41%
w/o skin	4 oz	4.0	180	20%
wing w/skin	4 oz	15.3	270	51%
young tom..roasted				
back w/skin	4 oz	15.5	270	52%
breast w/skin	4 oz	8.4	214	35%
dark meat				
w/skin	4 oz	12.3	245	45%
w/o skin	4 oz	8.0	210	34%
leg w/skin	4 oz	11.0	235	42%
light meat				
w/skin	4 oz	8.7	217	36%
w/o skin	4 oz	3.3	175	17%
wing w/skin	4 oz	13.0	251	47%

■ TURKEY & TURKEY PARTS/CANNED/BRAND NAME

(Armour)

Golden Star	1 oz	4.0	50	72%
loaf	2 oz	8.0	110	65%

Turkey Selects..boneless

Food and Description	Amount	Fat Grams	Total Calories	% Fat Calories
breast				
roast	3 oz	5.0	120	38%
slices	3 oz	1.0	90	10%
tenderloins	3 oz	1.0	90	10%
ground	3 oz	6.0	120	45%
strips	3 oz	4.0	100	36%
(Briar Street Market)				
chunk..smoked breast				
w/white meat	2 oz	1.5	50	27%
diced..white/dark meat				
½" pieces	¼ cup	3.5	70	45%
ground	4 oz	16.0	210	69%
logs..loaves				
cooked white turkey roll	2 oz	7.0	100	63%
cured dark picnic				
turkey log	2 oz	2.5	60	38%
roasted turkey breast roll	2 oz	1.0	45	20%
meatballs..Italian	3 oz	12.0	210	51%
	6 pieces	12.0	210	51%
pulled white turkey				
½" pieces	3 oz	2.5	120	19%
¾" pieces	3 oz	2.5	120	19%
turkey ham				
25% water added	2 oz	2.5	60	38%
(Butterball)				
fresh premium turkey cuts				
breast				
boneless roast	4 oz	3.0	110	25%
fillets..fresh prime cuts	2.85 oz	1.0	80	11%
ground 99% fat-free	4 oz	1.0	110	8%
London broil prime cuts	4 oz	1.0	110	8%
roast	4 oz	3.0	110	25%
strips	4 oz	1.0	120	8%
tenderloins..boneless	4 oz	1.0	110	8%
whole breast				
frozen	4 oz	8.0	170	42%
frozen..boneless	2 oz	10.0	140	64%
young				
stuffed	4 oz	5.0	130	35%
whole	4 oz	5.0	140	32%
burger patties	1 piece	9.0	170	48%
ground				
43% less fat	4 oz	17.0	220	70%
7% fat	4 oz	8.0	160	45%
(Honeysuckle White)				
turkey breast..fresh				
99% fat-free..for scallopini				
& Milanese	4 oz	0.5	120	4%
boneless roast	4 oz	3.0	110	25%
split breast	4 oz	9.0	190	43%
tenderloins..boneless	4 oz	1.0	110	8%

Food and Description	Amount	Fat Grams	Total Calories	% Fat Calories
whole breast				
fresh	4 oz	8.0	170	42%
frozen	4 oz	8.0	170	42%
frozen..boneless	2 oz	10.0	140	64%
drumstick	4 oz	8.0	180	40%
drumettes	3 oz	10.0	190	47%
ground				
93% lean..chub	4 oz	8.0	160	45%
43% less fat	4 oz	17.0	220	70%
7% fat	4 oz	8.0	160	45%
thighs	4 oz	9.0	190	43%
young				
stuffed	4 oz	5.0	130	35%
whole	4 oz	8.0	170	42%
whole turkey..frozen..boneless	2 oz	8.0	160	45%
whole turkey..hickory-smoked	3 oz	6.0	140	39%
wings	4 oz	14.0	220	57%
(Hormel)				
turkey breast..whole				
canned in water..chunk turkey				
mixed	2 oz	–	60	–
white premium	2 oz	1.5	50	27%
hickory-smoked	2 oz	1.0	60	15%
natural shape..boneless	2 oz	1.0	50	18%
(Jennie-O Turkey Store)				
turkey				
burger patties..lean..7% fat	4 oz	8.0	160	45%
burger patties..7% fat	4 oz	8.0	180	40%
burgers..original	4 oz	9.0	160	51%
burgers..savory..seasoned	4 oz	9.0	160	51%
drumsticks	4 oz	6.0	190	28%
ground	4 oz	10.0	180	50%
thighs	4 oz	6.0	190	28%
whole..smoked				
premium young	3 oz	6.0	110	49%
wings	4 oz	6.0	290	28%
young				
premium fresh	4 oz	10.0	180	50%
whole premium	4 oz	10.0	180	50%
turkey breast..97% fat-free..extra-lean				
hickory-smoked..half	2 oz	3.0	60	45%
honey-cured..half	2 oz	3.0	60	45%
oven-roasted..w/broth	2 oz	0.5	50	9%
slices..extra-lean	4 oz	8.0	180	40%
turkey breast				
tenderloins				
lemon garlic	4 oz	2.0	120	15%
seasoned pepper	4 oz	2.5	100	18%
tequila lime	4 oz	8.0	190	38%
(Louis Rich)				
breaded				

Food and Description	Amount	Fat Grams	Total Calories	% Fat Calories
nuggets	4 nuggets	16.0	260	55%
patties	1 patty	13.0	220	53%
sticks	3 sticks	15.0	230	59%
ground				
bulk	4 oz	12.0	190	57%
patties..white	1 patty	10.0	170	53%
portions				
hickory-smoked	2 oz	–	50	–
honey-roasted	2 oz	–	60	–
oven-roasted	2 oz	–	50	–
(Perdue)				
Carving Classics				
turkey breast..pan-roasted				
braised home-style	2 oz	2.0	70	26%
cracked pepper	2 oz	–	50	–
hickory smoked	2 oz	2.5	70	32%
oven-roasted	2 oz	2.0	70	26%
pan-roasted	2 oz	2.0	70	26%
pan-roasted hickory-smoked	2 oz	2.5	70	32%
skinless...pan-roasted	2 oz	0.5	60	8%
w/skin	2 oz	2.0	70	26%
carving turkey breast				
Cajun-style	2 oz	1.0	50	18%
honey	2 oz	1.0	50	18%
honey-smoked	2 oz	–	50	–
mesquite-smoked	2 oz	–	50	–
deli turkey				
breast				
oven-roasted	2 oz	1.0	50	18%
ham..hickory-smoked	2 oz	2.5	60	38%
Fit 'n' Easy..fresh lean ground..cooked				
turkey	3 oz	9.0	160	51%
turkey breast	3 oz	9.0	160	51%
turkey breast cutlets	2.5 oz	0.5	90	5%
turkey breast for London broil				
cooked	3 oz	0.5	110	4%
turkey breast tenderloins	3 oz	0.5	110	4%
turkey burgers	3 oz	9.0	160	51%
fresh..cooked				
burgers..lean	4 oz	9.0	170	48%
drumsticks	3 oz	7.0	150	42%
ground..lean				
turkey breast	3 oz	1.0	110	8%
ground..lean	3 oz	9.0	160	51%
thighs	3 oz	8.0	160	45%
whole hen turkey cooked				
dark	3 oz	11.0	180	55%
white	3 oz	7.0	150	42%

Food and Description	Amount	Fat Grams	Total Calories	% Fat Calories
whole tom turkey cooked				
dark	3 oz	9.0	160	51%
white	3 oz	5.0	140	32%
wing				
drumettes	3 oz	9.0	180	45%
portions	3 oz	8.0	160	45%
wing portions	3 oz	2.5	160	14%
wings	3 oz	2.5	160	14%
(Sara Lee)				
pre-sliced				
turkey breast				
roasted	2.25 oz	0.5	60	8%
smoked	4 oz	6.0	140	39%
premium turkey breast				
home-style seasoned	3 oz	2.5	100	23%
honey-roasted	2 oz	0.5	60	8%
mesquite-smoked	2 oz	0.5	60	8%
roasted & browned	2 oz	1.5	60	23%
smoked..natural	3 oz	2.5	100	23%
smoked..skinless	2 oz	0.5	60	8%
raw..ready-to-cook..cook-in-bag				
turkey breast				
netted	4 oz	4.0	130	28%
turkey breast & thigh	4 oz	6.0	140	39%
(Shady Brook)				
turkey..fresh..raw				
breast..99% fat-free..boneless				
for London broil	4 oz	0.5	130	3%
for scallopini	4 oz	0.5	110	4%
chops..boneless	4 oz	0.5	110	4%
cutlets..boneless	4 oz	0.5	110	4%
ground	4 oz	1.0	120	8%
split..natural	4 oz	9.0	190	43%
tenderloin..97% fat-free	4 oz	3.0	130	21%
tenderloin..97% fat-free				
lemon garlic	4 oz	3.5	130	24%
rotisserie	4 oz	3.5	130	24%
young..fresh	4 oz	9.0	190	43%
young..hotel-style	4 oz	9.0	180	45%
burgers..93% lean				
patties	4 oz	9.0	170	48%
drumstick	4 oz	9.0	170	48%
ground				
85% fat-free	4 oz	17.0	240	64%
93% lean	4 oz	8.0	160	45%
93% lean..family pack	4 oz	8.0	160	45%
(Shelton's)..free-range turkey				
cooked/frozen				
ground turkey..chub	4 oz	10.0	170	53%
meatballs	6 pieces	14.0	180	70%
(Wampler Longacre)				

Food and Description	Amount	Fat Grams	Total Calories	% Fat Calories
burgers				
100% pure turkey	4 oz	15.0	210	64%
BBQ	4 oz	10.0	220	41%
specially seasoned	4 oz	11.0	180	55%
ground turkey	4 oz	15.0	210	64%
The Diamond Line				
1 Diamond turkey breast				
oven-roasted	2 oz	2.0	50	36%
smoked	2 oz	1.5	50	27%
2 Diamond turkey breast				
oven-roasted	2 oz	1.5	50	27%
smoked	2 oz	2.5	60	38%
3 Diamond turkey breast				
fat-free	2 oz	–	45	–
oiled browned				
no skin	2 oz	0.5	45	10%
w/skin	2 oz	1.5	50	27%
oven-roasted	2 oz	1.0	50	18%
smoked	2 oz	1.0	45	20%
4 Diamond turkey breast				
honey-cured..smoked	2 oz	2.0	70	26%
mesquite-smoked				
honey-cured	2 oz	–	50	–
oiled browned	2 oz	1.5	60	23%
oven-browned	2 oz	1.0	50	18%
petite honey-cured				
smoked	2 oz	–	50	–
skinless	2 oz	1.5	60	23%
smoked	2 oz	2.0	60	30%
turkey breast..no salt				
skinless	2 oz	–	60	–
5 Diamond turkey breast				
oiled browned				
no skin	2 oz	0.5	45	10%
w/skin	2 oz	1.0	70	13%
skin on	2 oz	2.5	70	32%
skinless	2 oz	–	50	–
smoked..w/skin	2 oz	2.5	70	32%

TURKEY ALTERNATIVE (*See* VEGETARIAN FOODS)
TURKEY BACON (*See* BACON)
TURKEY ENTRÉE/DINNER (*See also* FROZEN ENTRÉE/DINNER; PASTA ENTRÉE/DINNER)

Food and Description	Amount	Fat Grams	Total Calories	% Fat Calories
can or microwave container				
(Dinty Moore)				
American Classics				
turkey & dressing w/gravy	1 bowl	8.0	290	25%
turkey stew..microwave	1 cup	2.5	130	17%

Food and Description	Amount	Fat Grams	Total Calories	% Fat Calories
frozen..refrigerated				
(Bob Evans)				
turkey breast w/gravy				
slow-roasted	5 oz	1.0	100	9%
(Schwan's) partially or fully cooked				
gourmet turkey breast	3 oz	1.0	90	10%
turkey breast fillet/unbreaded	1 fillet	–	70	–
ready-to-serve				
(Honeysuckle White)				
rotisserie turkey breast				
boneless Italian				
herb-flavored	4 oz	8.0	170	42%
rotisserie turkey breast				
original flavor	4 oz	8.0	170	42%
Tenderloin..97% fat-free				
home-style flavor	4 oz	3.5	130	24%
Tenderloin..97% fat-free				
garlic flavor	4 oz	–	130	–
Tenderloin..97% fat-free				
rotisserie flavor	4 oz	3.5	130	24%
(Hormel)				
fully cooked				
meatballs				
Italian-style	3 oz	10.0	190	47%
turkey breast w/gravy				
oven-roasted & sliced	5.6 oz	3.0	130	21%
turkey breast w/gravy				
roasted & sliced				
family pack	6 oz	3.0	135	20%
(Jennie-O Turkey Store)				
stuffed turkey breast				
cheddar cheese				
& broccoli	2 oz	3.0	60	45%
stuffed turkey breast				
pepper cheese & rice	2 oz	3.0	60	45%
stuffed turkey breast				
w/Swiss cheese				
& ham	2 oz	3.0	60	45%
turkey breast				
wing portions & neck				
w/ribs..skin..w/gravy	4 oz	7.0	170	37%
turkey roast				
white lean meat				
w/gravy in roasting pan	4 oz	7.0	150	42%
turkey whole..smoked				
premium young				
fully cooked	3 oz	6.0	110	49%
(Schwan's)				
turkey				
boneless breast of				
turkey w/gravy	4 oz	4.5	140	29%

Food and Description	Amount	Fat Grams	Total Calories	% Fat Calories
mignon	1 fillet	9.0	220	37%
potpie	1 pie	43.0	690	56%
(Shady Brooks)..Turkey meatballs.. fully cooked appetizer size				
w/sweet & sour sauce	3 oz	10.0	190	47%
family size..all flavors	3 oz	10.0	190	47%
(Shelton's) Free Range				
meat balls	6 pieces	14.0	180	70%
(Wampler)				
Deli Roast collection..fully cooked classic spiced turkey breast				
paprika	2 oz	0.5	70	6%
pan-roasted..all natural	2 oz	1.0	50	18%
pan-roasted	2 oz	–	50	–
turkey ham..Black Forest..boneless	2 oz	1.5	60	23%
TURKEY HAM (See HAM; LUNCHEON MEAT)				
TURKEY SAUSAGE (See SAUSAGE; TURKEY & TURKEY PARTS/FRESH, OR CANNED/BRAND NAME)				
TURKEY SUBSTITUTES (See VEGETARIAN FOODS)				
TURMERIC/ground	1 tsp	–	8	–
TURNIP				
fresh				
boiled	½ cup	–	14	–
raw	½ cup	–	18	–
TURNIP GREENS				
canned				
(Bush's Best)				
chopped	½ cup	–	25	–
chopped..w/diced turnips	½ cup	–	30	–
(Glory Foods)	½ cup	0.5	45	10%
(Luck's)				
w/diced turnips seasoned w/pork	½ cup	1.5	35	39%
(The Allens)				
seasoned Southern-style	½ cup	0.5	35	13%
seasoned Southern-style w/diced turnips	½ cup	0.5	35	13%
seasoned Southern-style mustard & turnip	½ cup	0.5	45	10%
Verduras de nabo chopped	½ cup	0.5	25	18%
Verduras de nabo picadas w/diced turnips	½ cup	0.5	30	15%
(The Allens Sunshine)				
all styles	½ cup	0.5	35	13%
fresh				
boiled-drained	½ cup	–	15	–
raw	½ cup	–	7	–

Food and Description	Amount	Fat Grams	Total Calories	% Fat Calories
frozen				
(Birds Eye)				
chopped..w/diced	1 cup	–	25	–
(Lowes Foods)				
chopped..w/diced				
turnips	1 cup	–	25	–
(Pictsweet) w/diced turnips	3.3 oz	–	20	–
TURTLE/green				
canned	3 oz	0.6	91	6%
raw	3 oz	<1.0	76	6%

V

Food and Description	Amount	Fat Grams	Total Calories	% Fat Calories
VEAL				

(NOTE: All serving sizes are for cooked portions, unless otherwise stated. "Lean" means veal trimmed of separable fat before cooking. "Lean & fat" means untrimmed and cooked or eaten as purchased. In most cases, 4 ounces of raw veal yields approximately 3 ounces cooked.)

Food and Description	Amount	Fat Grams	Total Calories	% Fat Calories
chop				
lean w/bone/raw	6.5 oz	5.0	170	26%
cutlet, steak				
lean/boneless/braised or broiled	3 oz	4.0	170	21%
ground/broiled	3 oz	6.0	146	37%
loin				
lean				
braised or broiled	3 oz	8.0	195	37%
roasted	3 oz	6.0	150	36%
lean & fat				
braised or broiled	3 oz	15.0	240	56%
roasted	3 oz	11.0	185	54%
organs				
brain				
braised	3 oz	8.0	120	60%
fried	3 oz	14.0	180	70%
heart/braised	3 oz	6.0	160	34%
kidney/braised	3 oz	5.0	140	32%
liver				
braised	3 oz	6.0	140	39%
fried	3 oz	10.0	210	43%
spleen/braised	3 oz	3.0	110	25%
sweetbreads/braised	3 oz	3.0	145	19%
tongue/braised	3 oz	9.0	170	48%

Food and Description	Amount	Fat Grams	Total Calories	% Fat Calories
rib roast				
lean				
braised or broiled	3 oz	7.0	185	34%
roasted	3 oz	6.0	150	36%
lean & fat				
braised or broiled	3 oz	11.0	214	46%
roasted	3 oz	12.0	195	55%
round w/rump				
roasts & leg cutlets/lean/braised				
or broiled	3 oz	4.0	175	20%
sirloin				
lean				
braised or broiled	3 oz	6.0	175	31%
braised or broiled/chopped	1 cup	9.0	290	28%
roasted	3 oz	5.0	145	31%
roasted/chopped	1 cup	9.0	235	34%
lean & fat				
braised or broiled	3 oz	11.0	220	46%
braised or broiled/chopped	1 cup	18.0	355	45%
roasted	3 oz	9.0	175	46%
roasted/chopped	1 cup	15.0	285	47%
top round				
lean				
roasted	4 oz	6.0	230	23%
roasted/chopped	1 cup	5.0	210	21%
lean & fat				
braised or broiled	4 oz	6.0	230	23%
braised or broiled/chopped	1 cup	7.0	285	22%
roasted	4 oz	5.0	180	25%
roasted/chopped	1 cup	7.0	225	28%
VEAL DISH (*See* FROZEN ENTRÉE/DINNER)				
VEGETABLE JUICE/JUICE COCKTAIL/JUICE DRINK				
bottled, boxed, or canned				
(Campbell's)				
Invigor8				
Energy Boost	8 fl oz	–	110	–
Nutrition Boost	8 fl oz	–	110	–
V8 Splash Juice Drink				
all flavors	1 cup	–	110	–
V8 Splashy Juice Drink..diet				
all flavors	1 cup	–	10	–
V8 Splash Vegetable Juice				
100% juice..100% A-C-E Vitamin-rich..100% vegetable juice				
all flavors	8 fl oz	–	50	–
(DelMonte)				
vegetable blended cocktail				
Snap-E-Tom..tomato & chile cocktail	6 fl oz	–	40	–
	10 fl oz	–	60	–

Food and Description	Amount	Fat Grams	Total Calories	% Fat Calories
(Hain) veggie juice				
w/lutein	1 cup	0.5	45	10%
(Knudsen)				
Very Veggie				
100% juice..all styles	8 fl oz	–	50	–
Vita Juice	8 fl oz	–	120	–
(Muir Glen) organic..all styles	5.5 gl oz	–	50	–
(Red Gold)..Sacramento..from concentrate				
vegetable cocktail	8 fl oz	–	50	–
vegetable juice	8 fl oz	–	50	–

VEGETABLE OIL (*See* COOKING SPRAY; OIL)
VEGETABLE SOUP (*See* SOUP)
VEGETABLES, MIXED (*See also* ASIAN FOOD; FROZEN ENTRÉE/DINNER; SUCCOTASH)
■ **CANNED OR JARRED**

Food and Description	Amount	Fat Grams	Total Calories	% Fat Calories
(Allen)				
green beans & potatoes	½ cup	–	35	–
okra & tomatoes	½ cup	–	30	–
okra, tomatoes & corn	½ cup	–	30	–
(Bush's Best)				
mixed greens	½ cup	–	20	–
(Del Monte)				
mixed vegetables				
regular	½ cup	–	40	–
w/potatoes	½ cup	–	45	–
peas & carrots	½ cup	–	60	–
(Freshlike)				
mixed vegetables				
no salt	½ cup	0.5	45	10%
no salt or sugar	½ cup	0.5	45	10%
sweet corn & diced				
peppers				
Freshlike Selects	½ cup	1.0	80	11%
sweet peas & carrots	½ cup	–	60	–
(Green Giant)				
garden medley	½ cup	–	40	–
Mexicorn	⅓ cup	–	60	–
mixed vegetables	½ cup	–	60	–
peas & carrots	½ cup	–	50	–
sweet peas				
w/tiny pearl onions	½ cup	–	60	–
3-bean salad	½ cup	–	90	–
yellow & white corn	⅓ cup	–	50	–
(LeSueur)..early peas..w/mushrooms				
& pearl onions	½ cup	–	60	–
(Libby's)				
mixed vegetables	½ cup	–	45	–
peas & carrots	½ cup	–	60	–
vegetables for stew	½ cup	–	45	–
(S&W)				
peas & carrots	⅔ cup	–	50	–

Food and Description	Amount	Fat Grams	Total Calories	% Fat Calories
peas & onions	⅔ cup	–	40	–
summer harvest	½ cup	–	35	–
(Trappey)				
okra & tomatoes	½ cup	–	30	–
okra..tomatoes				
& corn	½ cup	–	30	–
(Veg-All)				
Cajun	½ cup	–	50	–
chunky vegetables				
mixtos en Trocitos	½ cup	–	45	–
chicharos y zanahorias	½ cup	–	60	–
hot 'n' spicy	½ cup	–	40	–
home-style..large	½ cup	–	40	–
original				
no salt added	½ cup	–	40	–
regular	½ cup	–	40	–
peas..sweet & carrots	⅓ cup	–	60	–
(Vlasic)				
hot & spicy garden mix	1 oz	–	5	–
■ FROZEN				
(Big Valley)				
California Blend	¾ cup	–	25	–
Italian Blend	¾ cup	–	30	–
Oriental Blend	¾ cup	–	25	–
stew vegetables	¾ cup	–	25	–
Winter Blend	¾ cup	–	25	–
(Birds Eye)				
Baby Vegetable Blends				
baby bean & carrot	1 cup	–	30	–
baby broccoli	1 cup	1.5	70	19%
baby corn	⅔ cup	–	60	–
baby corn & bean	¾ cup	0.5	60	8%
baby gold and white corn	⅔ cup	0.5	60	8%
baby pea	¾ cup	–	40	–
baby sweet peas				
& pearl onions	⅔ cup	0.5	60	8%
Farm Fresh Mixtures				
brocoli & cauliflower	1 cup	–	15	–
broccoli..carrots				
& water chestnuts	1 cup	–	35	–
broccoli..cauliflower				
& carrots	1 cup	–	25	–
broccoli..cauliflower				
& red peppers	1 cup	–	20	–
broccoli..corn				
& red peppers	1 cup	–	60	–
broccoli..green beans				
& pearl onions				
& red peppers	1 cup	–	25	–

Food and Description	Amount	Fat Grams	Total Calories	% Fat Calories
broccoli..red pepper				
onions & mushrooms	1 cup	–	25	–
brussel sprouts				
cauliflower & carrots	1 cup	–	35	–
cauliflower..carrots				
& snow pea pods	1 cup	–	30	–
Sauce Vegetables..boxed				
broccoli..cauliflower				
& carrots				
in cheese sauce	½ cup	4.0	70	51%
French-style broccoli				
red potatoes				
& carrots				
'n' butter sauce	⅔ cup	6.0	110	49%
gold & white corn blend	½ cup	1.0	60	15%
Oriental-style vegetables	1 cup	8.0	190	38%
peas & potatoes				
in real cream sauce	½ cup	2.5	90	25%
roasted potatoes				
& broccoli	⅔ cup	3.5	100	32%
stir-fry vegetables	½ cup	4.0	60	60%
tender peas				
& pearl onions	⅔ cup	0.5	90	5%
Simply Grillin' Vegetables				
garden herb	¼ box	6.0	140	30%
potatoes & onions	¼ box	7.0	180	35%
roasted corn				
& potatoes	⅕ box	5.0	140	32%
roasted garlic	⅕ box	4.5	120	34%
Southern vegetables				
gumbo blend	¾ cup	–	40	–
okra & tomatoes	¾ cup	–	25	–
seasoning blend	¾ cup	–	20	–
turnip greens w/diced turnips	1 cup	–	25	–
vegetables for stew	¾ cup	–	40	–
vegetable blends				
Asian blend				
in sesame sauce	½ box	1.0	60	15%
Szechuan vegetables				
in sesame sauce	½ box	1.5	60	23%
teriyaki & vegetables	⅓ box	2.5	150	15%
Tuscan vegetables				
in herbed tomato sauce	½ box	2.0	50	36%
(C&W)				
plain				
baby pea pods				
w/water chestnuts	⅔ cup	–	40	–
petite peas..w/pearl onions	⅔ cup	–	70	–
petite peas & baby carrots	⅔ cup	–	60	–
rancho fiesta blend	⅔ cup	–	60	–

Food and Description	Amount	Fat Grams	Total Calories	% Fat Calories
Vegetable Stand combinations				
broccoli florets..julienne red peppers..sugar snap peas & water chestnuts	1 cup	–	40	–
corn..broccoli & red peppers	⅔ cup	0.5	60	8%
Early Harvest corn.. broccoli florets & julienne red peppers	⅔ cup	0.5	60	8%
fancy mixed vegetables Farmer's Harvest	¾ cup	–	60	–
Healthy Garden vegetables Farmer's Harvest	1 cup	–	25	–
peas..corn & carrots	⅔ cup	0.5	60	8%
sugar snap peas, baby carrots cauliflower & broccoli florets	1 cup	–	30	–
Ultimate petite mixed vegetables	¾ cup	–	60	–
Ultimate Southwest Blend	⅔ cup	1.0	90	10%
Ultimate Stir Fry	¾ cup	–	30	–
(Cascadian Farm)..as packaged				
California blend	⅔ cup	–	20	–
gardener's blend	¾ cup	–	57	–
hearty stew veggies	⅔ cup	–	45	–
peas & carrots	⅔ cup	–	50	–
peas & pearl onions	¾ cup	–	60	–
Santa Fe blend	¾ cup	0.5	60	8%
stir-fry blends Chinese	1 cup	–	25	–
Thai	¾ cup	–	25	–
vegetable medley w/cheddar cheese sauce	½ cup	2.5	60	38%
(Full Circle)..mixed vegetables				
100% organic	½ cup	0.5	55	8%
(Green Giant) as packaged				
Boil-in-Bag broccoli..carrots cauliflower & cheese	⅔ cup	3.0	80	34%
Italian-style vegetables	1 cup	3.5	90	35%
rice medley	10 oz pkg	4.0	280	13%
roasted potatoes w/broccoli & cheese	¾ cup	3.5	120	26%
roasted potatoes w/garlic & herbs	1¼ cups	14.0	270	47%
Southwest corn & roasted red peppers	¾ cup	0.5	80	6%
sweet peas & pearl onions	½ cup	–	50	–
Szechuan vegetables	¾ cup	0.5	50	9%
teriyaki vegetables	1¼ cups	5.0	80	56%
Create a Meal!				
vegetables				

Food and Description	Amount	Fat Grams	Total Calories	% Fat Calories
beefy noodle	1¾ cups	1.5	170	8%
chicken Alfredo	2 cups	6.0	230	23%
garlic herb chicken	2⅓ cups	9.0	230	35%
home-style stew	1¼ cups	3.0	140	19%
lemon pepper chicken	1½ cups	0.5	140	3%
Parmesan herb	1¾ cup	2.5	160	14%
stir-fry				
garlic & ginger	1⅔ cups	1.5	130	10%
lo mein	2⅓ cups	1.5	170	8%
sweet & sour	1½ cups	–	180	–
Szechuan	1¼ cups	5.0	150	30%
teriyaki	1¾ cup	0.5	100	5%
Select vegetables..as packaged				
broccoli..carrots & cauliflower	⅔ cups	–	25	–
broccoli..carrots & water chestnuts	⅔ cup	–	25	–
gold & white corn	¾ cup	1.0	70	13%
(McKenzie's)				
soup mix..w/tomatoes	3 oz	–	40	–
vegetable gumbo mixture	2.66 oz	–	35	–
(Pictsweet) as packaged				
mixed vegetables for stir-fry				
California	1 cup	–	35	–
Chinese	1¼ cups	–	50	–
Singapore	1¼ cups	–	45	–
teriyaki	1¼ cups	0.5	45	10%
premium mixed vegetables				
carrots..green beans & corn	⅔ cup	–	50	–
(Schwan's)				
California blend	1 cup	–	25	–
fire-roasted vegetable blend	1 cup	1.5	60	23%
herb garlic roasted Yukon gold potato & vegetable blend	1 cup	2.0	90	20%
mini bow tie pasta & vegetable blend	1 cup	1.0	120	8%
stir-fry vegetables	1 cup	–	40	–
(Seneca)				
broccoli				
Italian blend	¾ cup	–	30	–
Normandy	1 cup	–	30	–
stir-fry blend	1 cup	–	30	–
Oriental blend..all styles	¾ cup	–	25	–
Scandinavian blend	¾ cup	–	40	–
soup mix	¾ cup	–	40	–
winter blend	1 cup	–	25	–
(Veg-All)				
soup vegetables/potato	3.5 oz	–	50	–
stew vegetables				
4-ways	3.5 oz	–	55	–
5-ways	3.5 oz	–	50	–

Food and Description	Amount	Fat Grams	Total Calories	% Fat Calories
vegetable blends				
country	3.5 oz	–	50	–
Scandinavian	3.5 oz	–	45	–

VEGETARIAN FOODS

(NOTE: Some of the foods listed in this category were designed to be substitutes for meat and foods traditionally made with meat, and their names may therefore reflect the items they are intended to replace. However, all products listed here are meatless.)

(Amy's)..organic

Food and Description	Amount	Fat Grams	Total Calories	% Fat Calories
can or jar				
chili				
black bean	1 cup	2.0	200	9%
other styles..all regular	1 cup	6.0	190	28%
pasta sauces				
family marinara				
low sodium	½ cup	1.0	40	23%
regular	½ cup	1.0	50	18%
garlic mushroom	½ cup	7.0	120	53%
puttanesca	½ cup	2.0	40	45%
pomodoro zucca	½ cup	0.5	30	15%
tomato basil	½ cup	6.0	110	49%
soups				
alphabet	1 cup	0.5	80	6%
black bean vegetable	1 cup	1.5	130	10%
butternut squash				
light in sodium	1 cup	2.5	100	23%
regular	1 cup	2.5	100	23%
cream of mushroom	1 cup	9.0	140	58%
cream of tomato				
low sodium	1 cup	2.0	100	18%
regular	1 cup	2.0	100	18%
lentil				
light in sodium	1 cup	4.0	150	27%
regular	1 cup	4.5	150	27%
vegetable				
low sodium	1 cup	4.0	150	24%
regular	1 cup	4.0	150	24%
minestrone	1 cup	1.5	90	15%
no chicken noodle	1 cup	3.0	90	30%
pasta & 3-bean	1 cup	5.0	130	35%
split pea	1 cup	–	100	–
tomato bisque..chunky	1 cup	3.5	130	24%
vegetable barley	1 cup	1.0	70	13%
frozen				
bowls				
brown rice				
& vegetable	1 bowl	8.0	240	30%
country cheddar	1 bowl	19.0	400	43%
pesto tortellini	1 bowl	19.0	470	36%
Santa Fe enchilada	1 bowl	9.0	340	24%
stuffed pasta shells	1 bowl	12.0	300	36%
teriyaki	1 bowl	2.0	300	6%

Food and Description	Amount	Fat Grams	Total Calories	% Fat Calories
entrées				
black bean vegetable				
enchilada	4.75 oz	5.0	170	26%
cheese enchilada	4.75 oz	12.0	220	49%
cheese lasagna	10.25 oz	12.0	330	33%
classic lasagna	10.25 oz	12.0	330	33%
garden vegetable				
lasagna	10.25 oz	9.0	290	28%
macaroni & cheese	9 oz	16.0	410	35%
macaroni & soy cheese	9 oz	15.0	370	36%
pasta primavera	9.5 oz	11.0	300	33%
ravioli w/sauce	8 oz	12.0	340	32%
rice mac & cheese	9 oz	16.0	410	35%
tofu vegetable lasagna	9.5 oz	10.0	300	30%
vegetable lasagna	9.5 oz	12.0	300	36%
family-size				
black bean vegetable				
enchilada	5 oz	5.0	170	26%
cheese enchilada	5 oz	13.0	240	49%
macaroni & cheese..20 oz	1 cup	14.0	360	20%
vegetable lasagna	7 oz	8.0	200	36%
veggie loaf	5.7 oz	7.0	220	29%
pizzas				
cheese pizza	⅓ pizza	12.0	300	36%
mushroom & olive	⅓ pizza	9.0	250	32%
pesto w/tomato & broccoli	⅓ pizza	12.0	310	35%
rice crust cheese	⅓ pizza	14.0	300	42%
roasted vegetable	⅓ pizza	8.0	260	26%
soy cheese	⅓ pizza	11.0	290	34%
spinach	⅓ pizza	12.0	300	36%
veggie combo	⅓ pizza	11.0	290	34%
pocket sandwiches				
broccoli & cheese	4.5 oz	10.0	270	33%
Mediterranean vegetables	4.5 oz	7.0	220	29%
Mexican tamale	4.5 oz	7.0	250	25%
spinach feta	4.66 oz	12.0	300	36%
vegetable pie	5 oz	9.0	300	27%
vegetarian pizza	4.5 oz	6.0	250	22%
potpies				
broccoli	1 pie	22.0	430	46%
country vegetable	1 pie	16.0	370	39%
Mexican tamale	1 pie	3.0	150	18%
shepherd's	1 pie	4.0	160	23%
vegetable				
non-dairy	1 pie	13.0	360	37%
regular	1 pie	19.0	420	41%
whole meals..burgers..sandwiches				
all-American veggie burger	1.5 oz	3.0	120	23%
bean & cheese burrito	6 oz	8.0	280	26%
bean & rice burrito	6 oz	6.0	280	19%

Food and Description	Amount	Fat Grams	Total Calories	% Fat Calories
bean..rice & cheese burrito	6 oz	8.0	280	26%
black bean burrito	6 oz	8.0	320	23%
black bean enchilada	10 oz	8.0	320	23%
black bean & vegetable enchilada	6.0 oz	8.0	280	26%
breakfast burrito	6 oz	6.0	230	23%
broccoli & cheese in a pocket	1 pocket	10.0	270	33%
burrito especial	6 oz	6.0	260	21%
California veggie burger	2.5 oz	5.0	130	35%
cannelloni dinner	9 oz	11.0	260	38%
cheese enchilada	9 oz	14.0	330	38%
cheese ravioli	8 oz	12.0	340	32%
Chicago Veggie Burger	2.5 oz	5.0	160	28%
chili & cornbread	10.5 oz	6.0	340	16%
country dinner	10 oz	12.0	390	28%
enchilada dinner	10 oz	8.0	250	29%
Indian Mattar Paneer	10 oz	8.0	320	23%
macaroni & cheese	1 serving	19.0	450	38%
macaroni & soy cheese	1 serving	14.0	360	35%
Mexican tamale pie	1 pie	3.0	220	12%
pizza pocket				
cheese	1 pocket	9.0	300	27%
soy cheese	1 pocket	8.0	260	28%
spinach feta	1 pocket	9.0	250	32%
vegetarian	1 pocket	6.0	250	22%
roasted vegetables in a pocket	1 pocket	8.0	220	33%
stir-fry				
Asian noodle	10 oz	4.5	240	17%
Thai	9.5 oz	11.0	310	32%
tofu scramble in a pocket	1 pocket	6.0	180	30%
tofu-vegetable lasagna	9.5 oz	10.0	300	30%
vegetable lasagna w/cheese	9.5 oz	10.0	300	30%
vegetable pie in a pocket	1 pocket	9.0	300	27%
veggie loaf dinner	10 oz	7.0	280	23%
■ **(Boca Burgers)** (*See* Oscar Mayer, within this category)				
■ **(Bonavita)** vegetarian pâté/canned				
herb	1 Tbs	2.0	30	60%
garlic	1 Tbs	2.0	30	60%
green pepper	1 Tbs	2.0	30	60%
mushroom	1 Tbs	2.0	30	60%
■ **(Cascadian Farm)** frozen				
Meals for a Small Planet				
Aztec	3½ cups	4.0	290	12%
Indian	3½ cups	5.0	340	13%
Moroccan	3½ cups	5.0	310	15%

Food and Description	Amount	Fat Grams	Total Calories	% Fat Calories
Organic meals				
fettuccini Alfredo w/mushrooms	1 meal	16.0	360	40%
fiesta vegetarian enchiladas	1 meal	12.0	370	29%
spaghetti marinara w/vegetables	1 meal	4.0	230	16%
spinach lasagna	1 meal	13.0	330	35%
3-cheese pasta w/red peppers	1 meal	13.0	340	34%
vegetable blends				
California	⅔ cup	–	20	–
Chinese stir-fry	1 cup	–	25	–
gardener's	¾ cup	–	57	–
Santa Fe	¾ cup	–	60	–
Thai stir-fry	¾ cup	–	25	–
veggie & chicken bowls				
Caribbean veggies & rice	1 bowl	5.0	280	16%
Cascade veggies au gratin	1 bowl	6.0	170	32%
Fiesta casserole	1 bowl	11.0	340	29%
garden calzone	1 bowl	10.0	340	26%
Japanese noodles & vegetables	1 bowl	2.5	180	13%
pasta marinara	1 bowl	3.0	180	15%
pasta primavera	1 bowl	8.0	270	27%
Szechuan rice	1 bowl	1.5	210	6%
Teriyaki rice	1 bowl	7.0	270	23%
■ (CedarLane) Natural Cuisine..organic				
APPETIZERS, SIDES & SNACKS				
3-cheese quesadilla	1	11.0	250	40%
5-layer Mexican dip	2 Tbs	3.0	60	45%
mini bistro pizza	3 pizzas	15.0	280	48%
pesto, mozzarella & tomato bruschetta	1 piece	5.0	100	45%
BURRITOS & WRAPS				
low-fat				
beans, rice & cheese–style burrito	1	1.0	260	6%
couscous & vegetable veggie wraps	1	3.0	220	12%
vegetarian pizza veggie wraps	1	3.0	220	12%
roasted vegetable & cheese burrito	1	8.0	330	22%
vegetable & rice teriyaki veggie wrap	1	6.0	320	17%
veggie ham & cheese veggie wrap	1	10.0	350	26%

Food and Description	Amount	Fat Grams	Total Calories	% Fat Calories
CARB BUSTER ENTRÉES				
chili relleno pie	1 pkg	40.0	520	68%
eggplant Parmesan	1 pkg	15.0	220	61%
quiche				
broccoli cheddar	1 pkg	24.0	320	68%
4-cheese	1 pkg	38.0	500	68%
spinach artichoke	1 pkg	25.0	330	68%
spinach and				
feta enchiladas	1 pkg	37.0	490	68%
vegetable lasagna	1 pkg	40.0	504	71%
FOCACCIA/stuffed				
Mediterranean stuffed	⅓ focaccia	10.0	296	30%
roma tomato & basil	⅓ focaccia	9.0	275	29%
veggie pepperoni	⅓ focaccia	6.0	250	22%
SPECIALTY DINNER ENTRÉES				
3-layer enchilada pie	½ pie	7.0	215	29%
cheese enchiladas	1	17.0	270	57%
garden vegetable				
enchiladas low-fat	1	3.0	140	19%
lasagna	½ pkg	3.0	180	15%
grande burrito				
w/lasagna w/meatless				
ground round	1 pkg	12.0	380	28%
w/salsa roja	½ burrito	4.0	220	16%
■ **(Fantastic Foods)**				
entrées				
Carb'tastic Fast Naturals				
penne Alfredo	1 pkg	15.0	280	48%
Carb'tastic meal cups				
Asian ginger broccoli	1 pkg	1.5	80	11%
broccoli cheddar	1 pkg	3.0	110	25%
hot & sour	1 pkg	2.5	70	32%
shiitake mushroom	1 pkg	2.0	80	23%
sun-dried tomato basil	1 pkg	1.0	70	13%
vegetarian beef..w/barley	1 pkg	1.0	70	13%
vegetarian chicken gumbo	1 pkg	1.5	90	15%
vegetarian mandarin				
chicken	1 pkg	1.0	90	10%
Carb'tastic Ready Meals				
penne..w/ "meat" sauce	1 pkg	14.0	240	53%
vegetarian				
chili mac	1 pkg	18.0	290	56%
ginger shiitake				
w/rice noodles	1 pkg	10.0	340	26%
pad Thai..w/rice noodles	1 pkg	11.0	400	25%
pesto primavera	1 pkg	13.0	270	43%
Spanish paella	1 pkg	5.0	280	16%
teriyaki	1 pkg	10.0	220	41%
Thai lemon				
grass w/rice noodles	1 pkg	10.0	340	26%

Food and Description	Amount	Fat Grams	Total Calories	% Fat Calories
3-bean chili	1 pkg	4.0	180	20%
Tuscan mushroom				
risotto	1 pkg	1.5	310	4%
International Dishes..dry mix only				
black beans				
instant	⅓ cup	1.5	160	8%
falafel	¼ cup	2.0	120	15%
hummus				
original	2 Tbs	3.0	80	34%
pesto	2 Tbs	4.0	90	40%
spinach & Parmesan	2 Tbs	3.0	80	34%
polenta	¼ cup	5.0	260	17%
refried beans				
instant	¼ cup	1.5	130	10%
tabouli	2 Tbs	–	70	–
vegetarian meatless main dish mixes				
mix only..dry				
Nature's burger	¼ cup	3.0	170	16%
sloppy Joe	¼ cup	0.5	70	6%
taco filling	¼ cup	1.0	80	11%
tofu burger	3 Tbs	2.5	80	28%
tofu scrambler	2 Tbs	–	35	–
vegetarian chili/mix only	¼ cup	1.0	100	9%
■ (Forkless Gourmet)				
Filled Bun Meals				
beef & broccoli	1 bun	8.0	300	24%
beef asada	1 bun	7.0	280	23%
black bean adobo	1 bun	7.0	270	23%
chicken sesame teriyaki	1 bun	8.0	320	23%
chipotle chicken	1 bun	7.0	280	23%
kung pao shrimp	1 bun	9.0	320	25%
margarita chicken	1 bun	5.0	260	17%
pork & vegetables				
w/five fortune BBQ sauce	1	8.0	310	23%
pork w/ancho				
honey BBQ sauce	1	7.0	270	23%
Thai-style chicken	1	9.0	310	26%
vegetarian feast				
w/tofu & edamame	1	9.0	320	25%
■ (Gardenburger)				
frozen burgers				
classic Greek	1 burger	3.0	120	23%
dinner deluxe	1 burger	5.0	110	41%
fire-roasted vegetable	1 burger	2.5	120	19%
flame-grilled				
hamburger-style	1 burger	4.0	120	30%
garden vegan	1 burger	–	90	–
hamburger-style/fat-free	1 burger	–	90	–
Lifeburger/fat-free	1 burger	–	100	–
original	1 burger	3.0	110	25%

Food and Description	Amount	Fat Grams	Total Calories	% Fat Calories
roasted-garlic/fat-free	1 burger	–	90	–
Santa Fe	1 burger	2.5	130	17%
sautéed onion/fat-free	1 burger	–	100	–
savory portabello	1 burger	2.5	120	19%
smoked cheddar	1 burger	3.0	140	19%
veggie medley	1 burger	–	90	–
meatless, other				
BBQ chick'n	1 patty			
+ sauce		8.0	250	29%
buffalo chick'n wings	3 pieces	12.0	170	64%
chick'n grill	1 patty	2.5	100	23%
country fried chick'n	1 patty			
+ gravy		9.0	190	43%
herb-crusted cutlet	1 cutlet	9.0	170	48%
meatballs	6 pieces	4.5	110	37%
meat loaf w/gravy	1 slice	3.5	130	24%
riblets w/sauce	1 riblet	5.0	210	21%
soy BBQ ribs in smokey BBQ sauce	5 oz	5.0	210	21%
soy breakfast patties 6-count package	1 pattie	3.5	50	63%
soy herb patty	2.5 oz	9.0	170	48%
sweet 'n' sour pork	½ pouch	2.0	170	11%
veggie nuggets crispy 'n' crunchy pizza-spiced	2.66 oz	9.0	180	45%
■ (Lightlife)				
frozen				
Grilles				
BBQ	1 patty	3.5	120	26%
lemon	1 patty	6.0	140	39%
tamari	1 patty	5.0	130	35%
hot dogs				
Deli Jumbos..Smart	1 link	–	80	–
Dogs..Smart	1 link	–	40	–
Tofu Pups	1 link	2.5	60	38%
Lightburgers..2-count pkg	1 patty	–	100	–
Links..Smart				
Dog				
grill-ready brats	1 link	5.0	120	38%
grill-ready..2 oz	1 link	4.5	110	37%
links				
country breakfast– style	2 links	2.0	80	23%
Old World Italian–style	1 link	3.0	90	30%
breakfast	1 link	3.0	60	45%
lean Italian	1 link	2.0	60	38%
meatless..slices				
3 peppercorn–style pastrami	2 oz	–	60	–

Food and Description	Amount	Fat Grams	Total Calories	% Fat Calories
bologna.. Old World–style	2 oz	–	60	–
franks..1½ oz	1 link	–	45	–
ham..country-style	2 oz	–	90	–
Italian-style..Smart Links	2 oz	5.0	120	38%
pepperoni-style	1 oz	–	45	–
roast-style turkey	2 oz	–	80	–
Seitan..organic				
BBQ	3 oz	1.5	130	10%
teriyaki	3 oz	1.5	120	11%
Smart ground burgers				
& sausage				
Gimme Lean	2 oz	–	50	–
ground beef–style	2 oz	–	50	–
ground..meatless				
original	2 oz	1.0	80	11%
taco & burrito	2 oz	–	170	–
Smart Menu				
burger	1 burger	1.0	110	8%
Chick'n Nuggets	4 nuggets	11.0	220	45%
crumbles	⅓ cup	1.0	80	11%
cutlets				
Salisbury steak				
w/mushroom gravy	4.5 oz	1.0	130	7%
seasoned chicken	4.0 oz	3.5	180	18%
ground				
original	⅓ cup	–	70	–
taco burrito	⅓ cup	–	60	–
meatballs	5 pieces	7.0	160	39%
veggie burger	1 burger	1.0	80	11%
tempeh..organic				
Fakin' Bacon strips	3 slices	2.5	80	28%
garden veggie	4 oz	9.0	240	34%
soy	4 oz	9.0	210	39%
3-grain	4 oz	9.0	240	34%
wild rice	4 oz	11.0	280	35%
■ (Linda McCartney)..frozen meals				
butternut squash ravioli	1 meal	7.0	450	45%
Caribbean-style ragout	1 meal	12.0	310	35%
cheese enchiladas.. w/Mexican-style				
corn risotto	1 meal	11.0	250	40%
fettuccini Alfredo	1 meal	13.0	360	33%
fire-grilled vegetarian				
chicken & vegetables	1 meal	11.0	340	29%
macaroni & cheese	1 meal	21.0	420	45%
portabello mushroom				
barley pilaf	1 meal	6.0	250	22%
spicy peanut pasta				
w/vegetarian chicken	1 meal	5.0	340	13%
vegetarian chicken fajita	1 meal	9.0	320	25%
vegetarian chicken				

Food and Description	Amount	Fat Grams	Total Calories	% Fat Calories
Parmesan	1 meal	23.0	510	41%
■ (Loma Linda)				
canned or dry-packed				
Big Franks				
low-fat	1 link	3.0	80	34%
original	1 link	6.0	110	49%
chicken supreme/mix only	⅓ cup	1.0	90	10%
dinner cuts	2 slices	1.5	90	15%
Fried Chik'n..w/gravy	2 pieces	10.0	150	60%
Gravy Quik				
dry mix only	1 Tbs	–	20	–
brown	1 Tbs	–	20	–
chicken-style	1 Tbs	–	20	–
country-style	1 Tbs	0.5	20	23%
mushroom	1 Tbs	–	15	–
onion	1 Tbs	–	15	–
Linketts	1 link	4.5	70	58%
Little Links	2 links	6.0	90	60%
Nuteena luncheon loaf	⅜" slice	13.0	160	73%
ocean platter mix/mix only	⅓ cup	1.0	90	10%
patty mix/mix only	⅓ cup	1.0	90	10%
Redi-Burger	⅝" slice	2.5	120	19%
sandwich spread	¼ cup	4.5	80	51%
savory dinner loaf/mix only	⅓ cup	1.5	90	15%
Swiss Stake	1 piece	6.0	120	45%
Tender Bits	6 pieces	4.5	110	37%
Tender Rounds	8 pieces	4.5	120	34%
Vege-Burger	¼ cup	1.5	70	19%
Vitaburger..dry mix only				
chunks	¼ cup	1.0	70	13%
granules	3 Tbs	1.0	70	13%
frozen				
Chik Nuggets	5 pieces	15.0	240	56%
corn dog	1 piece	4.0	150	24%
mix..Soyagen..mix..only..all styles	¼ cup	6.0	130	42%
■ (Morningstar Farms)				
dry				
roasted soy butter	2 Tbs	11.0	170	58%
veggie burger kits				
Garden Grille	¼ pkg	–	80	–
Southwestern	¼ pkg	–	90	–
frozen or refrigerated				
America's original veggie dog	1 link	0.5	80	6%
Better 'n Burgers	1 pattie	2.0	100	18%
Better 'n Eggs	¼ cup	–	20	–
breakfast sausage links	2 links	3.0	80	34%
breakfast sausage patties	1 pattie	3.0	80	34%
breakfast sandwiches				
English muffin				
Scramblers..patty	1 sandwich	2.5	240	9%

Food and Description	Amount	Fat Grams	Total Calories	% Fat Calories
English muffin				
Scramblers				
w/cheese	1 sandwich	3.0	280	10%
breakfast strips	2 strips	4.5	60	68%
burger-style recipe crumbles	⅔ cup	3.0	90	30%
Chik patties				
Parmesan ranch	1 patie	7.0	170	37%
regular	1 pattie	6.0	150	34%
Chik'n				
buffalo wings	5 pieces	9.0	200	41%
nuggets	4 nuggets	7.0	190	33%
potpie	1 pie	14.0	350	36%
chili & cornbread potpie				
home-style	1 pie	9.0	330	25%
corn dogs				
mini	4 pieces	4.5	170	24%
regular	1	4.0	150	24%
deli franks	1 link	7.0	110	57%
fajita burger	1 burger	7.0	130	48%
garden grille patty	1 patty	2.5	120	19%
garden veggie patties	1 patty	2.5	100	23%
Grillers				
burger-style recipe crumbles	⅔ cup	2.5	80	28%
patties	1 patty	7.0	140	45%
Prime	1 patty	9.0	170	48%
veggie burgers	1 patty	6.0	140	39%
ground meatless crumbles	½ cup	–	60	–
Harvest burgers				
patties..original	1 patty	4.0	140	26%
oven-roasted veggie burgers	1 patty	4.0	120	30%
pizza..supreme	½ pizza	10.0	360	25%
portabello mushrooms & oven-roasted				
peppers veggie burgers	1 burger	4.0	120	30%
Quarter Prime Patties	1 patty	2.0	140	13%
sausage-style recipe crumbles	⅔ cup	3.0	90	30%
Scramblers	¼ cup	–	35	–
spicy black bean burger	1 patty	4.5	150	27%
tomato & basil pizza burger	1 patty	6.0	130	42%
■ (Natural Touch)				
canned				
vegetarian chili	1 cup	1.0	170	5%
frozen or refrigerated				
breakfast patty				
made w/organic soy	1 patty	3.0	80	34%
classic burger	1 burger	7.0	150	24%
corn dog..veggie	1	6.0	170	32%
dinner entrée	1 patty	15.0	220	61%
garden veggie patty	1 patty	2.5	110	20%
Herb Chik'n made w/organic soy	1 patty	2.5	110	20%
lentil rice loaf	1" slice	7.0	160	39%
9-bean loaf	1" slice	8.0	160	45%

Food and Description	Amount	Fat Grams	Total Calories	% Fat Calories
okra patty	1 patty	5.0	120	38%
spicy black bean burger	1 patty	1.0	100	9%
Tex Mex burger				
made w/organic soy	1 patty	1.5	120	11%
Thai burger	1 burger	3.5	100	32%
vegan burger				
made w/organic soy	1 patty	–	100	–
vegan burger crumbles	½ cup	–	60	–
vegan sausage crumbles	½ cup	–	60	–
Vege Frank	1 link	6.0	100	54%
Vegetarian Tuno tuna				
fish substitute	⅓ cup	2.0	60	30%
veggie medley				
made w/organic soy	1 patty	4.0	120	30%
zesty tomato basil burger	1 burger	6.0	130	42%
mix..dry mix only				
Kaffree Roma	1 rounded tsp	–	10	–
loaf	4 Tbs	0.5	100	5%
roasted soy butter	2 Tbs	11.0	170	58%
Roma Cappuccino	3 Tbs	3.0	50	54%
Stroganoff	4 Tbs	3.5	90	35%
taco	3 Tbs	1.0	60	15%
Veggie Burger Kit				
original	¼ pkg	–	80	–
Southwestern	¼ pkg	–	90	–
(Nasoya)				
marinated tofu				
refrigerated				
ginger sesame	½ pkg	6.0	210	26%
sweet & sour	½ pkg	4.0	190	19%
teriyaki	½ pkg	4.0	190	19%
Thai peanut	½ pkg	9.0	240	34%
(Near East)				
falafel				
vegetable patty mix				
dry mix only	¼ cup	1.00	100	9%
prepared	2½ patties	15.0	230	59%
taboule salad				
dry mix only	2½ Tbs	–	80	–
prepared	⅔ cup	3.0	110	25%
■ (NewMenu)..refrigerated				
Vegi-Burger	1 patty	1.0	110	8%
Vegidogs	1 link	–	45	–
■ (Oscar Mayer)..Boca soy				
breakfast links				
10-count package	2 links	4.0	100	36%
links				
70% less fat				
10-count package	2 links	3.5	90	35%
patties, 6-count package	⅙ pkg	4.0	80	45%

Food and Description	Amount	Fat Grams	Total Calories	% Fat Calories
patties, 10-count package				
70% less fat	2 patties	3.5	90	35%
burgers				
All American Classic				
55% less fat	¼ pkg	5.0	150	30%
70% less fat	¼ pkg	3.5	110	29%
cheese	¼ pkg	6.0	130	42%
garden vegetable				
70% less fat	¼ pkg	3.0	120	23%
grilled vegetable	¼ pkg	1.0	90	10%
roasted garlic				
70% less fat	¼ pkg	3.5	140	23%
80% less fat	¼ pkg	2.0	100	18%
roasted onion				
75% less fat	¼ pkg	2.5	140	16%
90% less fat	¼ pkg	1.0	90	10%
vegan				
75% less fat	¼ pkg	2.5	130	17%
original	¼ pkg	1.0	90	10%
ground				
burger..meatless..				
original	2 oz	0.5	70	6%
95% less fat	2 oz	0.5	70	6%
sausage..Italian	2 oz	0.5	60	8%
nuggets				
Original Chik'n				
65% less fat	2.85 oz	7.0	190	33%
patties				
Original Chik'n				
50% less fat	¼ pkg	6.0	150	36%
Spicy Chik'n				
50% less fat	¼ pkg	6.0	150	36%
pizza..meatless				
pepperoni				
regular	4 oz	8.0	240	30%
tomato & herb	4 oz	8.0	240	30%
supreme..w/pepperoni				
& sausage	4 oz	8.0	250	29%
sausages				
bratwurst				
60% less fat	¼ pkg	7.0	130	48%
natural ingredients	¼ pkg	6.0	120	45%
Italian				
65% less fat	¼ pkg	6.0	120	45%
natural ingredients	¼ pkg	7.0	130	48%
smoked..65% less fat	¼ pkg	5.0	130	35%

■ (Quorn)
cutlets
  garlic & herb

Food and Description	Amount	Fat Grams	Total Calories	% Fat Calories
chicken-style	1 cutlet	8.0	200	36%
naked	1 cutlet	2.5	80	28%
ground				
beef-style recipe	⅔ cup	2.5	80	28%
links..meat-free	2 links	3.0	70	39%
meatballs..meat-free	4 pieces	3.0	110	25%
pasta meals				
fettuccini Alfredo	1 pkg	16.0	360	40%
lasagna..meat-free	1 pkg	12.0	360	30%
nuggets..chicken-style	3-4 nuggets	8.0	180	40%
patties..chicken-style	1 patty	7.0	160	39%
roast..turkey-style	⅕ pkg	2.5	90	25%
Simply Sauté				
Indian	½ pack	4.0	240	15%
Mexican	½ pack	7.0	340	19%
Thai	½ pack	9.0	240	34%
tenders..chicken-style recipe	1 cup	2.0	90	20%
■ (Tamarind Tree)				
shelf stable				
low-fat				
Alu Chole	1 meal	6.0	350	15%
Channa Dal Masla	1 meal	5.0	340	13%
Dal Makhani	1 meal	6.0	330	16%
Dhingri Mutter				
vegan	1 meal	5.0	290	16%
regular				
Navratan Korma	1 meal	16.0	430	33%
Palak paneer	1 meal	15.0	380	36%
Saag Chole				
vegan	1 meal	10.0	370	24%
Vegetable Jalfrazi				
vegan	1 meal	6.0	310	17%
■ (Turtle Island Foods)				
Tofurky				
deli slices				
cranberry & stuffing	3 slices	3.0	103	26%
hickory-smoked	3 slices	3.0	103	26%
Italian	3 slices	4.0	103	35%
original	3 sices	3.0	103	26%
peppered	3 slices	3.0	10	26%
Philly style	3 slices	3.0	110	25%
gourmet sausages				
Beerbrats	3.5 oz	11.0	250	40%
kielbasa	3.5 oz	12.0	240	45%
sweet Italian sausage	¾ oz	13.0	260	45%
Jurky				
ginger teriyaki	4 pieces	2.0	110	16%
original	4 pieces	2.0	100	18%
peppered	4 pieces	2.0	100	18%
Super Burgers				
original	1 burger	2.0	120	15%

Food and Description	Amount	Fat Grams	Total Calories	% Fat Calories
smoked	1 burger	2.0	120	15%
Tex Mex	1 burger	2.0	120	15%
■ (Van's)..Frozen Waffles..eggless..dairy-free				
Belgian				
blueberry	2 waffles	3.5	184	17%
original	2 waffles	3.5	172	18%
7-grain	2 waffles	4.0	180	20%
Carb Manager				
butter pecan	2 waffles	12.0	200	54%
home-style	2 waffles	12.0	200	54%
flax	2 waffles	13.0	200	59%
gourmet				
97% fat free	2 waffles	2.0	180	9%
blueberry	2 waffles	3.5	157	20%
buckwheat	2 waffles	11.0	260	38%
flax	2 waffles	8.0	230	31%
multigrain	2 waffles	3.0	190	14%
original	2 waffles	3.5	145	22%
Mini..2 sets of 4				
blueberry	1 serving	3.5	119	26%
chocolate chip	1 serving	4.0	119	30%
home-style	1 serving	3.5	107	29%
wheat-free	1 serving	4.5	160	25%
organic				
blueberry	2 waffles	4.5	202	20%
original	2 waffles	4.5	190	21%
soy..flax	2 waffles	7.0	190	33%
wheat-free				
apple cinnamon	2 waffles	5.0	220	20%
blueberry	2 waffles	5.0	232	19%
flax	2 waffles	6.0	230	23%
mini	2 sets of 4	4.5	160	25%
original	2 waffles	5.0	220	20%
■ (White Wave)..refrigerated Tofu Tenders				
Havana black bean	½ pkg	8.0	200	36%
Mediterranean tahini	½ pkg	14.0	240	53%
sesame ginger..teriyaki	½ pkg	9.0	220	37%
tamari	⅓ pkg	8.0	150	48%
■ (Worthington)				
canned or dry-packed				
Chik				
diced/drained	¼ cup	–	50	–
sliced/drained	3 slices	6.0	90	60%
chili				
low-fat	1 cup	1.0	170	5%
original	1 cup	15.0	290	47%
choplets	2 slices	1.5	90	15%
corned beef meatless	4 slices	9.0	140	26%
country stew	1 cup	9.0	210	34%
cutlets	1 slice	1.0	70	13%
cutlets..multigrain	2 slices	2.0	100	18%

Food and Description	Amount	Fat Grams	Total Calories	% Fat Calories
FriChik				
low-fat	2 pieces	2.5	80	28%
original	2 pieces	8.0	140	51%
GranBurger	3 Tbs	0.5	60	8%
meatless				
chicken..diced	¼ cup	–	60	–
chicken roll	⅜" slice	4.5	90	45%
chicken slices	3 slices	4.5	90	45%
corned beef				
roll	⅜" slice	9.0	140	58%
slices	3 slices	9.0	140	58%
salami	3 slices	7.0	120	53%
smoked beef	3 slices	7.0	130	48%
smoked turkey				
vegetable protein slices	3 slices	9.0	140	58%
smoked turkey.. vegetable & grain				
protein roll	⅜" slice	9.0	140	58%
multigrain cutlets	2 slices	1.0	100	18%
Numete	⅜" slice	10.0	130	69%
Prime Stakes	1 piece	7.0	120	53%
Prosage				
links	2 links	3.0	80	34%
patties	1 patty	3.0	80	34%
vegetable & grain				
protein roll	⅝" slice	10.0	140	64%
Protose	⅜" slice	7.0	130	48%
Saucettes	1 link	6.0	90	60%
savory slices	3 slices	8.0	150	48%
sliced chik	3 slices	0.5	80	56%
sloppy joe	½ cup	2.0	140	13%
Stakelets patties	1 piece	7.0	150	42%
Stripples	2 strips	4.0	40	90%
Stroganoff	½ cup	3.5	110	29%
Super Links	1 link	8.0	110	65%
Tuno				
drained	⅓ cup	4.0	80	45%
tuna substitute..frozen	½ cup	6.0	80	68%
turkee slices	3 slices	12.0	180	60%
vegetable skallops	½ cup	1.5	90	15%
vegetable steaks	2 pieces	1.5	80	17%
vegetarian burger	¼ cup	2.0	60	30%
vegetarian cutlets	1 slice	1.0	70	13%
Veja-Links				
low-fat	1 link	1.5	40	34%
original	1 link	3.0	50	54%
Wham				
vegetable protein roll	⅜" slice	6.0	110	49%
vegetable protein slices	3 slices	7.0	110	57%
frozen				
BBQ FriChik				
w/5 Tbs BBQ sauce	2 pieces	9.0	240	34%

Food and Description	Amount	Fat Grams	Total Calories	% Fat Calories
Bolono	3 slices	3.0	80	34%
Chic-ketts roll	2⅝" slice	7.0	120	53%
ChikStiks	1 piece	6.0	100	54%
corned beef meatless	4 slices	9.0	140	58%
Crispy Chik	1 patty	6.0	150	36%
dinner roast	¾" slice	12.0	180	60%
fillet	2 fillets	9.0	180	45%
Fripats	1 patty	6.0	130	42%
golden croquettes	4 pieces	11.0	210	47%
Leanies..vegetable & grain protein links	1 link	7.0	100	63%
multigrain cutlets	2 slices	2.0	100	18%
■ (Yves)..Veggie Dogs				
hot 'n' spicy chili	1.85 oz	1.0	74	12%
original..jumbo	1.7 oz	1.3	104	11%
tofu dogs	1.35 oz	0.5	47	10%
veggie	1.6 oz	–	56	–
VENISON/boneless				
cured	3 oz	5.0	151	30%
raw				
ground/antelope	3.5 oz	2.0	110	16%
lean meat	3 oz	3.0	107	25%
steak	3 oz	5.0	153	29%
stew meat				
antelope	3.5 oz	2.0	110	16%
nilgai	3.5 oz	2.0	110	16%
roasted	3 oz	3.0	135	20%
stewed	3 oz	5.0	153	29%
VICHYSSOISE (See SOUP)				
VINE SPINACH				
fresh/raw	4 oz	–	22	–
VINEGAR				
(Bertolli)				
balsamic of Modena	1 Tbs	–	15	–
red wine	1 Tbs	–	3	–
white wine	1 Tbs	–	3	–
(China Bowl)				
white rice	1 Tbs	–	–	–
(Consorzio)				
balsamic..organic	1 Tbs	–	–	–
red wine	1 Tbs	–	–	–
(Eden)..all styles	1 Tbs	–	–	–
(Filippo Berio)				
balsamic of Modena	1 Tbs	–	–	–
sherry..cooking wine	2 Tbs	–	40	–
wine vinegar pure extra-strength	1 Tbs	–	–	–
(Four Monks)..all styles	1 Tbs	–	–	–
(Grey Poupon)				
balsamic	1 Tbs	–	–	–

Food and Description	Amount	Fat Grams	Total Calories	% Fat Calories
garden herb	1 Tbs	–	10	–
raspberry	1 Tbs	–	10	–
(Hain)				
apple cider				
raw/unpasteurized	1 Tbs	–	2	–
balsamic..from Italy	1 Tbs	–	10	–
cider	1 Tbs	–	2	–
red wine..from Italy	1 Tbs	–	–	–
white wine..from Italy	1 Tbs	–	–	–
(Heinz)..all styles	1 Tbs	–	2	–
(Indian Summer)				
apple cider	1 Tbs	–	3	–
	1 cup	–	40	–
white	1 Tbs	–	2	–
	1 cup	–	30	–
(Nakano)				
rice vinegar				
balsamic blend	1 Tbs	–	15	–
basil & oregano	1 Tbs	–	20	–
Italian herb	1 Tbs	–	20	–
natural	1 Tbs	–	–	–
roasted garlic				
original..seasoned	1 Tbs	–	20	–
pesto	1 Tbs	–	20	–
seasoned red pepper	1 Tbs	–	20	–
(Progresso)				
balsamic	1 Tbs	–	10	–
other styles..all	1 Tbs	–	–	–
(Regina) wine	1 oz	–	4	–
(S&W)..all styles	1 Tbs	–	–	–
(Spectrum Naturals) organic				
brown rice	1 Tbs	–	–	–
wine..raspberry	1 Tbs	–	10	–
(White House)				
apple cider	2 Tbs	–	2	–
red wine	2 Tbs	–	4	–

VODKA (See LIQUOR, DISTILLED)

W

Food and Description	Amount	Fat Grams	Total Calories	% Fat Calories
WAFFLE (*See also* PANCAKE & WAFFLE MIX)				
(Aunt Jemima) frozen				
blueberry	2 waffles	5.0	190	24%
buttermilk	2 waffles	5.0	200	23%
low-fat	2 waffles	2.5	160	14%
home-style				
10-count pkg	2 waffles	5.0	190	24%
16-count pkg	2 waffles	6.0	200	27%
(Belgian Chef)				
frozen				
Belgian waffles	2 waffles	2.0	180	10%
(Kashi)				
GoLean Waffles				
blueberry	2 waffles	3.0	170	16%
original	2 waffles	3.0	170	16%
(Kellogg's) frozen				
Eggo Waf-Fulls				
apple cinnamon	1 piece	5.0	150	30%
blueberry	1 piece	5.0	150	30%
strawberry	1 piece	5.0	150	30%
Eggo Waffles				
apple cinnamon	2 waffles	7.0	200	32%
banana bread	2 waffles	6.0	190	28%
blueberry	2 waffles	7.0	200	32%
buttermilk	2 waffles	7.0	190	33%
chocolate chip	2 waffles	7.0	200	32%
cinnamon toast	2 waffles	10.0	290	31%
Froot Loops	2 waffles	7.0	200	32%
home-style				
mini—3 sets	4 waffles	9.0	260	31%
regular	2 waffles	7.0	190	33%
Minis..2 sets of 4				
chocolate chip				
cookie dough	4 waffles	5.0	180	25%
Nutri-Grain				
low-fat				
blueberry	2 waffles	2.5	150	15%
whole wheat	2 waffles	2.5	140	16%
multi-bran	2 waffles	5.0	160	28%
whole wheat	2 waffles	5.0	170	26%

Food and Description	Amount	Fat Grams	Total Calories	% Fat Calories
Special K	2 waffles	–	120	–
SpongeBob Square Pants				
strawberry banana	2 waffles	7.0	190	33%
strawberry	2 waffles	7.0	200	32%
(Krusteaz)				
frozen				
Belgian	1 waffle	7.0	190	33%
golden	1 waffle	2.5	110	20%
mix/prepared				
Belgian waffle/7" round	1 waffle	19.0	440	39%
Supreme waffle/4x4" square	3 waffles	21.0	420	45%
(Nature's Path)				
natural waffles				
8-grain	2 waffles	9.0	240	34%
buckwheat wild berry	2 waffles	5.0	230	20%
flax plus	2 waffles	9.0	240	34%
hemp plus	2 waffles	9.0	240	34%
mesa sunrise	2 waffles	8.0	240	30%
soy plus	2 waffles	8.0	230	31%
organic waffles				
Envirokidz Gorilla				
banana	2 waffles	6.0	220	25%
Envirokidz Koala Choco	2 waffles	7.0	240	26%
Optimum Power	2 waffles	4.0	190	19%
(Thomas)..fresh				
blueberry	2 waffles	9.0	230	35%
buttermilk	2 waffles	8.0	220	33%
carb-counting				
home-style	1 waffle	5.0	110	41%
home-style	1 waffle	4.0	110	33%

(Van's) *See* VEGETARIAN FOODS
WAFFLE SYRUP (*See* MAPLE SYRUP; PANCAKE & WAFFLE SYRUP)
WAKAME (*See* SEAWEED)
WALNUT

Food and Description	Amount	Fat Grams	Total Calories	% Fat Calories
(Ann's House of Nuts)				
English	1 oz	18.0	180	90%
(Arroyo Seco)..all styles	1 oz	19.0	190	90%
(Azar)..English..pieces	1 oz	19.0	190	90%
(Diamond)..English..all styles	¼ cup	19.0	190	90%
(Diamond of California)				
black walnuts	¼ cup	18.0	200	81%
chopped	¼ cup	20.0	210	86%
finely diced	¼ cup	20.0	210	86%
ground	¼ cup	20.0	210	86%
halves & pieces	¼ cup	20.0	210	86%
shelled	¼ cup	20.0	210	86%
toasted walnut topping	2 Tbs	10.0	110	82%
	¼ cup	20.0	210	86%
(Fisher Chef's Naturals)				
walnuts				
chopped	1 oz	19.0	200	86%

Food and Description	Amount	Fat Grams	Total Calories	% Fat Calories
ground..fine	1 oz	19.0	200	86%
halves & pieces	1 oz	20.0	200	90%
in the shell..shelled	1 oz	20.0	200	90%
(Planters)				
black	2 oz	31.0	340	82%
English or Persian				
halves				
Gold Measure	2 oz	38.0	380	90%
regular	⅓ cup	22.0	220	90%
WATER (See also SOFT DRINK; COCKTAIL/COCKTAIL MIXERS)				
(Cascadia)..sparkling water w/juice				
all flavors	6 fl oz	–	2	–
grapefruit	6 fl oz	–	2	–
(Clearly Canadian)				
sparkling water				
blackberry	8 fl oz	–	100	–
cherry	8 fl oz	–	90	–
cranberry	8 fl oz	–	90	–
peach	8 fl oz	–	90	–
raspberry	8 fl oz	–	80	–
(Crystal Geyser)..seltzer water..light				
all flavors	6 fl oz	0	60	0
(Evian) spring water	8 fl oz	–	–	–
(Perrier)..mineral water with-a-twist				
all flavors	12 fl oz	–	–	–
(Propel) fitness water/all styles	8 fl oz	0	10	0
(San Francisco)				
sweetened seltzer				
almond cream	8 fl oz	–	100	–
black cherry	8 fl oz	–	110	–
peach	8 fl oz	–	100	–
raspberry	8 fl oz	–	110	–
WATER CHESTNUT (See also ASIAN FOOD)				
canned				
(3 Diamonds)				
sliced	½ cup	–	40	–
whole..peeled	½ cup	–	40	–
(Geisha)				
sliced	4.6 oz	–	50	–
whole..peeled	4.6 oz	–	45	–
(La Choy)				
sliced	1.33 oz	–	10	–
fresh..raw..sliced	½ cup	–	66	–
WATERCRESS/fresh/raw				
chopped	½ cup	–	2	–
whole	1 sprig	–	–	–
WATERMELON (See also WATERMELON RIND)				
fresh				
wedges/10" dia	1/16 wedge	2.0	152	12%
cubed	1 cup	0.7	50	12%

Food and Description	Amount	Fat Grams	Total Calories	% Fat Calories
WATERMELON RIND				
(Old South)	2 cubes	–	70	–
(Reese)	2 cubes	–	70	–
WATERMELON SEEDS/KERNELS				
dried	1 oz	13.0	158	74%
	1 cup	51.0	602	76%
WAX BEAN				
canned				
(Blue Boy).. cut wax beans	½ cup	–	25	–
(Del Monte)..cut..golden	½ cup	–	20	–
(Libby's)..cut wax	½ cup	–	80	–
(S&W)..all styles	½ cup	–	20	–
(Seneca) cuts	½ cup	–	25	–
WAX GOURD/fresh				
boiled	1 cup	–	23	–
raw	1 cup	–	17	–
WEAKFISH				
broiled w/butter or margarine	3 oz	9.6	177	49%
WELSH RAREBIT (*See also* FROZEN ENTRÉE/DINNER; SAUCE)				
WHALE/raw	3 oz	6.0	130	42%
WHEAT (*See also* BULGUR/HARD RED WINTER WHEAT; FLOUR; CEREAL; WHEAT GERM)				
(Arrowhead Mills)				
flakes	⅓ cup	0.5	110	4%
whole grain	¼ cup	1.0	160	6%
(Grain Gourmet) cracked wheat/mix only				
Side Dish Solutions	⅒ box	0.5	150	3%
(Hodgson Mill) vital wheat gluten				
w/vitamin C	4 tsp	–	40	–
(White Wave)				
seitan	¼ pkg	–	140	–
traditional	3 oz	1.0	140	6%
vegetarian stir-fry strips	3 oz	1.0	100	9%
WHEAT GERM (*See also* CEREAL)				
(Arrowhead Mills).. raw	3 Tbs	1.5	50	27%
(Bob's Red Mill) natural..raw	⅛ cup	1.0	52	17%
(Hodgson Mill)..untoasted	2 Tbs	1.0	55	16%
(Kretschmer)				
honey crunch	2 Tbs	1.0	50	18%
plain	1⅔ Tbs	1.0	50	18%
(Mother's)..toasted	2 Tbs	1.0	50	18%
(Stone-Buhr)..untoasted	2 Tbs	2.0	60	30%
WHELK (*See* SNAIL)				
WHEY				
dried				
acid	1 Tbs	–	10	–
	1 cup	–	193	–
sweet	1 Tbs	–	26	–
	1 cup	–	512	–
fluid				
acid	1 Tbs	–	4	–
	1 cup	<1.0	60	8%

Food and Description	Amount	Fat Grams	Total Calories	% Fat Calories
sweet	1 Tbs	–	4	–
	1 cup	0.7	65	10%

WHIPPED TOPPING (*See also* CREAM)
(Note: Unless specified otherwise, 1 serving of mix = the amount in 2 Tbs prepared)

Food and Description	Amount	Fat Grams	Total Calories	% Fat Calories
(Cool Whip)				
extra-creamy	2 Tbs	2.0	25	72%
free	2 Tbs	–	15	–
light	2 Tbs	1.0	20	45%
whipped topping				
original	2 Tbs	1.5	25	54%
(Dream Whip)..mix only	1 serving	0.5	10	45%
(Gay Lea)..real whipped cream				
light	3 oz	3.0	43	63%
regular	3 oz	4.8	72	60%
(Hood)				
whipped cream				
aerosol..instant				
light	2 Tbs	0.5	15	30%
regular	2 Tbs	1.5	20	68%
whipping cream	1 Tbs	4.5	45	90%
(Kraft)				
free..fat-free	2 Tbs	–	15	–
light cream/whipped	2 Tbs	1.0	10	90%
(LaCreme) light	2 Tbs	1.0	15	60%
(RediWhip)				
chocolate	2 Tbs	1.0	15	60%
deluxe/extra-creamy	2 Tbs	1.5	15	90%
fat-free	2 Tbs	–	5	–
original	2 Tbs	1.0	15	60%
real whipped				
heavy cream	2 Tbs	3.0	30	90%
light cream	2 Tbs	2.0	20	90%
(Rich's)				
non-dairy				
aerosol	2 Tbs	2.0	25	72%
bowl	2 Tbs	1.5	25	54%
Richwhip				
liquid	2 Tbs	2.0	25	72%
whipped	2 Tbs	2.0	25	72%
(Rockview Farms)..ultra-pasteurized				
sweetened..aerosol	2 Tbs	1.5	20	68%

WHISKEY (*See* LIQUOR, DISTILLED)

WHITE BEAN
canned

Food and Description	Amount	Fat Grams	Total Calories	% Fat Calories
(Goya)..Spanish-style	½ cup	0.5	125	4%
(S&W)..lightly seasoned				
low-fat	½ cup	0.5	80	6%
(Trappey's).. flavored w/slab bacon				
white lima beans	½ cup	1.5	130	10%

Food and Description	Amount	Fat Grams	Total Calories	% Fat Calories
dried				
boiled				
regular	½ cup	–	125	–
small	½ cup	0.5	127	4%
raw				
regular	½ cup	1.0	340	30%
small	½ cup	1.5	365	4%
WHITE PERCH/raw	3 oz	3.0	100	27%
WHITE SAUCE (*See* SAUCE)				
WHITEFISH/mixed species				
fresh				
cooked—dry heat	3 oz	5.5	145	34%
raw	3 oz	5.0	115	39%
jarred				
(Manischewitz)				
jellied..14.5-oz jar	1 ball	2.0	60	30%
regular..24-oz jar	1 ball	1.5	40	34%
(Mother's)				
jellied				
12-oz jar	1 ball	<1.0	50	14%
24-oz jar	1 ball	1.0	60	15%
regular				
12-oz jar	1 ball	<1.0	55	13%
24-oz jar	1 ball	1.0	70	13%
smoked				
(Ducktrap River)	2 oz	2.0	70	26%
	4 oz	1.0	122	7%
WHITEFISH & PIKE				
jarred				
(Manischewitz)				
jellied..14.5-oz jar	1 ball	1.5	60	23%
regular..14.5-oz jar	1 ball	1.5	50	27%
sweet	1 ball	1.5	70	19%
(Mother's)				
jellied in broth..12-oz jar	1 ball	<1.0	50	14%
regular	1 ball	1.0	70	13%
(Rokeach) jellied	1 ball	1.0	60	15%
WHITING (*See also* SEAFOOD ENTRÉE/DINNER)				
breaded & fried	3 oz	9.7	171	51%
cooked—dry heat	3 oz	1.0	98	9%
raw	3 oz	1.0	77	12%
WIENER (*See* FRANKFURTER; FRANKFURTER, VEGETARIAN; SAUSAGE; VEGETARIAN FOODS)				
WILD CELERY (*See* CELERIAC)				
WINE (Note: For the calories in a 4-ounce glass of wine, simply multiply calorie figures by 4.)				
(Andre) Champagne				
blush	1 fl oz	–	22	–
brut	1 fl oz	–	25	–
cold duck	1 fl oz	–	25	–
extra-dry	1 fl oz	–	24	–

Food and Description	Amount	Fat Grams	Total Calories	% Fat Calories
(Carl Jung) white/alcohol removed	1 fl oz	–	20	–
(Carlo Rossi)				
blush	1 fl oz	–	21	–
Burgundy	1 fl oz	–	22	–
chablis	1 fl oz	–	21	–
paisano	1 fl oz	–	23	–
red sangria	1 fl oz	–	24	–
Rhine	1 fl oz	–	21	–
vin rose	1 fl oz	–	21	–
white grenache	1 fl oz	–	20	–
(Eden Roc)				
brut	1 fl oz	–	21	–
brut rose	1 fl oz	–	22	–
extra-dry	1 fl oz	–	21	–
(Four Monks)..cooking sherry	1 fl oz	–	40	–
(Gallo)				
Ernest & Julio Gallo Vineyards				
cabernet sauvignon	1 fl oz	–	23	–
cafe zinfadel	1 fl oz	–	19	–
chardonnay	1 fl oz	–	24	–
classic Burgundy	1 fl oz	–	22	–
hearty Burgundy	1 fl oz	–	24	–
sauvignon blanc	1 fl oz	–	20	–
Malvasia chardonnay	1 fl oz	–	19	–
merlot	1 fl oz	–	24	–
white grenache	1 fl oz	–	21	–
white zinfandel	1 fl oz	–	20	–
Gallo of Sonoma				
barbera/Barrelli Creek—'95	1 fl oz	–	25	–
cabernet sauvignon				
Frei Ranch Vineyards				
all years	1 fl oz	–	24-25	–
Sonoma City..all years	1 fl oz	–	24-25	–
Stefani Vineyards				
all years	1 fl oz	–	24-25	–
chardonnay				
Laguna Ranch Vineyards				
all years	1 fl oz	–	24-25	–
Sonoma County—'95	1 fl oz	–	24	–
Stevani Vineyards				
all years	1 fl oz	–	24-25	–
merlot				
Frei Ranch Vineyards				
all years	1 fl oz	–	23-24	–
Sonoma City..all years	1 fl oz	–	25	–
Sonoma County	1 fl oz	–	24	–
pinot noir/Russian River Valley				
all years	1 fl oz	–	24-25	–
sangiovese/Alexander				
Valley—'97	1 fl oz	–	26	–

Food and Description	Amount	Fat Grams	Total Calories	% Fat Calories
valdiquie/Barrelli Creek Vineyards				
all years	1 fl oz	–	22-23	–
zinfandel				
Chiotti Vineyards—'95	1 fl oz	–	24	–
Frei Ranch Vineyards				
all years	1 fl oz	–	24-26	–
Sonoma County				
all years	1 fl oz	–	25-27	–
Sheffield label				
sherry				
cream	1 fl oz	–	44	–
very dry	1 fl oz	–	32	–
tawny port	1 fl oz	–	45	–
Turning Leaf				
cabernet sauvignon	1 fl oz	–	24	–
chardonnay	1 fl oz	–	22	–
fume blanc	1 fl oz	–	23	–
Johannesburg Riesling—'96	1 fl oz	–	22	–
merlot—'95	1 fl oz	–	23	–
white zinfandel—'96	1 fl oz	–	20	–
zinfadel	1 fl oz	–	23	–
Turning Leaf Sonoma Reserve				
cabernet sauvignon				
all years	1 fl oz	–	22-24	–
chardonnay..all years	1 fl oz	–	23-25	–
chardonnay fume—'95	1 fl oz	–	22	–
merlot..all years	1 fl oz	–	22-24	–
pinot noir..all years	1 fl oz	–	22-24	–
zinfandel..all years	2 fl oz	–	23-24	–
general				
barbera/white	4 fl oz	–	91	–
Beaujolais—12% alcohol	4 fl oz	–	96	–
Bordeaux/red—12% alcohol	4 fl oz	–	96	–
Burgundy				
cooking	¼ cup	–	2	–
red—12% alcohol	4 fl oz	–	96	–
sparkling—12% alcohol	4 fl oz	–	116	–
white—12% alcohol	4 fl oz	–	90	–
cabernet sauvignon	4 fl oz	–	88	–
chablis	4 fl oz	–	84	–
emerald	4 fl oz	–	102	–
gold	4 fl oz	–	97	–
pink	4 fl oz	–	98	–
ruby	4 fl oz	–	104	–
Champagne				
brut	4 fl oz	–	100	–
domestic	4 fl oz	–	84	–
extra-dry	4 fl oz	–	105	–
pink	4 fl oz	–	98	–
chardonnay	4 fl oz	–	88	–
chenin blanc	4 fl oz	–	86	–

Food and Description	Amount	Fat Grams	Total Calories	% Fat Calories
Chianti	4 fl oz	–	100	–
cold duck	4 fl oz	–	108	–
dessert	4 fl oz	–	180	–
Dubonnet	4 fl oz	–	160	–
French colombard	4 fl oz	–	88	–
Liebfraumilch—10% alcohol	4 fl oz	–	84	–
Madeira—19% alcohol	4 fl oz	–	160	–
muscatel	3.5 fl oz	–	158	–
port				
ruby—20% alcohol	4 fl oz	–	184	–
tawny—20% alcohol	4 fl oz	–	184	–
white	4 fl oz	–	172	–
Riesling—12% alcohol	4 fl oz	–	90	–
Rhone—12% alcohol	4 fl oz	–	96	–
rosé	4 fl oz	–	90	–
sake/saki	1.5 fl oz	–	36	–
sauvignon blanc	4 fl oz	–	80	–
sherry				
cooking	¼ cup	–	20	–
cream—19.5% alcohol	4 fl oz	–	200	–
dry—19% alcohol	4 fl oz	–	162	–
sweet	4 fl oz	–	165	–
table				
red	3.5 fl oz	–	74	–
rosé	3.5 fl oz	–	73	–
white	3.5 fl oz	–	70	–
Tokay	4 fl oz	–	164	–
vermouth				
dry—17% alcohol	4 fl oz	–	136	–
sweet—17% alcohol	4 fl oz	–	180	–
wine spritzer	5 fl oz	–	61	–
zinfandel				
red	4 fl oz	–	92	–
white	4 fl oz	–	82	–
(Grey Poupon) cooking wine				
Burgundy	1 fl oz	–	20	–
sherry	1 fl oz	–	35	–
white	1 fl oz	–	20	–
(Holland House) cooking wine				
Marsala	1 fl oz	–	45	–
red	1 fl oz	–	20	–
sherry	1 fl oz	–	45	–
vermouth	1 fl oz	–	35	–
white	1 fl oz	–	20	–
white..w/lemon flavor	1 fl oz	–	20	–
(Regina)				
cooking wine				
Burgundy	2 Tbs	–	20	–
sauterne..white	2 Tbs	–	20	–
sherry	2 Tbs	–	35	–

Food and Description	Amount	Fat Grams	Total Calories	% Fat Calories
WINE COOLER				
(Bartles & Jaymes)				
malt-based coolers				
black cherry	12 fl oz	–	200	–
Classic Original	12 fl oz	–	190	–
Exotic Berry	12 fl oz	–	210	–
Fuzzy Navel	12 fl oz	–	230	–
hard lemonade	12 fl oz	–	230	–
Juicy Peach	12 fl oz	–	210	–
kiwi strawberry	12 fl oz	–	214	–
Luscious Blackberry	12 fl oz	–	228	–
margarita	12 fl oz	–	260	–
original	12 fl oz	–	190	–
peach	12 fl oz	–	210	–
piña colada	12 fl oz	–	270	–
raspberry daiquiri	12 fl oz	–	216	–
raspberry hard lemonade	12 fl oz	–	226	–
strawberry cosmopolitan	12 fl oz	–	219	–
strawberry daiquiri	12 fl oz	–	220	–
tropical burst	12 fl oz	–	230	–
wine-based coolers				
Brazilian Mist Berry	12 fl oz	–	210	–
Classic Original	12 fl oz	–	200	–
Exotic Berry	12 fl oz	–	220	–
Fuzzy Navel	12 fl oz	–	250	–
hard lemonade	12 fl oz	–	240	–
kiwi strawberry	12 fl oz	–	230	–
Luscious Blackberry	12 fl oz	–	240	–
original	12 fl oz	–	200	–
raspberry hard lemonade	12 fl oz	–	230	–
strawberry daiquiri	12 fl oz	–	230	–
Tropical Burst	12 fl oz	–	240	–
(Boone's)				
Country Quencher	1 fl Oz	–	24	–
Delicious Apple	1 fl Oz	–	21	–
Sangria	1 fl Oz	–	22	–
Snow Creek Berry	1 fl Oz	–	18	–
Strawberry Hill	1 fl Oz	–	22	–
Sun Peak Peach	1 fl Oz	–	18	–
Wild Island	1 fl oz	–	18	–
WINGED BEAN				
cooked	½ cup	5.0	126	36%
raw	½ cup	15.0	375	36%
WOLFFISH				
Atlantic/fresh				
cooked—dry heat	3 oz	2.0	105	17%
raw	3 oz	2.0	80	23%
WONTON (See ASIAN FOOD)				
WONTON WRAPPER (See ASIAN FOOD)				
WORCESTERSHIRE SAUCE (See SAUCE)				

Food and Description	Amount	Fat Grams	Total Calories	% Fat Calories
YAM (*See also* SWEET POTATO)				
can or bag				
(Bruce's)..cut				
yams in syrup	⅔ cup	0.5	150	3%
yams in heavy syrup	⅔ cup	–	190	–
(McCain)..Roasters				
oven-roasted sweet potatoes	½ cup	4.0	120	30%
(Princella)				
candied	½ cup	–	240	–
in heavy syrup	½ cup	–	130	–
in light syrup	⅔ cup	0.5	160	3%
in pineapple-orange sauce	½ cup	–	210	–
in water	½ cup	–	90	–
(Royal Prince)				
candied	½ cup	–	210	–
in heavy syrup	6.3 oz	0.5	200	2%
in light syrup	½ cup	–	100	–
(S&W) candied/old-fashioned	½ cup	–	170	–
(Trappey's)				
golden sweet..whole yams				
in heavy syrup	6.3 oz	0.5	200	2%
Sugary Sam Golden				
mashed yams	⅔ cup	–	120	–
Sugary Sam Golden				
cut yams in syrup	⅔ cup	–	160	–
fresh				
Hawaii/mountain				
cooked/cubed	½ cup	–	59	–
raw				
cubed	½ cup	–	46	–
whole/ 8¼" long..2½ dia	1 yam	0.5	280	2%
regular				
boiled or baked..cubed	1 cup	–	158	–
raw..cubed	1 cup	–	177	–
YAM BEAN-TUBER (*See* JICAMA/YAM BEAN-TUBER)				
YARDLONG BEAN				
dried				
boiled	½ cup	<1.0	100	4%
raw	½ cup	1.0	290	3%
fresh				
boiled/drained/sliced	½ cup	–	25	–

Food and Description	Amount	Fat Grams	Total Calories	% Fat Calories
raw/sliced	½ cup	–	22	–
YEAST				
baker's				
(Fleischmann's) active dry & rapid rise				
packet or jar	¼ oz	–	–	–
fresh active	⅓ pkt	–	–	–
household	0.5 oz	–	–	–
(Red Star)				
active dry	¼ oz	–	15	–
	4 Tbs	–	45	–
flakes	3 Tbs	–	45	–
brewer's				
(Louis Laboratories)	2 Tbs	1.0	114	8%
torula	1 oz	–	79	–
YELLOWTAIL				
mixed species/fresh				
cooked—dry heat	3 oz	5.5	160	31%
raw	3 oz	4.5	125	32%
YOGURT, DAIRY				
(Alta Dena)				
fat-free..most flavors	1 cup	–	190	
fat-free..other flavors				
strawberry	1 cup	–	180	–
vanilla	1 cup	–	180	–
wildberries	1 cup	–	180	–
low-fat				
black cherry	1 cup	2.0	220	8%
peach	1 cup	2.0	220	8%
raspberry	1 cup	2.0	110	8%
strawberry	1 cup	2.5	210	11%
strawberry banana	1 cup	2.5	210	11%
(Blue Bunny)				
Carb Freedom..all flavors	6 oz	3.0	90	30%
Disney				
Swirl'n Magic cotton candy				
& bubblegum	1 cup	1.0	80	11%
strawberry & cherry	1 cup	1.0	80	11%
Yo-pals..all flavors	1 cup	3.0	120	23%
Lite 85..all flavors	6 oz	–	80	–
Lite 85..multipacks..all flavors	4 oz	–	50	–
(Breyers)				
Creme Savers ..all flavors	4 oz	1.5	120	11%
low-fat yogurt 4-oz cups				
all flavors	4 oz	1.5	120	11%
low-fat yogurt 8-oz cups				
all flavors	8 oz	3.0	240	11%
smoothie..all flavors	10 fl oz	3.0	190	14%
Fruit on the Bottom				
low-fat..all flavors	8 oz	2.0	240	8%
light..non-fat..4-oz cups				
all flavors	4 oz	–	60	–

Food and Description	Amount	Fat Grams	Total Calories	% Fat Calories
non-fat..8-oz cups				
all flavors	8 oz	–	120	–
Smooth & Creamy				
4-oz cups				
black cherry parfait	4 oz	1.0	110	8%
classic strawberry	4 oz	1.0	115	8%
peaches 'n' cream	4 oz	1.0	120	8%
raspberries 'n' cream	4 oz	1.0	120	8%
strawberry and banana	4 oz	1.0	120	8%
8-oz cups				
apple cobbler	8 oz	2.0	230	8%
black cherry parfait	8 oz	2.0	230	8%
classic strawberry	8 oz	2.0	230	8%
peaches 'n' cream	8 oz	2.0	240	8%
raspberries 'n' cream	8 oz	2.0	240	8%
strawberry and banana	8 oz	2.0	240	8%
strawberry cheesecake	8 oz	2.0	230	8%
vanilla	8 oz	2.0	240	8%
(Colombo)				
light..blended—6-count multipack				
all flavors	4 oz	1.0	110	8%
light..fat-free..all flavors	8 oz	–	120	–
low-fat..99% fat-free				
most flavors	8 oz	2.0	220	8%
vanilla	8 oz	2.0	180	10%
low-fat..32-oz container				
French vanilla	1 cup	2.5	180	13%
plain	1 cup	2.5	130	17%
strawberry	1 cup	3.0	190	14%
(Crowley)				
non-fat..all flavors	8 oz	1.5	130	10%
Swiss-style..all flavors	8 oz	2.5	240	9%
(Dannon)				
blended..all flavors	4 oz	–	100	–
Carb Control				
Light 'n' Fit..all flavors	4 oz	3.0	160	17%
Danimals..Super Creamy				
all flavors	4 oz	3.0	130	21%
Dannon Sprinklin's..low-fat				
Sprinklin's..multipack				
all flavors	4.1 oz	1.5	120	11%
fruit blends				
4-oz cups..mini pack				
all flavors	4 oz	1.0	110	8%
fruit blends..6-oz cups				
all flavors	6 oz	1.5	170	8%
Fruit on the Bottom..low-fat				
all flavors	6 oz	1.5	160	8%
La Crème				
banana	4 oz	5.0	150	30%

Food and Description	Amount	Fat Grams	Total Calories	% Fat Calories
other flavors..all	4 oz	5.0	140	32%
Light 'n' Fit Creamy..multipack				
all flavors	4 oz	–	60	–
Light 'n' Fit..Creamy Yogurt				
all flavors	6 oz	–	100	–
Light 'n' Fit..non-fat yogurt				
all flavors	6 oz	–	90	–
non-fat yogurt..mini pack				
raspberry..blueberry	4 oz	–	60	–
strawberry..peach	4 oz	–	60	–
strawberry..peach raspberry	4 oz	–	90	–
natural flavors..low-fat				
all flavors	6 oz	2.5	150	15%
original yogurt				
plain				
low-fat	6 oz	2.5	110	20%
natural	6 oz	8.0	160	45%
non-fat	6 oz	–	90	–
whipped..Low-fat				
all flavors	4.6 oz	3.0	160	17%
(Go-Gurt)..all flavors	1 tube	2.0	80	23%
(Hood)				
Carb Countdown				
all flavors	6 oz	1.5	80	17%
(Horizon)..organic				
baby yogurt..all flavors	½ cup	3.0	120	23%
blended..all flavors	¾ cup	2.0	160	11%
fat-free..all flavors	¾ cup	–	130	–
fat-free..32-oz carton				
plain	1 cup	–	170	–
vanilla	1 cup	–	170	–
Tubes..low-fat yogurt				
all flavors	1 tube	1.0	70	13%
Yo Yo's..all flavors	4 oz	1.0	110	8%
(Kemp's)				
Classic yogurt..low-fat				
all flavors	6 oz	1.5	160	8%
JR's yogurt..4-oz cups				
all flavors	1 cup	1.0	130	7%
non-fat yogurt				
all flavors	6 oz	–	90	–
100 Calorie yogurt				
all flavors	5 oz	–	100	–
(La Yogurt)				
blended..low-fat..6-oz cups				
light				
all flavors	6 oz	–	90	–
mixed berry	6 oz	2.0	160	11%

Food and Description	Amount	Fat Grams	Total Calories	% Fat Calories
original				
blueberry	6 oz	1.5	150	9%
cherry	6 oz	2.0	150	12%
cherry cheesecake	6 oz	1.5	160	8%
cherry vanilla	6 oz	2.0	170	11%
cinnamon bun	6 oz	2.0	160	11%
peach	6 oz	2.0	130	14%
pina colada	6 oz	1.5	150	9%
strawberry	6 oz	1.5	150	9%
strawberry banana	6 oz	1.5	150	9%
strawberry fruit cup	6 oz	2.0	150	12%
vanilla	6 oz	2.5	150	15%
blended..low-fat..8-oz cups				
blueberries 'n' cream	8 oz	2.0	200	9%
peaches 'n' cream	8 oz	2.0	200	9%
raspberries 'n' cream	8 oz	2.0	190	9%
strawberries 'n' cream	8 oz	2.0	200	9%
vanilla 'n' cream	8 oz	2.0	200	9%
blended..low-fat..enriched				
peach	6 oz	2.0	130	14%
piña colada	6 oz	2.0	160	11%
strawberry	6 oz	2.0	160	11%
Fruit on the Bottom yogurt..low-fat				
blueberry	8 oz	2.5	220	10%
mixed berry	8 oz	2.5	230	10%
peach	8 oz	2.0	220	8%
raspberry	8 oz	2.5	230	10%
strawberry	8 oz	2.0	220	8%
strawberry banana	8 oz	2.5	230	10%
vanilla	8 oz	3.0	200	14%
(Mountain High)				
Classic..low-fat..all flavors	6 oz	1.0	140	6%
European Delight				
all flavors	4 oz	2.0	110	16%
fat-free				
most flavors	6 oz	–	120	–
plain	6 oz	–	110	–
vanilla	1 cup	–	170	–
low-fat				
plain	1 cup	2.0	150	12%
vanilla	1 cup	2.0	200	9%
natural..fat-free..all flavors	6 oz	–	110	–
naturally nutritious				
all flavors	4 oz	0.5	100	5%
original				
plain	1 cup	8.0	190	38%
vanilla	1 cup	7.0	240	26%
(New Country) low-fat				
all flavors	6 oz	2.0	150	12%

Food and Description	Amount	Fat Grams	Total Calories	% Fat Calories
(Stonyfield Farm)				
organic yogurt				
32-ounce cups				
Banilla	1 cup	2.5	200	11%
plain	1 cup	2.0	120	15%
strawberry	1 cup	2.5	200	11%
vanilla	1 cup	2.0	190	9%
99% fat-free				
most all flavors	6 oz	1.5	130	10%
plain	6 oz	1.5	90	15%
vanilla	6 oz	1.5	140	10%
all natural..fat-free				
apricot mango	6 oz	–	130	–
Berry Bash	6 oz	–	130	–
black cherry	6 oz	–	130	–
blackberry	6 oz	–	140	–
blueberry	6 oz	–	130	–
Chocolate Underground	6 oz	–	180	–
French vanilla	6 oz	–	140	–
key lime	6 oz	–	140	–
Lotsa Lemon	6 oz	–	140	–
peach	6 oz	–	120	–
plain	6 oz	–	80	–
raspberry	6 oz	–	130	–
strawberry	6 oz	–	130	–
strawberry cheesecake	6 oz	–	140	–
for kids				
6-pack..4-oz cups				
all flavors	4 oz	1.0	110	8%
8-pack..2-oz tubes				
all flavors	1 tube	1.0	60	15%
Moo-La-La				
double chocolate	4 oz	5.0	150	30%
lemon chiffon	4 oz	5.0	140	32%
strawberry cheesecake	4 oz	6.0	140	39%
white chocolate				
raspberry	4 oz	6.0	140	39%
O'Soy..6 pack..6-oz cups				
most all flavors	6 oz	2.0	170	11%
vanilla	6 oz	2.0	150	12%
whole milk..6-oz cups				
French vanilla	6 oz	6.0	170	32%
strawberries & cream	6 oz	6.0	170	32%
vanilla truffle	6 oz	5.0	220	20%
wild blueberry	6 oz	6.0	170	32%
whole milk..32-oz cups				
French vanilla	1 cup	8.0	250	29%
plain	1 cup	9.0	180	45%
(TCBY)				
light				
all flavors	8 oz	–	100	–

Food and Description	Amount	Fat Grams	Total Calories	% Fat Calories
low-fat..all flavors	8 oz	2.0	220	8%
(Trix)..all flavors	4 oz	1.5	120	11%
(Weight Watchers) Ultimate 90				
all flavors	1 cup	–	90	–
(White Wave)..cultured soy				
apricot mango	6 oz	2.0	160	11%
banana strawberry	6 oz	2.0	160	11%
black cherry	6 oz	2.0	150	12%
blueberry	6 oz	2.0	160	11%
key lime	6 oz	2.0	160	11%
lemon	6 oz	2.0	160	11%
peach	6 oz	2.0	160	11%
plain	6 oz	3.0	120	23%
raspberry	6 oz	2.0	160	11%
strawberry	6 oz	2.0	160	11%
vanilla	6 oz	2.0	120	15%
(Yami)				
Yami-Free..all flavors	8 oz	–	100	–
Yami..low-fat..strawberry	8 oz	3.0	240	11%
(Yoplait)				
custard-style				
all flavors	6 oz	3.5	190	17%
all flavors	4 oz	2.0	120	15%
Go-Gurt..all flavors	1 tube	2.0	80	23%
light..fat-free				
most flavors	6 oz	–	100	–
other flavors				
Boston cream pie	6 oz	–	110	–
very cherry	6 oz	–	110	–
original..99% fat-free*				
(*except for coconut cream pie)				
all flavors..6 oz	6 oz	1.5	170	8%
other flavors				
coconut cream pie	6 oz	3.0	190	14%
plain	6 oz	–	100	–
white chocolate raspberry	6 oz	1.0	170	5%
all flavors..4 oz	4 oz	1.0	110	8%
Ultra..low-carb				
blueberry	6 oz	2.5	90	25%
peach	6 oz	2.5	90	25%
raspberry	6 oz	2.5	90	25%
strawberry crème	6 oz	2.5	170	13%
Whips..all flavors				
Yumsters..all flavors	4 oz	2.0	120	15%

YOGURT, FROZEN
■ BARS & NOVELTIES

Food and Description	Amount	Fat Grams	Total Calories	% Fat Calories
(Ben & Jerry's) Cherry Garcia pop	1 pop	13.0	250	47%
(Häagen-Dazs)				
raspberry & vanilla bar	1 bar	–	90	–
(Yoplait)				
Breakfast Bar				

Food and Description	Amount	Fat Grams	Total Calories	% Fat Calories
double fruit smoothie	1 bar	–	45	–
strawberry	1 bar	1.5	120	11%
orange vanilla	1 bar	4.5	180	23%
triple-dipped	1 bar	6.0	110	49%
■ REGULAR & SOFT-SERVE/CARTON OR PACKAGE				
(Baskin-Robbins)				
low-fat				
Maui Brownie Madness	½ cup	4.0	210	17%
Perils of Praline	½ cup	3.5	190	17%
Raspberry Cheese Louise	½ cup	4.0	190	19%
non-fat				
vanilla scoop	4 oz	–	150	–
non-fat..soft-serve				
chocolate	½ cup	–	120	–
peppermint	½ cup	–	110	–
red raspberry	½ cup	–	110	–
vanilla	½ cup	–	110	–
non-fat..soft-serve..no sugar added				
Truly Free				
most flavors	½ cup	–	90	–
other..chocolate	½ cup	–	80	–
(Ben & Jerry's)				
Cherry Garcia				
chocolate	½ cup	4.0	190	19%
original	½ cup	3.0	170	16%
Chocolate Fudge Brownie	½ cup	2.5	190	12%
Half Baked	½ cup	3.5	210	15%
Phish Food	½ cup	5.0	230	20%
(Blue Bunny)				
Brownie Fudge Fantasy	½ cup	–	110	–
all other flavors	½ cup	–	100	–
(Breyers)				
all-natural				
chocolate	½ cup	3.0	130	21%
strawberry	½ cup	2.5	120	19%
vanilla				
natural	½ cup	3.0	120	23%
no sugar added	½ cup	8.0	150	48%
vanilla..chocolate				
& strawberry	½ cup	2.5	120	19%
Carb Smart..all flavors	½ cup	4.5	90	45%
(Cascadian Farm)				
organic				
chocolate	½ cup	3.0	130	21%
lemon chiffon	½ cup	2.0	120	15%
mocha fudge	½ cup	2.0	120	15%
raspberry				
& chocolate swirl	½ cup	2.0	110	16%
vanilla	½ cup	3.0	130	21%
(Columbo) soft-serve				
low-fat				

Food and Description	Amount	Fat Grams	Total Calories	% Fat Calories
Old World Chocolate	½ cup	2.0	110	16%
peanut butter	½ cup	2.5	120	19%
strawberry	½ cup	1.5	110	12%
vanilla..all types	½ cup	1.5	110	12%
non-fat				
cookies'n cream	½ cup	–	120	–
German chocolate fudge	½ cup	–	110	–
all other flavors	½ cup	–	100	–
Slender Sensations				
chocolate	½ cup	–	70	–
all other flavors	½ cup	–	60	–
(Dannon) soft				
fat-free..all flavors	½ cup	–	100	–
low-fat				
chocolate	½ cup	3.0	120	23%
peanut butter	½ cup	3.0	120	23%
vanilla	½ cup	2.0	110	16%
(Dreyer's)				
fat-free				
black cherry vanilla swirl	½ cup	–	90	–
caramel praline crunch	½ cup	–	100	–
vanilla	½ cup	–	90	–
vanilla chocolate swirl	½ cup	–	90	–
regular				
cookies 'n' cream	½ cup	3.5	120	26%
Heath Toffee Crunch	½ cup	4.0	120	30%
raspberry vanilla	½ cup	2.5	100	23%
(Edy's)				
fat-free				
caramel praline crunch	½ cup	–	100	–
all other flavors	½ cup	–	90	–
regular				
cookies 'n' cream	½ cup	3.5	120	26%
Heath Toffee Crunch	½ cup	4.0	120	30%
raspberry vanilla	½ cup	2.5	100	23%
(Elan)				
Andes Mint Drift	½ cup	5.0	160	28%
black raspberry	½ cup	2.5	130	17%
chocolate	½ cup	3.0	130	21%
chocolate almond	½ cup	6.0	160	34%
coffee	½ cup	2.5	130	17%
decaf cappuccino	½ cup	2.5	130	17%
chocolate chip	½ cup	4.0	140	26%
strawberry	½ cup	2.5	120	19%
vanilla	½ cup	2.5	130	17%
(Friendly's)				
Apple Bettie	½ cup	3.0	140	19%
Fabulous Fudge Swirl	½ cup	3.0	140	19%
Fudge Berry Swirl	½ cup	4.0	150	24%
Strawberry Cheesecake Blast	½ cup	4.0	140	26%
Toffee Almond Crunch	½ cup	5.0	160	28%

Food and Description	Amount	Fat Grams	Total Calories	% Fat Calories
(Häagen-Dazs)				
pints				
low-fat				
chocolate fudge				
brownie	½ cup	2.5	200	11%
coffee	½ cup	4.5	200	20%
dulce de leche	½ cup	2.5	190	12%
strawberry	½ cup	–	140	–
strawberry banana	½ cup	2.0	160	11%
strawberry banana yogurt				
& sorbet	½ cup	2.0	160	11%
vanilla	½ cup	4.5	200	20%
vanilla raspberry				
swirl	½ cup	2.5	170	13%
soft-serve..at shops-non-fat				
chocolate mousse	½ cup	–	80	–
vanilla mousse	½ cup	–	70	–
all other flavors	½ cup	–	110	–
(Hood)				
non-fat				
caramel & brownie sundae	½ cup	–	120	–
double raspberry	½ cup	–	110	–
mocha fudge	½ cup	–	110	–
old-fashioned vanilla	½ cup	–	110	–
strawberry	½ cup	–	100	–
vanilla	½ cup	–	120	–
vanilla fudge	½ cup	–	120	–
regular				
chocolate almond praline	½ cup	3.0	140	19%
Classic Trio	½ cup	2.5	120	19%
coffee toffee chunk sundae	½ cup	3.0	150	18%
cookies 'n' cream	½ cup	3.5	140	26%
vanilla Swiss almond sundae	½ cup	4.0	150	24%
(Kemp's)				
fat-free				
caramel praline crunch	½ cup	–	110	–
chocolate	½ cup	–	90	–
cookies 'n' cream	½ cup	–	110	–
peach	½ cup	–	90	–
strawberry	½ cup	–	80	–
strawberry shortcake	½ cup	–	100	–
vanilla	½ cup	–	90	–
low-fat				
caramel brownie	½ cup	4.0	140	26%
chocolate almond	½ cup	5.0	140	32%
chocolate chip	½ cup	4.5	140	29%
Moose Lake fudge	½ cup	7.0	170	37%
peach	½ cup	2.0	110	16%
raspberry	½ cup	2.0	110	16%
strawberry	½ cup	2.0	110	16%

Food and Description	Amount	Fat Grams	Total Calories	% Fat Calories
vanilla	½ cup	3.0	120	23%
no sugar added..fat-free				
strawberry	½ cup	–	70	–
vanilla	½ cup	–	70	–
no sugar added..light				
butter pecan	½ cup	8.0	120	60%
chocolate caramel				
brownie	½ cup	5.0	110	41%
peanut butter	½ cup	8.0	130	55%
vanilla	½ cup	5.0	90	50%
(Schwan's)				
premium..low-fat				
black cherry	½ cup	2.5	120	19%
chocolate	½ cup	3.0	120	23%
chocolate fudge brownie	½ cup	3.0	130	21%
orange pineapple	½ cup	2.5	110	20%
peach	½ cup	2.0	110	16%
vanilla	½ cup	3.0	110	25%
wild berry	½ cup	2.5	120	19%
(Stonyfield Farm)				
organic				
chocolate	½ cup	–	100	–
chocolate mint chip	½ cup	3.0	130	21%
crème caramel	½ cup	1.5	120	11%
decaf coffee	½ cup	–	90	–
mocha almond fudge	½ cup	2.5	130	17%
raspberry	½ cup	–	100	–
vanilla	½ cup	–	110	–
vanilla fudge swirl	½ cup	–	110	–
(TCBY)				
soft-serve..all flavors				
96% fat-free	½ cup	3.0	140	19%
non-fat	½ cup	–	110	–
non-fat..no sugar added	½ cup	–	90	–
non-fat & non-dairy sorbet	½ cup	–	100	–
(Turkey Hill)				
low-fat				
mint cookies 'n' cream	½ cup	1.5	110	12%
vanilla bean	½ cup	1.5	110	12%
non-fat				
chocolate cherry cordial	½ cup	–	110	–
chocolate marshmallow	½ cup	–	120	–
fudge ripple	½ cup	–	100	—
Neapolitan	½ cup	–	90	–
orange swirl	½ cup	–	100	–
regular				
chocolate chip cookie dough	½ cup	3.5	130	24%
Graham Canyon	½ cup	7.0	160	39%

YOGURT BAR (*See* CANDY; YOGURT, FROZEN)

Food and Description	Amount	Fat Grams	Total Calories	% Fat Calories
YOGURT DRINK				
(Breyers)..Creme Savers				
Smoothies..all flavors	10 fl oz	3.0	190	14%
(Dannon)				
Actimel				
cultured dairy drink				
orange	3.3 fl oz	1.5	100	14%
original	3.3 fl oz	1.5	90	15%
vanilla	3.3 fl oz	1.5	100	14%
DanActive				
cultured dairy drink				
orange	3.3 fl oz	1.5	100	15%
original	3.3 fl oz	1.5	90	15%
strawberry	3.3 fl oz	1.5	100	14%
vanilla	3.3 fl oz	1.5	100	14%
Danimals drinkable				
all flavors	3.1 fl oz	1.5	90	15%
Danimals drinkable..multipacks				
all flavors	3.1 fl oz	1.5	90	15%
Danimals XL drinkable				
all flavors	5.75 oz	3.0	170	16%
Frusion smoothies..blends				
banana berry	10 fl oz	3.5	270	12%
cherry berry	10 fl oz	3.5	280	11%
peach passionfruit	10 fl oz	3.5	270	12%
strawberry kiwi	10 fl oz	3.5	270	12%
tropical fruit	10 fl oz	3.5	270	12%
wild berry	10 fl oz	3.5	280	11%
(Hood) yogurt smoothies				
all flavors	10 fl oz	3.0	100	27%
(Stonyfield Farm)..organic				
peach	1 bottle	3.0	250	11%
raspberry	1 bottle	3.0	240	11%
strawberry	1 bottle	3.0	250	11%
tropical banana	1 bottle	3.0	250	11%
vanilla	1 bottle	3.0	250	11%
wild berry	1 bottle	3.0	250	11%
(TCBY)				
Fruithead Smoothies				
20 oz..w/yogurt				
A Lotta Colada	1	17.0	550	28%
Berry Slim	1	3.0	410	6%
Healthy Balance	1	3.0	410	6%
Holy-Cal	1	3.0	470	6%
Peachy Lean	1	3.0	470	6%
Raspberry				
DeLite	1	3.0	360	8%
Revitalizer	1	3.0	370	7%
Tropical Replenisher	1	3.0	370	7%

Food and Description	Amount	Fat Grams	Total Calories	% Fat Calories
Workout Whey	1	3.0	460	6%
32 oz..w/yogurt				
A Lotta Coloda	1	17.0	710	22%
Berry Slim	1	4.0	600	6%
Healthy Balance	1	4.0	590	6%
Holy-Cal	1	3.5	610	5%
Peachy Lean	1	3.5	620	5%
Raspberry				
DeLite	1	4.5	510	8%
Revitalizer	1	3.5	530	6%
Tropical Replenisher	1	4.0	520	7%
Workout Whey	1	4.5	600	7%
(Tropicana)..smoothies				
all flavors	11 fl oz	–	250	–
(Yoplait)..Nouriche Smoothies				
light..all flavors	11 fl oz	–	170	–
regular..all flavors	11 fl oz	–	290	–
(Yonique)				
low-fat..all flavors	6 fl oz	1.5	150	9%

Z

Food and Description	Amount	Fat Grams	Total Calories	% Fat Calories

ZABAGLIONE (*See* CUSTARD)
ZUCCHINI (*See* SQUASH)
ZWIEBACK (*See* COOKIE)

FAST FOOD

Food and Description	Amount	Fat Grams	Total Calories	% Fat Calories
A&W				
fries				
cheese	1 order	16.0	350	41%
chili	1 order	16.0	370	39%
chili cheese	1 order	19.0	400	43%
regular	large	18.0	430	38%
hot dogs				
plain	1	17.0	280	55%
Coney..chili	1	18.0	310	52%
Coney..chili..cheese	1	21.0	350	54%
cheese	1	29.0	500	52%
onion rings	1 order	17.0	350	38%
sandwiches				
Deluxe				
bacon double cheeseburger	1	49.0	830	53%
double cheeseburger	1	42.0	750	50%
1¼ pound				
bacon cheeseburger	1	33.0	600	50%
¼ pound hamburger	1	26.0	500	47%
¼ pound cheeseburger	1	24.0	500	43%
Jr. hamburger	1	21.0	430	44%
Jr. cheeseburger	1	22.0	470	42%
Chicken sandwich				
crispy	1	25.0	580	39%
grilled	1	15.0	430	31%
chicken strips	3 pieces	29.0	500	52%
Sweet Treats				
float..A&W Root Beer	1	4.5	300	14%
freeze..A&W Root Beer	1	10.0	480	19%
milk shakes				
A&W Root Beer	1			
chocolate	1	29.0	700	37%
strawberry	1	29.0	670	39%
vanilla	1	31.0	720	39%
Polar Swirls..Sundaes				
chocolate	1	8.0	320	23%
hot caramel	1	9.0	340	24%
hot fudge	1	11.0	350	28%
strawberry	1	8.0	300	24%

Food and Description	Amount	Fat Grams	Total Calories	% Fat Calories
vanilla	1	8.0	310	23%

ARBY'S

■ BEVERAGES

shakes

chocolate	large	17.0	660	23%
	regular	14.0	510	25%
Jamocha	large	17.0	650	24%
	regular	13.0	500	23%
strawberry and vanilla	large	17.0	650	24%
	regular	13.0	500	23%

■ BREAKFAST

biscuit..plain	1	12.0	230	47%
add butter	1 Tbs	11.0	100	99%
add scrambled eggs	1 serving	6.0	80	68%
add Swiss cheese	1 slice	3.0	40	68%

biscuits..other

bacon	1	17.0	300	51%
ham	1	13.0	270	43%
sausage	1	27.0	390	62%

croissant

bacon 'n' egg	1	26.0	410	57%
ham 'n' cheese	1	26.0	410	57%
sausage 'n' egg	1	36.0	510	64%

sourdough

bacon..egg 'n' Swiss	1	29.0	500	52%
egg 'n' cheese	1	16.0	330	44%
ham..egg 'n' Swiss	1	23.0	450	46%

■ CHICKEN

fingers

4-pack	1 order	38.0	640	53%
combo.. w/curly fries	1 order	60.0	1050	51%
snack..w/curly fries	1 order	34.0	590	52%

■ DESSERT

Gourmet Chocolate Cookie	1 cookie	10.0	200	45%

■ SALADS..SALAD DRESSINGS

salad

chicken club salad	1 salad	33.0	530	56%
Martha's Vineyard	1 salad	8.0	250	29%
Santa Fe	1 salad	29.0	520	50%

salad dressing

buttermilk ranch

light	2 oz	6.0	100	54%
regular	2.28 oz	34.0	330	93%
Santa Fe	2.28 oz	31.0	300	93%
raspberry vinaigrette	2.28 oz	12.0	170	64%

■ SANDWICHES

chicken

bacon 'n' Swiss	1	27.0	550	44%
breast fillet	1	24.0	490	44%
Cordon Bleu	1	29.0	570	46%

Food and Description	Amount	Fat Grams	Total Calories	% Fat Calories
grilled chicken deluxe	1	12.0	380	28%
hot ham 'n' cheese	1	8.0	270	27%
hot ham 'n' Swiss melt	1	8.0	270	27%
roast chicken club	1	25.0	470	48%
roast beef				
Arby-Q				
in BBQ sauce	1	11.0	360	28%
Arby's melt w/cheddar	1	19.0	380	45%
beef 'n' cheddar	1	21.0	440	43%
Big Montana	1	29.0	590	44%
French Dip 'n' Swiss	1	25.0	320	70%
original				
giant	1	19.0	450	38%
junior	1	25.0	320	70%
regular	1	13.0	320	37%
super	1	19.0	440	39%
Philly beef supreme	1	37.0	450	74%
other sandwiches				
Market Fresh				
chicken salad	1	44.0	860	46%
roast turkey	1	38.0	830	41%
Ultimate BLT	1	46.0	780	53%
roast beef & Swiss	1	39.0	790	44%
roast ham & Swiss	1	31.0	700	40%
roast turkey & Swiss	1	27.0	720	34%
Market Fresh..Low Carbys..wraps				
chicken Caesar	1	27.0	520	47%
roast turkey				
& bacon	1	39.0	710	49%
Southwest chicken	1	30.0	550	49%
Ultimate BLT	1	47.0	540	65%
■ SIDE ORDERS				
baked potato				
broccoli 'n' cheddar	1 potato	23.0	460	45%
deluxe	1 potato	34.0	570	54%
plain	1 potato	–	200	–
chicken fingers				
meal	1 meal	47.0	880	48%
snack	1 snack	32.0	610	47%
curly fries				
regular	small	16.0	340	42%
	medium	22.0	410	48%
	large	34.0	630	49%
home-style fries	small	13.0	300	39%
	medium	16.0	380	38%
	large	24.0	570	38%
jalapeño bites				
large	10 bites	37.0	610	55%
regular	5 bites	19.0	310	55%

Food and Description	Amount	Fat Grams	Total Calories	% Fat Calories
mozzarella sticks				
large	8 sticks	45.0	850	48%
regular	4 sticks	23.0	430	48%
onion petals				
large	1 order	48.0	830	52%
regular	1 order	19.0	330	52%
potato cakes	2 cakes	14.0	220	57%
AU BON PAIN				
■ BAGELS				
bagels				
Asiago cheese	1 bagel	8.0	380	19%
cinnamon crisp	1 bagel	6.0	430	13%
cinnamon raisin	1 bagel	1.0	330	3%
cranberry walnut	1 bagel	4.0	460	8%
Dutch apple				
w/walnut streusel	1 bagel	3.5	470	7%
Everything	1 bagel	3.0	330	8%
French toast	1 bagel	7.0	420	15%
honey 9-grain	1 bagel	2.0	360	5%
jalapeño double cheddar	1 bagel	6.0	350	15%
onion	1 bagel	1.0	360	3%
plain	1 bagel	1.0	300	3%
sesame	1 bagel	4.0	380	9%
■ BREADS & LOAVES				
apple spice loaf	1 slice	8.0	190	38%
artisan				
baguette	1 slice	–	150	–
ficele	1 slice	–	150	–
Asiago flat bread	1 slice	29.0	330	79%
braided roll	1 roll	14.0	420	30%
bread bowl	1 bowl	3.0	640	4%
chocolate cherry bread	1 slice	2.5	170	13%
country white loaf	1 slice	–	110	–
focaccia	10.3 oz	9.0	740	11%
4-grain	1 slice	3.0	310	9%
French sandwich roll	1 roll	1.0	290	3%
hearth roll	1 roll	2.0	240	8%
Lahvash	1 roll	2.0	240	8%
multigrain loaf	1 slice	1.0	130	7%
Parisienne loaf	1 slice	–	120	–
petit pain roll	1 roll	–	200	–
rosemary garlic breadstick	1 slice	5.0	200	23%
3-seed sandwich roll	1 roll	2.0	330	5%
tomato herb loaf	1 slice	1.0	140	6%
■ BROWNIES & COOKIES				
brownies				
blonde..w/nuts	1	36.0	570	57%
cheesecake	1	26.0	470	50%
chocolate chip	1	25.0	480	47%
pecan	1	31.0	510	55%

Food and Description	Amount	Fat Grams	Total Calories	% Fat Calories
rocky road	1	33.0	550	54%
cookies				
chocolate chip	1 cookie	13.0	270	43%
chocolate-dipped				
cranberry almond	1 cookie	16.0	320	45%
double chocolate				
shortbread	1 cokie	19.0	340	50%
English toffee	1 cookie	11.0	210	47%
macaroon..chocolate-				
dipped shortbread	1 cookie	10.0	300	30%
oatmeal raisin	1 cookie	9.0	250	32%
shortbread				
plain	1 cookie	22.0	340	58%
white chocolate				
dipped chocolate	1 cookie	21.0	380	50%
■ MUFFINS				
apple spice	1 muffin	15.0	420	32%
banana walnut	1 muffin	19.0	440	39%
blueberry	1 muffin	19.0	510	34%
carrot nut	1 muffin	27.0	550	44%
chocolate cake..low-fat	1 muffin	2.0	320	6%
chocolate chunk	1 muffin	20.0	590	31%
corn	1 muffin	18.0	440	37%
cranberry walnut	1 muffin	26.0	560	42%
pumpkin	1 muffin	20.0	580	31%
raisin bran	1 muffin	13.0	530	22%
triple berry..low-fat	1 muffin	2.0	290	6%
■ PASTRY & CAKE				
cake				
apple crumble	1 piece	30.0	540	50%
butter crumb	1 piece	42.0	790	48%
raspberry crumb	1 piece	41.0	770	48%
pastry				
cinnamon roll	1 roll	15.0	340	13%
crème de fleur	1 piece	26.0	550	43%
Danish				
cranberry	1 Danish	10.0	370	24%
cranberry cheese	1 Danish	23.0	460	45%
lemon	1 Danish	20.0	430	42%
sweet cheese	1 Danish	18.0	420	39%
pecan roll	1 roll	29.0	750	35%
strudel				
apple	1 piece	18.0	410	40%
cherry	1 piece	19.0	390	44%
■ SALADS				
Caesar salad	1 serving	16.0	320	45%
Cobb	1 serving	22.0	460	43%
field green, gorgonzola				
& roasted walnuts	1 serving	34.0	400	77%
Thai chicken salad	1 serving	2.5	140	16%

Food and Description	Amount	Fat Grams	Total Calories	% Fat Calories
tomato mozzarella				
w/basil pesto	1 serving	19.0	280	61%
tuna garden salad	1 serving	25.0	420	54%
turkey medallion Cobb	1 serving	24.0	440	49%
■ **SANDWICHES & WRAPS**				
baguette sandwiches				
Dijon albacore tuna	1	10.0	450	20%
grilled chicken club				
w/chili dressing	1	29.0	670	39%
honey Dijon Cordon Bleu	1	12.0	590	18%
roast beef				
& Emmental Swiss	1	36.0	690	47%
Tucsan	1	39.0	710	49%
fresh sandwiches				
chicken				
Arizona chicken	1	19.0	580	29%
chicken tarragon				
w/field greens	1	42.0	800	47%
honey Dijon	1	12.0	630	17%
grilled w/mozzarella focaccia	1	24.0	740	29%
honey Dijon chicken salad	1	18.0	730	22%
Thai	1	6.0	420	13%
mozzarella..tomato & pesto	1	43.0	820	47%
Thai chicken	1	7.0	490	13%
turkey..ham & provolone	1	26.0	1030	23%
turkey..smoked				
hot-roasted club	1	34.0	360	85%
wraps				
chicken Caesar	1 wrap	25.0	600	38%
Cobb turkey	1 wrap	21.0	570	33%
fields & feta	1 wrap	17.0	560	27%
Mediterranean	1 wrap	23.0	580	36%
Southwestern tuna	1 wrap	26.0	650	36%
■ **SOUP**				
baked stuffed potato	8 oz	15.0	240	56%
broccoli cheddar	8 oz	16.0	230	63%
chicken Florentine	8 oz	9.0	170	48%
chicken noodle..low-fat	8 oz	2.0	90	20%
clam chowder	8 oz	15.0	220	61%
corn chowder	8 oz	13.0	240	49%
curried rice				
& lentil..low-fat	8 oz	1.0	100	9%
French Moroccan				
tomato lentil..low-fat	8 oz	1.0	110	8%
French onion				
soup..low-fat	8 oz	3.0	80	34%
garden vegetable..low-fat	8 oz	1.0	40	23%
Harvest Pumpkin	8 oz	7.0	140	45%
Italian Wedding	8 oz	4.0	100	36%

Food and Description	Amount	Fat Grams	Total Calories	% Fat Calories
Jamaican black bean				
low-fat..reduced-sodium	8 oz	0.5	110	4%
potato cheese	8 oz	9.0	180	40%
potato leek	8 oz	12.0	190	57%
red beans..rice	8 oz			
& sausage	8 oz	4.0	180	20%
Southern black-eyed pea				
low-fat	8 oz	1.0	190	5%
Southwest tortilla	8 oz	6.0	140	39%
Southwestern vegetable				
reduced-sodium..low-fat	8 oz	3.0	150	18%
wild mushroom bisque	8 oz	5.0	110	41%

BLIMPIE

■ SANDWICHES..SANDWICH BREAD..COOKIES

Food and Description	Amount	Fat Grams	Total Calories	% Fat Calories
9 grams of fat or less				
buffalo chicken sub	6" reg	7.4	320	21%
grilled chicken sub	6" reg	9.0	425	19%
MexiMax sub	6" reg	9.0	425	19%
roast beef sub	6" reg	7.5	388	17%
seafood sub	6" reg	7.7	355	20%
turkey sub	6" reg	7.4	320	21%
VegiMax sub	6" reg	7.0	395	16%
9 grams of fat or less..cookie				
oatmeal raisin cookie	1 cookie	8.0	190	43%
9 grams of fat or less..salads				
chef	regular	9.0	212	38%
grilled chicken	regular	5.2	139	34%
seafood	regular	4.4	122	32%
BCC IT! Café Sandwiches				
Cable Car Club	6" reg	10.0	300	30%
Fisherman's Wharf				
tuna melt	6" reg	12.0	300	36%
Golden Gate Gourmet	6" reg	16.0	350	41%
Union Square Ultimate Veggie	6" reg	17.0	280	55%
breads				
garden Italian	6" reg	4.0	268	13%
honey oat	6" reg	7.4	298	22%
LoCarb wrap	10"	3.0	127	21%
marbled rye	6" reg	3.0	297	9%
Mediterranean				
flat bread	1 piece	9.0	270	30%
tortilla				
flour	1 wrap	8.2	323	23%
spinach	1 wrap	8.0	308	23%
wheat	6" reg	3.7	233	14%
w/poppy seed	6" reg	4.2	240	16%
w/sesame seed	6" reg	5.0	247	18%
white	6" reg	3.4	238	13%
w/poppy seed	6" reg	4.0	245	15%
w/sesame seed	6" reg	4.7	252	17%
zesty Parmesan	6" reg	4.0	268	13%

Food and Description	Amount	Fat Grams	Total Calories	% Fat Calories
café sandwiches				
Cable Car Club	6" reg	9.0	350	23%
Fisherman's Wharf tuna melt	6" reg	11.0	350	28%
Golden Gate Gourmet	6" reg	14.0	400	32%
Union Square Ultimate Veggie	6" reg	15.0	330	41%
cold subs				
Blimpie Best	6" reg	16.0	476	30%
club	6" reg	12.0	440	25%
ham & cheese	6" reg	12.5	436	26%
roast beef	6" reg	13.5	468	26%
seafood	6" reg	7.7	355	20%
tuna	6" reg	23.0	493	42%
turkey	6" reg	11.0	424	23%
desserts..cookies				
chocolate chunk	1	10.0	200	45%
macadamia white chunk	1	10.0	210	43%
oatmeal raisin	1	8.0	190	38%
peanut butter	1	12.0	220	49%
sugar	1	17.0	330	46%
grilled subs				
beef, turkey & cheddar	6" reg	31.0	600	47%
Cuban	6" reg	12.0	462	23%
Pastrami Special	6" reg	14.0	462	27%
Reuben	6" reg	33.0	630	47%
Ultimate Club	6" reg	42.0	724	52%
hot subs				
BLT	6" reg	32.0	588	50%
chicken				
grilled	6" reg	9.0	373	22%
buffalo	6" reg	13.4	400	30%
ChikMax	6" reg	13.2	511	23%
meatball	6" reg	27.0	572	42%
MexiMax	6" reg	9.0	425	19%
pastrami	6" reg	17.0	507	30%
steak & onion melt	6" reg	15.0	440	32%
VegiMax	6" reg	7.0	395	16%
wraps				
beef & cheddar	reg	37.0	714	47%
chicken Caesar	reg	35.0	646	49%
Southwestern	reg	35.0	674	47%
steak & onion	reg	37.0	716	47%
Ultimate BLT	reg	50.0	831	54%
Zesty Italian	reg	33.0	638	47%
BOSTON MARKET				
■ BAKED GOODS				
apple pie	1 slice	31.0	550	51%
brownie				
caramel pecan	1	47.0	900	47%
family-size	1	24.0	500	43%
chocolate brownie	1	23.0	580	36%

Food and Description	Amount	Fat Grams	Total Calories	% Fat Calories
family-size	1	8.0	160	45%
chocolate				
cake	1 slice	32.0	650	44%
Mania	1	33.0	490	61%
cookies				
chocolate chip	1 cookie	19.0	390	44%
oatmeal scotchie	1 cookie	20.0	390	46%
cornbread	1 loaf	6.0	200	27%
■ ENTRÉES				
chicken				
crispy-baked country	1 serving	22.0	420	47%
mango..grilled	1 serving	12.0	390	28%
marinated..grilled	1 serving	10.0	230	39%
potpie	1 pie	46.0	750	55%
ham..honey-glazed	1 serving	8.0	210	34%
meat loaf..Angus				
w/beef gravy	1 serving	23.0	360	58%
w/chunky Creole sauce	1 serving	19.0	350	49%
w/double sauce	1 serving	19.0	310	55%
rotisserie chicken				
¼ chicken				
dark meat				
garlic				
skinless	1 serving	10.0	190	47%
w/skin	1 serving	21.0	320	59%
white meat				
garlic				
skinless..w/o wing	1 serving	4.0	170	21%
w/skin & wing	1 serving	12.0	280	39%
½ chicken..sweet garlic				
w/skin	1 serving	33.0	590	50%
turkey breast rotisserie				
skinless	1 serving	1.0	170	5%
■ SALADS				
Caesar				
chicken..marinated grilled	1 salad	62.0	800	70%
entrée	1 salad	40.0	470	77%
side	1 salad	26.0	300	78%
w/o dressing	1 salad	12.0	230	47%
Oriental grilled chicken				
w/dressing & noodles	1 salad	20.0	570	32%
w/o dressing or noodles	1 salad	9.0	300	27%
Southwest grilled chicken				
w/dressing & chips	1 salad	58.0	890	59%
w/o dressing & chips	1 salad	23.0	470	44%
tossed/individual				
w/Caesar dressing	1 salad	31.0	380	73%
w/fat-free ranch	1 salad	2.5	160	14%
w/Old Venice dressing	1 salad	27.0	340	71%

Food and Description	Amount	Fat Grams	Total Calories	% Fat Calories
■ SANDWICHES				
chicken carver				
marinated..grilled	1	36.0	670	48%
w/no mayo	1	13.0	470	25%
w/cheese & sauce	1	29.0	640	41%
w/no cheese & no sauce	1	6.0	400	14%
meat loaf carver..w/cheese	1	29.0	730	36%
turkey carver				
w/cheese & sauce	1	26.0	630	37%
w/no cheese & no sauce	1	4.5	400	10%
■ SIDE DISHES				
butternut squash	¾ cup	6.0	150	36%
coleslaw	¾ cup	22.0	310	64%
creamed spinach	¾ cup	20.0	260	69%
garlic new potatoes	¾ cup	2.5	130	17%
green bean casserole	¾ cup	4.5	80	51%
green beans	¾ cup	4.0	70	51%
macaroni & cheese	¾ cup	11.0	280	35%
mashed potatoes				
home-style w/gravy	¾ cup	9.0	230	35%
plain	⅔ cup	9.0	210	39%
poultry gravy	1 oz	0.5	15	30%
rice pilaf	⅔ cup	4.0	140	26%
savory stuffing	¾ cup	8.0	190	38%
sesame broccoli	½ cup	2.5	80	28%
squash casserole	¾ cup	24.0	330	65%
steamed vegetables/low-fat	⅔ cup	0.5	35	13%
sweet corn	¾ cup	4.0	180	20%
sweet potato casserole	¾ cup	13.0	280	42%
tomato au gratin	¾ cup	10.0	160	56%
vegetable medley	¾ cup	–	30	–
■ SOUPS				
chicken tortilla	1 cup	11.0	220	45%
tomato bisque	1 cup	29.0	380	69%
tortilla..w/topping	1 cup	8.0	170	42%
BURGER KING				
■ BEVERAGES				
shakes				
chocolate shake	1 medium	16.0	600	24%
	1 large	27.0	850	29%
strawberry shake	1 medium	17.0	590	26%
	1 large	26.0	840	28%
vanilla shake	1 medium	20.0	540	33%
	1 large	29.0	800	33%
■ BREAKFAST				
biscuit				
bacon, egg & cheese	1 biscuit	21.0	380	50%
plain	1 biscuit	15.0	300	45%
sausage	1 biscuit	33.0	490	61%
sausage, egg & cheese	1 biscuit	43.0	620	62%

Food and Description	Amount	Fat Grams	Total Calories	% Fat Calories
Cini-Minis w/o icing	4 rolls	23.0	440	47%
Croissan'wich				
w/bacon..egg..cheese	1	22.0	360	55%
w/egg & cheese	1	19.0	320	53%
w/ham..egg..cheese	1	20.0	360	50%
w/sausage & cheese	1	31.0	420	66%
w/sausage..egg..cheese	1	39.0	520	68%
French toast sticks	5 pieces	20.0	390	46%
hash browns	small	15.0	230	59%
	large	25.0	390	58%
sourdough breakfast sandwich				
w/bacon..egg..cheese	1	22.0	380	52%
w/ham..egg..cheese	1	20.0	380	47%
w/sausage..egg..cheese	1	39.0	540	65%
■ BURGERS				
bacon cheeseburger				
double	1 burger	31.0	530	53%
regular	1 burger	20.0	390	46%
BK VEGGIE burger	1 burger	16.0	380	38%
fire-grilled burgers				
cheeseburger..regular	1 burger	17.0	350	44%
double cheeseburger	1 burger	31.0	530	53%
hamburger	1 burger	23.0	440	47%
hamburger..regular	1 burger	13.0	310	38%
Whopper				
double sandwich				
low-carb	1 burger	40.0	540	67%
w/mayo	1 burger	61.0	970	57%
w/o mayo	1 burger	44.0	810	49%
double w/cheese sandwich				
low-carb	1 burger	47.0	630	67%
w/mayo	1 burger	69.0	1060	59%
w/o mayo	1 burger	50.0	850	53%
original sandwich				
low-carb	1 burger	20.0	280	64%
w/mayo	1 burger	42.0	700	54%
w/o mayo	1 burger	24.0	540	40%
original w/cheese sandwich				
low-carb	1 burger	28.0	370	68%
w/mayo	1 burger	49.0	800	55%
w/o mayo	1 burger	31.0	640	44%
Whopper Jr. sandwich				
low-carb	1 burger	0.0	140	64%
w/mayo	1 burger	22.0	390	51%
w/o mayo	1 burger	13.0	310	38%
Whopper Jr. w/cheese sandwich				
low-carb	1 burger	14.0	190	66%
w/mayo	1 burger	26.0	430	54%
w/o mayo	1 burger	19.0	370	46%

Food and Description	Amount	Fat Grams	Total Calories	% Fat Calories
■ CHICKEN & FISH				
chicken				
sandwich				
grilled Caesar club	1	14.0	480	26%
original				
w/mayo	1	28.0	560	45%
w/o mayo	1	17.0	460	33%
Santa Fe..fire-grilled				
baguette	1	4.5	370	11%
savory mustard				
fire-grilled baguette	1	4.5	380	11%
TenderCrisp				
w/mayo	1	47.0	810	52%
w/o mayo	1	23.0	600	35%
Whopper				
low-carb	1	3.5	160	20%
w/mayo	1	25.0	570	39%
w/o mayo	1	7.0	410	15%
Tenders	4 pieces	9.0	170	48%
	5 pieces	12.0	210	51%
	8 pieces	19.0	340	50%
fish sandwich/BK Big Fish				
w/tartar sauce	1	30.0	520	52%
w/o tartar sauce	1	13.0	360	33%
■ DESSERT				
Nestlé Toll House				
chocolate chip cookies	2 cookies	16.0	440	33%
■ SIDE ORDERS				
chili	1 serving	8.0	190	38%
French fries				
salted/unsalted	small	11.0	230	43%
	medium	18.0	230	70%
	large	25.0	500	45%
	king-size	30.0	600	45%
onion rings	small	9.0	180	45%
	medium	16.0	320	45%
	large	23.0	480	43%
	king size	27.0	550	44%
CHICK-FIL-A				
■ BEVERAGES				
■ CHICKEN & CHICKEN SANDWICHES				
chicken..no bun..no pickle				
char-grilled	1 fillet	1.5	100	5%
regular	1 fillet	11.0	230	43%
chicken				
nuggets	4 pieces	13.0	290	40%
	8-pack	12.0	260	42%
sandwiches				
char-grilled				
club sdw..no sauce	1	11.0	380	26%
regular sdw	1	3.5	270	12%

Food and Description	Amount	Fat Grams	Total Calories	% Fat Calories
Chick-fil-A	1	16.0	410	35%
no butter	1	13.0	380	31%
Chick-fil-A deluxe	1	16.0	420	34%
chicken salad	1	15.0	350	39%
wraps..Cool Wraps				
Caesar	1 wrap	10.0	460	20%
regular	1 wrap	7.0	390	16%
spicy	1 wrap	6.0	380	14%
■ DESSERT				
cheesecake..plain	1 slice	21.0	340	56%
fudge nut brownie	1 brownie	15.0	330	41%
ice cream				
cone	1 small	4.0	160	23%
cup	1 small	6.0	230	23%
■ SALADS & SOUP				
salad toppings				
croutons				
garlic and butter	1 pkt	3.0	50	54%
sunflower kernels				
honey-roasted	1 pkt	7.0	80	79%
tortilla strips	1 pkt	3.5	70	45%
salads and slaw				
carrot & raisin	1 salad	6.0	170	32%
char-grilled chicken				
garden salad	1 salad	6.0	180	30%
Southwest	1 salad	8.0	240	30%
chicken Caesar salad	1 salad	10.0	230	39%
Chick-fil-A Chick-n				
strips salad	1 salad	18.0	390	42%
coleslaw	small	21.0	260	73%
■ SIDE ORDERS (See also SALADS & SOUP in this section)				
waffle potato fries	small	14.0	280	45%
CHURCH'S CHICKEN				
■ CHICKEN				
with batter and skin removed				
breast	2.5 oz	5.5	145	34%
leg	2 oz	6.2	118	47%
thigh	2.25 oz	11.0	180	55%
wing	2.25 oz	7.5	160	42%
with skin				
breast	2.8 oz	12.4	200	56%
leg	2 oz	9.0	140	58%
tender crunchers	6-8 pieces	15.0	411	33%
tender strip	2 oz	5.0	137	33%
thigh	2.8 oz	16.0	230	63%
wing	3.1 oz	16.0	250	58%
■ DESSERT				
apple pie	1 piece	12.0	280	39%
Edward's double-lemon pie	1 pie	12.0	380	39%

Food and Description	Amount	Fat Grams	Total Calories	% Fat Calories
Edward's strawberry cream cheese pie	1 pie	15.0	280	48%
■ SIDE ORDERS				
biscuit..honey butter	1 biscuit	16.0	250	58%
Cajun rice	1 serving	7.0	130	48%
coleslaw	1 serving	6.0	92	59%
collard greens	1 serving	–	25	–
corn on the cob	1 piece	3.0	139	19%
French fries	1 serving	11.0	210	47%
jalapeño cheese bombers	1 serving	10.0	113	80%
macaroni & cheese	1 serving	11.0	210	47%
okra	1 serving	16.0	210	69%
potatoes & gravy	1 serving	3.0	90	30%
steak..country-fried w/white gravy	1 serving	28.0	470	54%
sweet corn nuggets	regular	12.0	250	43%
whole jalapeño peppers	2	–	10	–
COUSINS SUBS				
■ BREADS				
15" rolls				
Italian	1	3.0	420	6%
Parmesan-Asiago	1	18.0	620	26%
wheat	1	3.0	420	6%
ciabatta bread	1	1.0	230	4%
low-carb wraps	1 wrap	8.0	188	38%
■ SALADS, SAUCE & SOUPS				
salads				
tuna	1 salad	28.0	369	68%
salads..lower fat & calories				
chef	1 salad	11.5	280	37%
garden	1 salad	13.0	195	60%
w/chicken breast	1 salad	17.0	335	46%
seafood	1 salad	35.0	440	72%
side	1 salad	7.0	103	61%
soups				
cheese	regular	16.0	240	60%
	large	24.0	360	60%
chicken dumpling	regular	5.0	170	26%
	large	8.0	255	28%
chicken noodle	regular	3.0	120	23%
	large	4.0	180	20%
chicken w/rice	regular	12.0	230	47%
	large	18.0	340	48%
chili	regular	9.0	250	32%
	large	14.0	375	34%
cream of broccoli	regular	12.0	190	57%
	large	18.0	285	57%
cream of potato	regular	9.0	190	43%
	large	14.0	285	44%
New England clam chowder	regular	5.0	150	30%
	large	8.0	225	32%

Food and Description	Amount	Fat Grams	Total Calories	% Fat Calories
tomato basil				
w/ravioli	regular	1.0	110	8%
	large	2.0	165	11%
vegetable beef	regular	2.0	80	23%
	large	2.0	120	15%
■ SUBS & SANDWICHES				
ciabatta sandwiches				
Classic Cubano pork	1 sdw	34.0	592	52%
Spicy chicken Sedona	1 sdw	23.0	480	43%
Tucsan Market club	1 sdw	23.0	438	47%
cold subs..mini..4"				
ham & provolone	1 sub	23.0	382	54%
Italian special	1 sub	27.0	431	56%
meatball & provolone	1 sub	14.0	329	38%
provolone	1 sub	27.0	422	58%
seafood w/crab	1 sub	16.0	311	46%
tuna	1 sub	33.0	476	62%
turkey breast	1 sub	19.0	347	49%
cold subs 7½"				
BLT	1 sub	42.0	613	62%
cappacola				
& cheese	1 sub	39.0	637	55%
& Genoa	1 sub	40.0	630	57%
cheesesteak	1 sub	24.0	540	40%
chicken breast	1 sub	34.0	618	50%
club	1 sub	43.0	744	52%
double cheesesteak	1 sub	46.0	851	48%
garden veggie	1 sub	11.0	365	27%
Genoa & provolone	1 sub	49.0	730	60%
gyro	1 sub	40.0	680	53%
ham & provolone	1 sub	39.0	644	55%
hot veggie	1 sub	23.0	491	42%
Italian				
Cousins' Special	1 sub	53.0	797	60%
regular	1 sub	44.0	683	58%
meatball & provolone	1 sub	27.0	586	41%
pepperoni melt	1 sub	52.0	784	60%
Philly cheesesteak	1 sub	36.0	680	48%
pizza sub	1 sub	49.0	771	57%
provolone	1 sub	45.0	686	59%
roast beef	1 sub	36.0	618	52%
seafood w/crab	1 sub	32.0	554	52%
tuna salad	1 sub	60.0	832	65%
turkey breast	1 sub	32.0	559	52%
cold subs..lower fat..no mayo or cheese				
4" mini				
ham	1 sub	3.0	189	14%
turkey breast	1 sub	2.0	194	9%
7½"				
BLT	1 sub	14.0	358	35%
chicken breast	1 sub	6.0	363	15%

Food and Description	Amount	Fat Grams	Total Calories	% Fat Calories
club	1 sub	6.0	369	15%
garden veggie	1 sub	2.0	245	7%
ham	1 sub	5.0	309	15%
hot veggie	1 sub	7.0	289	22%
roast beef	1 sub	6.0	363	15%
steak	1 sub	15.0	420	32%
turkey breast	1 sub	3.0	304	9%
hot subs				
cheesesteak	½ sub	17.0	470	33%
chicken breast	½ sub	31.8	556	51%
double cheesesteak	½ sub	26.0	550	43%
gyro	½ sub	23.0	550	38%
Italian sausage	½ sub	57.5	816	63%
meatball & cheese	½ sub	43.3	685	57%
pepperoni melt				
w/mayo	½ sub	46.1	702	59%
w/o mayo	½ sub	19.8	466	38%
Philly cheesesteak	½ sub	23.0	510	41%
steak	½ sub	12.0	425	25%
veggie	½ sub	14.3	380	34%
DAIRY QUEEN				
■ BEVERAGES				
malt				
chocolate	small	16.0	640	23%
	medium	22.0	870	23%
	large	35.0	1320	24%
Misty Slush	small	–	220	–
	medium	–	290	–
shakes				
chocolate	small	15.0	560	24%
	medium	20.0	760	24%
	large	33.0	1140	26%
■ BURGERS & HOT DOGS				
hamburger..DQ home-style				
double				
deluxe				
plain	1 burger	17.0	340	45%
w/bacon & cheese	1 burger	36.0	610	53%
w/cheese	1 burger	31.0	540	52%
single				
plain	1 burger	12.0	290	37%
w/cheese	1 burger	17.0	340	45%
Ultimate	1 burger	43.0	670	58%
hot dog				
chili 'n' cheese	1 hot dog	21.0	330	57%
plain	1 hot dog	14.0	240	53%
Super Dog				
chili 'n' cheese	1 hot dog	47.0	710	60%
plain	1 hot dog	37.0	580	57%

Food and Description	Amount	Fat Grams	Total Calories	% Fat Calories
■ **CHICKEN..BEEF..PORK**				
beef				
BBQ beef sandwich	1	9.0	300	27%
chicken				
basket				
strip basket	1 basket	50.0	1000	45%
sandwiches				
breaded chicken	1	27.0	510	48%
pork				
BBQ pork sandwich	1	8.0	280	26%
■ **FROZEN DESSERT SPECIALTIES**				
banana split	1 serving	12.0	510	21%
Blizzard				
banana split	small	14.0	460	27%
	medium	17.0	580	26%
	large	23.0	810	26%
chocolate chip				
cookie dough	small	28.0	720	35%
	medium	40.0	1030	35%
	large	52.0	1320	35%
Oreo cookies	small	21.0	570	33%
	medium	26.0	700	33%
	large	37.0	1010	33%
cone				
chocolate	small	8.0	240	30%
	regular	11.0	340	29%
dipped	small	17.0	340	45%
	medium	24.0	490	44%
	large	36.0	710	46%
vanilla	small	7.0	230	27%
	medium	9.0	330	25%
	large	15.0	460	29%
Brownie Earthquake	1	27.0	740	33%
Dilly Bar..chocolate	1 bar	13.0	210	56%
DQ				
cake..undecorated				
frozen 8" round	⅛ cake	13.0	370	32%
fudge bar				
no sugar added	1 bar	–	50	–
lemon Freez'r	½ cup	–	80	–
sandwich	1	6.0	200	27%
soft serve				
chocolate	½ cup	5.0	150	30%
vanilla	½ cup	4.5	140	29%
Starkiss	1	–	80	–
vanilla orange bar				
no sugar added	1 bar	–	60	–
Peanut Buster Parfait	1 serving	31.0	730	38%
Pecan Praline Parfait	1 serving	29.0	720	36%
Starkiss	1 serving	–	80	–

Food and Description	Amount	Fat Grams	Total Calories	% Fat Calories
strawberry shortcake sundae	1 serving	14.0	430	29%
chocolate	small	7.0	280	23%
	medium	10.0	400	23%
	large	15.0	580	23%
strawberry	small	7.0	240	26%
	medium	9.0	340	24%
	large	15.0	500	27%
Triple Chocolate Utopia	1 serving	39.0	770	46%
■ SIDE ORDERS				
French fries	small	12.0	200	54%
	medium	15.0	300	45%
	large	19.0	400	43%
onion rings	1 serving	30.0	470	57%
DAVANNI'S				
calzones				
chicken tomato	1	28.0	660	38%
pepperoni sausage	1	38.0	730	47%
sausage green pepper	1	32.0	696	41%
3-cheese	1	35.0	700	45%
garlic cheese bread				
half order..w/sauce	½ order	25.5	369	62%
whole order..w/sauce	1 order	48.0	687	63%
hoagies				
cheese	½ hoagie	29.0	401	65%
chicken				
breast	½ hoagie	33.0	495	60%
Parmigana	½ hoagie	19.0	383	45%
club	½ hoagie	27.0	400	61%
ham	½ hoagie	25.0	379	59%
Italian sausage	½ hoagie	37.0	522	64%
meatball	½ hoagie	31.0	464	60%
Mediterranean	½ hoagie	38.0	511	67%
pastrami	½ hoagie	27.0	459	53%
pizza	½ hoagie	18.0	315	51%
roast beef	½ hoagie	25.0	385	58%
salami	½ hoagie	38.0	484	71%
tuna	½ hoagie	44.0	563	70%
turkey	½ hoagie	24.0	372	58%
veggie	½ hoagie	29.0	445	59%
lasagna				
half lasagna..w/toast	1 serving	36.0	547	59%
whole lasagna..w/toast	1 serving	66.0	989	60%
DEL TACO				
■ BURGERS				
Bun Taco	1	21.0	440	43%
Cheeseburger	1 burger	13.0	330	35%
Del cheeseburger				
bacon	1 burger	39.0	610	58%
double	1 burger	35.0	560	56%

Food and Description	Amount	Fat Grams	Total Calories	% Fat Calories
regular	1 burger	13.0	330	35%
single	1 burger	25.0	430	52%
hamburger	1 burger	9.0	280	29%
■ BREAKFAST				
bacon	2 slices	4.0	50	72%
burritos				
egg & cheese	1 burrito	24.0	450	48%
Macho bacon & egg	1 burrito	60.0	1030	52%
regular breakfast	1 burrito	11.0	250	40%
steak & egg	1 burrito	34.0	580	53%
hash brown sticks	1 order	19.0	250	68%
quesadillas				
bacon & egg	1	23.0	450	46%
■ BURRITOS				
beef				
Del Beef				
regular	1 burrito	30.0	550	49%
deluxe	1 burrito	33.0	590	50%
Macho	1 burrito	62.0	1170	48%
carnitas	1 burrito	21.0	440	43%
chicken				
Del Classic	1 burrito	36.0	560	58%
Macho	1 burrito	33.0	930	32%
spicy	1 burrito	16.0	480	30%
Works	1 burrito	23.0	520	40%
combination				
deluxe	1 burrito	25.0	570	39%
Macho	1 burrito	44.0	1050	38%
regular..Del Combo	1 burrito	22.0	530	37%
green				
bean & cheese	1 burrito	8.0	280	26%
half pound	1 burrito	12.0	430	25%
red				
bean & cheese	1 burrito	8.0	270	27%
half pound	1 burrito	12.0	430	25%
Steak Works	1 burrito	31.0	590	47%
Veggie Works	1 burrito	18.0	490	33%
■ COMBO MEALS..regular fries and drink included				
#1 Combo burrito	1 meal	44.0	1020	30%
#2 Del Classic chicken burrito	1 meal	59.0	1050	51%
#3 steak taco, fries	1 meal	45.0	940	43%
#3 chicken tacos	1 meal	33.0	830	36%
#4 two chicken soft tacos	1 meal	46.0	910	45%
#5 Ultimate taco..chicken				
chicken quesadilla	1 meal	48.0	980	44%
#6 two tacos, quesadilla	1 meal	47.0	960	44%
#7 Macho combo burrito	1 meal	67.0	1540	39%
#8 Two Big Fat steak tacos	1 meal	60.0	1270	43%
#8 Two Big Fat chicken tacos	1 meal	49.0	802	55%
#9 Double Del cheeseburger	1 meal	58.0	1050	50%

Food and Description	Amount	Fat Grams	Total Calories	% Fat Calories
#10 Big Fat chicken taco				
& soft chicken taco	1 meal	48.0	1040	42%
#11 Del beef burrito, taco	1 meal	63.0	1200	47%
#12 spicy chicken burrito				
& soft taco	1 meal	50.0	1180	38%
■ COMBO MEALS..LARGE				
large fries and drink included				
#1 combo burrito	1 meal	54.0	1250	39%
#2 Del Classic chicken burrito	1 meal	68.0	1280	48%
#3 steak tacos Del Carbon	1 meal	54.0	1170	42%
#3 chicken tacos Del Carbon	1 meal	42.0	1050	36%
#4 two chicken soft tacos	1 meal	55.0	1130	44%
#5 two Ultimate tacos				
chicken quesadilla	1 meal	65.0	1340	44%
#6 three tacos, quesadilla	1 meal	57.0	1200	43%
#7 Macho combo burrito	1 meal	76.0	1760	39%
#8 Two Big Fat steak tacos	1 meal	69.0	1500	41%
#8 Two Big Fat chicken tacos	1 meal	59.0	1400	38%
#9 Double Del cheeseburger	1 meal	67.0	1280	47%
#10 Big Fat chicken taco				
soft chicken taco	1 meal	57.0	1270	40%
#11 Del beef burrito, taco	1 meal	72.0	1430	45%
#12 spicy chicken burrito				
chicken soft taco	1 meal	59.0	1400	38%
■ NACHOS				
Macho nachos	1 order	63.0	1100	52%
regular nachos	1 order	24.0	380	57%
■ QUESADILLAS				
chicken cheddar	1	31.0	580	48%
plain	1	12.0	257	42%
regular	1	27.0	500	49%
spicy jack	1	12.0	254	43%
chicken	1	30.0	570	47%
regular	1	26.0	490	48%
■ SALADS				
chicken salad..deluxe	1 salad	34.0	740	41%
taco salad				
deluxe	1 salad	40.0	780	46%
regular	1 salad	30.0	350	77%
tostada	1 tostada	9.0	210	39%
■ TACOS				
Big Fat taco				
chicken	1 taco	13.0	340	34%
crispy chicken	1 taco	38.0	620	55%
steak	1 taco	19.0	390	44%
taco	1 taco	11.0	320	31%
carnitas	1 taco	6.0	170	32%
chicken				
Del Carbon	1 taco	5.0	170	26%
soft	1 taco	12.0	210	51%

Food and Description	Amount	Fat Grams	Total Calories	% Fat Calories
steak taco Del Carbon	1 taco	11.0	220	45%
taco				
regular	1 taco	10.0	160	56%
soft	1 taco	8.0	160	45%
Ultimate taco	1 taco	17.0	260	59%
potpie dinner	1 serving	55.0	1065	46%
grilled dinner	1 serving	4.0	130	28%
grilled stir-fry	1 serving	10.0	864	10%
strips	1 serving	25.0	635	35%
onion rings	1 serving	23.0	381	54%
tomatoes/sliced	3 slices	–	13	–
vegetable rice pilaf	1 serving	1.0	85	11%
Southern	1 meal	84.0	1,065	71%

DOMINO'S PIZZA
■ BUFFALO WINGS & BREAD

Food and Description	Amount	Fat Grams	Total Calories	% Fat Calories
bread				
cheesy	1 piece	6.0	142	38%
Cinna Stix	1 piece	5.0	111	41%
sweet icing	2.5 oz cup	5.0	283	16%
sticks	1 piece	4.0	116	31%
dipping sauce				
blue cheese	1.5 oz	23.5	223	95%
hot	1.5 oz	–	15	–
ranch	1.5 oz	20.5	197	94%
wings..Kickers				
BBQ	1 piece	2.5	50	43%
Hot Buffalo	1 piece	2.5	45	50%

■ 12" MEDIUM PIZZA

Food and Description	Amount	Fat Grams	Total Calories	% Fat Calories
America's Favorite Feast				
deep-dish	⅛ pizza	17.0	309	50%
hand-tossed	⅛ pizza	11.5	257	40%
thin crust	⅛ pizza	13.5	208	58%
Bacon Cheeseburger Feast				
deep-dish	⅛ pizza	18.5	325	51%
hand-tossed	⅛ pizza	13.0	273	43%
thin crust	⅛ pizza	14.5	224	58%
barbecue				
deep-dish	⅛ pizza	15.0	304	44%
hand-tossed	⅛ pizza	10.0	252	36%
thin crust	⅛ pizza	11.5	203	51%
beef				
deep-dish	⅛ pizza	14.5	277	47%
hand-tossed	⅛ pizza	9.0	225	36%
thin crust	⅛ pizza	10.5	175	54%
cheese				
deep-dish	⅛ pizza	11.0	238	42%
hand-tossed	⅛ pizza	5.5	186	27%
thin crust	⅛ pizza	7.0	137	46%
Deluxe Feast				
deep-dish	⅛ pizza	15.0	287	47%

Food and Description	Amount	Fat Grams	Total Calories	% Fat Calories
hand-tossed	⅛ pizza	5.5	234	21%
thin crust	⅛ pizza	11.5	185	56%
ExtravaganZZa Feast				
deep-dish	⅛ pizza	19.5	341	51%
hand-tossed	⅛ pizza	14.0	289	44%
thin crust	⅛ pizza	.15.5	240	58%
green pepper..onion..mushroom				
deep-dish	⅛ pizza	11.0	244	41%
hand-tossed	⅛ pizza	5.5	191	26%
thin crust	⅛ pizza	7.5	142	48%
ham				
deep-dish	⅛ pizza	11.5	250	41%
hand-tossed	⅛ pizza	6.0	198	27%
thin crust	⅛ pizza	7.5	148	46%
ham & pineapple				
deep-dish	⅛ pizza	11.5	252	41%
hand-tossed	⅛ pizza	6.0	230	23%
thin crust	⅛ pizza	7.5	150	45%
Hawaiian Feast				
deep-dish	⅛ pizza	13.0	275	43%
hand-tossed	⅛ pizza	8.0	223	32%
thin crust	⅛ pizza	9.5	174	49%
MeatZZa Feast				
deep-dish	⅛ pizza	19.0	333	51%
hand-tossed	⅛ pizza	13.5	281	43%
thin crust	⅛ pizza	15.0	232	58%
pepperoni				
deep-dish	⅛ pizza	14.0	275	46%
hand-tossed	⅛ pizza	9.0	223	36%
thin crust	⅛ pizza	10.5	174	54%
pepperoni & sausage				
deep-dish	⅛ pizza	17.0	307	50%
hand-tossed	⅛ pizza	11.5	255	41%
thin crust	⅛ pizza	13.5	206	59%
Pepperoni Feast				
deep-dish	⅛ pizza	17.5	317	50%
hand-tossed	⅛ pizza	12.5	265	42%
thin crust	⅛ pizza	5.5	216	23%
sausage				
deep-dish	⅛ pizza	15.0	283	48%
hand-tossed	⅛ pizza	9.5	231	37%
thin crust	⅛ pizza	11.0	191	52%
Veggie Feast				
deep-dish	⅛ pizza	13.5	270	45%
hand-tossed	⅛ pizza	8.0	218	33%
thin crust	⅛ pizza	9.5	168	51%
■ 14" MEDIUM PIZZA				
America's Favorite Feast				
deep-dish	⅛ pizza	23.5	433	49%
hand-tossed	⅛ pizza	15.0	353	38%

Food and Description	Amount	Fat Grams	Total Calories	% Fat Calories
thin crust	⅛ pizza	18.5	285	58%
Bacon Cheeseburger Feast				
deep-dish	⅛ pizza	25.5	459	50%
hand-tossed	⅛ pizza	18.0	379	43%
thin crust	⅛ pizza	20.5	311	59%
barbecue				
deep-dish	⅛ pizza	20.5	424	44%
hand-tossed	⅛ pizza	13.5	344	35%
thin crust	⅛ pizza	15.5	276	51%
beef				
deep-dish	⅛ pizza	20.0	392	46%
hand-tossed	⅛ pizza	12.5	312	36%
thin crust	⅛ pizza	15.0	243	56%
cheese				
deep-dish	⅛ pizza	15.0	336	40%
hand-tossed	⅛ pizza	8.0	256	28%
thin crust	⅛ pizza	10.0	188	48%
Deluxe Feast				
deep-dish	⅛ pizza	20.0	397	45%
hand-tossed	⅛ pizza	12.5	316	36%
thin crust	⅛ pizza	15.0	247	54%
ExtravaganZZa Feast				
deep-dish	⅛ pizza	25.5	468	49%
hand-tossed	⅛ pizza	18.5	388	43%
thin crust	⅛ pizza	20.5	320	58%
green pepper..onion..mushroom				
deep-dish	⅛ pizza	15.0	343	39%
hand-tossed	⅛ pizza	8.0	263	27%
thin crust	⅛ pizza	10.0	201	45%
ham				
deep-dish	⅛ pizza	15.5	352	40%
hand-tossed	⅛ pizza	8.5	272	28%
thin crust	⅛ pizza	10.5	204	46%
ham & pineapple				
deep-dish	⅛ pizza	15.5	355	39%
hand-tossed	⅛ pizza	8.5	275	28%
thin crust	⅛ pizza	10.5	207	46%
Hawaiian Feast				
deep-dish	⅛ pizza	18.0	389	42%
hand-tossed	⅛ pizza	11.0	309	32%
thin crust	⅛ pizza	13.0	240	49%
MeatZZa Feast				
deep-dish	⅛ pizza	25.0	458	49%
hand-tossed	⅛ pizza	18.0	378	43%
thin crust	⅛ pizza	20.0	310	58%
pepperoni				
deep-dish	⅛ pizza	19.5	385	46%
hand-tossed	⅛ pizza	12.0	305	35%
thin crust	⅛ pizza	14.5	237	55%

Food and Description	Amount	Fat Grams	Total Calories	% Fat Calories
pepperoni & sausage				
deep-dish	⅛ pizza	23.0	430	48%
hand-tossed	⅛ pizza	16.0	350	41%
thin crust	⅛ pizza	18.5	282	59%
Pepperoni Feast				
deep-dish	⅛ pizza	24.0	443	49%
hand-tossed	⅛ pizza	17.0	363	42%
thin crust	⅛ pizza	19.0	295	58%
sausage				
deep-dish	⅛ pizza	20.5	400	46%
hand-tossed	⅛ pizza	13.5	320	38%
thin crust	⅛ pizza	15.5	252	55%
Veggie Feast				
deep-dish	⅛ pizza	18.0	380	43%
hand-tossed	⅛ pizza	11.0	300	33%
thin crust	⅛ pizza	13.5	231	53%

DUNKIN' DONUTS (*See also* BAGEL; COOKIE; CROISSANT; DONUT; PASTRY)

■ BAGELS

Food and Description	Amount	Fat Grams	Total Calories	% Fat Calories
bagels				
Berry Berry	1 bagel	3.0	340	8%
blueberry	1 bagel	3.0	350	8%
cinnamon raisin	1 bagel	3.0	330	8%
everything	1 bagel	7.0	430	15%
garlic	1 bagel	3.5	410	8%
onion	1 bagel	4.0	370	9%
plain	1 bagel	3.0	360	8%
poppyseed	1 bagel	10.0	440	20%
salsa	1 bagel	3.0	320	8%
salt	1 bagel	3.0	360	8%
sesame	1 bagel	11.0	450	22%
sourdough	1 bagel	3.0	340	8%
wheat	1 bagel	4.5	350	12%

■ BEVERAGES

Food and Description	Amount	Fat Grams	Total Calories	% Fat Calories
Coolatta				
flavored				
lemonade Coolatta	16 fl oz	–	240	–
orange mango	16 fl oz	–	270	–
strawberry	16 fl oz	–	290	–
vanilla bean	16 fl oz	17.0	440	35%
Dunkaccino	10 fl oz	10.0	230	39%
hot chocolate	10 fl oz	8.0	220	33%
hot espresso drinks				
cappuccino				
plain	10 oz	4.5	80	51%
w/sugar	10 oz	4.5	130	31%
espresso				
plain	2 oz	–	–	–
w/sugar	2 oz	–	30	–
latte				
caramel swirl	10 oz	6.0	230	23%

Food and Description	Amount	Fat Grams	Total Calories	% Fat Calories
mocha swirl	10 oz	7.0	230	27%
plain	10 oz	6.0	120	45%
w/sugar	10 oz	6.0	160	34%
iced latte				
caramel swirl	16 oz	7.0	240	26%
mocha swirl	16 oz	8.0	240	30%
plain	16 oz	7.0	120	53%
w/sugar	16 oz	7.0	170	37%
■ BREAKFAST SANDWICHES				
bagel				
egg..bacon..cheese	1	13.0	500	23%
egg..sausage..cheese	1	28.0	670	38%
ham..egg..cheese	1	11.0	500	20%
biscuit				
egg & cheese	1	20.0	360	50%
egg..sausage..cheese	1	38.0	560	61%
croissant				
egg..ham..cheese	1	27.0	470	52%
English muffin				
bacon..egg..cheese	1	11.0	310	32%
egg..cheese	1	8.0	270	27%
ham..egg..cheese	1	10.0	310	29%
New England maple cheddar	1	47.0	700	60%
■ CROISSANTS				
plain	1	18.0	330	48%
reduced-carb	1	24.0	370	57%
■ DONUTS & PASTRIES				
CRULLER..French	1	8.0	150	48%
DANISH				
apple	1 danish	10.0	250	36%
cheese	1 danish	14.0	270	47%
strawberry cheese	1 danish	12.0	250	43%
DONUTS				
apple crumb	1 donut	10.0	230	39%
apple 'n' spice	1 donut	8.0	200	36%
Bavarian Kreme	1 donut	9.0	210	39%
black raspberry	1 donut	8.0	210	34%
blueberry				
cake	1 donut	16.0	290	50%
crumb	1 donut	10.0	240	
Boston Kreme	1 donut	9.0	240	35%
chocolate				
coconut cake	1 donut	19.0	300	57%
frosted				
cake donut	1 donut	20.0	360	50%
donut	1 donut	9.0	200	41%
Kreme-filled	1 donut	13.0	270	43%
cinnamon cake	1 donut	20.0	330	55%
double chocolate				
cake	1 donut	17.0	310	49%

Food and Description	Amount	Fat Grams	Total Calories	% Fat Calories
glazed				
cake donut	1 donut	19.0	350	49%
donut	1 donut	8.0	180	40%
jelly-filled	1 donut	8.0	210	34%
lemon cake				
burst	1 donut	14.0	300	42%
frosted	1 donut	14.0	240	53%
glazed	1 donut	14.0	240	53%
maple-frosted	1 donut	9.0	210	39%
marble-frosted	1 donut	9.0	200	41%
old-fashioned cake	1 donut	19.0	300	57%
powdered cake	1 donut	19.0	330	51%
strawberry				
donut	1 donut	8.0	210	34%
frosted	1 donut	9.0	210	39%
sugar raised	1 donut	8.0	170	42%
Vanilla Kreme–filled	1 donut	13.0	270	43%
whole wheat				
glazed cake	1 donut	19.0	310	55%
FANCIES				
apple fritter	1	14.0	300	42%
bowtie donut	1 donut	17.0	300	51%
chocolate-iced				
Bismarck	1	15.0	340	40%
coffee-frosted				
coffee roll	1 roll	15.0	290	68%
coffee roll	1 roll	14.0	270	47%
éclair	1	11.0	270	37%
glazed fritter	1	14.0	260	49%
maple-frosted				
coffee roll	1 roll	14.0	290	43%
vanilla-frosted				
coffee roll	1 roll	14.0	290	43%
MUNCHKINS				
cinnamon cake	4 pieces	15.0	270	50%
glazed				
cake	3 pieces	13.0	280	42%
chocolate cake	3 pieces	10.0	200	45%
jelly-filled	5 pieces	9.0	210	39%
lemon-filled	4 pieces	8.0	170	42%
Munchkin	5 pieces	9.0	200	41%
plain cake	4 pieces	14.0	270	47%
powdered cake	4 pieces	14.0	270	47%
sugar raised	7 pieces	12.0	220	49%
STICKS				
cinnamon cake	1 stick	30.0	450	60%
glazed				
cake	1 stick	29.0	490	53%
chocolate cake	1 stick	29.0	470	56%
jelly	1 stick	29.0	530	49%

Food and Description	Amount	Fat Grams	Total Calories	% Fat Calories
plain cake	1 stick	29.0	420	62%
powdered cake	1 stick	29.0	450	58%
■ MUFFINS				
English muffin	1 muffin	1.5	160	8%
other muffins				
banana walnut	1 muffin	23.0	540	38%
blueberry	1 muffin	18.0	490	33%
reduced-fat	1 muffin	13.0	450	26%
carrot walnut spice	1 muffin	27.0	600	41%
chocolate chip	1 muffin	23.0	590	35%
coffee cake..w/topping	1 muffin	29.0	710	37%
corn	1 muffin	17.0	510	30%
cranberry orange	1 muffin	16.0	460	31%
honey bran raisin	1 muffin	14.0	490	26%
■ OTHER BAKERY ITEMS				
apple pie	1 serving	28.0	610	41%
apple pie à la mode	1 serving	38.0	810	42%
biscuit..plain	1 biscuit	13.0	250	47%
croissant..plain	1	18.0	330	49%
scones				
maple walnut	1 scone	22.0	470	42%
raspberry white chocolate	1 scone	22.0	450	44%
EINSTEIN BROTHERS BAGELS				
■ BAGELS				
Asiago cheese	1 bagel	3.0	360	8%
chocolate chip	1 bagel	3.0	370	7%
chopped garlic	1 bagel	3.0	380	7%
chopped onion	1 bagel	1.0	330	3%
cinnamon raisin swirl	1 bagel	1.0	350	3%
cinnamon sugar	1 bagel	1.0	330	3%
cinnamon sugar				
Chicago-style	1 bagel	21.0	500	38%
cranberry	1 bagel	1.0	350	3%
dark pumpernickel	1 bagel	1.0	320	3%
egg	1 bagel	3.0	340	8%
everything	1 bagel	2.0	340	5%
honey whole wheat	1 bagel	1.0	320	3%
lower carb 9-grain	1 bagel	3.5	210	15%
w/cream cheese	1 bagel	13.0	310	38%
mango	1 bagel	1.0	360	3%
marble rye	1 bagel	2.0	340	5%
nutty banana	1 bagel	3.0	360	8%
peppercorn potato	1 bagel	4.0	350	10%
plain	1 bagel	1.0	320	3%
poppy dip'd	1 bagel	2.0	350	5%
potato	1 bagel	4.5	350	12%
Power	1 bagel	5.0	410	11%
w/peanut butter	1 bagel	34.0	750	41%
pumpkin	1 bagel	1.5	330	4%
salt	1 bagel	1.0	330	3%

Food and Description	Amount	Fat Grams	Total Calories	% Fat Calories
sesame dip'd	1 bagel	5.0	380	12%
sun-dried tomato	1 bagel	1.0	320	3%
wild blueberry	1 bagel	1.0	350	3%
■ BEVERAGES				
cafe latte..non-fat	12 fl oz	–	100	–
cappuccino				
low-fat	12 fl oz	1.0	130	7%
non-fat	12 fl oz	–	60	–
regular	12 fl oz	3.5	90	35%
mocha				
low-fat	12 fl oz	2.5	190	12%
regular	12 fl oz	6.0	230	23%
other beverages				
hot chocolate	12 fl oz	11.0	260	24%
lower-fat	12 fl oz	7.0	260	24%
smoothie..mocha	10 fl oz	5.0	470	10%
■ BREAD SPECIALTY				
artisan wheat	1 slice	2.0	120	15%
Bagel Shtick				
Asiago	1 shtick	9.0	450	18%
cinnamon sugar	1 shtick	24.0	570	38%
everything	1 shtick	4.5	380	11%
potato	1 shtick	4.5	350	12%
sesame	1 shtick	8.0	420	17%
baguette bread	2 oz	0.5	160	3%
challah				
loaf	1 slice	2.0	120	15%
roll	1 roll	4.5	300	14%
Club Mex	1 serving	45.0	750	54%
flat bread				
peanut sesame	1 piece	15.0	650	21%
rosemary & Asiago	1 piece	9.0	520	16%
focaccia				
cheese pizza	1 serving	11.0	500	20%
margherita	1 serving	17.0	400	38%
pepperoni pizza	1 serving	19.0	590	29%
Lahvash bread	1 serving	11.0	270	37%
rustic white	1 serving	–	140	–
■ SALADS				
Asiago				
Caesar	1 salad	53.0	660	72%
chicken Caesar	1 salad	54.0	740	66%
Bros. Bistro	1 salad	69.0	810	77%
chicken chipotle	1 salad	40.0	630	57%
Jamaican Jerk	1 salad	10.0	340	26%
■ SANDWICHES, etc.				
Bagel Dogs				
Chicago				
Asiago	1	34.0	740	41%

Food and Description	Amount	Fat Grams	Total Calories	% Fat Calories
chili cheese	1	38.0	810	42%
Everything	1	34.0	730	42%
onion..no cheese	1	30.0	680	40%
Frittata's				
Denver omelet				
breakfast panini	1	31.0	750	37%
egg				
Black Forest ham	1	21.0	660	29%
plain	1	20.0	590	31%
Santa Fe	1	28.0	720	35%
sausage	1	23.0	660	31%
thick-cut bacon	1	42.0	840	45%
panini sandwiches				
Cali club	1	56.0	990	51%
	½ sdw	28.0	495	51%
ham & cheese	1	23.0	640	32%
	½ sdw	11.5	320	32%
Italian chicken	1	27.0	690	35%
	½ sdw	13.5	345	35%
sandwiches				
100% albacore tuna				
on artisan wheat	1	9.0	400	20%
	½ sdw	4.5	200	20%
Black Forest ham				
on challah	1	23.0	620	33%
Calypso chicken salad	1	9.0	460	18%
Club Mex on challah	1	53.0	920	52%
Cobbie on challah	1	44.0	810	49%
Einstein club				
on rustic white	1	44.0	840	47%
Mediterranean hummus				
& feta on ciabatta	1	10.0	450	20%
roasted turkey				
on artisan wheat	1	28.0	610	41%
Tasty turkey on Asiago bagel	1	18.0	630	26%
Veg Out on sesame				
seed bagel	1	13.0	500	23%
New York lox & bagel	1	27.0	660	37%
■ SOUP/CHILI..Bowl				
broccoli..sharp cheddar	1	35.0	540	58%
butternut squash bisque	1	27.0	660	37%
Caribbean crab chowder	1	38.0	520	66%
chicken noodle	1	21.0	510	37%
chicken & wild rice	1	9.0	440	18%
clam chowder	1	25.0	370	61%
minestrone..low-fat	1	10.0	360	25%
tomato bisque	1	23.0	440	47%
tortilla	1	6.0	200	27%
turkey chili	1	11.0	330	18%

Food and Description	Amount	Fat Grams	Total Calories	% Fat Calories
■ SWEETS				
cake				
lemon..iced pound	1	28.0	510	49%
marble pound	1	20.0	370	67%
cake..coffee				
apple cinnamon	1	24.0	570	38%
blueberry	1	24.0	600	36%
chocolate chip	1	29.0	660	40%
cookie				
Heavenly Chocolate Chip	1	29.0	565	46%
honey-roasted peanut butter	1	35.0	610	52%
trail mix cookie	1	21.0	500	38%
muffins				
97% fat-free apple cinnamon	1	1.5	350	4%
banana nut	1	29.0	520	50%
blueberry	1	24.0	460	47%
chocolate chip	1	13.0	240	49%
lemon poppyseed/low-fat	1	7.0	370	17%
mocha chocolate chip	1	29.0	550	47%
Morning Harvest	1	19.0	460	37%
pastry				
cinnamon				
twists	1	21.0	370	51%
walnut strudel	1	31.0	550	51%
scones				
lemon currant	1 scone	17.0	490	31%
whole wheat w/fruit	1 scone	17.0	480	31%
FAZOLI'S				
■ DESSERT				
cheesecake				
chocolate chip	1 piece	22.0	300	66%
plain	1 piece	22.0	290	68%
Turtle	1 piece	34.0	420	73%
cookie..milk chocolate chunk	1	15.0	360	38%
■ ENTRÉES..Italian Specialties				
baked ziti				
classic meaty	1 small	27.0	500	49%
	1 regular	42.0	770	49%
twice baked				
w/meat sauce	1 serving	51.0	910	50%
baked				
chicken Alfredo	1 serving	29.0	790	33%
chicken Parmesan	1 serving	20.0	740	24%
pizza baked spaghetti	1 serving	31.0	750	37%
spaghetti Parmesan	1 serving	25.0	700	32%
broccoli				
fettuccini Alfredo				
regular	1 serving	23.0	830	25%
lasagna..6-layer	1 serving	30.0	690	39%
fettuccini				
shrimp & scallop	1 serving	16.0	610	24%

Food and Description	Amount	Fat Grams	Total Calories	% Fat Calories
lasagna				
broccoli..6-layer	1 serving	30.0	690	39%
classic..w/6 layers	1 serving	25.0	810	28%
six-layer..w/meat sauce	1 serving	26.0	630	37%
twice-baked	1 serving	40.0	820	44%
ravioli..cheese				
w/marinara	1 serving	17.0	510	30%
w/meat sauce	1 serving	17.0	510	30%
Ultimate sampler platter	1 serving	37.0	1030	32%
■ ENTRÉES..pasta				
fettuccini				
Alfredo	1 serving	15.0	530	25%
regular	1 serving	22.0	800	25%
broccoli	1 serving	15.0	560	24%
penne				
chicken..garden style	1 serving	28.0	830	30%
spicy marinara penne				
w/chicken	1 serving	13.0	990	12%
peppery chicken Alfredo	1 serving	16.0	610	24%
spaghetti				
w/marinara..regular	1 serving	8.0	620	12%
w/meatballs..regular	1 serving	42.0	1020	37%
w/meat sauce..regular	1 serving	11.0	670	15%
■ PIZZA				
cheese	dbl slice	15.0	460	29%
combination	dbl slice	25.0	570	39%
pepperoni	dbl slice	22.0	530	37%
■ SALADS & RELATED ITEMS				
breadstick				
regular	1	6.0	140	39%
dry	1	1.0	90	10%
salad				
chicken & pasta				
Caesar salad	1 salad	13.0	370	32%
chicken Caesar salad	1 salad	29.0	420	62%
chicken finger salad				
regular	1 salad	9.0	190	43%
w/bacon	1 salad	28.0	400	63%
garden salad	1 salad	–	30	–
Italian chef salad	1 salad	21.0	260	73%
side pasta salad	1 salad	10.0	240	38%
salad dressing				
honey French	1 pkt	12.0	150	72%
house Italian	1 pkt	9.0	110	74%
Italian..reduced calorie	1 pkt	5.0	50	90%
Thousand Island	1 pkt	13.0	130	90%
■ SUBMARINOS & PANINIS				
paninis				
chicken				
Caesar club	1	35.0	660	47%
pesto	1	20.0	510	35%

Food and Description	Amount	Fat Grams	Total Calories	% Fat Calories
4-cheese & tomato	1	43.0	720	54%
ham & Swiss	1	30.0	600	45%
Italian				
club	1	37.0	670	50%
deli	1	35.0	660	48%
smoked turkey	1	38.0	710	48%
subs				
Submarino				
club	½ sub	44.0	1100	36%
ham & Swiss	½ sub	37.0	1000	33%
original	½ sub	55.0	1160	43%
pepperoni pizza	½ sub	40.0	1060	34%
turkey	½ sub	59.0	1260	42%
w/meatballs	½ sub	34.0	990	31%
GODFATHER'S PIZZA				
■ **DESSERT PIZZA..Golden Crust**				
apple				
alum pan	⅙ pizza	2.0	139	13%
small	⅙ pizza	5.0	202	22%
medium	⅛ pizza	4.0	206	17%
large	⅒ pizza	5.0	229	20%
cherry				
alum pan	⅙ pizza	2.0	142	13%
small	⅙ pizza	5.0	206	22%
medium	⅛ pizza	4.0	210	17%
large	⅒ pizza	5.0	233	19%
cinnamon streusel				
alum pan	⅙ pizza	3.0	161	17%
small	⅙ pizza	6.0	226	24%
medium	⅛ pizza	6.0	228	24%
large	⅒ pizza	7.0	258	24%
M&M Streusel				
alum pan	⅙ pizza	4.0	173	21%
small	⅙ pizza	7.0	249	25%
medium	⅛ pizza	7.0	263	24%
large	⅒ pizza	8.0	300	24%
■ **GOLDEN CRUST**				
medium				
all-meat combo	⅛ pizza	13.0	285	41%
bacon cheeseburger	⅛ pizza	12.0	267	40%
cheese	⅛ pizza	8.0	221	37%
combo	⅛ pizza	13.0	288	41%
Hawaiian	⅛ pizza	8.0	238	31%
Hot Stuff	⅛ pizza	14.0	294	43%
Humble Pie	⅛ pizza	15.0	306	44%
pepperoni	⅛ pizza	11.0	255	39%
super combo	⅛ pizza	15.0	322	42%
super Hawaiian	⅛ pizza	8.0	235	31%
super taco	⅛ pizza	17.0	328	47%
taco	⅛ pizza	14.0	300	42%

Food and Description	Amount	Fat Grams	Total Calories	% Fat Calories
veggie	⅛ pizza	8.0	232	31%
large				
all-meat combo	⅒ pizza	15.0	325	42%
bacon cheeseburger	⅒ pizza	14.0	307	41%
cheese	⅒ pizza	9.0	252	32%
combo	⅒ pizza	15.0	328	41%
Hawaiian	⅒ pizza	10.0	268	34%
Hot Stuff	⅒ pizza	17.0	337	45%
Humble Pie	⅒ pizza	18.0	352	46%
pepperoni	⅒ pizza	13.0	289	40%
super combo	⅒ pizza	18.0	371	44%
super Hawaiian	⅒ pizza	10.0	268	34%
super taco	⅒ pizza	20.0	377	48%
taco	⅒ pizza	17.0	346	44%
veggie	⅒ pizza	10.0	264	34%
■ ORIGINAL CRUST PIZZA				
all-meat combo				
jumbo	⅒ pizza	23.0	566	37%
large	⅒ pizza	16.0	383	38%
medium	⅛ pizza	16.0	373	39%
mini	¼ pizza	8.0	201	36%
bacon cheeseburger				
jumbo	⅒ pizza	23.0	541	38%
large	⅒ pizza	15.0	266	51%
medium	⅛ pizza	13.0	328	36%
mini	¼ pizza	8.0	196	37%
cheese				
jumbo	⅒ pizza	13.0	431	27%
large	⅒ pizza	15.0	366	37%
medium	⅛ pizza	7.0	260	24%
mini	¼ pizza	4.0	150	24%
combo				
jumbo	⅒ pizza	24.0	578	37%
large	⅒ pizza	9.0	293	29%
medium	⅛ pizza	14.0	352	36%
mini	¼ pizza	8.0	207	35%
Hawaiian				
jumbo	⅒ pizza	13.0	465	25%
large	⅒ pizza	9.0	316	26%
medium	⅛ pizza	8.0	281	26%
mini	¼ pizza	4.0	162	23%
Hot Stuff				
jumbo	⅒ pizza	26.0	592	40%
large	⅒ pizza	18.0	401	40%
medium	⅛ pizza	16.0	360	40%
mini	¼ pizza	9.0	213	38%
Humble Pie				
jumbo	⅒ pizza	30.0	621	43%
large	⅒ pizza	20.0	420	43%
medium	⅛ pizza	18.0	379	43%

Food and Description	Amount	Fat Grams	Total Calories	% Fat Calories
mini	¼ pizza	11.0	225	44%
pepperoni				
jumbo	⅒ pizza	18.0	486	33%
large	⅒ pizza	12.0	330	33%
medium	⅛ pizza	10.0	294	31%
mini	¼ pizza	5.0	162	28%
super combo				
jumbo	⅒ pizza	28.0	634	40%
large	⅒ pizza	19.0	432	40%
medium	⅛ pizza	17.0	387	40%
mini	¼ pizza	9.0	220	37%
super Hawaiian				
jumbo	⅒ pizza	13.0	457	26%
large	½ pizza	9.0	311	26%
medium	⅛ pizza	8.0	277	29%
mini	¼ pizza	4.0	158	23%
super taco				
jumbo	⅒ pizza	31.0	643	43%
large	⅒ pizza	22.0	450	44%
medium	⅛ pizza	18.0	392	41%
mini	¼ pizza	11.0	234	42%
taco				
jumbo	⅒ pizza	27.0	594	41%
large	⅒ pizza	19.0	418	41%
medium	⅛ pizza	16.0	362	40%
mini	¼ pizza	9.0	214	38%
veggie				
jumbo	⅒ pizza	14.0	456	28%
large	⅒ pizza	8.0	310	23%
medium	⅛ pizza	8.0	275	26%
mini	¼ pizza	5.0	161	28%
■ THIN CRUST PIZZA				
medium				
all-meat combo	⅛ pizza	15.0	282	48%
bacon cheeseburger	⅛ pizza	13.0	246	48%
cheese	⅛ pizza	9.0	200	41%
combo	⅛ pizza	14.0	266	47%
Hawaiian	⅛ pizza	9.0	217	37%
Hot Stuff	⅛ pizza	15.0	272	50%
Humble Pie	⅛ pizza	16.0	285	51%
pepperoni	⅛ pizza	12.0	234	46%
super combo	⅛ pizza	16.0	301	48%
super Hawaiian	⅛ pizza	9.0	213	38%
super taco	⅛ pizza	18.0	306	53%
taco	⅛ pizza	15.0	278	49%
veggie	⅛ pizza	9.0	209	39%
HARDEE'S				
■ BEVERAGES				
shakes				
chocolate	regular	7.0	710	9%

Food and Description	Amount	Fat Grams	Total Calories	% Fat Calories
strawberry	regular	6.0	710	8%
vanilla	regular	8.0	580	12%
■ BREAKFAST				
Big Country Breakfast				
w/bacon	1 serving	43.0	740	52%
w/sausage	1 serving	61.0	930	59%
biscuits				
bacon	1 serving	38.0	560	61%
bacon, egg & cheese	1 serving	38.0	560	61%
bacon & egg	1 serving	27.0	490	50%
Big Country				
biscuit platter				
bacon	1 platter	56.0	980	51%
breakfast ham	1 platter	52.0	970	48%
chicken	1 platter	61.0	1140	48%
country ham	1 platter	53.0	970	48%
country steak	1 platter	68.0	1150	53%
sausage	1 platter	64.0	1060	54%
Biscuit 'n' Gravy	1 serving	34.0	530	58%
chicken fillet	1 serving	34.0	600	51%
country ham	1 serving	34.0	600	51%
country steak	1 serving	41.0	620	60%
ham	1 serving	20.0	410	44%
ham, egg & cheese	1 serving	35.0	560	56%
loaded omelet	1 serving	33.0	500	60%
low-carb breakfast bowl	1 serving	50.0	620	73%
Made from Scratch	1 serving	23.0	370	56%
pancakes	3	5.0	300	15%
sausage	1 serving	38.0	530	65%
sausage & egg	1 serving	44.0	610	65%
smoked sausage	1 serving	46.0	620	67%
Sunrise croissant				
w/bacon	1 serving	29.0	450	58%
w/ham	1 serving	26.0	430	54%
w/sausage patty	1 serving	38.0	550	62%
Frisco breakfast sandwich/ham	1 serving	13.0	360	33%
Tortilla Scrambler	1 serving	19.0	310	55%
■ BREAKFAST SIDES				
bacon	1½ strips	5.0	60	75%
biscuit gravy	5 oz	11.0	160	62%
cheese				
American	1 slice	4.0	50	72%
Swiss	1 slice	4.0	50	72%
cinnamon roll	1 roll	20.0	390	46%
croissant	1	10.0	210	43%
grits	1 serving	5.0	110	41%
ham				
breakfast	2 oz	3.0	60	45%
country	1.25 oz	3.0	60	45%

Food and Description	Amount	Fat Grams	Total Calories	% Fat Calories
hash browns	small	16.0	260	55%
	medium	22.0	350	57%
	large	29.0	460	57%
sausage				
patty	1	14.0	150	84%
smoked	2.78 oz	23.0	250	83%
scrambled egg	1 serving	12.0	160	68%
■ BURGERS & SANDWICHES				
burgers				
⅓-lb bacon cheese				
Thickburger	1	63.0	910	62%
⅓-lb cheeseburger	1	39.0	680	52%
⅓-lb chili cheese				
Thickburger	1	54.0	870	56%
⅓-lb low-carb Thickburger	1	32.0	420	69%
⅓-lb mushroom 'n' Swiss				
Thickburger	1	42.0	720	53%
⅓-lb Thickburger	1	57.0	850	60%
½-lb Six Dollar burger	1	73.0	1120	59%
½-lb grilled sourdough				
Thickburger	1	74.0	1100	61%
⅔-lb bacon cheese				
Thickburger	1	96.0	1340	64%
⅔-lb double Thickburger	1	90.0	1230	66%
⅔-lb double bacon cheese				
Thickburger	1	96.0	1300	66%
sandwiches				
chicken				
big	1	36.0	770	42%
charbroiled chicken				
low-carb	1	24.0	420	51%
regular	1	26.0	590	40%
spicy	1	22.0	430	46%
hot dog w/condiments	1	30.0	420	64%
hot ham 'n' cheese				
big	1	23.0	570	36%
regular	1	18.0	420	39%
roast beef				
big	1	23.0	470	44%
regular	1	16.0	330	44%
Slammer				
w/cheese	1	16.0	280	51%
w/o cheese	1	12.0	240	45%
■ CHICKEN...fried				
individual pieces				
breast	1 serving	15.0	370	36%
leg	1 serving	7.0	170	37%
thigh	1 serving	15.0	330	41%
wing	1 serving	8.0	200	36%

Food and Description	Amount	Fat Grams	Total Calories	% Fat Calories
Kid's Meal				
chicken strips..no sauce	1 order	25.0	500	45%
Slammers	1 order	35.0	720	44%
strips				
3-piece	1 order	21.0	380	50%
5-piece	1 order	34.0	630	49%
■ SALADS				
garden	1 serving	13.0	210	56%
grilled chicken	1 serving	3.0	150	18%
■ SIDES				
chili cheese fries	1 order	39.0	700	50%
coleslaw	small	10.0	170	53%
Crispy Curls potatoes	small	17.0	340	45%
	medium	20.0	410	44%
	large	23.0	480	43%
dipping sauce cups				
BBQ	1 oz	–	45	–
honey mustard	1 oz	9.0	110	74%
ranch dressing	1 oz	16.0	160	90%
sweet 'n' sour	1 oz	–	45	–
French fries	kid's	12.0	250	43%
	small	19.0	390	44%
	medium	24.0	520	42%
	large	28.0	610	41%
	monster	24.0	510	42%
gravy..chicken	1 serving	1.0	20	45%
mashed potatoes	small	2.0	90	20%
IN-N-OUT BURGER				
■ BEVERAGES				
shakes				
chocolate	15 oz	36.0	690	47%
strawberry	15 oz	33.0	690	43%
vanilla	15 oz	37.0	680	49%
■ CHEESEBURGERS				
protein-style	1 burger	25.0	330	68%
w/mustard & ketchup	1 burger	18.0	400	41%
w/onion	1 burger	27.0	480	51%
■ DOUBLE-DOUBLE HAMBURGERS				
protein-style	1 burger	39.0	520	68%
w/mustard & ketchup	1 burger	32.0	590	49%
w/onion	1 burger	41.0	670	55%
■ FRENCH FRIES	1 order	18.0	400	41%
■ HAMBURGERS				
protein-style	1 burger	17.0	240	64%
w/mustard & ketchup	1 burger	10.0	310	29%
w/onion	1 burger	19.0	390	44%
JACK-N-THE-BOX				
■ BEVERAGES				
shakes-w/ice cream				
banana	medium	38.0	900	38%
	large	56.0	1410	36%

Food and Description	Amount	Fat Grams	Total Calories	% Fat Calories
chocolate	medium	38.0	850	40%
	large	57.0	310	39%
creamy caramel	medium	40.0	860	42%
	large	59.0	1330	49%
Oreo cookie	medium	43.0	870	44%
	large	66.0	1350	44%
strawberry	medium	38.0	830	41%
	large	56.0	1270	40%
vanilla	medium	38.0	750	46%
	large	58.0	1140	46%
■ BREAKFAST				
Breakfast Jack	1	14.0	305	41%
Extreme Sausage Sandwich	1	50.0	690	65%
French toast sticks	1 serving	18.0	560	29%
hash browns	1 serving	10.0	150	60%
sausage biscuit	1	36.0	600	54%
sausage croissant	1	40.5	605	60%
sausage, egg & cheese biscuit	1	68.0	970	63%
Sourdough Breakfast Sandwich	1	26.0	445	53%
Supreme Croissant	1	27.0	475	51%
Ultimate Breakfast Sandwich	1	30.5	605	45%
■ BURGERS & SANDWICHES				
burgers				
cheeseburger				
Bacon Bacon	1 burger	50.0	780	58%
Bacon Ultimate	1 burger	70.5	1025	62%
Ultimate	1 burger	64.5	945	61%
hamburger				
deluxe burger				
regular	1 burger	21.0	370	51%
w/cheese	1 burger	28.0	460	55%
regular burger	1 burger	14.0	310	41%
w/cheese	1 burger	17.5	355	44%
Jumbo Jack				
Junior bacon	1 burger	36.0	525	62%
plain	1 burger	34.5	600	52%
w/cheese	1 burger	41.5	695	54%
Sourdough Jack	1 burger	51.0	715	64%
sandwiches				
Deli Trio Pannido	1	34.0	645	47%
Ham & Turkey Pannido	1	29.0	610	43%
Ultimate Club sandwich	1	29.0	630	41%
Zesty Turkey Pannido	1	43.5	740	53%
■ CHICKEN..FISH..MEXICAN ITEMS				
chicken				
breast strips	1 order	38.0	630	54%
sandwich				
Jack's spicy				
regular	1	30.5	615	45%
w/cheese	1	33.5	655	45%
regular	1	21.0	390	48%

Food and Description	Amount	Fat Grams	Total Calories	% Fat Calories
sourdough grilled club	1	27.0	505	48%
w/cheese	1	24.0	430	50%
fish & chips	1 serving	56.0	840	60%
Mexican				
chicken fajita pita	1 pita	9.0	315	26%
taco				
Monster	1 taco	14.0	240	53%
regular	1 taco	8.0	160	45%
■ DESSERTS & SNACKS				
desserts				
cheesecake	1 piece	16.0	310	46%
double fudge cake	1 slice	11.0	310	32%
snacks				
bacon cheddar potato				
wedges	1 order	41.0	620	60%
egg rolls	1 piece	6.0	175	31%
■ SALADS				
salads				
Asian chicken salad	1 salad	32.5	595	49%
chicken club	1 salad	61.5	825	67%
side salad	1 salad	7.5	155	44%
Southwest chicken	1 salad	43.5	735	53%
■ SIDE ORDERS				
Curly Fries	medium	23.0	400	52%
	large	31.0	550	51%
French fries	medium	20.0	410	44%
	large	28.0	580	43%
Onion rings	1 serving	30.0	500	54%
KENTUCKY FRIED CHICKEN				
■ CHICKEN				
Extra Crispy				
breast	1 piece	28.0	480	53%
drumstick	1 piece	10.0	160	56%
thigh	1 piece	26.0	370	63%
wing/whole	1 piece	12.0	190	57%
Hot & Spicy				
breast	1 piece	27.0	460	53%
drumstick	1 piece	9.0	150	54%
thigh	1 piece	28.0	400	63%
wing/whole	1 piece	11.0	180	55%
Nuggets & Sauce				
nuggets only	3.4 oz	18.0	284	57%
sauce				
barbecue	1 oz	<1.0	35	13%
honey	1 oz	–	49	–
mustard	1 oz	<1.0	36	23%
sweet & sour	1 oz	<1.0	58	9%
Original Recipe				
breast				
w/skin	1 piece	29.0	380	69%
w/o skin or breading	1 piece	3.0	140	19%

Food and Description	Amount	Fat Grams	Total Calories	% Fat Calories
drumstick	1 piece	8.0	140	51%
thigh	1 piece	25.0	360	63%
wing/whole	1 piece	9.0	150	54%
Popcorn chicken	Individual	30.0	450	60%
	kid's	18.0	270	60%
	large	44.0	660	90%
potpie..chunky chicken	1 pot pie	40.0	770	47%
strips..crispy	3 pieces	24.0	400	54%
wings..boneless				
honey BBQ	7 pieces	28.0	600	42%
hot	6 pieces	29.0	450	58%
■ **DESSERTS**				
cheesy cheesecake parfait	1	11.0	300	33%
Colonel's Pies				
apple	1 slice	9.0	279	29%
lemon meringue	1 slice	11.0	310	32%
pecan	1 slice	15.0	370	36%
strawberry creme	1 slice	12.0	270	40%
double chocolate chip cake	1 slice	29.0	400	65%
Little Bucket Parfaits				
fudge brownie	1 serving	9.0	270	30%
lemon creme	1 serving	14.0	400	32%
strawberry shortcake	1 serving	7.0	200	7%
■ **SANDWICHES/chicken**				
honey BBQ–flavored	1	6.0	300	18%
Original Recipe				
w/sauce	1	27.0	450	54%
w/o sauce	1	13.0	320	37%
Tender Roast				
w/sauce	1	19.0	390	44%
w/o sauce	1	5.0	260	17%
Triple Crunch				
w/sauce	1	40.0	670	54%
w/o sauce	1	28.0	540	47%
Zinger				
w/sauce	1	41.0	650	57%
w/o sauce	1	26.0	540	43%
■ **SIDE ORDERS**				
BBQ beans	1 serving	1.0	230	4%
buttermilk biscuit	1 biscuit	10.0	190	47%
coleslaw	1 serving	13.5	232	52%
corn on the cob..3"	1 piece	1.5	70	19%
green beans	1 order	1.5	80	17%
macaroni & cheese	1 serving	6.0	130	42%
mashed potatoes & gravy	1 serving	4.0	110	33%
potato salad	1 serving	9.0	180	45%
potato wedges	1 serving	12.0	240	42%
LITTLE CAESAR'S PIZZA				
■ **PIZZA**				
Baby Pan! Pan!	1 pizza	16.0	360	40%

Food and Description	Amount	Fat Grams	Total Calories	% Fat Calories
deep-dish				
14" ..⅙ pizza				
cheese only	1 slice	11.0	330	30%
pepperoni	1 slice	14.0	390	32%
med ..⅛ pizza				
cheese only	1 slice	9.0	230	35%
pepperoni	1 slice	11.0	260	38%
large ..⅛ pizza				
cheese only	1 slice	12.0	320	34%
pepperoni	1 slice	14.0	350	36%
round				
12" ..⅛ pizza				
cheese only	1 slice	6.0	180	30%
pepperoni	1 slice	8.0	210	34%
14" ..1/10 pizza				
cheese only	1 slice	6.0	200	27%
Meatsa	1 slice	13.0	279	42%
pepperoni	1 slice	8.0	230	31%
supreme	1 slice	10.0	270	33%
veggie	1 slice	8.0	240	30%
16" ..1/12 pizza				
cheese only	1 slice	7.0	220	29%
pepperoni	1 slice	9.0	240	34%
18" ..1/14 pizza				
cheese only	1 slice	7.0	230	27%
pepperoni	1 slice	9.0	260	31%
thin crust				
12" ..⅛ pizza				
cheese only	1 slice	7.0	140	45%
pepperoni	1 slice	8.0	240	30%
14" ..1/10 pizza				
cheese only	1 slice	7.0	160	39%
pepperoni	1 slice	9.0	180	45%
■ BREAD & SIDES				
bread				
Crazy breadstick	1 slice	2.5	90	25%
Italian cheese	1 piece	6.0	130	42%
chicken wings	1 wing	5.0	70	64%
Cinnamon Crazy	2 sticks	2.0	100	18%
sauce/crazy	1 serving	–	45	–
LONG JOHN SILVER'S				
■ DESSERTS				
pie				
chocolate cream	1 piece	22.0	310	64%
pecan	1 piece	15.0	370	36%
pineapple cream	1 piece	13.0	290	40%
■ ENTRÉES				
chicken				
batter-dipped plank	1 piece	8.0	140	51%
clams..breaded	1 order	13.0	240	49%

Food and Description	Amount	Fat Grams	Total Calories	% Fat Calories
fish				
baked cod	1 piece	4.5	120	34%
batter-dipped				
regular	1 piece	13.0	230	51%
country-style breaded	1 piece	10.0	200	45%
lemon crumb	2 pieces	12.0	240	45%
à la carte	2 fish w/rice	17.0	480	32%
Add-a-Piece	1 fish w/rice	7.0	150	42%
meal	1 meal	29.0	730	36%
shrimp				
battered	1 piece	2.5	45	50%
crunchy shrimp basket	1 basket	19.0	340	50%
giant	1 piece	5.0	80	56%
popcorn	1 serving	15.0	320	42%
■ SALADS				
chicken club	1 salad	30.0	510	53%
shrimp & seafood	1 salad	12.0	280	39%
■ SANDWICHES				
chicken	1	15.0	380	36%
fish				
batter-dipped w/o sauce	1	13.0	320	37%
plain	1	20.0	440	41%
Ultimate	1	25.0	500	45%
w/cheese	1	25.0	480	47%
■ SIDE ORDERS				
broccoli cheese soup	1 bowl	12.0	180	60%
cheese sticks	3 sticks	8.0	140	51%
clam chowder	1 bowl	10.0	220	41%
coleslaw	1 serving	7.0	170	37%
Corn Cobbette	1	3.0	90	30%
crumbles	1 oz	12.0	170	64%
fries	regular	10.0	230	39%
	large	17.0	390	39%
hush puppy	1 piece	2.5	60	38%
lobster-stuffed crab cake	1 piece	9.0	170	48%
rice pilaf	1 serving	3.5	180	18%
side salad	1 serving	–	25	–
slaw	1 serving	18.0	200	81%
McDONALD'S				
■ BREAKFAST				
bagels				
ham, egg & cheese	1 bagel	23.0	550	38%
plain	1 bagel	1.0	260	3%
Spanish omelet	1 bagel	40.0	710	51%
steak, egg & cheese	1 bagel	31.0	640	44%
Big Breakfast	1 serving	47.0	700	60%
biscuits				
bacon, egg & cheese	1 biscuit	26.0	430	54%
plain	1 biscuit	11.0	240	41%
sausage	1 biscuit	28.0	410	61%

Food and Description	Amount	Fat Grams	Total Calories	% Fat Calories
sausage & egg	1 biscuit	33.0	490	61%
breakfast burrito	1 burrito	20.0	320	56%
cinnamon roll				
deluxe..warm	1 roll	23.0	510	41%
warm	1 roll	19.0	440	39%
deluxe breakfast	1 serving	61.0	1190	46%
Egg McMuffin	1	12.0	300	36%
English muffin				
w/spread	1 muffin	2.0	150	8%
hash brown potatoes	1 serving	8.0	130	55%
hotcakes				
& sausage	1 serving	33.0	780	38%
plain	1 serving	8.0	340	21%
w/margarine & syrup	1 serving	17.0	600	26%
McGriddles				
bacon..egg..cheese	1 serving	21.0	440	43%
sausage	1 serving	23.0	420	49%
sausage..egg..cheese	1 serving	33.0	550	54%
sausage	1.5 oz	16.0	170	85%
sausage burrito	1 burrito	16.0	290	50%
Sausage McMuffin				
regular	1	23.0	370	56%
w/egg	1	28.0	450	56%
scrambled eggs	2 eggs	11.0	160	62%
■ BURGERS				
Big Mac	1 burger	33.0	600	50%
Big N' Tasty				
w/cheese	1 burger	36.0	590	55%
w/o cheese	1 burger	32.0	540	53%
cheeseburger	1 burger	14.0	330	38%
double	1 burger	26.0	490	48%
hamburger	1 burger	10.0	280	32%
Quarter Pounder				
double w/cheese	1 burger	47.0	770	55%
w/cheese	1 burger	29.0	540	48%
w/o cheese	1 burger	21.0	430	44%
■ CHICKEN & FISH				
Chicken McNuggets & sauce				
McNuggets	4 pieces	10.0	170	53%
	6 pieces	15.0	250	54%
	10 pieces	24.0	420	51%
	20 pieces	49.0	840	53%
sauce				
barbecue	1 pkt	–	45	–
honey	1 pkt	–	45	–
hot mustard	1 pkt	3.5	60	46%
sweet & sour	1 pkt	–	50	–
sandwiches				
chicken				
crispy	1	26.0	510	46%

Food and Description	Amount	Fat Grams	Total Calories	% Fat Calories
McChicken sandwich				
hot 'n' spicy	1	26.0	450	52%
original	1	23.0	430	48%
McGrilled				
w/mayonnaise	1	16.0	400	36%
Fillet-O-Fish sandwich	1	20.0	410	44%
■ DESSERTS & SHAKES				
Apple Dippers				
low-fat caramel dip	1 pkg	1.0	70	13%
w/low-fat caramel dip	1 serving	1.0	100	9%
w/o caramel dip	1 pkg	–	35	–
baked apple pie	1 pie	13.0	260	45%
cookies				
chocolate chip	1 cookie	10.0	170	53%
oatmeal raisin	1 cookie	6.0	150	36%
sugar	1 cookie	6.0	140	39%
cookies..McDonaldland				
chocolate chip	1 pkg	14.0	280	45%
cookies	1 pkg	8.0	230	31%
fruit 'n' yogurt parfaits				
w/granola	1	2.0	160	11%
w/o granola	1	2.0	130	14%
ice cream				
cone				
Kiddie	1 cone	1.5	45	30%
vanilla..reduced fat	1 cone	4.5	150	27%
sundaes				
hot caramel sundae	1 serving	10.0	360	25%
hot fudge	1 serving	12.0	340	32%
strawberry	1 serving	7.0	290	22%
sundae nuts	1 serving	3.5	40	79%
McFlurry				
M&M's	1	23.0	630	33%
Oreo	1	20.0	570	32%
Triple Thick Shake				
chocolate	12 fl oz	12.0	430	25%
	16 fl oz	17.0	580	26%
	21 fl oz	22.0	750	26%
	32 fl oz	33.0	1150	26%
strawberry	12 fl oz	12.0	420	26%
	16 fl oz	16.0	560	26%
	21 fl oz	21.0	730	26%
	32 fl oz	32.0	1120	26%
vanilla	12 fl oz	12.0	430	25%
	16 fl oz	16.0	570	25%
	21 fl oz	21.0	750	25%
	32 fl oz	32.0	1140	25%
■ SALADS				
bacon ranch..w/o dressing	1 salad	8.0	130	55%
Caesar salad	1 salad	4.0	90	40%

Food and Description	Amount	Fat Grams	Total Calories	% Fat Calories
California Cobb salad	1 salad	9.0	150	54%
chef salad	1 salad	8.0	150	48%
crispy chicken				
bacon ranch	1 salad	10.0	250	36%
Caesar	1 salad	16.0	310	46%
California Cobb	1 salad	21.0	370	51%
Fiesta salad				
w/salsa	1 salad	22.0	390	51%
w/sour cream	1 salad	27.0	420	58%
w/sour cream & salsa				
9.8 oz	1 salad	22.0	360	55%
14.0 oz	1 salad	27.0	450	54%
garden salad	1 salad	6.0	100	54%
grilled chicken				
bacon ranch	1 salad	10.0	250	36%
Caesar	1 salad	6.0	200	27%
California Cobb	1 salad	11.0	270	37%
side salad	1 serving	–	15	–
■ SIDE ORDERS				
French fries	small	11.0	220	45%
	medium	17.0	350	44%
	large	25.0	520	43%

MRS. FIELD'S COOKIES

Food and Description	Amount	Fat Grams	Total Calories	% Fat Calories
Breakfast Cookies				
banana nut	1	20.0	340	53%
blueberry	1	16.0	330	44%
chocolate chip	1	14.0	320	39%
mandarin orange	1	13.0	290	40%
raspberry	1	12.0	280	39%
Brownies				
cheesecake	1	37.0	520	64%
double fudge	1	19.0	360	48%
frosted fudge	1	21.0	440	43%
German chocolate	1	35.0	570	55%
Peanut Butter Dream Bar	1	42.0	670	56%
pecan				
fudge brownie	1	21.0	340	56%
pie brownie	1	7.0	140	45%
Rocky Mountain Mogul	1	35.0	610	52%
walnut fudge	1	20.0	340	53%
Cookie Cups				
butter	1 cup	9.0	220	37%
butter toffee	1 cup	18.0	420	39%
chewy fudge	1 cup	20.0	410	44%
coconut macadamia	1 cup	24.0	440	49%
Debra's Special	1 cup	17.0	410	37%
milk chocolate				
regular	1 cup	20.0	430	42%
milk chocolate macadamia	1 cup	24.0	450	48%
milk chocolate				
w/walnuts	1 cup	23.0	440	47%

Food and Description	Amount	Fat Grams	Total Calories	% Fat Calories
oatmeal raisin	1 cup	17.0	410	37%
peanut butter	1 cup	22.0	430	46%
Pumpkin Harvest	1 cup	19.0	370	46%
semi-sweet chocolate				
regular	1 cup	20.0	420	43%
w/walnuts	1 cup	23.0	440	47%
triple chocolate	1 cup	21.0	430	44%
white chunk macadamia	1 cup	24.0	460	47%
croissants				
apple-filled	1	14.0	260	48%
cheese	1	19.0	300	57%
chocolate	1	24.0	350	62%
original	1	16.0	310	46%
Jumbo Cookies				
snickerdoodle	1	29.0	640	41%
miscellaneous items				
carrot cake				
w/cream cheese icing	1 piece	22.0	420	47%
cinnamon roll				
w/cream cheese icing	1 roll	48.0	1070	40%
cinnamon roll				
w/sticky bun topping	1 roll	49.0	1100	40%
cookies				
Cookie Monster	1	17.0	370	41%
Elmo	1	18.0	400	41%
lemon..w/cream				
cheese icing	1	12.0	300	36%
muffins				
banana nut	1	25.0	420	54%
blueberry	1	20.0	400	45%
bran	1	16.0	400	36%
chocolate chip	1	17.0	390	39%
mandarin orange	1	16.0	360	40%
raspberry	1	15.0	340	40%
Nibblers..cookies				
butter	2	4.5	110	37%
chewy chocolate fudge	2	5.0	110	41%
cinnamon sugar	2	4.5	120	34%
Debra's Special	2	4.5	100	41%
milk chocolate				
regular	2	5.0	110	41%
w/walnuts	2	6.0	120	45%
peanut butter	2	6.0	110	49%
semi-sweet chocolate	2	5.0	110	41%
triple chocolate	2	6.0	110	49%
white chunk macadamia	2	7.0	120	53%
regular cookies				
butter	1	12.0	290	37%
butter toffee	1	13.0	290	40%
chewy fudge	1	14.0	300	42%

Food and Description	Amount	Fat Grams	Total Calories	% Fat Calories
cinnamon sugar	1	12.0	300	36%
coconut macadamia	1	13.0	280	42%
Debra's Special	1	12.0	280	39%
eggnog	1	13.0	300	39%
gingersnap	1	5.0	250	18%
M&M's	1	14.0	330	38%
milk chocolate				
regular	1	13.0	280	42%
w/ macadamia nuts	1	18.0	320	51%
w/walnuts	1	17.0	320	48%
oatmeal chocolate chip	1	13.0	280	42%
peanut butter				
regular	1	16.0	310	46%
w/milk chocolate chips	1	17.0	300	51%
Pumpkin Harvest	1	14.0	260	48%
semi-sweet chocolate				
regular	1	14.0	280	45%
w/pecans	1	16.0	300	48%
w/walnuts	1	16.0	310	46%
white chunk macadamia	1	17.0	310	49%
smoothies				
Banana Berry Blast-Off	20 fl oz	–	400	–
Colada Combustion	20 fl oz	3.0	420	6%
Latte Cooler	20 fl oz	–	410	–
Mighty Berry	20 fl oz	–	300	–
Outrageous Orange	20 fl oz	–	250	–
NATHAN'S				
burgers				
deluxe				
bacon cheeseburger	1	70.0	919	69%
cheeseburger	1	65.0	859	68%
regular	1	59.0	784	68%
cheesesteaks				
6" cheesesteaks				
classic	1	11.0	420	24%
original	1	11.0	408	24%
works	1	23.0	532	39%
chicken				
6" chicken Philly				
classic	1	27.0	551	44%
pitas				
chicken	1	13.0	392	30%
gyros	1	39.0	662	53%
platters				
chicken breast	1 platter	41.0	743	50%
gyros	1 platter	93.0	1420	59%
10 wings..w/fries	1 platter	67.0	1020	59%
salads				
Caesar..w/dressing	1 salad	34.0	459	67%
garden	1 salad	18.0	310	52%

Food and Description	Amount	Fat Grams	Total Calories	% Fat Calories
chicken Caesar				
w/dressing	1 salad	39.0	608	58%
chicken club	1 salad	25.0	490	46%
Greek	1 salad	15.0	294	46%
Greek side				
w/dressing	1 salad	5.0	79	57%
sides				
fries..spicy	regular	39.0	532	66%
	large	72.0	1042	62%
mozzarella sticks	1 order	57.0	757	68%
onion rings	1 order	68.0	869	70%
■ PANDA EXPRESS				
appetizers				
chicken egg roll	1 roll	8.0	190	38%
fried shrimp	6 pieces	12.0	260	42%
veggie spring roll	1 roll	2.5	80	28%
beef				
w/broccoli	1 serving	8.0	150	48%
w/string beans	1 order	9.0	170	48%
chicken				
black pepper	1 order	10.0	180	20%
mandarin	1 order	9.0	250	32%
orange-flavored	1 order	21.0	480	39%
sweet & sour	1 order	14.0	310	41%
w/mushrooms	1 order	7.0	130	48%
w/peanuts	1 order	7.0	200	32%
w/potato	1 order	11.0	220	45%
pork				
BBQ	1 order	19.0	350	49%
sweet & sour	1 order	30.0	410	66%
rice & noodles				
steamed rice	1 order	0.5	330	1%
vegetable				
chow mein	1 order	11.0	330	30%
fried rice	1 order	12.0	390	28%
sauces				
hot	2 tsp	0.5	10	45%
hot mustard	2 tsp	–	18	–
mandarin	1.5 oz	–	70	–
soy	1 tbs	–	16	–
sweet & sour	1.5 oz	–	60	–
tofu				
string beans w/fried tofu	1 order	11.0	180	55%
vegetables				
mixed vegetables	1 order	3.0	70	39%
PAPA JOHN'S PIZZA				
■ PIZZA/based on 14" pizza				
original crust				
All the Meats	⅛ pizza	15.0	348	39%

Food and Description	Amount	Fat Grams	Total Calories	% Fat Calories
BBQ chicken & bacon	⅛ pizza	14.0	369	34%
cheese	⅛ pizza	10.0	290	31%
chicken Alfredo	⅛ pizza	12.0	310	35%
garden fresh	⅛ pizza	9.0	287	28%
Hawaiian BBQ	⅛ pizza	14.0	376	34%
pepperoni	⅛ pizza	15.0	343	39%
sausage	⅛ pizza	14.0	335	38%
spinach Alfredo	⅛ pizza	12.0	303	36%
The Works	⅛ pizza	16.0	370	39%
thin crust				
All the Meats	⅛ pizza	18.0	298	54%
BBQ chicken & bacon	⅛ pizza	18.0	336	48%
cheese	⅛ pizza	13.0	238	51%
chicken Alfredo	⅛ pizza	15.0	276	49%
garden fresh	⅛ pizza	11.0	228	43%
Hawaiian BBQ	⅛ pizza	16.5	324	46%
pepperoni	⅛ pizza	18.0	294	55%
sausage	⅛ pizza	18.0	303	53%
spinach Alfredo	⅛ pizza	15.0	251	54%
The Works	⅛ pizza	18.0	315	51%
PIZZA HUT				
■ **APPETIZERS**				
bread stick				
cheese	1	10.0	200	45%
regular	1	6.0	150	36%
bread stick dipping sauce	1 serving	–	50	–
buffalo wings				
hot	2 pieces	6.0	110	49%
mild	2 pieces	7.0	110	49%
garlic bread	1 piece	8.0	150	48%
wing dipping sauce				
blue cheese	1.5 oz	24.0	230	94%
ranch	1.5 oz	22.0	210	94%
■ **DESSERT**				
apple dessert pizza	1 slice	3.5	260	12%
cherry dessert pizza	1 slice	3.5	240	13%
cinnamon sticks	2 pieces	5.0	170	26%
white icing dipping cup	2 oz	–	190	–
■ **P'ZONE**				
Classic	½	21.0	610	31%
Meat Lover's	½	28.0	680	37%
pepperoni	½	22.0	610	32%
P'zone marinara dipping sauce	3 oz	–	45	–
Cavatini				
■ **PIZZA**				
16" extra-large				
cheese	1 slice	15.0	420	32%
Chicken Supreme	1 slice	12.0	400	27%
ham..quartered	1 slice	12.0	380	28%
Meat Lover's	1 slice	22.0	500	40%

Food and Description	Amount	Fat Grams	Total Calories	% Fat Calories
pepperoni	1 slice	17.0	430	36%
Pepperoni Lover's	1 slice	24.0	520	42%
Sausage Lover's	1 slice	23.0	510	41%
Super Supreme	1 Slice	21.0	490	39%
Supreme	1 slice	19.0	460	37%
Veggie Lover's	1 slice	12.0	390	28%
Buffalo chicken pizza				
hand-tossed-style	1 slice	7.0	238	26%
pan	1 sice	12.0	281	38%
thin 'n' crispy	1 slice	7.0	200	32%
Buffalo chicken pizza				
dipping sauce..ranch	1.5 oz cup	22.0	210	94%
Fit 'n' Delicious..12" medium pizza				
diced chicken				
w/mushroom & jalapeño	1 slice	5.0	170	26%
w/red onion & green pepper	1 slice	4.5	170	24%
green pepper..red onion				
& diced red tomato	1 slice	4.0	150	24%
ham				
w/pineapple				
& diced red tomato	1 slice	4.0	160	23%
w/red onion & mushrooms	1 slice	4.0	150	24%
tomato..mushroom				
& jalapeño	1 slice	4.0	150	24%
Fit 'n' Delicious..14" large				
diced chicken				
w/red onion & green				
pepper	1 slice	4.0	160	23%
w/mushroom & jalapeño	1 slice	4.5	160	25%
green pepper..red onion				
& jalapeño	1 slice	3.5	140	23%
ham				
w/pineapple				
& diced red tomato	1 slice	4.0	150	24%
w/red onion & mushrooms	1 slice	4.0	150	24%
tomato..mushroom				
& jalapeño	1 slice	4.0	140	26%
hand-tossed				
12" medium pizza				
cheese	1 slice	8.0	240	30%
Chicken Supreme	1 slice	6.0	230	23%
ham..quartered	1 slice	6.0	220	25%
Meat Lover's	1 slice	13.0	300	39%
pepperoni	1 slice	9.0	250	32%
Pepperoni Lover's	1 slice	13.0	300	39%
Sausage Lover's	1 slice	12.0	280	39%
Super Supreme	1 Slice	13.0	300	39%
Supreme	1 slice	11.0	270	37%
Veggie Lover's	1 slice	6.0	220	25%

Food and Description	Amount	Fat Grams	Total Calories	% Fat Calories
hand-tossed				
14" large pizza				
cheese	1 slice	8.0	220	33%
Chicken Supreme	1 slice	6.0	210	26%
ham..quartered	1 slice	6.0	200	27%
Meat Lover's	1 slice	12.0	280	39%
pepperoni	1 slice	9.0	230	35%
Pepperoni Lover's	1 slice	13.0	280	42%
Sausage Lover's	1 slice	11.0	260	38%
Super Supreme	1 slice	20.0	440	41%
Supreme	1 slice	10.0	250	36%
Veggie Lover's	1 slice	6.0	200	27%
Pan..12" medium pizza				
cheese	1 slice	13.0	280	42%
Chicken Supreme	1 slice	12.0	280	39%
ham..quartered	1 slice	11.0	260	38%
Meat Lover's	1 slice	19.0	340	50%
pepperoni	1 slice	15.0	290	16%
Pepperoni Lover's	1 slice	19.0	340	50%
Sausage Lover's	1 slice	17.0	330	46%
Super Supreme	1 Slice	18.0	340	48%
Supreme	1 slice	16.0	320	45%
Veggie Lover's	1 slice	12.0	260	42%
Pan..14" large pizza				
cheese	1 slice	13.0	270	43%
Chicken Supreme	1 slice	11.0	260	38%
ham..quartered	1 slice	11.0	250	40%
Meat Lover's	1 slice	18.0	320	51%
pepperoni	1 slice	14.0	280	45%
Pepperoni Lover's	1 slice	18.0	330	49%
Sausage Lover's	1 slice	17.0	300	51%
Super Supreme	1 Slice	17.0	320	48%
Supreme	1 slice	16.0	300	48%
Veggie Lover's	1 slice	11.0	250	40%
Personal Pan..6" pizza				
cheese	1 pizza	7.0	160	39%
Chicken Supreme	1 pizza	6.0	160	34%
ham..quartered	1 pizza	6.0	150	36%
Meat Lover's	1 pizza	10.0	200	45%
pepperoni	1 pizza	8.0	170	42%
Pepperoni Lover's	1 pizza	10.0	200	45%
Sausage Lover's	1 pizza	10.0	190	47%
Super Supreme	1 Pizza	10.0	200	45%
Supreme	1 pizza	9.0	190	43%
Veggie Lover's	1 pizza	6.0	150	36%
Stuffed Crust..14" pizza				
cheese	1 slice	13.0	360	33%
Chicken Supreme	1 slice	13.0	380	31%
ham..quartered	1 slice	11.0	340	29%
Meat Lover's	1 slice	21.0	450	42%

Food and Description	Amount	Fat Grams	Total Calories	% Fat Calories
pepperoni	1 slice	15.0	370	36%
Pepperoni Lover's	1 slice	19.0	420	41%
Sausage Lover's	1 slice	19.0	430	40%
Super Supreme	1 slice	20.0	440	41%
Supreme	1 slice	16.0	400	36%
Veggie Lover's	1 slice	14.0	360	35%
Thin 'n' Crispy..12" medium pizza				
cheese	1 slice	8.0	200	36%
Chicken Supreme	1 slice	7.0	200	32%
ham..quartered	1 slice	6.0	180	30%
Meat Lover's	1 slice	14.0	270	47%
pepperoni	1 slice	10.0	210	43%
Pepperoni Lover's	1 slice	14.0	260	48%
Sausage Lover's	1 slice	13.0	240	11%
Super Supreme	1 slice	13.0	260	45%
Supreme	1 slice	11.0	240	41%
Veggie Lover's	1 slice	7.0	180	35%
PRETZELMAKER				
Pretzel Dog				
regular	1	30.0	490	55%
Pretzel Stix				
plain	1 order	2.5	360	6%
regular	1 order	6.0	390	14%
pretzels				
butter & salt	1	5.0	370	12%
caramel crunch	1	6.0	390	14%
cinnamon	1	5.0	380	12%
garlic	1	5.0	380	12%
original				
plain	1	2.0	340	5%
Parmesan	1	6.0	390	14%
poppy seed	1	6.0	380	14%
sesame	1	6.0	380	14%
sauces				
caramel	1.5 oz	1.5	100	14%
cheddar cheese	1.5 oz	10.0	130	69%
chili spice	1.5 oz	5.0	360	13%
cream cheese	1.5 oz	14.0	145	9%
nacho cheese	1.5 oz	–	105	–
pizza sauce	1.5 oz	–	135	–
Wrapzel				
ham & Swiss	1	15.0	540	25%
pepperoni	1	21.0	570	33%
turkey & Swiss	1	17.0	580	26%
ROUND TABLE PIZZA				
■ 14" PIZZA				
Original Crust				
cheese	1 slice	8.0	210	34%
chicken garlic gourmet	1 slice	10.0	240	38%
Chicken Roastadoro	1 slice	10.0	250	36%

Food and Description	Amount	Fat Grams	Total Calories	% Fat Calories
Gourmet Veggie	1 slice	9.0	220	37%
Guinevere's Garden Delight	1 slice	7.0	210	30%
Hawaiian	1 slice	7.0	210	30%
Hearty Bacon Supreme	1 slice	16.0	290	50%
Italian garlic	1 slice	14.0	270	47%
King Arthur's Supreme	1 slice	14.0	270	47%
Maui Zaui				
Polynesian sauce	1 slice	9.0	250	32%
zesty red sauce	1 slice	9.0	240	34%
Montague's All-Meat Marvel	1 slice	17.0	300	51%
pepperoni	1 slice	11.0	240	41%
Pepperoni Roastadoro	1 slice	12.0	270	40%
Roastin' Toastin' Chicken Club	1 slice	12.0	260	42%
Western BBQ				
Chicken Supreme	1 slice	9.0	230	35%
pan crust				
cheese	1 slice	10.0	290	31%
chicken garlic gourmet	1 slice	11.0	320	31%
Chicken Roastadoro	1 slice	10.0	220	41%
Gourmet Veggie	1 slice	11.0	310	32%
Guinevere's Garden Delight	1 slice	9.0	290	28%
Hawaiian	1 slice	9.0	290	28%
Hearty Bacon Supreme	1 slice	17.0	360	43%
Italian garlic	1 slice	16.0	360	40%
King Arthur's Supreme	1 slice	14.0	340	37%
Maui Zaui				
Polynesian sauce	1 slice	11.0	330	30%
zesty red sauce	1 slice	11.0	320	31%
Montague's All-Meat Marvel	1 slice	16.0	260	55%
pepperoni	1 slice	12.0	320	34%
Pepperoni Roastadoro	1 slice	14.0	350	36%
Roastin' Toastin' Chicken Club	1 slice	12.0	230	47%
Western BBQ				
Chicken Supreme	1 slice	11.0	320	31%
Skinny Crust				
cheese	1 slice	8.0	180	40%
Chicken Garlic Gourmet	1 slice	9.0	200	41%
Chicken Roastadoro	1 slice	10.0	220	41%
Gourmet Veggie	1 slice	8.0	190	38%
Guinevere's Garden Delight	1 slice	7.0	170	37%
Italian garlic	1 slice	14.0	240	53%
King Arthur's Supreme	1 slice	14.0	240	53%
Maui Zaui				
Polynesian sauce	1 slice	9.0	210	39%
zesty red sauce	1 slice	9.0	210	39%
pepperoni	1 slice	11.0	210	47%
Pepperoni Roastadoro	1 slice	14.0	350	36%
Roastin' Toastin' Chicken Club	1 slice	12.0	230	47%
Western BBQ				
Chicken Supreme	1 slice	9.0	200	41%

Food and Description	Amount	Fat Grams	Total Calories	% Fat Calories
RUBIO'S BAJA GRILL				
■ BAJA BOWLS				
asada				
grilled grande	1 bowl	37.0	770	43%
chicken				
grilled grande	1 bowl	31.0	710	39%
■ BAJA GOURMET				
SEAFOOD BURRITOS				
fish	1	41.0	780	47%
shrimp	1	25.0	650	35%
mahimahi	1	30.0	630	43%
lobster	1	26.0	660	35%
side served..w/burrito				
chips	1 serving	11.0	220	45%
rice	1 serving	1.5	110	12%
■ BURRITOS				
Baja Grill				
carnitas	1	30.0	660	41%
carne asada	1	33.0	710	42%
chicken	1	26.0	640	37%
cheesy bean	1	37.0	850	39%
Especial				
carne asada	1	37.0	970	34%
chicken	1	32.0	920	31%
Health-Mex				
chicken	1	11.0	520	19%
veggie	1	8.0	470	15%
■ COMBO PLATES				
Burrito Combo Plate				
original + pinto beans	1 plate	18.0	350	46%
dos tacos	1 plate	45.0	860	47%
Original No. 1	1 plate	45.0	870	47%
Pesky	1 plate	56.0	1000	50%
Street Tacos	1 plate	27.0	640	38%
■ KID'S MEALS				
burritos				
bean & cheese	1 meal	21.0	570	33%
cheese quesadilla	1 meal	21.0	490	39%
original fish taco	1 meal	21.0	570	33%
taquitos	1 meal	15.0	290	47%
ADD ON:				
chips/tortilla	1 serving	11.0	220	45%
"churro"/mini	1 churro	4.0	90	40%
rice	1 serving	1.0	80	11%
■ RUBIO'S FAVORITES				
nachos				
grande	1 order	79.0	1270	56%
grande carne asada	1 order	87.0	1430	55%
grande chicken	1 order	82.0	1380	53%

Food and Description	Amount	Fat Grams	Total Calories	% Fat Calories
quesadilla				
carne asada	1	61.0	1010	54%
cheese	1	53.0	860	55%
chicken	1	56.0	960	53%
taquitos..chicken	3	11.0	310	32%
■ **SALADS**				
grilled chicken chopped	1 salad	33.0	540	55%
HealthMex chicken	1 salad	3.5	220	14%
low-carb chicken	1 salad	34.0	480	64%
salad dressing				
Serrano grape..fat-free	1 pkt	–	10	–
■ **SIDES**				
black beans	1 serving	2.5	220	10%
carne asada	1 serving	8.0	160	45%
carnitas	1 serving	6.0	85	64%
chicken	1 serving	2.5	100	23%
chips	1 serving	22.0	430	46%
churro	1	8.0	170	42%
guacamole	small	16.0	170	85%
	large	32.0	340	85%
pinto beans	1 serving	3.0	190	14%
rice	1 serving	2.0	150	12%
■ **TACO MEAL DEALS**				
carne asada taco + sides	1 meal	21.0	600	32%
chicken taco + sides	1 meal	29.0	680	38%
fish taco + sides	1 meal	29.0	690	39%
■ **TACOS**				
carne asada	1	8.0	220	33%
chicken	1	16.0	300	48%
HealthMex	1	2.5	170	13%
fish tacos				
especial	1	21.0	370	51%
original	1	16.0	310	46%
mahimahi	1	16.0	310	46%
Street Tacos				
carnitas	1	5.0	110	41%
carne asada	1	3.5	100	32%
taquitos	1 serving	17.0	320	48%
	½ sdw	29.0	470	56%
SCHLOTSKY'S DELI				
■ **BREAD/BUNS**				
dark rye	small	1.0	218	4%
	regular	2.0	327	6%
jalapeño cheese	small	3.0	235	11%
	regular	4.0	353	10%
pizza crust	6.7 oz	2.0	332	5%
sourdough	small	1.0	225	4%
	regular	2.0	333	5%
	large	4.0	667	5%

Food and Description	Amount	Fat Grams	Total Calories	% Fat Calories
wheat	small	2.0	226	8%
	regular	4.0	336	11%
■ CHIPS & PRETZELS				
potato chips/deli-style..all styles	1.5 oz	11.0	210	47%
■ DESSERTS				
cake..fudge brownie	1 slice	25.0	410	55%
cheesecake -				
cookies & cream	1 slice	18.0	330	49%
New York cream-style	1 slice	18.0	310	52%
strawberry swirl	1 slice	17.0	300	51%
cookies				
chocolate chip	1 cookie	7.0	160	39%
cookies w/real M&M's	1 cookie	11.0	140	71%
fudge chocolate chip	1 cookie	8.0	170	42%
oatmeal raisin	1 cookie	5.0	150	30%
peanut butter	1 cookie	8.0	170	42%
chocolate chunk	1 cookie	8.0	170	42%
sugar	1 cookie	6.0	160	34%
white chocolate				
macadamia nut	1 cookie	8.0	170	42%
cranberry walnut crunch	1 serving	6.0	160	34%
golden oatmeal raisin	1 serving	7.0	160	39%
triple chocolate chip	1 serving	8.0	170	42%
■ KID'S DEALS				
pizza				
cheese	1 serving	11.0	460	22%
pepperoni	1 serving	16.0	507	28%
sandwich				
cheese	1 sdw	15.0	401	34%
ham & cheese	1 sdw	16.0	431	33%
PBJ (peanut butter & jelly)	1 sdw	16.0	470	31%
■ PIZZAS..8" sourdough crust pizzas				
BBQ chicken	1 pizza	15.0	683	21%
double cheese & pepperoni	1 pizza	32.0	721	40%
kid's				
cheese	1 pizza	11.0	460	22%
pepperoni	1 pizza	16.0	507	28%
kung pao chicken	1 pizza	20.0	718	25%
Thai chicken	1 pizza	17.0	663	23%
"The Original" combination	1 pizza	23.0	625	33%
3-meat	1 pizza	39.0	805	44%
Tuscan herb	1 pizza	15.0	541	25%
vegetarian special	1 pizza	17.0	551	28%
■ SALADS & SALAD EXTRAS				
deli salads				
Albacore tuna	1 salad	13.0	218	54%
California pasta	1 serving	3.0	58	47%
chicken & pesto	1 salad	15.0	454	30%
chicken salad	1 salad	21.0	376	50%

Food and Description	Amount	Fat Grams	Total Calories	% Fat Calories
coleslaw..home-style	1 serving	10.0	188	48%
fresh fruit	1 salad	1.0	123	7%
macaroni..elbow	1 serving	19.0	275	62%
potato				
choice	1 serving	15.0	288	47%
mustard & egg	1 serving	13.0	250	47%
leaf salads w/o salad extras				
Caesar	1 salad	1.0	30	30%
chicken Caesar	1 salad	3.0	111	24%
garden				
regular	1 salad	1.0	48	19%
smoked turkey..chef's	1 salad	10.0	199	45%
salad extras				
chow mein noodles	1 serving	4.0	74	49%
croutons..garlic cheese	1 serving	2.0	46	39%
dressings				
Greek balsamic vinaigrette	3 Tbs	17..0	170	90%
Italian..light	3 Tbs	8.0	90	80%
Olde World Caesar	3 Tbs	27.0	260	93%
ranch				
spicy..light	3 Tbs	11.0	140	71%
traditional ranch	3 Tbs	29.0	270	97%
sesame ginger vinaigrette	3 Tbs	15.0	170	79%
Thousand Island	3 Tbs	21.0	220	86%
■ SANDWICHES				
HOT				
albacore tuna	regular	10.0	496	18%
	large	20.0	970	19%
chicken breast	regular	4.0	499	7%
	large	9.0	981	8%
Fiesta Chicken	regular	36.0	839	39%
	large	63.0	1598	35%
original ham & cheese	regular	27.0	749	32%
	large	50.0	1423	32%
deluxe	regular	42.0	930	41%
	large	80.0	1785	40%
turkey	regular	32.0	822	35%
	large	60.0	1569	34%
pastrami & Swiss	regular	36.0	882	37%
	large	70.0	1748	36%
roast beef & cheese	regular	32.0	855	34%
	large	60.0	1641	33%
smoked turkey breast	regular	7.0	498	13%
	large	13.0	988	12%
turkey & bacon club	regular	35.0	834	38%
	large	64.0	1589	36%
■ WRAPS				
Asian almond chicken	1	7.0	459	14%
chicken Caesar	1	27.0	511	48%
salsa chicken..w/cheddar	1	17.0	460	33%

Food and Description	Amount	Fat Grams	Total Calories	% Fat Calories
zesty albacore tuna	1	7.0	311	20%
SONIC				
■ **BREAKFAST**				
breakfast burrito	1	37.0	616	54%
Sonic Sunrise	regular	–	224	–
	large	–	368	–
Sonic Toasters				
bacon..egg..cheese	1 order	29.0	500	52%
ham..egg..cheese	1 order	19.0	436	39%
sausage..egg..cheese	1 order	36.0	570	57%
■ **BURGERS & HOT DOGS..w/add-on's**				
add-on's				
bacon	1 serving	7.0	80	79%
BBQ sauce..Sonic hickory	1 oz	–	41	–
cheese	1 serving	6.0	70	77%
cheddar cheese..shredded	1 oz	9.0	104	78%
chili..Sonic	1 serving	4.0	52	69%
honey mustard dressing	1 oz	9.0	110	74%
ranch dressing	1 oz	16.0	147	98%
slaw	1 serving	3.0	45	60%
Thousand Island	1 oz	15.0	150	90%
burgers				
bacon cheeseburger	1	49.0	727	61%
Jr. burger	1	21.0	353	54%
Sonic				
burgers				
No. 1	1	36.0	577	56%
No. 2	1	25.0	481	47%
cheeseburger				
No. 1	1	42.0	647	58%
No. 2	1	31.0	551	51%
Super Sonic				
No. 1	1	66.0	929	64%
No. 2	1	5.0	839	59%
Coneys				
corn dog	1	17.0	262	58%
extra-long	1	27.0	483	50%
cheese Coney	1	42.0	666	57%
regular	1	16.0	262	55%
w/cheese	1	24.0	366	59%
■ **CHICKEN**				
chicken sandwich				
breaded	1	23.0	582	36%
grilled	1	13.0	343	34%
strip				
dinner	1 dinner	32.0	749	38%
snack	1 snack	13.0	272	43%
■ **FROZEN FAVORITES**				
banana split	1	11.0	467	21%

Food and Description	Amount	Fat Grams	Total Calories	% Fat Calories
floats				
Coca-Cola	regular	12.0	386	28%
	large	17.0	553	28%
Dr Pepper	regular	12.0	377	29%
ice cream				
cone	1	11.0	285	35%
dish	1	11.0	265	37%
malt..add to any shake	1 oz	1.0	104	9%
shakes				
banana cream pie	regular	27.0	775	31%
	large	35.0	1058	30%
chocolate	regular	18.0	564	29%
	large	25.0	752	30%
chocolate cream pie	regular	27.0	795	31%
	large	35.0	1151	27%
coconut cream pie	regular	26.0	721	32%
	large	35.0	1004	31%
strawberry	regular	18.0	510	32%
	large	24.0	680	32%
vanilla	regular	18.0	454	36%
	large	24.0	605	36%
shakes..Sonic Blast				
Butterfinger	regular	26.0	636	37%
	large	37.0	924	36%
M&M's	regular	27.0	641	38%
	large	39.0	931	38%
Oreo	regular	27.0	638	38%
	large	39.0	927	38%
Reese's	regular	30.0	658	41%
	large	45.0	963	42%
■ KID'S MEAL				
Wacky Pack				
chicken strips	2 pieces	9.0	184	44%
corn dog	1	17.0	262	58%
French fries	1 regular	11.0	195	51%
grilled cheese	1	12.0	282	38%
hot dog..plain	1	16.0	262	55%
Jr. burger	1	21.0	353	54%
Tots	regular	16.0	259	56%
■ SANDWICH				
steak..country-fried	9.78 oz	47.0	748	57%
■ SANDWICHES..TOASTER				
bacon cheddar burger	1	38.0	675	51%
BLT	1	41.0	581	64%
Chicken club	1	29.0	675	39%
grilled cheese	1	12.0	282	38%
steak..country-fried	1	45.0	708	57%
■ SIDE ORDERS..FAVE & CRAVES				
Ched 'R' Peppers	1 order	12.0	256	42%

Food and Description	Amount	Fat Grams	Total Calories	% Fat Calories
French fries				
cheese	regular	17.0	265	58%
	large	19.0	322	53%
chili cheese	regular	19.0	299	57%
	large	22.0	357	55%
plain	regular	11.0	195	51%
	large	13.0.	252	46%
Super Sonic	1 order	18.0	358	45%
Fritos chili pie	1	44.0	611	65%
mozzarella sticks	1 order	19.0	382	45%
onion rings	regular	25.0	331	68%
	large	37.0	507	66%
Tater Tots				
cheese	regular	22.0	329	60%
	large	27.0	437	56%
chili cheese	regular	25.0	363	62%
	large	36.0	547	59%
plain	regular	16.0	259	56%
	large	21.0	365	52%
Super Sonic	1 serving	28.0	485	52%
■ WRAPS				
Fritos chili cheese wrap	1 wrap	42.0	743	51%
grilled				
chicken				
strip wrap				
w/ranch dressing	1 wrap	29.0	574	45%
w/o ranch dressing	1 wrap	13.0	428	27%
w/ ranch dressing	1 wrap	27.0	539	45%
w/o ranch dressing	1 wrap	12.0	393	27%
STARBUCKS (*See also* ICE CREAM & ICE CREAM-LIKE FROZEN DESSERTS)				
■ BEVERAGES				
apple juice	16 fl oz	–	230	–
Café Misto..café au lait	16 fl oz	8.0	140	51%
Caffe Americano	16 fl oz	–	15	–
caffe latte	16 fl oz	14.0	260	48%
caffe mocha				
no whip-cream	16 fl oz	12.0	300	36%
w/whip-cream	16 fl oz	22.0	400	50%
caffe vanilla				
Frappuccino blended coffee (see more Frappuccino products next page)				
caramel				
light..no whip-cream	16 fl oz	1.5	180	8%
w/whip-cream	16 fl oz	14.0	310	41%
regular..no whip-cream	16 fl oz	3.5	280	11%
w/whip-cream	16 fl oz	16.0	430	33%
java chip				
light..no whip-cream	16 fl oz	7.0	260	24%
w/whip-cream	16 fl oz	19.0	400	43%

Food and Description	Amount	Fat Grams	Total Calories	% Fat Calories
regular..no whip-cream	16 fl oz	9.0	370	22%
w/whip-cream	16 fl oz	22.0	510	39%
mocha				
light..no whip-cream	16 fl oz	1.5	180	8%
w/whip-cream	16 fl oz	14.0	310	41%
regular..no whip-cream,	16 fl oz	4.0	290	12%
w/whip-cream	16 fl oz	16.0	420	34%
original				
light..no whip-cream	16 fl oz	1.0	230	4%
w/whip-cream	16 fl oz	13.0	360	33%
regular..no whip-cream	16 fl oz	3.5	340	9%
w/whip-cream	16 fl oz	16.0	470	31%
white chocolate mocha				
no whip-cream	16 fl oz	2.5	200	11%
w/whip-cream	16 fl oz	15.0	340	40%
cappuccino	16 fl oz	8.0	150	48%
caramel apple cider				
no whip-cream	16 fl oz	–	300	–
w/whip-cream	16 fl oz	10.0	410	22%
caramel macchiato	16 fl oz	12.0	310	35%
caramel mocha				
no whip-cream	16 fl oz	11.0	370	27%
w/whip-cream	16 fl oz	21.0	470	40%
chocolate milk	16 fl oz	15.0	340	40%
cinnamon spice mocha				
no whip-cream	16 fl oz	12.0	330	33%
w/whip-cream	16 fl oz	22.0	430	46%
coffee Frappuccino blended coffee				
light				
no whip-cream	16 fl oz	1.0	150	6%
w/whip-cream	16 fl oz	13.0	280	42%
regular				
no whip-cream	16 fl oz	3.5	260	12%
double chocolate chip Frappuccino				
blended crème..				
no whip-cream	16 fl oz	12.0	460	23%
w/whip-cream	16 fl oz	24.0	590	37%
espresso Frappuccino				
blended coffee	16 fl oz	3.0	230	12%
light..				
no whip-cream	16 fl oz	1.0	140	6%
w/whip-cream	16 fl oz	13.0	270	43%
gingerbread latte..				
no whip-cream	16 fl oz	13.0	270	43%
w/whip-cream	16 fl oz	22.0	430	46%
hot chocolate				
peppermint..				
no whip-cream	16 fl oz	14.0	410	31%
w/whip-cream	16 fl oz	24.0	510	42%

Food and Description	Amount	Fat Grams	Total Calories	% Fat Calories
peppermint mocha				
no whip-cream	16 fl oz	12.0	370	29%
w/whip-cream	16 fl oz	22.0	470	42%
regular..				
no whip-cream	16 fl oz	15.0	340	40%
w/whip-cream	16 fl oz	24.0	440	49%
white hot chocolate				
no whip-cream	16 fl oz	18.0	480	34%
w/whip-cream	16 fl oz	28.0	580	43%
iced				
Caffe Americano	16 fl oz	–	20	–
Caffe Latte	16 fl oz	8.0	160	45%
mocha..				
no whip-cream	16 fl oz	8.0	220	33%
w/whip-cream	16 fl oz	20.0	350	51%
caramel macchiato	16 fl oz	10.0	270	33%
shaken coffee	16 fl oz	–	80	–
syrup-flavored latte	16 fl oz	7.0	210	30%
Tazo chai tea latte	16 fl oz	7.0	270	23%
vanilla latte	16 fl oz	7.0	210	30%
white chocolate mocha				
no whip-cream	16 fl oz	11.0	360	28%
w/whip-cream	16 fl oz	24.0	490	44%
latte..syrup-flavored	16 fl oz	10.0	280	32%
peppermint mocha Frappuccino				
blended coffee.no whip-cream	16 fl oz	4.0	310	12%
w/whip-cream	16 fl oz	16.0	440	33%
pumpkin spice creme				
no whip-cream	16 fl oz	14.0	400	32%
w/whip-cream	16 fl oz	24.0	500	43%
pumpkin spice Frappuccino				
blended coffee				
light..no whip-cream	16 fl oz	1.0	190	5%
w/whip-cream	16 fl oz	13.0	320	37%
regular..no whip-cream	16 fl oz	3.5	300	11%
w/whip-cream	16 fl oz	16.0	430	33%
pumpkin spice latte				
no whip-cream	16 fl oz	12.0	380	28%
w/whip-cream	16 fl oz	22.0	480	41%
strawberries & cream Frappuccino				
blended creme..no whip-cream	16 fl oz	5.0	450	10%
w/whip-cream	16 fl oz	17.0	580	26%
Tazo Chai Creme Frappuccino				
blended tea..no whip-cream	16 fl oz	5.0	380	12%
w/whip-cream	16 fl oz	17.0	510	30%
■ FRESH FOOD ITEMS				
almond-filled croissant	1	18.0	330	49%
apple danish..w/mocha swirls	1	19.0	370	46%
Apple Harvest torte	1	15.0	350	39%
apple walnut coffee cake	1	17.0	320	48%

Food and Description	Amount	Fat Grams	Total Calories	% Fat Calories
apricot currant scone	1	17.0	450	34%
bagel..plain	1	1.0	430	2%
banana pound cake	1	18.0	360	45%
banana pullman	1	17.0	400	38%
black & white cookie	1	17.0	430	36%
blueberry muffin	1	19.0	380	45%
blueberry scone	1	18.0	460	35%
blueberry walnut coffee cake	1	18.0	340	48%
butter croissant w/apricot glaze	1	17.0	320	48%
butterscotch pecan scone	1	27.0	520	47%
caramel apple bar	1	16.0	310	46%
caramel brownie	1	36.0	580	56%
caramel pecan sticky roll	1	40.0	730	49%
carrot cake bar	1	25.0	420	54%
cheese Danish w/mocha swirls	1	28.0	460	55%
chocolate big baby bundt cake	1	15.0	330	41%
chocolate cream cheese muffin	1	24.0	450	48%
chocolate-filled croissant	1	19.0	350	49%
chocolate hazelnut biscotti	1	3.0	110	25%
chocolate pullman	1	17.0	380	40%
cinnamon chip scone w/icing	1	23.0	510	41%
cinnamon-flavored twist	1	17.0	320	48%
cinnamon raisin bagel	1	1.0	440	42%
cinnamon roll	1	29.0	620	42%
cinnamon walnut coffee cake	1	18.0	360	45%
classic coffee cake	1	28.0	570	44%
Cranberry Bliss bar	1	18.0	320	51%
cranberry orange muffin	1	20.0	410	44%
cranberry walnut pound cake	1	21.0	390	48%
cranberry walnut pullman	1	15.0	360	38%
crisp cinnamon twist	1	2.0	60	30%
crumb cake	1	32.0	670	43%
crumble berry coffee cake	1	26.0	420	56%
dark chocolate graham	1	8.0	140	51%
double chocolate chunk cookie	1	21.0	430	44%
enrobed espresso brownie	1	25.0	430	52%
espresso brownie	1	21.0	370	51%
hazelnut coffee cake	1	35.0	630	50%
holiday gingerbread	1	16.0	480	30%
home-style oatmeal raisin cookie	1	15.0	390	35%
iced carrot pound cake	1	13.0	540	22%
iced lemon pound cake	1	23.0	500	41%
key lime crumb cake				
lemon bar	1	27.0	550	44%

Food and Description	Amount	Fat Grams	Total Calories	% Fat Calories
lemon glazed pullman	1	15.0	370	36%
lemon yogurt bundt cake	1	13.0	350	33%
madeleine	1	3.5	80	39%
maple oat scone				
w/icing	1	22.0	490	40%
marble chocolate chip				
pullman	1	20.0	440	41%
marble pound cake	1	21.0	400	47%
milk chocolate graham	1	8.0	140	51%
milk chocolate peanut				
butter brownie	1	29.0	460	57%
Morning Sunrise muffin	1	12.0	330	33%
oatmeal cranberry mountain	1	24.0	430	50%
orange poppy cheese				
pullman	1	22.0	450	44%
orange poppy pound cake	1	27.0	490	50%
oreo dream bar	1	30.0	420	64%
pecan diamond	1	37.0	490	68%
peppermint brownie	1	27.0	440	55%
pumpkin pound cake	1	12.0	310	35%
pumpkin pullman	1	17.0	370	41%
raspberry and cream cheese–				
filled croissant	1	12.0	260	42%
raspberry Danish				
w/mocha swirls	1	19.0	370	46%
raspberry Sammy	1	14.0	300	42%
raspberry scone	1	18.0	40	37%
sesame bagel	1	3.0	142	19%
shortbread	1	6.0	100	54%
sour cream coffee cake	1	25.0	420	54%
toffee cream cheese chew	1	31.0	440	63%
toffee crunch bar	1	21.0	430	44%
vanilla almond biscotti	1	5.0	110	49%
white chocolate macadamia				
nut cookie	1	27.0	470	52%
zucchini pound cake	1	19.0	370	46%

STEAK & SHAKE

shakes (See Fountain & Desserts within this section)

■ **BREAKFAST**

à la carte

bacon strips	4 strips	20.0	220	82%
bagel..plain	1	1.0	350	3%
biscuit				
buttermilk				
no margarine	1 biscuit	16.0	360	40%
w/margarine	1 biscuit	24.0	428	50%
cinnamon roll	1 roll	54.0	800	61%
egg..cooked w/margarine	1 egg	12.5	142	79%
egg..Healthy Morning				
cholesterol-free egg product	2 eggs	16.0	197	73%

Food and Description	Amount	Fat Grams	Total Calories	% Fat Calories
English muffin				
no margarine	1	1.0	130	–
w/o magarine	1	16.0	265	54%
French toast..cinnamon				
swirl	3 slices	7.0	263	24%
hash browns				
regular	1 serving	25.0	372	60%
w/cheese sauce	1 serving	30.5	449	61%
pancakes..buttermilk	3	4.0	240	15%
	2	2.5	160	14%
sausage gravy	1 serving	13.5	178	68%
sausage patties	2	40.0	420	86%
toast				
rye..no margarine	2 slices	2.0	140	13%
w/margaine	2 slices	17.0	275	56%
sourdough.. no margarine	2 slices	3.0	180	15%
w/margarine	2 slices	18.0	315	51%
wheat..no margarine	2 slices	2.0	104	17%
w/margarine	2 slices	17.0	239	64%
white..no margarine	2 slices	3.0	200	14%
w/margarine	2 slices	18.0	335	48%
biscuits..gravy 'n'				
hash browns	1 serving	99.0	1584	56%
breakfast sandwiches				
egg & cheese	1	20.0	366	49%
egg..cheese..bacon	1	30.0	476	57%
egg..cheese..sausage	1	40.0	576	63%
sausage & biscuit	1	44.0	638	62%
steak..egg..cheese	1	36.0	546	59%
breakfast specials				
sausage patty	1 patty	20.0	210	86%
The Number 1				
eggs only	1 serving	25.0	291	77%
The Number 2	1 serving	60.0	918	59%
The Number 3	1 serving	62.0	897	62%
The Number 4	1 serving	49.0	663	67%
The Number 5	1 serving	62.0	978	57%
The Number 6	1 serving	25.0	291	77%
The Number 7	1 serving	39.0	668	53%
The Number 8	1 serving	68.0	1010	61%
The Number 9	1 serving	30.0	676	40%
two bacon strips	1 serving	10.0	110	82%
Cheddar Scrambler	1 serving	90.0	1283	63%
Country Scrambler				
cakes 'n' eggs..bacon				
& sausage	1 serving	78.0	1029	68%
eggs				
w/the works				
& bacon	1 serving	70.0	876	72%
& bacon..hold the				
hash browns	1 serving	46.0	504	82%

Food and Description	Amount	Fat Grams	Total Calories	% Fat Calories
& sausage	1 serving	90.0	1076	75%
& sausage..hold the hash browns	1 serving	65.0	704	83%
French toast,.strawberry	3 slices	11.0	470	21%
Just biscuits 'n' gravy	1 serving	74.0	1212	55%
one egg				
w/the works				
& bacon	1 serving	47.0	624	68%
& sausage	1 serving	57.0	724	71%
pancakes				
Classic Stack 'o Cakes	1 serving	4.0	240	15%
strawberry stack	1 serving	8.0	447	16%
Steak 'n' Eggs				
breakfast	1 serving	80.0	1016	71%
■ BURGERS & CHILI				
chili 3-way	1 serving	35.5	662	48%
chili 5-way	1 serving	66.5	1033	58%
chili Deluxe				
bowl	10 oz	64.0	861	67%
cub	6 oz	35.5	480	67%
chili mac				
regular	1 serving	29.5	696	38%
supreme	1 serving	59.5	1067	50%
chili & oyster crackers	1 serving	14.0	337	37%
chili mac & 4 saltines	1 serving	12.4	311	36%
chili 3 ways & 4 saltines	1 serving	16.0	402	36%
genuine chili				
bowl	10 oz	34.0	490	62%
cup	6 oz	21.0	294	64%
steakburger				
BBQ 'n' bacon	1	49.0	875	50%
bacon 'n' cheese double	1	48.0	697	62%
deluxe cheddar 'n' bacon	1	49.0	809	55%
mushroom Swiss	1	46.5	812	52%
original..double				
plain	1	32.0	510	56%
w/cheese	1	38.0	680	50%
original..single				
plain	1	17.0	330	46%
w/cheese	1	23.0	400	52%
Philadelphia	1	52.0	848	55%
triple				
regular	1	47.0	690	61%
w/double cheese	1	59.0	830	64%
■ DINNERS				
Steak 'n' Shake	1 dinner	32.0	510	56%
chicken fingers	1 dinner	62.0	818	68%
chicken melt dinner	1 dinner	70.0	950	66%
Chili Mac Supreme	1 dinner	93.0	1496	56%

Food and Description	Amount	Fat Grams	Total Calories	% Fat Calories
fish dinner	1 dinner	52.0	704	67%
Frisco melt	1 dinner	93.0	1173	71%
■ **FOUNTAIN & DESSERTS**				
desserts..à la mode				
apple cobbler	1	33.0	699	42%
w/o ice cream	1	22.0	504	39%
Berry Berry cobbler	1	31.0	663	42%
w/o ice cream	1	20.0	468	38%
blackberry cobbler	1	33.0	681	44%
w/o ice cream	1	22.0	486	41%
blueberry cobbler	1	33.0	681	44%
w/o ice cream	1	22.0	486	41%
brownie fudge sundae	1	43.5	871	45%
cherry cobbler	1	33.0	741	40%
w/o ice cream	1	22.0	545	36%
hot fudge				
brownie	1	23.0	492	42%
sundae	1	26.0	511	46%
Outrageous Parfait	1	40.0	769	47%
peach cobbler à la mode	1	33.0	681	44%
w/o ice cream	1	22.0	486	41%
pumpkin pie				
w/whipped topping	⅛ pie	14.0	393	32%
strawberry cobbler à la mode	1	20.0	468	38%
strawberry				
shortcake	1	25.0	563	40%
sundae	1	19.5	363	48%
vanilla ice cream	½ cup	14.0	244	52%
The Fountain				
float..root beer	1	22.0	557	36%
freeze..orange	regular	19.0	615	28%
	large	24.5	774	28%
milk shakes & malt				
banana	regular	21.0	667	28%
chocolate	regular	21.5	684	28%
chocolate mint	regular	23.0	717	29%
mocha	regular	21.0	666	28%
peach	regular	21.0	660	28%
strawberry	regular	21.0	631	30%
vanilla	regular	21.0	664	28%
Shakes Alive				
cookies 'n' cream	1	23.5	713	30%
double chocolate chip	1	25.0	753	30%
very very strawberry	1	17.5	515	31%
■ **SALADS**				
beef taco	1 salad	59.0	940	56%
beef taco..double beef	1 salad	65.5	1047	56%
chicken chef	1 salad	32.0	463	62%
chicken taco	1 salad	70.0	1072	59%

Food and Description	Amount	Fat Grams	Total Calories	% Fat Calories
deluxe garden	1 salad	15.0	226	60%
fried chicken	1 salad	81.0	1048	70%
■ SANDWICHES				
melts				
All-American	1 sdw	103.0	1298	71%
Frisco	1 sdw	93.0	1173	71%
patty	1 sdw	83.0	1013	74%
chicken	1 sdw	69.0	988	63%
pepper Jack	1 sdw	91.0	1122	73%
turkey	1 sdw	70.0	950	66%
tuna	1 sdw	77.0	919	75%
specialties				
bacon..lettuce..tomato	1 sdw	34.0	528	58%
chicken fingers 'n' fries	1 serving	59.0	873	61%
chicken fingers only	1 serving	46.0	613	68%
fish fillet	1 sdw	52.0	753	62%
grilled cheese	1 sdw	51.0	680	68%
grilled cheese 'n' bacon	1 sdw	61.0	790	69%
grilled chicken breast	1 sdw	26.0	471	50%
spicy chicken	1 sdw	31.5	542	52%
tuna salad	1 sdw	30.0	445	61%
■ SOUPS 'N' SIDES				
sides				
baked beans				
old-fashioned	1 crock	1.0	372	2%
cheddar cheese fries	large	45.0	838	48%
	regular	34.5	626	93%
	small	18.5	336	50%
chili..genuine	1 cup	21.0	294	64%
chili cheese fries	1 order	72.5	1279	51%
coleslaw..creamy	1 order	24.0	306	71%
cottage cheese	3.5 oz	2.0	103	17%
French fries	large	33.5	684	44%
	regular	23.0	472	44%
	small	12.0	260	42%
onion rings	regular	39.5	668	53%
	small	19.5	334	53%
soup..bowl				
chicken gumbo	12 oz	4.5	172	24%
chicken noodle	12 oz	2.5	141	16%
cream of broccoli	12 oz	15.5	286	49%
vegetable beef	12 oz	12.5	234	48%
SUBWAY				
Atkins-Friendly Salads				
classic club..w/ranch dressing	1 salad	43.0	590	66%
grilled chicken & baby spinach w/Atkins sweet as honey dressing	1 salad	48.0	620	70%
Atkins-Friendly Wraps				
chicken bacon ranch	1 wrap	26.0	440	53%

Food and Description	Amount	Fat Grams	Total Calories	% Fat Calories
turkey bacon melt	1 wrap	27.0	430	57%
turkey breast & ham	1 wrap	23.0	390	53%
■ BREADS				
bread..6" except roll & wrap				
Atkins-Friendly wrap	1 wrap	4.5	120	34%
deli-style roll	1 roll	2.5	170	8%
honey oat	3 oz	3.5	250	13%
Italian white bread	2.5 oz	2.5	200	11%
hearty	2.78 oz	2.5	210	11%
herb & cheese	3.4 oz	6.0	240	23%
Monterey cheddar	3 oz	6.0	240	23%
Parmesan oregano	2.8 oz	3.5	210	15%
wheat	2.67 oz	2.5	200	11%
■ COOKIES				
Atkins-Friendly				
double chocolate	1	6.0	100	54%
chocolate chip	1	10.0	210	43%
chocolate chunk	1	10.0	220	41%
double chocolate chip	1	10.0	210	43%
M&M's	1	10.0	210	43%
oatmeal raisin	1	8.0	200	36%
peanut butter	1	12.0	220	49%
sugar	1	12.0	230	47%
white macadamia nut	1	11.0	220	45%
■ OMELETS & FRENCH TOAST				
French toast				
w/syrup	1 serving	8.0	350	21%
omelets				
bacon & egg	1	17.0	240	64%
cheese & egg	1	17.0	240	64%
ham & egg	1	14.0	230	55%
vegetable & egg	1	14.0	210	60%
Western & egg	1	14.0	220	57%
■ SALADS..DRESSINGS				
salad dressings				
Atkins honey mustard	1 pkt	22.0	200	99%
Greek vinaigrette	1 pkt	21.0	200	95%
Italian fat-free	1 pkt	–	35	–
ranch regular	1 pkt	22.0	200	99%
red wine vinaigrette	1 pkt	1.0	80	11%
salads				
Classic Club	1 salad	21.0	390	48%
Garden Fresh salad	1 salad	1.0	60	15%
grilled chicken				
& baby spinach	1 salad	26.0	420	56%
Mediterranean chicken	1 salad	4.5	170	24%
■ SANDWICHES & SUBS				
6" 6 grams of fat or less sandwiches				

Food and Description	Amount	Fat Grams	Total Calories	% Fat Calories
chicken				
oven-roasted breast	1	5.0	330	14%
teriyaki..sweet onion	1	5.0	370	12%
ham	1	5.0	290	16%
honey mustard ham	1	5.0	310	15%
roast beef	1	5.0	290	16%
turkey breast				
ham & roast beef	1	6.0	320	17%
savory	1	4.5	280	14%
savory & ham	1	5.0	290	16%
Veggie Delite	1	3.0	230	12%
6" cold sandwiches				
Classic Italian BMT	1	21.0	450	42%
cold cut combo	1	17.0	410	37%
Subway Seafood Sensation	1	22.0	450	44%
tuna	1	31.0	530	53%
6" double meat (DM)				
cheesesteak	1	14.0	450	28%
chicken	1	8.0	430	17%
chicken..sweet onion				
teriyaki	1	7.0	450	14%
cold cut combo	1	28.0	550	46%
ham	1	7.0	350	18%
Italian BMT	1	35.0	630	50%
meatball marinara	1	38.0	740	46%
roast beef	1	7.0	360	18%
Seafood Sensation	1	20.0	490	37%
Southwest chipotle				
cheesesteak	1	22.0	530	37%
tuna..classic	1	42.0	610	62%
turkey				
breast	1	5.0	330	14%
breast & ham	1	7.0	360	18%
breast..ham & roast beef	1	8.0	410	18%
breast..ham				
& bacon melt	1	17.0	490	31%
6" hot sandwiches				
cheesesteak	1	10.0	360	25%
chipotle Southwest				
cheesesteak	1	19.0	440	39%
Dijon turkey..ham				
& bacon melt	1	21.0	470	40%
meatball marinara	1	22.0	500	40%
turkey breast..ham				
& bacon melt	1	12.0	380	28%
Breakfast Sandwiches				
6" Italian or wheat bread				
bacon & egg	1	19.0	450	38%
cheese & egg	1	19.0	440	39%
ham & egg	1	17.0	430	36%

Food and Description	Amount	Fat Grams	Total Calories	% Fat Calories
steak & egg	1	18.0	460	35%
vegetable & egg	1	16.0	410	35%
Western & egg	1	17.0	430	36%
Deli Round				
bacon & egg	1	15.0	320	42%
cheese & egg	1	15.0	320	42%
ham & egg	1	13.0	310	38%
steak & egg	1	14.0	330	38%
vegetable & egg	1	12.0	290	37%
Western & egg	1	12.0	300	36%
■ SOUPS				
broccoli				
& cheese..golden	1 cup	11.0	180	55%
cream of	1 cup	6.0	130	42%
cheese..w/ham & bacon	1 cup	15.0	240	56%
chicken				
& dumpling	1 cup	4.5	130	31%
& rice..Spanish-style	1 cup	2.0	90	20%
roasted noodle	1 cup	1.5	60	23%
w/brown & wild rice	1 cup	11.0	190	52%
chili con carne	1 cup	10.0	240	38%
minestrone	1 cup	4.0	90	40%
New England clam chowder	1 cup	3.5	110	29%
potato..cream of..w/bacon	1 cup	11.0	200	50%
tomato garden vegetable				
w/rotini	1 cup	0.5	100	5%
vegetable beef	1 cup	1.0	90	10%
■ WRAPS				
chicken bacon ranch	1 wrap	26.0	440	53%
Mediterranean chicken	1 wrap	18.0	350	46%
turkey				
bacon melt	1 wrap	27.0	430	57%
breast & ham	1 wrap	23.0	390	53%
TACO BELL				
■ BREAKFAST				
burrito	1	25.0	510	44%
Gordita	1	24.0	380	57%
quesadilla	1	20.0	400	45%
steak				
burrito	1	26.0	500	47%
quesadilla				
w/green sauce	1	23.0	480	43%
■ BURRITOS				
7-layer	1	22.0	530	37%
bean	1	10.0	370	24%
Burrito Supreme				
beef	1	18.0	440	37%
chicken	1	14.0	410	31%
steak	1	16.0	420	34%
chili cheese	1	18.0	390	42%

Food and Description	Amount	Fat Grams	Total Calories	% Fat Calories
Fiesta Burrito				
beef	1	15.0	390	35%
chicken	1	12.0	370	29%
steak	1	13.0	370	32%
Grilled Stuft Burrito				
beef	1	33.0	730	41%
chicken	1	26.0	680	34%
steak	1	28.0	680	37%
■ CHALUPAS				
Baja				
beef	1 chalupa	27.0	430	57%
chicken	1 chalupa	24.0	400	54%
steak	1 chalupa	25.0	400	56%
Nacho Cheese				
beef	1 chalupa	22.0	380	52%
chicken	1 chalupa	18.0	350	46%
steak	1 chalupa	19.0	350	49%
Supreme				
beef	1 chalupa	24.0	390	55%
chicken	1 chalupa	20.0	370	49%
steak	1 chalupa	22.0	370	54%
■ GORDITAS				
Baja				
beef	1 gordita	19.0	350	49%
chicken	1 gordita	15.0	320	42%
steak	1 gordita	16.0	320	45%
Nacho Cheese				
beef	1 gordita	13.0	300	39%
chicken	1 gordita	12.0	290	37%
steak	1 gordita	11.0	270	37%
Supreme				
beef	1 gordita	16.0	310	46%
chicken	1 gordita	12.0	290	37%
steak	1 gordita	13.0	290	40%
■ NACHOS & SIDES				
Cinnamon Twists	1 twist	5.0	160	28%
Mexican rice	1 serving	10.0	210	43%
nachos				
BellGrande	1 serving	39.0	760	46%
regular	1 serving	19.0	320	53%
supreme	1 serving	24.0	440	49%
pintos 'n' cheese	1 serving	7.0	180	35%
■ SAUCES AND CONDIMENTS				
creamy				
jalapeño sauce	1 oz	14.0	140	90%
lime sauce	1 oz	19.0	180	95%
guacamole	1 oz	4.0	50	72%
nacho cheese sauce	1 oz	4.0	50	72%
pepper Jack cheese sauce	1 oz	15.0	150	90%
zesty dressing	1 oz	16.0	160	90%

Food and Description	Amount	Fat Grams	Total Calories	% Fat Calories
■ SPECIALTY ITEMS				
Enchirito				
beef	1	18.0	380	43%
chicken	1	14.0	350	36%
steak	1	16.0	360	40%
Express taco salad				
w/chips	1 salad	31.0	620	45%
Mexican pizza	1 pizza	31.0	550	51%
Meximelt	1 serving	16.0	290	49%
quesadilla				
cheese	1	28.0	490	51%
Extreme Cheese	1	25.0	470	48%
chicken	1	30.0	540	50%
steak	1	31.0	540	52%
Southwest Steak Bowl	1 bowl	32.0	700	41%
taco salad				
w/salsa	1 salad	42.0	790	48%
w/salsa..w/o shell	1	21.0	420	45%
tostada	1 tostada	10.0	250	36%
Zesty Border Bowl				
chicken				
w/dressing	1 bowl	42.0	730	52%
w/o dressing	1 bowl	19.0	500	34%
■ TACOS				
Taco				
Double Decker				
regular	1 taco	13.0	340	34%
Taco Supreme	1 taco	18.0	380	43%
plain..original	1 taco	10.0	170	53%
soft				
beef	1 taco	10.0	210	43%
chicken	1 taco	6.0	190	28%
grilled steak	1 taco	17.0	280	55%
Supreme				
original..regular	1 taco	14.0	220	57%
soft	1 taco	13.0	260	45%
beef	1 taco	14.0	260	48%
chicken	1 taco	10.0	230	39%
TACO JOHN'S				
■ BURRITOS				
bean	1	12.0	380	28%
no cheese	1	7.0	320	20%
Beefy	1	20.0	430	42%
chicken & potato	1	19.0	460	37%
combination	1	16.0	400	36%
meat & potato	1	23.0	490	42%
super	1	20.0	450	40%
■ DESSERTS				
Apple Grande	1	9.0	240	34%
churro	1	11.0	230	43%

Food and Description	Amount	Fat Grams	Total Calories	% Fat Calories
Choco Taco	1	15.0	300	45%
Elf Grahams..Kid's Meal	1 bag	2.0	60	30%
Taco John's				
Cinnamon Mint Swirl	1	–	10	–
cookies..Kid's Meal	1 bag	6.0	130	42%
■ LOCAL FAVORITES				
Beefy Cheesy Taco Bravo	1	22.0	410	48%
Cheese Crisp	1	14.0	210	60%
Chicken Festiva burrito	1	24.0	530	41%
chili enchilada	1	38.0	740	46%
Chili Potato Olés	1 order	36.0	610	53%
Chilito	1	22.0	430	46%
double enchilada	1	40.0	720	50%
El Grande Taco	1	32.0	510	56%
burrito	1	36.0	720	45%
chicken	1	20.0	380	47%
fajita burrito..chicken	1	11.0	340	29%
Mexi Rolls				
regular	1 order	30.0	480	56%
w/nacho cheese	1 order	21.0	370	51%
platters				
beef & bean chimi	1 platter	34.0	760	40%
beef enchilada	1 platter	37.0	780	43%
chicken enchiladas	1 platter	32.0	700	41%
smothered burrito	1 platter	33.0	830	36%
ranch burrito				
beef	1	22.0	420	47%
chicken	1	18.0	390	42%
smothered burrito	1	21.0	500	38%
Taco John's Mexican pizza	1 pizza	25.0	500	45%
tostada	1	10.0	180	50%
bean	1	6.0	160	34%
■ SPECIALTIES				
chicken				
Festiva Salad.. no dressing	1 salad	23.0	400	52%
taco salad..no dressing	1 salad	27.0	530	46%
Potato Olés				
Bravo	1 order	36.0	580	56%
Super	1 order	62.0	980	57%
quesadilla				
cheese	1	28.0	480	53%
chicken	1	29.0	540	48%
Super Nachos				
chicken	1 order	45.0	780	52%
regular	1 order	51.0	830	55%
taco salad..no dressing	1 salad	32.0	580	50%
■ TACOS				
Bravo	1	14.0	340	37%
burger	1	12.0	280	39%

Food and Description	Amount	Fat Grams	Total Calories	% Fat Calories
no cheese	1	9.0	250	32%
chicken soft shell	1	6.0	190	28%
crispy	1	10.0	180	50%
Sierra				
beef	1	23.0	430	48%
chicken	1	17.0	390	39%
soft shell	1	10.0	220	41%
WENDY'S				
■ **BURGERS**				
Big Bacon Classic				
on kaiser bun	1 burger	29.0	580	45%
cheeseburger				
bacon..junior	1 burger	19.0	380	45%
deluxe..junior	1 burger	15.0	350	39%
junior..plain	1 burger	12.0	310	35%
kid's meal	1 burger	12.0	310	35%
hamburger				
junior	1 burger	9.0	270	30%
kid's meal	1 burger	9.0	270	30%
hamburger.. patty only				
junior	2 oz patty	7.0	100	63%
¼ lb	1 patty	13.0	200	68%
single..classic				
w/everything	1 burger	19.0	410	42%
■ **CHICKEN**				
Chicken Nuggets & sauce				
chicken	5 pieces	14.0	220	57%
kid's meal	4 pieces	11.0	180	55%
sauce				
BBQ sauce only	1 pkt	–	40	–
honey mustard only	1 pkt	12.0	130	83%
sweet & sour	1 pkt	–	45	–
Chicken Strip Sauce				
deli honey mustard	1 pkt	16.0	170	85%
heartland ranch	1 pkt	21.0	200	95%
spicy Southwest chipotle	1 pkt	13.0	140	84%
Chicken Strips				
home-style	3 pieces	18.0	410	40%
Chicken Temptations Sandwiches				
home-style chicken fillet	1	22.0	540	37%
spicy chicken fillet	1	19.0	510	34%
Ultimate Chicken Grill	1	7.0	360	18%
■ **CHILI..CHEESE**				
cheese..cheddar..shredded	2 tbs	6.0	70	77%
chili.. small	1 serving	5.0	200	23%
large	1 serving	7.0	300	21%
■ **DESSERT**				
Frosty, dairy	6 oz	4.0	160	23%
	12 oz	8.0	330	22%
■ **FRENCH FRIES**				
Biggie	1 order	19.0	440	39%

Food and Description	Amount	Fat Grams	Total Calories	% Fat Calories
Great Biggie	1 order	23.0	530	39%
kid's meal	1 order	11.0	250	40%
medium	1 order	17.0	390	39%
■ POTATOES..baked				
bacon & cheese	1	25.0	560	40%
broccoli & cheese	1	15.0	440	31%
plain	1	–	270	–
sour cream & chives	1	6.0	340	20%
spread...Country Crock	1 pkt	7.0	60	100%
■ SALADS..DRESSINGS				
fresh salads				
chicken BLT	1 salad	19.0	360	48%
home-style chicken strips	1 salad	22.0	450	44%
mandarin chicken	1 salad	3.0	190	14%
spring mix	1 salad	11.0	180	55%
Taco Supreme	1 salad	16.0	360	40%
side salads				
Caesar	1 salad	2.5	70	32%
traditional	1 salad	–	35	–
salad dressings				
Caesar	1 pkt	16.0	150	96%
creamy ranch				
reduced-fat	1 pkt	8.0	100	72%
French..fat-free	1 pkt	–	80	–
honey mustard				
low-fat	1 pkt	3.0	110	25%
regular	1 pkt	26.0	280	84%
honey vinaigrette	1 pkt	18.0	190	85%
Oriental sesame	1 pkt	19.0	250	68%
■ SIDE ORDERS				
baked potato				
bacon & cheese	1 serving	18.0	530	31%
broccoli & cheese	1 serving	14.0	470	27%
cheese	1 serving	23.0	570	36%
chili & cheese	1 serving	24.0	630	34%
plain	1 serving	–	310	–
sour cream & chives	1 serving	6.0	380	14%
sour cream only	1 pkt	6.0	60	90%
whipped margarine only	1 pkt	7.0	60	100%
chili				
	small	7.0	210	30%
	large	10.0	310	29%
cheddar cheese only	2 Tbs	6.0	70	77%
crackers only	2 crackers	0.5	25	18%
French fries	small	13.0	270	43%
	biggie	23.0	470	44%
	great biggie	27.0	570	43%

WHATABURGER
■ BEVERAGES
shakes

Food and Description	Amount	Fat Grams	Total Calories	% Fat Calories
chocolate	medium	25.0	904	25%
	large	33.0	1216	24%
strawberry	medium	24.0	909	24%
	large	32.0	1159	25%
vanilla	medium	26.0	834	28%
	large	34.0	1118	27%
■ **BREAKFAST**				
biscuit..buttermilk	1 biscuit	16.0	300	48%
biscuit..w/				
bacon	1 biscuit	21.0	375	50%
egg & cheese	1 biscuit	29.0	475	49%
egg & cheese	1 biscuit	27.0	445	55%
egg, cheese & bacon	1 biscuit	33.0	515	58%
egg, cheese & sausage	1 biscuit	46.0	662	63%
gravy..sausage	1 biscuit	33.0	490	61%
sausage	1 biscuit	35.0	517	61%
breakfast platter				
w/bacon	1 platter	43.0	697	56%
w/sausage	1 platter	56.0	839	60%
breakfast on a bun				
w/bacon	1	23.0	398	52%
w/sausage	1	36.0	539	60%
breakfast on a bun..Ranchero				
w/bacon	1	23.0	403	51%
w/sausage	1	36.0	545	59%
cinnamon roll	1 roll	34.0	860	36%
egg omelet sandwich	1	17.0	322	48%
hash brown sticks	1 order	8.0	140	51%
Mexican breakfast				
taquito				
bacon & egg	1 taquito	22.0	387	51%
bacon..egg & cheese	1 taquito	25.0	432	52%
potato & egg	1 taquito	20.0	382	47%
potato..egg & cheese	1 taquito	24.0	427	51%
sausage & egg	1 taquito	24.0	390	55%
sausage..egg & cheese	1 taquito	27.0	434	56%
pancakes				
pancakes only	1 order	8.0	614	12%
w/bacon	1 serving	13.0	689	17%
w/sausage	1 serving	27.0	831	29%
Texas toast	1 slice	15.0	328	41%
■ **BURGERS & FAJITAS**				
Justaburger	1 burger	15.0	309	44%
Whataburger				
double meat	1 burger	42.0	823	46%
junior	1 burger	16.0	315	46%
regular	1 burger	30.0	607	44%
small bun, w/o oil	1 burger	19.0	410	42%
special request				
no bun	1 burger	18.0	270	60%

Food and Description	Amount	Fat Grams	Total Calories	% Fat Calories
small bun..no bun oil	1 burger	22.0	428	46%
triple meat	1 burger	66.0	1108	54%
w/bacon & cheese	1 burger	45.0	810	50%
special request..no bun w/cheese	1 burger	34.0	473	65%
special request..no bun	1 burger	25.0	360	63%
■ CHICKEN & FISH				
chicken strips	2 pieces	24.0	382	57%
	3 pieces	36.0	574	56%
	4 pieces	49.0	765	58%
grilled chicken fajita taco	1	13.0	363	32%
grilled chicken sandwich				
regular	1	20.0	473	38%
special request				
no bun	1	7.0	190	33%
small bun..dry	1	13.0	367	32%
small bun..no bun oil				
w/MLT	1	8.0	334	22%
w/o oil or salad dressing	1	5.5	358	14%
w/o salad dressing	1	8.5	385	20%
Whatacatch sandwich	1	26.0	472	50%
Whatachick'n sandwich	1	21.0	523	36%
special request..4" small				
white bun	1	20.0	473	38%
■ SALADS & RELATED ITEMS				
garden salad	1 salad	0.5	49	92%
w/cheddar cheese	1 salad	15.0	218	62%
w/cheddar cheese & bacon	1 salad	20.0	293	61%
grilled chicken salad	1 salad	7.0	229	28%
w/cheddar cheese	1 salad	21.0	398	47%
w/cheddar cheese & bacon	1 salad	27.0	473	51%
salad dressing				
ranch				
low-fat	1 pkt	4.0	66	55%
regular	1 pkt	33.0	310	96%
Thousand Island	1 pkt	13.0	150	78%
vinaigrette..low-fat	1 pkt	1.5	35	39%
■ SIDE ORDERS				
French fries	regular	18.0	332	49%
	large	124.5	445	50%
onion rings	medium	11.0	200	50%
	large	16.0	304	47%
■ COOKIES				
chocolate chunk	1	8.0	210	34%
oatmeal raisin	1	3.5	185	17%
peanut butter	1	9.5	215	40%
white chocolate macadamia	1	11.0	230	43%

WHITE CASTLE
■ BEVERAGES

Food and Description	Amount	Fat Grams	Total Calories	% Fat Calories
shake..chocolate or vanilla	14 oz	7.0	220	29%
■ BREAKFAST				
breakfast sandwich	1	25.0	340	66%
■ BURGERS				
cheeseburger				
bacon	1 burger	13.0	200	59%
double	1 burger	18.0	285	57%
single	1 burger	9.0	160	51%
hamburger				
double	1 burger	14.0	235	54%
single	1 burger	7.0	135	47%
■ CHICKEN & FISH				
chicken				
rings	1 order	21.0	310	61%
sandwich	1	8.0	190	38%
fish sandwich				
w/o tartar sauce	1	6.0	160	34%
■ CONDIMENTS				
onion chips	3.3 oz	17.0	329	47%
tartar sauce	1 Tbs	8.0	72	100%
■ SIDE ORDERS				
cheese sticks	1 order	17.0	290	53%
chicken rings	1 order	21.0	310	61%
chili	1 bowl	15.0	375	36%
French fries	1 order	6.0	115	47%
onion rings	1 order	26.0	540	43%

Personal Food Diary

Date	Food	Amount	Fat Grams	Total Calories	% Fat Calories

Personal Food Diary

Date	Food	Amount	Fat Grams	Total Calories	% Fat Calories

Personal Food Diary

Date	Food	Amount	Fat Grams	Total Calories	% Fat Calories

Personal Food Diary

Date	Food	Amount	Fat Grams	Total Calories	% Fat Calories

Personal Food Diary

Date	Food	Amount	Fat Grams	Total Calories	% Fat Calories

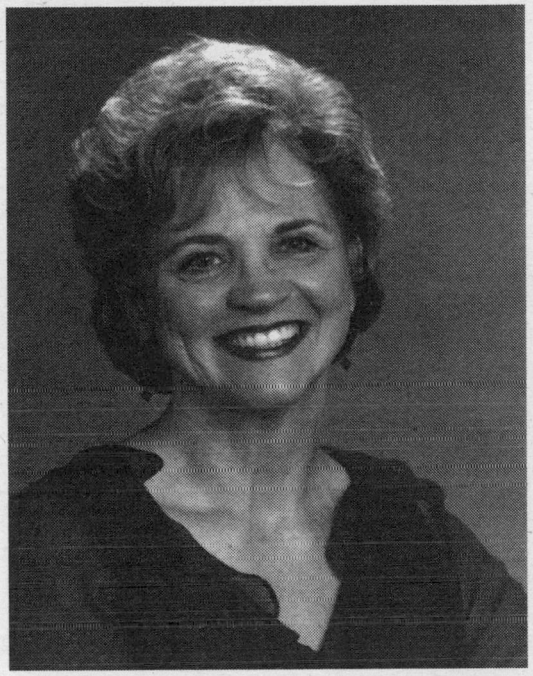

Karen J. Bellerson is the author of *The Shopper's Guide to Fat in Your Food* and *Low-Fat, No-Fat Cookbook*. She has been a nutritional consultant for more than twenty years and makes her home in the Southwest.